Paediatric Haematology

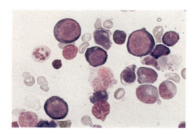

A. Megaloblastic Marrow in Juvenile Pernicious Anaemia × 540

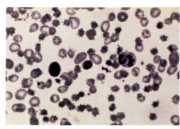

B. Infantile Pycnocytosis. Peripheral blood × 540

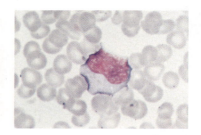

C. Glandular Fever Cell. Peripheral blood × 1,000

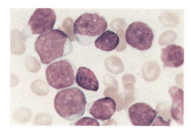

D. Leukaemic Lymphoblasts. Marrow × 1,000

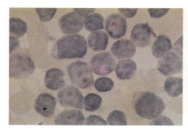

E. PAS positive Leukaemic Lymphoblasts. Marrow × 1,000

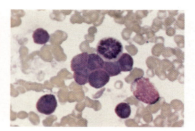

F. Neuroblastoma Cells in Marrow × 540

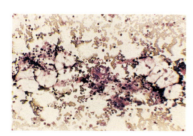

G. Reticulum Cells in Marrow. Histiocytosis X. × 100

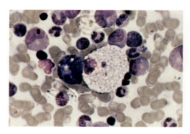

H. Sea-blue Histiocyte (Lt.) and Nieman-Pick-like Cell (Rt.) in Marrow of child with bizarre neurological syndrome. × 540

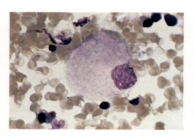

I. Gaucher-like Cell in Marrow × 540

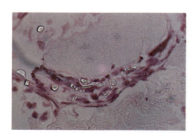

J. Cystine Crystals. Marrow in Cystinosis. × 540

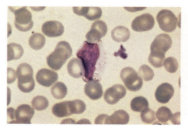

K. Reilly Bodies in Lymphocytes in Hurler's syndrome. Peripheral blood × 1,000

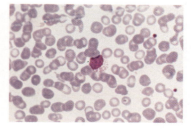

L. Vacuolated Lymphocytes in Gm1 Type 1 Gangliosidosis. Peripheral blood × 540

Leishman's stain, apart from PAS stain in E and Neutral Red in J.

Paediatric Haematology

Michael L. N. Willoughby MA, MD, MRC Path.
Consultant Haematologist
to the Royal Hospital for Sick Children
and Queen Mother's Hospital, Glasgow

CHURCHILL LIVINGSTONE
Edinburgh London and New York 1977

CHURCHILL LIVINGSTONE
Medical Division of Longman Group Limited

Distributed in the United States of America by
Longman Inc., 19 West 44th Street, New York,
N.Y. 10036 and by associated companies,
branches and representatives throughout
the world.

© Longman Group Limited 1977

All rights reserved. No part of this publication
may be reproduced, stored in a retrieval system,
or transmitted in any form or by any means,
electronic, mechanical, photocopying, recording
or otherwise, without the prior permission of the
publishers (Churchill Livingstone, 23 Ravelston
Terrace, Edinburgh, EH4 3TL).

ISBN 0 443 01442 6

Library of Congress Cataloging in Publication Data
Willoughby, Michael L N
    Paediatric haematology.

    Includes bibliographies.
    1. Pediatric hematology.   I.   Title.
RJ411.W55   618.9′21′5   76–49038

Printed in Great Britain by
Cox & Wyman Ltd
London, Fakenham and Reading

Preface

This book is written for all those concerned with the diagnosis and management of blood disorders in children, whether they are primarily paediatricians or haematologists. I have tried to integrate the fundamental molecular, genetic and cell kinetic aspects of each group of disorders with their clinical and haematological manifestations where this is contributory to an understanding of their pathogenesis and management.

A considerable body of documented information has accumulated in these fields over the past few years and I have attempted to provide access to this by reference to key papers and selected reviews or annotations throughout the text, together with a bibliography designed to give 'the way in' to the literature for the worker wishing to pursue some point in greater depth. Where there are divergent or currently unresolved views on a particular topic I have indicated this. On most issues, however, I have stated my own opinion and practice.

The bibliography also serves to give acknowledgement to the many investigators who have contributed to our better understanding of this complex and rapidly changing subject, including in particular that small band of paediatric haematologists whose contributions recur in chapter after chapter throughout the book.

I am personally indebted to Dr Rosemary Biggs, Professor R. G. Macfarlane and Dr A. A. Sharp of the Radcliffe Infirmary, Oxford, who initiated my interest in haematology, and to my colleagues at the Royal Hospital for Sick Children, Glasgow, who have taught me a little paediatrics! Mr J. Devlin and members of his department of Medical Illustration have generously given much time and effort in the preparation of the original clinical photographs and charts, as well as assisting in the preparation of the photomicrographs. The original X-ray plates have been reproduced by the courtesy of Dr Phillip Rawson and Dr Elizabeth Sweet of the department of Radiology. I especially wish to thank my secretary Mrs Catherine Walker who meticulously decoded my illegible notes into the text which follows.

Glasgow, 1976   M.L.N.W.

To my Wife Fiona,
and our children
Jonathan, James and Henry,
partially neglected
during the writing of this book

Contents

1. Iron Deficiency Anaemia 1
Pathogenesis 1
  Iron endowment at birth 1
  Iron in the diet 2
  Gastrointestinal function and iron deficiency 3
Incidence of iron deficiency 4
Clinical features 5
Diagnosis and laboratory findings 5
  Additional haematological findings 5
  Biochemical tests of iron deficiency 7
  Tests for intestinal blood loss 7
Treatment 8

2. Folate Metabolism and Deficiency 13
  Biochemistry of folic acid and its derivatives 13
  Dietary sources of folate 14
  Absorption of folates 15
Determination of folate status 16
  Folate assays in blood 16
  Figlu test 17
  Haematological changes 18
    Peripheral blood 18
    Marrow 18
Folate balance in infancy and childhood 19
  Daily folate requirements 19
  Folate status in the newborn 20
Conditions associated with folate deficiency in childhood 21
  Prematurity 21
  Infection 22
  Malabsorption 23
  Haemolysis 24
  Nutritional deficiency 25
  Anticonvulsants and other drugs associated with megaloblastic anaemia 26
  Inborn errors related to folate metabolism 28
  Conditions with increased folate loss 29
Clinical features and treatment 29

3. Vitamin B_{12} Metabolism and Deficiency 35
Biochemistry 35
Absorption and transport 35
Assessment of B_{12} status 36
B_{12} balance in infancy 37

Classification of B_{12} deficiency in infancy and childhood 38
  Intrinsic factor deficiency 38
  Selective ileal malabsorption of B_{12} 39
  Other causes of malabsorption 39
  Nutritional B_{12} deficiency 40
  Transcobalomin II deficiency 40

4. Aplastic Anaemia 43
  Introduction 43
  Classification 44
Constitutional aplastic anaemia 45
  Aetiology 45
  Clinical features 46
  Laboratory diagnosis 48
  Treatment and prognosis 50
Acquired aplastic anaemia 53
  Aetiology 53
  Clinical features 56
  Laboratory diagnosis 56
  Association of haemolysis, including PNH 57
  Treatment 58
    Androgens 58
    Prognostic features 60
    Marrow transplantation 60
    Miscellaneous therapy 60
Pure red-cell aplasia 61
  Aetiology 61
  Clinical features 62
  Laboratory diagnosis 63
  Course and treatment 64

5. Haemolytic Anaemias: General Features 71
Red-cell changes 71
  Spherocytes 71
  Red-cell fragmentation, 73
  Red-cell survival 73
Compensatory marrow activity 73
Pigment metabolism 74

6. Hereditary Haemolytic Anaemias with Characteristic Red-cell Morphology 77
Hereditary spherocytosis (HS) 78
  Aetiology and Pathogenesis 78

viii CONTENTS

Clinical features 78
Jaundice 78
Anaemia 78
Splenomegaly 78
Laboratory findings 79
Treatment 80
Hereditary elliptocytosis (HE) 80
Aetiology 80
Clinical features 81
Laboratory findings 81
Treatment 81
Stomatocytosis 81
Congenital haemolytic anaemia with dehydrated
red cells 82
Acanthocytosis 83
Congenital dyserythropoietic anaemias (CDA) 83

**7. Hereditary Non-spherocytic
Haemolytic Anaemias 89**
Introduction 89
Biochemical considerations 90
Disorders of the hexose monophosphate shunt 92
Glucose-6-phosphate dehydrogenase (G-6-PD) 92
Clinical manifestations of G-6-PD deficiency
Drug-induced haemolysis 94
Favism 96
Neonatal jaundice and kernicterus 96
Chronic non-spherocytic haemolytic
anaemia 97
Other defects affecting availability of reduced
glutathione (GSH) 97
6-phosphogluconate dehydrogenase (6-PGD) 97
Glutathione reductase (GSSG-R) 98
Glutathione peroxidase (GSH-Px) 98
Defects of glutathione (GSH) synthesis 98
Disorders of the glycolytic pathway (Embden-
Meyerhof) 100
Pyruvate kinase (PK) 101
Hexokinase (HK) 102
Phosphohexose isomerase (PHI) 103
Phosphofructokinase (PFK) 103
Triosephosphate isomerase (TPI) 104
Glyceraldehyde-3-phosphate dehydrogenase
(G-3-PD) 104
Phosphoglycerate kinase (PGK) 104
2, 3-Diphosphoglyceromutase (2, 3-
DPGase) 105
Adenosine triphosphatase (ATP-ase) 105

**8. Abnormalities of Haemoglobin
Synthesis 111**
Basic considerations 111
Chemical structure of haemoglobin 111
Normal variants of haemoglobin 112

Haemoglobins present at birth 113
Detection of foetal haemoglobin 113
Physiological significance of foetal
haemoglobin 113
Postnatal changes in Hb. F concentration 115
Genetically determined abnormalities of Haemo-
globin structure: the Haemoglobinopathies 116
Inheritance 117
Geographic distribution and incidence 117
Sickling states 118
Pathogenesis of sickling phenomena and
related haemolysis 118
Haematological diagnosis 120
Clinical manifestations of sickling
diseases 121
Treatment of sickling disorders 123
Unstable Haemoglobins 124
Pathogenesis of anaemia in UHHA 125
Clinical and haematological features of the
unstable haemoglobinopathies 126
Management 127
M-Haemoglobinopathies, and other causes of
Methaemoglobinaemia 127
Haematological aspects 127
Clinical features 128
Diagnosis 129
Treatment 129
Thalassaemia syndromes 129
Biochemical lesions in thalassaemia 129
Genetics of different forms of
thalassaemia 130
Pathogenesis of the anaemia 131
Haematological findings and diagnosis 132
Age of presentation and early diagnosis 133
Clinical features of thalassaemia 134
Management 135

9. Acquired Haemolytic Anaemias 145
Microangiopathic haemolytic anaemia
(MAHA) 145
Mechanism of burr cell formation. Pathogenesis
of MAHA 146
Haematological diagnosis 146
Red cell membrane disorders 147
Lipid accumulation and stagnation 147
Acanthocytosis 148
Spur cell haemolytic anaemia 148
Target cells in liver disease 148
Lipid peroxidation and haemolysis 148
Relationship to infantile pycnocytosis 149
Changes in membrane plasticity 149
Structural defects of red-cell membrane,
including dyserythropoietic anaemias 150
Autoimmune haemolytic anaemias 150
Pathogenesis of the anaemia 151

CONTENTS ix

Relationship of autoantibodies to underlying disease 151
Clinical manifestations 152
Haematological features 152
Treatment 153
Drug-induced and toxic haemolysis 154
Immune drug-induced haemolytic anaemia 154
'Immune' or drug-haptene type 156
'Autoimmune' drug-induced type 156
Haemolytic anaemias due to infection 156
Hypersplenism 157
Haemolytic anaemia secondary to systemic disease 157

10. Anaemias in the Neonatal Period. 1. Rhesus Disease (Rhesus Isoimmunisation) 163
Synonyms 163
Pathogenesis and Prevention 163
Antenatal detection and prediction of severity of Rh disease 164
Clinical findings 168
Laboratory findings 169
Management and treatment 170
Intrauterine transfusion 172

11. Anaemias in the Neonatal Period. 2. Abo Haemolytic Disease of the Newborn (Abo Hdnb) 181
Pathogenesis 181
Clinical features 182
Laboratory findings 182
Management 183
Phototherapy and phenobarbitone therapy 183
Phenobarbitone 183
Phototherapy 183
Other blood group incompatibilities 184

12. Non-immune Anaemias in the Neonatal Period 187
Infantile pycnocytosis 188
Neonatal haemolysis due to infection 190
Syphilis 190
Toxoplasmosis and cytomegalovirus 190
Rubella, Coxsackie B, Herpes simplex, malaria 191
Bacterial infections 191
Heinz-body anaemias in the newborn 191
Neonatal manifestations of hereditary haemolytic anaemias 194
Hereditary spherocytosis (HS) 194
Hereditary elliptocytosis (HE) 195
Hereditary red-cell enzyme defects 195
Thalassaemias and haemoglobinopathies 195

Neonatal anaemia due to blood loss 196
Chronic foetal blood loss 197
Aplastic anaemia in the neonatal period 198

13. Secondary Anaemias 203
Anaemias of prematurity 203
Anaemias due to chronic infections 204
Rheumatoid arthritis and collagen diseases 206
Renal failure 207
Liver disease 208
Endocrine disorders 208
Malignant disease and bone marrow encroachment 209
Marble-bone disease 210
Sideroblastic anaemias 212

14. Polycythaemia 217
Primary polycythaemia 217
Polycythaemia rubra vera 217
Benign familial polycythaemia (Erythrocytosis) 218
Secondary polycythaemia 218
Cyanotic congenital heart disease 218
Abnormal haemoglobins 219
Tumours and renal disease 219
Neonatal polycythaemia 219

15. Disorders of Granulocytes, Monocytes and Lymphocytes 223
Neutropenia and Agranulocytosis 223
Granulocyte kinetics and distribution 223
Hereditary forms of neutropenia and agranulocytosis 225
Infantile genetic agranulocytosis (IGA) 225
Familial benign chronic neutropenia 227
Reticular dysgenesis (congenital aleucocytosis) 227
Chronic benign granulocytopenia of childhood (CG) 227
Ineffective myelopoiesis 229
Cyclic Neutropenia 229
Lazy-leucocyte syndrome 231
Neutropenia associated with agammaglobulin-aemia and dysglobulinaemia 231
Neutropenia associated with pancreatic insufficiency 231
Neutropenia associated with inborn errors of metabolism 232
Drug-induced neutropenia 232
Neutropenia secondary to peripheral sequestration 233
Immunoneutropenias 233
Other causes of neutropenia 233

Disorders of phagocyte function 234
Physiology of neutrophil granulocytes 234
The biochemical defect in CGD and related disorders 235
NBT test in diagnosis of CGD and related conditions 236
Pathology of CGD 236
Clinical features of CGD and related disorders 236
Inheritance of CGD 237
Other abnormalities of phagocytic function 237
Myeloperoxidase deficiency 237
Job's syndrome 237
Leukocyte glutathione peroxidase deficiency 238
G-6-PD deficiency in leucocytes 238
Chédiak-Higashi disease 238
Congenital abnormality of specific granule formation 238
Acquired disorders of leukocyte function 238
Leukocyte changes secondary to infection 239
Infectious mononucleosis and related conditions 242
Infectious lymphocytosis 245
Eosinophilia 245

16. Thrombocytopenia 253
The platelet count 253
Normal platelet life-span and sequestration 254
Kinetics of thrombopoiesis 255
Morphological aspects of thrombopoiesis 256
Platelet size as a measure of thrombopoiesis 256
Classification of thrombocytopenias 257
Idiopathic thrombocytopenic purpura (ITP) 257
Nature of ITP 257
Difficulty in consistent demonstration of autoantibody 258
Site of platelet destruction in vivo 259
Course of ITP in children 260
Clinical features 260
Haematological findings 261
Diagnosis 261
Management of childhood ITP 262
Thrombocytopenia in the neonatal period 264
1. Secondary to maternal ITP 264
2. Isoimmune neonatal purpura 265
3. Secondary to maternal drug ingestion 267
4. Intrauterine or neonatal infection 267
5. Other causes of platelet consumption 268
6. Congenital megakaryocytic hypoplasia 268
(a) Bilateral absent radii (TAR) 268
(b) Fanconi's anaemia 271
(c) Trisomy syndromes 271
7. Hereditary thrombocytopenias 271

(a) Wiscott-Aldrich syndrome (WAS) 271
(b) Sex-linked recessive thrombocytopenia 272
(c) Autosomal thrombocytopenias 273
May-Hegglin 273
Dominant 274
Recessive 274
8. Metabolic causes of neonatal thrombocytopenia 275
9. Congenital leukaemia 275
Drug-induced thrombocytopenia 275
Mechanism of drug-haptene disease 275
Post transfusion thrombocytopenic purpura 278
Thrombopoietin deficiency 278
Cyclical thrombocytopenia 278
Hypersplenism 279
MAHA and DIC 279
Marrow encroachment 279
Thrombocytosis 279

17. Defects of Platelet and Capillary Function 287
Normal platelet function 287
Tests of platelet function 288
Bleeding time 288
Platelet size and morphology 289
Platelet aggregation and ADP release in vitro 290
Platelet adhesion to glass beads 291
Clot retraction 292
Platelet factor 3 (PF-3) availability 292
Inherited disorders of platelet function 293
Glanzmann's thrombasthenia 293
Thrombopathia (or defects of ADP release) 293
Bernard-Soulier syndrome 294
May-Hegglin anomaly 295
Von Willebrand's disease 295
Congenital afibrinogenaemia 298
Acquired defects of platelet function 298
Drug ingestion 298
Platelet function in the newborn 299
Uraemia 300
Liver disease, dysproteinaemia 300
Platelet transfusion 301
Non-thrombocytopenic purpura 302
Anaphylactoid purpura (Henoch-Schönlein syndrome) 302
Scurvy 303
Drugs, foods and infections 303
Inherited vascular and connective tissue disorders 303
Hereditary haemorrhagic telangiectasia (Rendu-Osler-Weber disease) 303
Ehler-Danlos syndrome 303

Pseudoxanthoma elasticum and osteogenesis
imperfecta 304

18. Coagulation Disorders. I. Hereditary 309
Physiology of blood coagulation 309
Investigation of disorders of coagulation 311
Hereditary coagulation defects 313
Haemophilia 313
Incidence 314
Inheritance 315
Newer knowledge regarding the nature of
antihaemophilic factor 315
Clinical manifestations 316
Diagnosis 317
Management 319
Correction of the coagulation deficiency 319
Use of plasma, cryoprecipitate and
concentrates 320
1. Fresh or fresh-frozen plasma 320
2. Cryoprecipitate 320
3. Concentrates of factors VIII and IX 321
Management of specific problems 321
1. Cuts and lacerations 321
2. Soft tissue bleeding 322
3. Haemarthrosis 322
4. Nosebleeds 322
5. Haematuria 323
6. Gastrointestinal bleeding 323
7. CNS bleeding 323
8. Dental treatment 323
9. Surgery in haemophilia 324
10. Injections and immunization 324
11. Home transfusion and prophylactic
treatment 324
12. Treatment of pain in haemophilia 325
13. Treatment of patients who have
developed inhibitors 326
Other hereditary coagulation disorders 327
Defects of the contact phase of coagulation
(factors XI and XII) 327
Deficiencies of factors in the prothrombin
complex (factors II, V, VII and X) 327
Defects of fibrinogen and fibrin stabilization
(factors I and XIII) 329

19. Coagulation Disorders II. Acquired 335
Impaired hepatic synthesis 335
Vitamin K 335
Coagulation status in the newborn 336
Haemorrhagic disease of the newborn 338
Intrapartum and perinatal bleeding 339
Maternal drug ingestion 339
Diagnosis 340

Treatment 340
Vitamin K deficiency beyond the neonatal
period 341
Hepatocellular disease 342
Disseminated intravascular coagulation (DIC) 343
Fibrin degradation products (FDPs) 344
Diagnosis of DIC 345
General considerations 346
Specific therapy for DIC 346
Heparin therapy 347
Control and dosage of Heparin 347
DIC in the neonatal period 349
Prematurity 350
Asphyxia and acidosis 350
Hypothermia 350
Infection 350
Severe rhesus disease 350
Respiratory distress syndrome 351
Maternal and intrauterine causes of
neonatal DIC 352
Causes of intravascular coagulation beyond the
newborn period 352
Renal vein thrombosis and hypertonic
dehydration 352
Giant haemangioma (Kasabach-Merritt
syndrome) 353
Congenital heart disease (CHD) 354
Post-operative haemorrhage after cardiac
surgery 355
Other vascular disorders 355
The haemolytic uraemic syndrome
(HUS) 356
Age incidence 356
Clinical features 356
Haematological findings 356
Coagulation investigations 357
Treatment 358
Thrombotic thrombocytopenic purpura
(TTP) 359
Septicaemia—bacterial, viral, fungal,
rickettsial, protozoal 359
Purpura fulminans 361
Miscellaneous causes of DIC:
Acute liver failure, disseminated malignancy,
acute intravascular haemolysis 362
Acquired inhibitors of coagulation 363

20. Leukaemia and Related Disorders 373
Incidence of leukaemia in childhood 373
Aetiology of leukaemia 374
Cell kinetic considerations 377
Diagnosis of acute leukaemia 379
Haematological findings in acute leukaemia 380
Management of acute leukaemia 383

xii CONTENTS

Remission induction 383
Supportive treatment during remission
induction 387
CNS prophylaxis 391
Treatment of overt meningeal leukaemia 391
Maintenance therapy 394
Factors affecting prognosis 397
Age at diagnosis 397
Race 397
White-cell count at diagnosis 397
Degree of tissue infiltration 398
Cytological features 398
Unusual types of childhood leukaemia 399
Chronic myelocytic leukaemia (CML) 399
Erythroleukaemia (Di Guglielmo's
syndrome) 401
Promyelocytic leukaemia 402
Chronic lymphocytic leukaemia (CLL) 402

Eosinophilic and basophilic leukaemia 402
Chronic monocytic leukaemia (CMOL) 403
Leukaemia reticuloendotheliosis 403
Leukaemic transformation of reticuloses 403
Congenital leukaemia 404
Non-leukaemic disorders with infiltration of the
marrow 405
Metastatic malignant infiltration of the
marrow 405
Myelomatosis 406
Letterer-Siwe disease 406
Familial erythrophagocytic lymphohistiocytosis
(FEL) 408
Histiocytic medullary reticulosis (HMR) 408
Storage diseases 409
Sea-blue histiocyte syndrome 410
Myelofibrosis 411
Familial myeloproliferative disease 411

Introduction

HAEMATOLOGICAL ASSESSMENT IN CHILDHOOD

Intrinsic handicaps in the practice of paediatric haematology are that 'clean' venepunctures are less dependable than in adults and that it is seldom justifiable to use radioactive isotope techniques to study red cell survival or iron metabolism. In fact almost all haematological investigations can be performed on capillary blood samples including coagulation tests such as the thromboplastin screening test or Factor VIII Assay (Hardisty and Ingram, 1965) providing the technical staff are adequately trained and the laboratory properly orientated to paediatric work. The relative ease of capillary blood sampling makes sequential observations more practical whether at intervals of hours, in monitoring the correction of coagulation disorders, at intervals of days, in assessing the response to haematinics, or at intervals of weeks in the surveillance of chemotherapy as in leukaemia. Many such children can be followed both in remission and relapse for periods of 3 to 5 years with frequent blood tests without recourse to a single diagnostic venepuncture. This policy permits the reservation of veins for therapeutic purposes. A further advantage is that the artefacts of red cell and white cell morphology often seen in anticoagulated blood collected some hours previously is avoided when freshly made blood films from capillary blood are used, and the spurious thrombocytopenia frequently found in 'difficult' venepuncture specimens is obviated. A modification of capillary blood collection using small plastic tubes containing EDTA rather than pipettes has recently been described for paediatric work by Stuart, Barrett and Pragnell (1974). It permits the use of automated cell counting as well as ESR determination by a micromethod. Only 0·5 ml of blood is collected for a number of tests.

It is strikingly informative to graph the therapy and relevant haematological measurements in patients with blood diseases; for example the platelet count in idiopathic thrombocytopenic purpura (ITP), the granulocytes, blast cells and platelets in leukaemia, and the reticulocytes plus haemoglobin in haemolytic or deficiency anaemias. Consideration of the graph may disclose trends and relationships not otherwise apparent, at the same time giving a better guide as to the appropriate intervals at which future tests should be performed; for instance reticulocyte peaks, response to Factor VIII therapy or the existence of cyclic neutropenia could be entirely missed by haphazard timing of tests.

Marrow examinations are frequently needed in the elucidation of abnormalities of the peripheral blood including all cases of thrombocytopenia, neutropenia, unexplained anaemia or leuco-erythroblastic anaemia. It is seldom profitable to examine the bone marrow before considering the peripheral blood findings since few diseases extensively involve the marrow without producing some abnormality of the peripheral blood. Also it may be impossible to evaluate the significance of the marrow findings without a knowledge of the peripheral blood picture and the clinical features (e.g. in ITP). Particularly in leukaemia repeated marrow examinations are of value to assess the response to therapy. The posterior iliac crest is the most consistently useful site over the age of 6–8 weeks; below this age the tibial puncture is used, taking great care to avoid damaging the upper tibial ossification centre.

Normal values

Table 1 shows the range of normal haemoglobin, PCV and MCV over the first 12 weeks of life. At 9 weeks the haemoglobin may fall as low as 9·5 g/100 ml in full-term infants. In premature infants even lower levels are seen viz. mean 9·4 g/100 ml ±1·0 (S.D.) at 10 weeks (Gorten and Cross, 1964). In a recent annotation on the subject Oski and Stockman (1974) state that apparently healthy premature infants weighing 1·2 kg or less show average haemoglobin levels of 8·0 g/100 ml between 6 and 8 weeks, and that values of 7·0 g/100 ml are frequently seen without recognizable haematological or other disease. From 6 months to puberty there is a gradual rise in haemoglobin and PCV to adult levels (Table 2).

xiv INTRODUCTION

Table 1   Haemoglobin, PCV and MCV in normal full-term infants

Days	No. Cases	Hb g/100 ml ± S.D.	PCV per cent ± S.D.	MCV μ^3 ± S.D.
1	19	19·0 ± 2·2	61 ± 7·4	119 ± 9·4
2	19	19·0 ± 1·9	60 ± 6·4	115 ± 7·0
3	19	18·7 ± 3·4	62 ± 9·3	116 ± 5·3
4	10	18·6 ± 2·1	57 ± 8·1	114 ± 7·5
5	12	17·6 ± 1·1	57 ± 7·3	114 ± 8·9
6	15	17·4 ± 2·2	54 ± 7·2	113 ± 10·0
7	12	17·9 ± 2·5	56 ± 9·4	118 ± 11·2
Weeks				
2nd	32	17·3 ± 2·3	54 ± 8·3	112 ± 19·0
3rd	11	15·6 ± 2·6	46 ± 7·3	111 ± 8·2
4th	17	14·2 ± 2·1	43 ± 5·7	105 ± 7·5
5th	15	12·7 ± 1·6	36 ± 4·8	101 ± 8·1
6th	10	11·9 ± 1·5	36 ± 6·2	102 ± 10·2
7th	10	12·0 ± 1·5	36 ± 4·8	105 ± 12·0
8th	17	11·1 ± 1·1	33 ± 3·7	100 ± 13·0
9th	13	10·7 ± 0·9	31 ± 2·5	93 ± 12·0
10th	12	11·2 ± 0·9	32 ± 2·7	91 ± 9·3
11th	11	11·4 ± 0·9	34 ± 2·1	91 ± 7·7
12th	13	11·3 ± 0·9	33 ± 3·3	88 ± 7·9

Note the physiological macrocytosis at birth.
Data reproduced by permission of Professor Matoth and the editor, from the paper by Matoth et al. (1971) Acta Paediat. Scand., 60, 317.

Table 2   Haemoglobin and PCV in children after the age of 6 months

Age	Hb g/100 ml ± S.D.	PCV per cent ± S.D.
6 Months	11·5 ± 0·7	38 ± 2
12 ,,	11·9 ± 0·6	39 ± 2
1½–3 Years	11·8 ± 0·5	39 ± 2
5 ,,	12·7 ± 1·0	37 ± 3
10 ,,	13·2 ± 1·0	39 ± 3
14 ,,	16·0 ± 2·0	40 ± 3
Adult male	16·0 ± 2·0	47 ± 5
Adult female	14·0 ± 2·0	42 ± 5

Data from Lascari (1973), p. 112.
Reproduced by permission of the author and publishers.

Table 3   Normal leucocyte values and differential counts in childhood

Age	Total WBC 10^3/mm³	Neutrophils Bands	Segmented	Mean per cent Lymphocytes	Monocytes	Eosinophils
Birth	9–30	9	52	31	6	2
12 hours	13–38	10	58	24	5	2
1 week	5–21	7	39	41	9	4
6 months	6–18	4	28	61	5	3
1 year	6–18	3	28	61	5	3
2 years	6–17	3	30	59	5	3
4 years	6–16	3	39	50	5	3
6 years	5–15	3	48	42	5	3
12 years	5–14	3	52	38	4	3
16 years	5–13	3	54	35	5	3

Data from Lascari (1973), p. 112, and Dittmar and Altman (1961).
Reproduced by permission of Professor Lascari and the publishers.

White cell counts show an absolute and relative lymphocytosis until the age of 4 years, after which adult proportions pertain (Table 3). The absolute number of neutrophils, however, normally remain above 1,500/mm³ during the first 4 years in spite of the relative lymphocytosis at this time.

Platelet counts are normal throughout infancy and childhood (Chap. 16).

Marrow findings are essentially normal through-out childhood apart from a marked erythroid depression with as low as 7 per cent of normo-blasts at the age of 1 month, rising to 15 per cent at 3 months, 16 per cent at 6 months and 19 per cent at 1 year, thereafter being indistinguishable from normal (Gairdner *et al.*, 1952; Glaser *et al.*, 1970). Marrow plasma cell counts are low in normal infants and young children, but approach adult levels at 5 years (Steiner and Pearson, 1966).

REFERENCES

Dittmer, E. S. & Altman, P. L. (1961) *Blood and other fluids*, p. 109, 125. Washington, D.C.: Federation of American Societies for Experimental Biology.

Gairdner, D., Marks, J. & Roscoe, J. P. (1952) Blood formation in infancy. Part I. The normal bone marrow. *Arch. Dis. Childh.*, **27**, 128.

Glaser, K., Limarzi, L. R. & Poncher, H. G. (1950) Cellular composition of the bone marrow in normal infants and children. *Pediatrics*, **6**, 789.

Gorten, M. K. & Cross, E. R. (1964) Iron metabolism in premature infants. II. Prevention of iron deficiency. *J. Pediat.* **64**, 569.

Hardisty, R. M. & Ingram, G. I. C. (1965) *Bleeding disorders: Investigations and management*. Oxford: Blackwell.

Lascari, A. D. (1973) *Leukemia in childhood*. p. 112. Springfield, Illinois: Charles C. Thomas.

Matoth, Y., Zaizor, R. & Varsano, I. (1971) Postnatal changes in some red-cell parameters. *Acta Paediat. Scand.*, **60**, 317.

Oski, F. A. & Stockman, J. A. (1974) Annotation: Anaemia in early infancy. *Brit. J. Haemat.*, **27**, 195.

Steiner, M. L. & Pearson, H. A. (1966) Bone marrow plasmacyte values in childhood. *J. Paediat.*, **68**, 562.

Stuart, J., Barrett, B. A. & Pragnell, D. R. (1974) Capillary blood collection in haematology. *J. clin. Path.*, **27**, 869.

1. Iron Deficiency Anaemia

Pathogenesis, *Iron endowment at birth, Iron in the diet, Gastrointestinal function* | Incidence of iron deficiency | Clinical features | Diagnosis and laboratory findings, *Additional haematological findings, Biochemical tests of iron deficiency, Tests for intestinal blood loss* | Treatment

---

This is the commonest form of anaemia seen in paediatric practice. The maximum incidence occurs between 6 months and 3 years of age.

PATHOGENESIS

The prime cause is exhaustion of the neonatal iron stores at a time when the demands of an increasing blood volume and red cell mass are exceeding dietary intake and absorption.

Iron endowment at birth

Over 75 per cent of the total body iron of the newborn is accounted for by its circulating haemoglobin (Table 1.1). This in turn is dependent upon

weight, Osgood, 1955). After birth there is a relatively more rapid growth rate and increase in blood volume in premature as compared to full-term infants (e.g. the birth weight is doubled much earlier in the premature infant). Schulman (1961) has calculated (Table 1.2) that the full-term infant requires a total of 156 mg of absorbed iron over its first year if it is to have an 'ideal' haemoglobin level 12·3 g/100 ml at the age of 1 year. A premature infant of 1·5 kg would require nearly twice this amount of iron over the year in order to achieve the same level of haemoglobin. (The figure of 12·3 g haemoglobin/100 ml used in this calculation was derived from earlier work by Sturgeon (1956) showing that this was the mean haemoglobin level at one year in a group of children

Table 1.1   Total body iron at birth in term and premature infants

Maturity	B.wt.	Hb g/100 ml	Hb mass	Hb Fe	Storage Fe	Tissue Fe	Total Fe
Full term	3·3 kg	19·0	55 g	185 mg	34 mg	23 mg	242 mg
Premature	1·5 kg	19·0	30 g	97 mg	15 mg	10 mg	122 mg
						Deficit at birth =	120 mg

From Schulman (1961) *J.A.M.A.*, **175,**, 118.

two factors: (a) the blood volume, which is proportional to the birth weight (85 ml/kg body wt.), and (b) the haemoglobin concentration at birth, polycythaemic by normal standards. Either low birth weight or a low haemoglobin concentration in the neonatal period result in a proportionately impoverished iron endowment for the newborn infant. Instead of the neonatal iron stores being adequate to meet haemopoietic requirements for 4–6 months, as in the normal infant, they become prematurely exhausted leading to iron deficiency.

In premature or multiple births the iron stores are diminished in direct proportion to the birth weight (75 mg of elemental iron per kg body

rendered iron-sufficient by the administration of 250 mg parenteral iron at 9 months.)

In fact there are two main periods when the premature infant may experience a fall in haemoglobin concentration. The early phase begins in the first week of life and may last to 4 months of age. Very little erythropoiesis is occurring during the first two months of either normal or premature infants and this 'early' anaemia of prematurity is caused by the disproportionately rapid increase in blood volume occurring at a time when there is little red cell production (Gairdner, Marks and Roscoe, 1955). The red cells are normochromic and normocytic (Hadley and Chinnook, 1954).

Table 1.2. Total body iron at 1 year compared to endowment at birth

B.wt.	Hb g/100 ml	Hb mass	Hb Fe	Storage Fe	Tissue Fe	Total Fe
10.5 kg	12.3	103 g	325 mg	0	73 mg	398 mg

Full-term infant required 398 − 242 = 156 mg over year
Premature infant required 398 − 112 = 276 mg over year

From Schulman *J.A.M.A.*, **175**, 118 (1961).

The second fall in haemoglobin concentration begins in the fourth or fifth months and has the features of a hypochromic iron deficiency anaemia. This 'late' anaemia of prematurity can be prevented by prophylactic iron supplementation (Gorten and Cross, 1964).

A low haemoglobin level in the neonatal period, similarly leading to a reduced endowment of iron stores, can be caused by a large foeto-maternal haemorrhage at delivery, by haemorrhage from one twin to another (twin transfusion syndrome between monochorial foetuses) or by intrapartum foetal blood loss from such causes as rupture of the umbilical cord, anomalous placental vessels, *placenta previa* or *abruptio placentae*. Exchange transfusion may also cause a reduction in the infant's red cell mass by replacing the normally polycythaemic infant's blood by banked blood having a lower haematocrit. Over-enthusiastic diagnostic venepunctures may occasionally cause anaemia, bearing in mind that the blood volume of the newborn is in the region of 250 ml. Chronic foeto-maternal haemorrhage is the unique cause of a hypochromic anaemia due to established iron deficiency at birth. Maternal iron deficiency probably never causes anaemia in the newborn infant (Lanzkowsky, 1961), although extreme degrees of maternal iron deficiency anaemia, e.g. 5.2 g/100 ml, may be associated with the development of anaemia in the infant at about one year (Strauss, 1933), presumably due to a reduction of foetal storage iron in these exceptional circumstances.

The Committee of Nutrition of the American Academy of Paediatrics (1969) have emphasized that it is a simple matter to identify the infants who are poorly endowed with iron stores from a consideration of (a) their birth weight and (b) their haemoglobin levels at the age of a few days. There is a greater need for iron supplements in the poorly endowed infant than in the well-endowed infant and therapeutic recommendations are given for these two groups (*vide infra*).

Iron in the diet

Milk, the natural food of the infant, contains negligible amounts of iron. The concentration is 0.5 mg/l for cow's milk and 1.5 mg/l for human. About 15 litres (or US Quarts) of milk per day would have to be consumed to provide for the iron requirements of normal infants during their first year of life. (Committee on Nutrition, 1969). Most of the naturally occurring dietary iron is derived from fruit, eggs, meat and vegetables and it is only when mixed feeding is introduced that natural

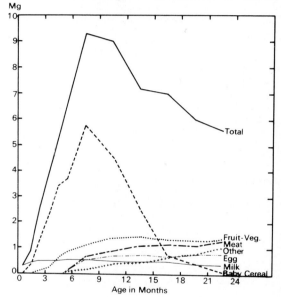

Fig. 1.1 Median total daily dietary iron intake and amounts contributed by various foods during infant development. (Reproduced by permission of Dr Beal and the Editor from the paper by Beal, Myers and McCammon (1962) *Paediatrics*, **30**, 518).

dietary iron becomes appreciable (Fig. 1.1). Only approximately 10 per cent of this dietary iron is absorbed (Schulz and Smith, 1958). The dietary requirement of elemental iron at 6 months has been estimated at 7–8 mg per day by Schulman (1961). This is similar to the recommendation of 1.0 mg/kg per day for well-endowed normal infants (Committee on Nutrition, 1969). It can be seen that this figure is seldom achieved from natural sources alone (Fig. 1.1). The current availability of iron-fortified infant cereals and milk formulae (Table 1.3) simplifies the satisfaction of these iron requirements. Up to 80 per cent of the total iron ingested over the first 6 months of life may be

Table 1.3 Iron content of certain infant feeds

Milk product	Iron in mg/100 ml*
National Dried Milk ($\frac{1}{2}$ cream or full cream)	0·66
Cow and Gate Babymilk 1 and 2	0·50
Cow and Gate 'Premium'	0·65
Cow and Gate 'Ready to Feed' ($\frac{1}{2}$ cream or full cream)	0·40
Ostermilk One	1·03
Ostermilk Two or 'Golden'	1·20
Ostermilk 'Ready to Feed' ('Golden' or 'New')	1·00
SMA 'Ready to Feed' or SMA S26	0·80
Human milk	0·15
Cow's milk	0·10

* Made up according to manufacturer's instructions. Around 150 to 200 ml/kg body wt./day taken in first 5–6 months.
Data largely from D.H.S.S. Report No. 9 (1974) 'Present-Day Practice in Infant Feeding'. London: H.M.S.O.

derived from these enriched sources. Although these products are available they are not always used. Ordinary cow's milk is often given instead. In the opinion of Diamond and Naiman (1967) continued or excessive milk administration, 'milkomania', due to poverty or ignorance, is the single most important cause of iron deficiency developing in the full-term infant.

An excellent recent commentary upon iron-fortified formulas in infancy, the incidence of iron deficiency and inter-relation between iron therapy and vitamin E deficiency is that of Pearson (1971).

Gastrointestinal function and iron deficiency

Occult gastrointestinal blood loss, accompanied by hypoproteinaemia, hypocupraemia and microscopic changes in the duodenal villi have been shown to occur in association with iron deficiency anaemia by the use of ^{51}Cr or ^{59}Fe-labelled red cells, this technique being more sensitive than direct chemical tests on the stools (Hoag, Wallerstein and Pollycove, 1961). Such blood loss may be attributed to the diffuse enteropathy described in children with nutritional iron deficiency by Naiman, Oski, Diamond, Vawter and Schwachman (1964). These authors demonstrated that children with iron deficiency had a high incidence of achlorhydria, impaired absorption of xylose and vitamin A with steatorrhoea and histological evidence of chronic duodenitis and mucosal atrophy. Following treatment with oral iron most of the abnormalities disappeared, suggesting that these were the effect rather than the cause of the iron deficiency.

An alternative theory has followed from the work of Wilson, Heiner and Lahey (1962) who found precipitins to milk protein in the sera of 75–80 per cent of iron deficient infants aged 6–24 months, together with loss of serum proteins into the gut. Subsequently Lahey and Wilson (1966) have presented evidence that gastro-intestinal blood loss may be induced by ingestion of whole cow's milk in infants possessing antibodies to milk proteins. In some of their patients the administration of milk was the triggering factor leading to a recurrence of blood loss in spite of previous correction of the anaemia by iron therapy. Milk-induced gastrointestinal loss of ^{131}I-labelled serum albumen was similarly found in 7 of 12 iron deficient infants (7–17 months) by an independent group (Woodruff, Wright and Wright, 1972). Further observations by Wilson, Lahey and Heiner (1974) suggest that enteropathy induced by cow's milk occurs in about 50 per cent of young children (6–25 months) with severe iron deficiency anaemia (Hb 2·4–7·7 g/100 ml). Transient allergy to bovine serum protein related to development of gastrointestinal immunity appears to be the cause. This subject has recently been reviewed (*B.M.J.*, 1972).

An unexpected role of acute gastroenteritis in the genesis of infantile anaemia and iron deficiency has been suggested by Elian, Bar-Shani, Liberman and Matoth (1966). Using ^{51}Cr-labelled red cells they found considerably greater blood loss in infants with gastroenteritis (0·7 to 4·8 ml/day, mean 1·85 ml) compared to controls (mean 0·64 ml) or infants with other infections (mean 0·43 ml). (One ml of blood contains approximately 0·5 mg of elemental iron.) They found that anaemia at the age of 1 year was more closely correlated with a history of recurrent diarrhoea than with a poor diet. Intestinal infestation, particularly with hookworm in appropriate geographical areas, can similarly be an important cause of blood loss and anaemia.

It is also well recognized that lesions of the gastrointestinal tract such as intestinal tumours, duplications, polyposis, oesophageal varices, peptic ulcers, telangiectasis, Meckel's diverticulae and ulcerative colitis can cause chronic or intermittent haemorrhage leading to anaemia. All occur in children on rare occasions (Cases 1 and 2). The blood loss need not be occult or confined to the gastrointestinal tract; iron deficiency is common among children with haemophilia or severe von Willebrand's disease and can occur in the rare chronic or paroxysmal haemoglobinurias. In older children and adolescents episodes of iron deficiency anaemia may be seen following periods of rapid growth, during which demands exceed supply.

Malabsorption, as part of the coeliac syndrome, becomes a major cause of iron deficiency after the first year of life. Although iron deficiency is almost invariably present in untreated coeliac disease (Dormandy, Waters and Mollin, 1963) it is not certain that malabsorption is the only mechanism involved. Webb, Taylor and Gattenby (1967) found that absorption of ^{59}Fe-labelled rabbit-haemoglobin was impaired in only one out of nine coeliac patients off therapy and with the active disease. They suggested that the malabsorption might be intermittent or that there might be an increased loss of iron by epithelial desquamation. Sutton et al. (1970) have recently shown such an excessive loss of iron from the gut in adult coeliac

disease when intestinal cell turnover is rapid. The magnitude of this iron loss is sufficient to contribute to the high incidence of iron deficiency in this condition. Croft (1970) has pointed out that the combination of a high mucosal cell loss plus impaired reabsorption of the lost iron could be a potent cause of iron deficiency (Fig. 1.2).

INCIDENCE OF IRON DEFICIENCY

A survey in Glasgow showed mild anaemia (Hb less than 11 g/100 ml) between the ages of 6 and 24 months in 32 per cent of a random group of children and in 59 per cent of last-borns from slum areas (Arneil, McKilligan and Lobo, 1965). Later-born children show a higher incidence of iron deficiency than first-borns (Guest and Brown, 1957). The incidence of more marked anaemia in some other surveys is given in Table 1.4. In children up to 3 years of age the incidence is related to socio-economic conditions and hospitalization. Above that age the incidence of anaemia drops in all social groups.

CLINICAL FEATURES

Irritability, decreased exercise tolerance, listlessness, gastrointestinal upsets, pica (Crosby, 1971) or intercurrent infection may bring the presence of iron deficiency anaemia to light. There

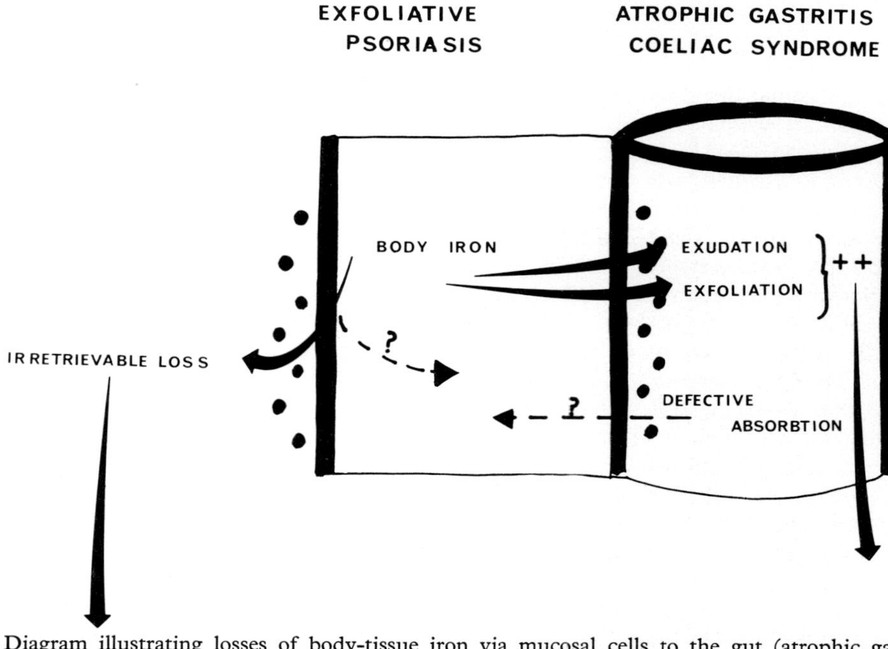

Fig. 1.2 Diagram illustrating losses of body-tissue iron via mucosal cells to the gut (atrophic gastritis coeliac syndrome) and by passage to the blood plasma (exfoliative psoriasis). (Reproduced by permission of the author and editor from the paper by Croft (1970) Proc. Roy. Soc. Med., 63, 1224).

IRON DEFICIENCY ANAEMIA

Table 1.4 Incidence of iron deficiency anaemia

Age	Population	Criteria	Anaemic per cent	Authors
9 months	Private practice	Hb < 10g/100 ml	3·2	Fuerth (1971)
1–2 years	Cross section of US pre-school children	,,	6·0	Owen, Nelson and Garry (1970)
0–3 years	Impoverished, black	,,	28	Zee, Walters and Mitchell (1970)
$\frac{1}{2}$–2 years	Hospitalized, Chicago	,,	44	Schulman (1961)
$4\frac{1}{2}$–$6\frac{1}{2}$ years	Random, 95 per cent black	PCV < 31 per cent	1·5	Brigety and Pearson (1970)

may be a history of low birth weight or blood loss at birth. Pallor of the palpebral conjunctivae, mucous membranes, nail beds and palms are more dependable signs of anaemia than pallor of skin. Atrophic glossitis, dysphagia and koilonychia are seldom seen in children; but slight splenomegaly is found in 10 per cent of children with iron deficiency, unlike the situation in adults. Soft apical systolic 'haemic' murmurs may be present and even cardiac enlargement. Other deficiencies may co-exist when the anaemia is nutritional or due to malabsorption. Milder degrees of iron deficiency may be discovered fortuitously in relatively asymptomatic children. A significant association between 'beeturia', i.e. the passing of red urine after eating beetroots, and iron deficiency has recently been described by Tunnessen, Smith and Oski (1969). Where the iron deficiency is secondary to blood loss or malabsorption there may be clinical evidence of the underlying disease (Cases 1 and 2).

There is conflicting evidence regarding the effect of iron deficiency upon susceptibility to infection (Lancet, 1974). On the one hand an *increased* liability to respiratory infection in iron-deficient children has been found in unsupplemented infants in the first year of life (Andelman and Sered, 1966) perhaps due to a decrease in the iron-containing enzyme myeloperoxidase causing impaired intracellular bacterial killing (Chandra, 1973). Also a defect in cell-mediated immunity has been demonstrated in iron deficiency (Joynson, Jacobs, Walker and Dolby, 1972) which may explain the beneficial effect of iron therapy in certain patients with mucocutaneous candidiasis (Higgs and Wells, 1972). On the other hand there is experimental evidence that the unsaturated transferrin, or siderophilin, inhibits the growth of bacteria by virtue of its iron-binding activity (Fletcher, 1971) and that iron injections in laboratory animals render them more susceptible to relatively avirulent bacteria (Jackson and Burrows, 1956). Clinically the liability to systemic moniliasis in patients with acute leukaemia is correlated with

their high serum iron and saturation of transferrin (Caroline, Rosner and Kozinn, 1969), while a reduced incidence of bacterial infections in the presence of iron deficiency has been reported by Masawe, Muindi and Swai (1974) working in Dar es Salaam. Clearly there are unresolved differences among these observations.

DIAGNOSIS AND LABORATORY FINDINGS

The minimum necessary investigations are a haemoglobin estimation and examination of a stained blood film. In established iron deficiency anaemia the haemoglobin level will usually be below 10 g/100 ml and the blood film will show characteristic elongated cigar-shaped red cells together with microcytosis and a variable degree of hypochromia. In iron deficiency the elongated cells never reach the 25 per cent or more seen in hereditary elliptocytosis. A useful feature may be anisochromia, viz. some red cells are paler than others in the same field. Also there is anisocytosis, viz. greater variation in cell diameter than normal, but this is a quite non-specific feature, occurring in all anaemias other than due to haemodilution or acute blood loss. A diagnosis of iron deficiency *should not be made on anisocytosis alone*.

Additional haematological findings

While it is true that the MCHC, MCH and MCV are low in established iron deficiency anaemia when these are calculated from the PCV determined by centrifugation (Bainton and Finch, 1964) this is not necessarily so when the PCV is determined by red cell sizing with the Coulter 'S' (Coulter Electronics Inc). The explanation is that the variation in size and shape of red cells in iron deficiency impairs centrifugal packing, giving rise to a spuriously high PCV (Rose, 1971). A further reason for not relying upon red cell indices in the screening for iron deficiency in young children is that these normally require a venepuncture (see, however, Introduction, Stuart et al., 1974).

Usually it is possible to say whether the morphological changes are consistent with the severity of the anaemia. If this is not so it may suggest an additional factor, such as chronic infection or renal failure, as contributing to the cause of the anaemia. The presence of polychromasia, viz. bluish staining red cells, or normoblasts in the blood film, or an elevated reticulocyte count (over 2 per cent) raise the possibility of recent blood loss or haematinic therapy.

In a typical case of iron deficiency these simple tests (i.e. Hb plus film) are all that are required *providing the response to iron therapy is subsequently established* by repeating the haemoglobin at weekly or fortnightly intervals until normal. The response can be determined sooner by performing serial reticulocyte counts, when a 'peak' value of over 5 per cent should occur on the 8th to 10th day after starting therapy.

Fuller haematological investigations should be performed in the atypical case. The platelet count* and white cell distribution are usually normal in simple iron deficiency, the reticulocyte count less than 2 per cent. The ESR is elevated in many secondary anaemias but seldom in simple iron deficiencies. The marrow shows a mild degree of erythroid hyperplasia but normal myeloid and megakaryocyte series with an increase in small polychromatic normoblasts with shrunken cytoplasm. Stainable iron (marrow haemosiderin) is absent from the reticulum cells, and below 10 per cent of nucleated red cells stain as sideroblasts in true iron deficiency (Bainton and Finch, 1964). In chronic infection there is an increased amount of haemosiderin in the reticulum cells, but still a relatively low percentage of sideroblasts (less than 20 per cent), due to 'reticuloendothelial iron block' (Freireich, Miller, Emerson and Ross, 1957). In other hypochromic anaemias such as thalassaemias, sideroblastic, lead poisoning or in the presence of associated folic acid deficiency

* See, however Chapter 16, last page.

both reticulum cell iron and sideroblast iron are increased.

During the early stage of iron therapy a striking macrocytosis may appear in the peripheral blood, accompanying a reticulocytosis (Leventhal and Stohlman, 1966), (Fig. 1.3). This 'pseudomacrocytosis' may falsely suggest a dimorphic anaemia due to iron plus folic acid deficiency unless the phenomenon is recognized.

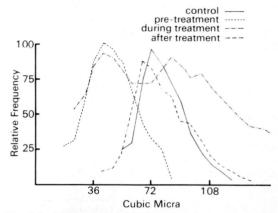

Fig. 1.3 Macrocytic response of an infant with dietary iron-deficiency anaemia, treated with large (12 mg/kg/day) doses of parenteral iron. (Reproduced by permission from the department of the late Dr F. Stohlman, and of the Editor of *Paediatrics*, from the paper by Leventhal and Stohlman (1966)).

Shortened red cell survival has been demonstrated in patients with severe iron deficiency without blood loss (Layrisse, Linares and Roche, 1965). This was thought to be due to the deformity of the hypochromic RBCs. It has, however, more recently been found that the activities of red cell glutathione peroxidase and catalase were decreased in children with iron deficiency increasing red cell susceptibility to hydrogen peroxide (Macdougall, 1972). None had vitamin E deficiency. The clinical significance of these observations is not clear but Macdougall points out that the possibility of haemolysis should be borne in mind when such children receive antipyretic, analgesic or antibiotic medication.

Table 1.5 Causes of hypochromic anaemia

1. Iron deficiency
2. Chronic infection or inflammation
3. Thalassaemias (alpha, beta, delta)
4. Sideroblastic anaemias, including lead and arsenic poisoning
5. Pulmonary haemosiderosis, including Goodpastures syndrome (Matsaniotis et al., 1968)
6. Congenital transferring deficiency (Heilmeyer et al., 1961)
7. Congenital metabolic defect with parenchymal hepatic accumulation of iron (Shahidi et al., 1964)
8. Copper deficiency (Karpel and Peden, 1972)

Biochemical tests of iron deficiency

Although iron deficiency constitutes by far the most frequent cause of hypochromic anaemia other less frequent causes also exist (Table 1.5) and should be considered in the atypical case, especially if there is no obvious cause of iron deficiency or if there is a failure of response to iron. A fasting serum iron and total iron-binding concentration (TIBC), collected at least 4 hours after the last meal and after ceasing all haematinics or iron-fortified foods for 2 days, is the single most useful test. In anaemia due to nutritional iron deficiency or blood loss the serum iron level is less than 60 µg/100 ml, the percentage saturation of transferrin is 16 per cent or less and the TIBC is usually above 300 µg/100 ml (Baintin and Finch, 1964). In the hypochromic anaemia of chronic infection or inflammation the serum iron is similar, percentage saturation may be somewhat higher (up to 20 per cent) but the TIBC is usually below 300 µg/100 ml (Fig. 1.4). High serum iron levels

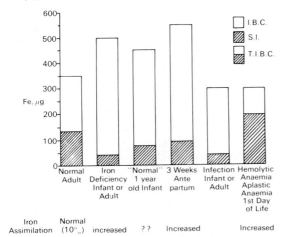

Fig. 1.4 Iron concentration of blood plasma from normal and clinically abnormal subjects. (After Sturgeon (1956)). (Reproduced by permission of the author and editor from the paper of Sturgeon (1956), *Paediatics*, **18**, 267).

are found in other hypochromic anaemias such as thalassaemias, lead poisoning and sideroblastic anaemias as well as in the very rare cases of hypochromic anaemia due to a congenital defect of iron metabolism (Shahidi, Nathan and Diamond, 1964) or due to copper deficiency (Karpel and Peden, 1972). If there is a possibility of coeliac disease or multiple dietary deficiencies as in gross malnutrition then the serum folate and B_{12} estimation can usefully be estimated on the same fasting sample of serum.

Total iron stores have recently been shown to be reflected by the serum ferritin level (Jacobs, Miller, Wormwood, Beamish and Wardrop, 1972). Ferritin is normally thought of as a storage compound in equilibrium with the transferrin-bound iron pool. It is mainly found in the reticuloendothelial cells and liver cells, but a little is also present in normoblasts. Traces can be detected in serum by using a sensitive immunoradiometric assay (Addison, Beamish, Hales, Hodkins, Jacobs and Llewelin, 1972). Because of the wide range and logarithmic distribution it is more appropriate to express group results as geometric means or median values (Table 1.6). Not only are the values low in iron deficiency and high in iron overload but they are also high in chronic haemolysis, in liver disease and in the anaemia of infection or inflammation. Siimes, Addiego and Dallman (1974) point out the value of serum ferritin in distinguishing hypochromic anaemia of infection from that of iron deficiency, since both may have low serum iron and reduced percentage of transferrin (Bainton and Finch, 1964). Siimes *et al.* (1974) also used the serum ferritin assay to confirm the known pattern of iron status in the newborn. At birth the levels were slightly elevated compared to later life, rising at the age of 1 month to higher than normal values reflecting the contribution of the neonatal red cell mass to iron stores. Thereafter there was a steady decrease in serum ferritin between 2 and 6 months at which time the lower levels of later childhood were reached. Practical advantages of the serum ferritin assay in paediatric practice are that only 0·1 ml of capillary blood are needed and that diurnal variation does not occur.

Tests for intestinal blood loss

Tests for faecal occult blood are valuable in that they may draw attention to bleeding from a Meckel's diverticulum, intestinal polyp or peptic ulcer. It has, however, recently been recognized that iron deficiency *per se* may be associated with intestinal blood loss (*vide supra*).

In the presence of probable occult intestinal bleeding radiological investigations are performed including barium meal and follow-through with special attention to small bowel views and supplemented by barium enema and sigmoidoscopy in an effort to detect polyposis of the colon (Case 2). Recently ^{99m}Tc pertechnetate scintillation scanning has proved a simple, safe and effective means of detecting Meckel's diverticula containing ectopic gastric mucosa and therefore prone to ulceration (Kilpatrick and Aseron, 1972; Jaros, Schussheim

8 PAEDIATRIC HAEMATOLOGY

Table 1.6 Serum ferritin levels

Adults	in μg/ml Geometric means	Range
Normal	59	12–300*
Fe deficiency	4·0	1–14
Fe overload	2930	1350–6800
Liver disease	509	25–3239
Anaemia due to inflammation	305	10–1650
	from Lipschitz *et al.* (1974)	

Children	Medians	Range
At birth	101	12–200 (approx)
At 1 month	356	60–600 (approx)
6 months to 15 years	30	7–142*
Fe defic anaemia	3·4	1·5–9
Latent Fe defic.	10·6	4·5–41
Thalassaemia major	850	590–1830
Chronic haemolysis	242	96–920
	from Siimes *et al.* (1974)	

* = 95 per cent confidence limits

and Levy, 1972; Leonidas and German, 1974). The technetium is concentrated in acid-secreting mucosa and juice whether ectopic or normal.

Case 1. A boy of $3\frac{1}{2}$ (No. 171486) developed loose stools and his mother thought these contained traces of blood. Three weeks later he developed colicky abdominal pains and was admitted to hospital. He was found to be pale with a Hb of 6·0 g/100 ml. The blood film showed hypochromia plus polychromasia suggesting blood loss, which was confirmed by consistently positive faecal occult tests (Okokit: Hughes and Hughes, Ltd.). Serum iron was 15 μg/100 ml and whole blood folate normal (104 ng/ml). He was transfused and put on oral iron (Sytron—5 ml t.d.s.).

A Meckel's diverticulum was suspected but barium meal and follow-through, and repeated barium enemas failed to show any intestinal abnormality. The FOBs remained strongly positive. A laparotomy showed lymphosarcoma of the ileum with massive enlargement of the mesenteric glands. Right hemicolectomy was performed excising about 2 ft of terminal ileum but it was impossible to remove all the involved lymph glands.

A week after laparotomy the wound was healing well and he was commenced on chemotherapy consisting of weekly I.V. vincristine, adriamycin, and cyclophosphamaide plus oral prednisolone. A marrow examination at the time of starting chemotherapy was normal, excluding leukaemic transformation of the lymphosarcoma. After 4 weeks on the above therapy this was changed to maintenance chemotherapy consisting of daily 6-mercaptopurine plus weekly methotrexate and cyclophosphamide and 3-monthly vincristine plus prednisolone. He is remaining well 28 months later.

Case 2. A girl aged 12 (No. 170211) was referred from the family doctor as a matter of urgency as he suspected leukaemia. She had become increasingly pale over 6 months but there were no other symptoms or specific clinical features. The haemoglobin was 7·0 g/100 ml with normal white cells and platelet count. The blood film showed hypochromia plus polychromasia (retics. 3 per cent). Serum iron was 6 μg/100 ml and TIBC 520. Marrow smears showed a mild degree of erythroid hyperplasia with absence of stainable iron in reticulum cells and erythroblasts. Serum folate and B_{12} were normal, As she was well outside the age of nutritional iron deficiency (6 months to 3 years) and had no clinical features to suggest malabsorption subacute blood loss was suspected as the cause of the anaemia. This was supported by the presence of hypochromic polychromatic red cells on the initial blood film. She had not been given iron therapy at that time. Menstruation had not commenced and there was no question of overt blood loss. Investigations for occult intestinal bleeding showed 6 negative faecal occult blood tests, followed by 3 giving 'trace' results and then 3 positive results. Barium meal and follow-through was normal apart from suggesting ileal polyposis, which was confirmed by special small bowel examination on a repeat barium follow-through. The polyps were mainly ileal. No definite large bowel polyps were seen with barium enema. Neither were any found on sigmoidoscopy.

Careful examination of her mouth showed a single pigmented spot in the middle of the lower lip, which, together with the small bowel polyposis, suggested the Peutz-Jegher's syndrome. She was transfused and put on oral iron for 3 months. No recurrence of anaemia has occurred over 18 months follow-up. The small intestinal polyps of Peutz-Jegher's syndrome are not thought to be premalignant, and surgery was not considered.

TREATMENT

The presence of iron deficiency anaemia indicates not only a deficit of circulating haemoglobin iron but also a total exhaustion of all iron stores (Bainton and Finch, 1964). Occurring at a time of growth and expanding blood volume the mere institution of a normal dietary intake is insufficient to replenish the stores fully. Additional therapeutic iron administration is essential and the objective should be both that of correcting the anaemia and providing adequate iron stores to meet future demands. With the latter objective in mind oral medicinal iron should be continued for approximately 3 months (Woodruff, 1961).

Oral iron is preferable to parenteral iron therapy unless patient intolerance or lack of parental co-operation make the oral route unreliable (Sitarz, Wolff, and Van Hofe, 1960). There is no evidence that the rate of haemoglobin response is greater with parenteral iron (Fig. 1.5). Fatal reactions to parenteral iron have been reported in patients with the malabsorption syndrome (Karhunen et al., 1970).

Ferrous iron is more efficient than ferric iron. The dosage of preparations should be considered in terms of mg of elemental iron per day. Only iron compounds of known efficacy should be used since highly palatable but ineffective preparations have been marketed (Diamond, Naiman, Allen and Oski, 1963). An elemental oral iron dose of 4·5 to 6·0 mg/kg/day in 3 divided doses is adequate for therapy of established iron deficiency. Percentage absorption falls off above this dose and no additional benefit is achieved from higher doses (Woodruff, 1961). It is advisable to build up to this dose gradually in order to reduce gastrointestinal intolerance.

Prophylactic administration of iron involves lower doses than those given for therapy. The Committee on Nutrition (1969) recommended 1 mg/kg/day from the age of 2 months for normally endowed infants (this being obtained from iron-enriched foodstuffs) and 2 mg/kg/day from the age of 2 months for poorly endowed infants of low birth weight or low haemoglobin in the neonatal period. To achieve this higher intake medicinal iron is usually needed.

The simplest oral preparation is ferrous sulphate which can be given in solution (ferrous sulphate mixture paediatric, BPC) for infants, or in tablet form for older children. Iron absorption was thought to be superior when administered between feeds (Schulz and Smith, 1958) but this timing is liable to produce intolerance in some infants. However, it has been found that administration of iron simultaneously with milk or cereal feeds results in adequate absorption with less intestinal intolerance (Marsh, Long and Steirwalt, 1959). Alternatively a chelated iron preparation such as Plesmet (iron-glycinate, 25 mg elemental iron/5 ml), Sytron (iron-EDTA, 55 mg elemental iron/10 ml) or Niferex (non-ionic polysaccharide iron complex, 100 mg elemental iron/5 ml) syrups

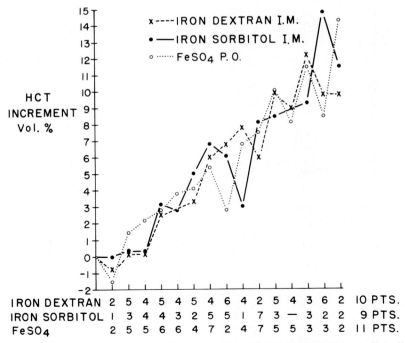

Fig. 1.5 Comparison of the HCT increment (vol. per cent) on administration of three clinically-approved iron compounds, orally or i.m. (Reproduced by permission of the author and editor from the paper by McCurdy (1965) *J. Am. Med. Assoc.*, **191**, 859).

are well tolerated although a little more expensive than ferrous sulphate. I routinely use a chelated iron preparation.

The total dose of parenteral iron (Imferon: iron dextran) is 100 mg for infants under 6 months, 200 mg between the ages of 6 and 12 months, 300 mg from 12–24 months and 400 mg over 24 months. The injections are given in 50 mg (1 ml) I.M. doses at daily or weekly intervals. Alternatively the following formula may be used: mg of iron to be injected = desired rise in Hb g/100 ml × kg body wt × 3.

The response to therapy, whether oral or parenteral, should be followed. After a lag period of 7–10 days the haemoglobin level should then rise at the rate of approximately 1 g/100 ml every 10 days. If this rise is not achieved the possibilities of continuing blood loss, coexisting infection, renal failure, folic acid deficiency or thalassaemia should be considered.

Blood transfusion is not recommended for simple iron deficiency unless the anaemia is sufficiently severe (e.g. 3–4 g/100 ml) to cause cerebral or cardiopulmonary symptoms, there is associated blood loss, or correction of the anaemia becomes a matter of urgency in such circumstances as serious infection or prior to surgery. Transfusion in a patient with severe anaemia should be with packed cells, given slowly over 6–12 hours aiming only to partially correct the anaemia in the first instance. 6 ml of whole blood (or 4 ml of packed red cells) per kg body weight raises the haemoglobin level by approximately 1 g/100 ml. A diuretic such as lasix (Frusemide) may be given during the transfusion if there is thought to be a risk of cardiopulmonary embarrassment.

REFERENCES

Addison, G. M., Beamish, M. R., Hales, C. N., Hodkins, M., Jacobs, A. & Llewellin, P. (1972) An immunoradiometric assay for ferritin in the serum of normal subjects and patients with iron deficiency and iron overload. *J. clin. Path.*, **25**, 326.

American Academy of Paediatrics (1969) Iron balance and requirements in infancy. *Pediatrics*, **43**, 134.

Andelman, M. & Sered, B. R. (1966) Utilization of dietary iron by term infants: A study of 1,048 infants from a low socioeconomic population. *Am. J. Dis. Child.*, **111**, 45.

Arneil, G. C., McKilligan, H. R. & Lobo, E. (1965) Malnutrition in Glasgow children. *Scot. med. J.*, **10**, 480.

Bainton, D. F. & Finch, C. A. (1964) The diagnosis of iron deficiency anemia. *Am J. Med.*, **37**, 62.

Beal, V. A., Meyers, A. J. & McCammon, R. W. (1962) Iron intake, hemoglobin, and physical growth during the first 2 years of life. *Pediatrics*, **30**, 518.

Brigety, R. E. & Pearson, H. A. (1970) Effects of dietary and iron supplementation on haematocrit levels of preschool children. *J. Pediat.*, **76**, 757.

British Medical Journal (1972) Editorial: Problems of iron-deficiency anaemia in infancy. *Brit. med. J.*, **i**, 437.

Caroline, L., Rosner, F. & Kozinn, P. J. (1969) Elevated serum iron, low unbound transferrin and candidiasis in acute leukemia. *Blood*, **34**, 441.

Chandra, R. K. (1973) Reduced bactericidal capacity of polymorphs in iron deficiency. *Arch. Dis. Childh.*, **48**, 864.

Committee on Nutrition, American Academy of Pediatrics (1969) Iron balance and requirements in infancy. *Pediatrics*, **43**, 134.

Croft, D. N. (1970) Body iron loss and cell loss from epithelia. *Proc. Roy. Soc. Med.*, **63**, 1221.

Crosby, W. H. (1971) Editorial: Food pica and iron deficiency. *Arch. Intern. Med.*, **127**, 960.

Diamond, L. K., Naiman, J. L., Allen, D. M. & Oski, F. A. (1963) The treatment of iron-deficiency anaemia—palatable but ineffective iron medication. *Pediatrics*, **31**, 1041.

Diamond, L. K. & Naiman, J. L. (1967) More on iron deficiency anemia. *J. Pediat.*, **70**, 304.

Dormandy, K. M., Waters, A. H. & Mollin, D. L. (1963) Folic acid deficiency in coeliac disease. *Lancet*, **i**, 632.

Elian, E., Ban-Shani, S., Liberman, A. & Matoth, Y. (1966) Intestinal blood loss: A factor in calculations of body iron in late infancy. *J. Pediat.*, **69**, 215.

Fletcher, J. (1971) The effect of iron and transferrin on the killing of *Escherichia coli* in fresh serum. *Immunology*, **20**, 493.

Freireich, E. J. Miller, A., Emerson, C. P. & Ross, J. F. (1957) The effect of inflammation on the utilization of erythrocyte and transferrin bound radioiron for red cell production. *Blood*, **12**, 972.

Fuerth, J. H. (1971) Incidence of anemia in full-term infants seen in private practice. *J. Pediat.*, **79**, 560.

Gairdner, D., Marks, J. & Roscoe, J. D. (1955) Blood formation in infancy. *IV*. The early anemia of prematurity. *Arch. Dis. Childh.*, **30**, 203.

Gorten, M. K. & Cross, E. R. (1964) Iron metabolism in premature infants. *II*. Prevention of iron deficiency. *J. Pediat.*, **64**, 509.

Guest, G. & Brown, E. (1957) Erythrocytes and hemoglobin of the blood in infancy and childhood. *Am. J. Dis. Child.*, **93**, 486.

Hadley, G. C. & Chinnock, R. F. (1954) A study of hemograms in premature infants. *J. Pediat.*, **45**, 413.

Haehunen, P., Hartel, G., Kivikangas, V. & Reinikainen, M. (1970) Reaction to iron Sorbitol injection in three cases of malabsorption. *Brit. med. J.*, **ii**, 521.

Heilmeyer, L., Keller, W., Vivell, O., Keiderling, W., Betke, K., Wohler, F. & Schultze, H. E. (1961) Kongenitale Atransferrinämie bei einem sieben Jahre alten Kind. *Deutsche med. Wchnschr.*, **86**, 1745.

Higgs, J. M. & Wells, R. S. (1972) Chronic mucocutaneous candidiasis: associated abnormalities of iron metabolism. *Brit. J. Derm.*, **86**, Suppl. 888.

Hoag, M. S., Wallerstein, R. O. & Pollycove, M. (1961) Occult blood loss in iron deficiency anemia of infanty. *Pediatrics*, **27**, 199.

Jackson, S. & Burrows, T. N. (1956) The virulence-enhancing effect of iron on nonpigmented mutants of virulent strains of *Pasteurella pestis. Br. J. Exp. Path.*, **37**, 577.

Jacobs, A., Miller, F., Wormwood, M., Beamish, M. R. & Wardrop, C. A. (1972) Ferritin in the serum of normal subjects and patients with iron deficiency and iron overload. *Brit. med. J.*, **4**, 206.

Jaros, R., Schussheim, A. & Levy, L. M. (1973) Diagnosis of bleeding Meckel's diverticulum utilising 99m technetium pertechnetate scinti-imaging. *J. Pediat.*, **82**, 45.

Joynson, D. H. M., Jacobs, A., Murray Walker, D. & Dolby, A. E. (1972) Defect of cell-mediated immunity in patients with iron-deficiency anaemia. *Lancet*, **ii**, 1058.

Karpel, J. T. & Peden, V. H. (1972) Copper deficiency in long-term parenteral nutrition. *J. Pediat.*, **80**, 32.

Kilpatrick, Z. M. & Aseron, C. A. (1972) Radioisotope detection of Meckel's diverticulum causing acute rectal hemorrhage. *New Eng. J. Med.*, **287**, 653.

Lahey, M. E. & Wilson, J. F. (1966) The etiology of iron deficiency anemia in infants—a reappraisal. *J. Pediat.*, **69**, 339.

Lancet (1974) Editorial: Iron and resistance to infection. *Lancet*, **ii**, 325.

Lanzkowsky, P. (1961) The influence of maternal iron deficiency on the haemoglobin of the infant. *Arch. Dis. Childh.*, **36**, 205.

Layrisse, M., Linares, J. & Roche, M. (1965) Excess hemolysis in subjects with severe iron deficiency anaemia and non-associated with hookworm infection. *Blood*, **25**, 73.

Leonidas, J. C. & Germann, D. R. (1974) Technetium-99m pertechnetate imaging in diagnosis of Meckel's diverticulum. *Arch. Dis. Childh.*, **49**, 21.

Leventhal, B. & Stohlman, F. (1966) Regulation of erythropoiesis *XVII*: The determinants of red-cell size in iron-deficiency states. *Pediatrics*, **37**, 62.

Lipschitz, D. A., Cook, J. D. & Finch, C. A. (1973) A clinical evaluation of serum ferritin as an index of iron stores. *New Eng. J. Med.*, **290**, 1213.

Macdougall, L. G. (1972) Red cell metabolism in iron deficiency anemia. *III*. The relationship between glutathione peroxidase, catalse, serum vitamin E, and susceptibility of iron-deficient red cells to oxidative hemolysis. *J. Pediat.*, **80**, 775.

Marsh, A. K., Long, H. & Stierwalt, E. (1959) Comparative hematological response to iron fortification of a milk formula for infants. *Pediatrics*, **24**, 404.

Masawe, A. E., Muindi, J. M. & Swai, G. B. R. (1974) Infections in iron deficiency and other types of anaemia in the tropics. *Lancet*, **ii**, 314.

Matsaniotis, N., Karpouzas, J., Apostolopoulou, E. & Messaritakis, J. (1968) Idiopathic pulmonary haemosiderosis in children. *Arch. Dis. Childh.*, **43**, 307.

Naiman, J. L., Oski, F. A., Diamond, L. K., Vawter, G. F. & Shwachman, H. (1964) The gastrointestinal effects of iron deficiency anemia. *Pediatrics*, **33**, 83.

Osgood, E. E. (1955) Development and growth of hematopoietic tissues. *Pediatrics*, **15**, 733.

Owen, G. M., Nelson, C. E. & Garry, P. J. (1970) Nutritional status of preschool children: Hemoglobin, hematocrit, and plasma iron values. *J. Pediat.*, **76**, 761.

Pearson, H. A. (1971) Iron-fortified formulas in infancy. *J. Pediat.*, **79**, 557.

Rose, M. S. (1971) Epitaph for the M.C.H.C. *Brit. med. J.*, **iv**, 169.

Schulman, I. (1961) Iron requirements in infancy. *J. Am. Med. Assoc.*, **175**, 118.

Schulz, J. & Smith, N. J. (1958) A quantitative study of the absorption of food iron in infants and children. *Amer. J. Dis. Child.*, **95**, 109.

Shahidi, N. T., Nathan, D. G. & Diamond, L. K. (1964) Iron-deficiency anemia associated with an inborn error of iron metabolism in two siblings. *J. Clin. Invest.*, **45**, 510.

Siimes, M. A., Addiego, J. E. & Dallman, P. R. (1974) Ferritin in serum: Diagnosis of iron deficiency and iron overload in infants and children. *Blood*, **43**, 581.

Sitarz, A. L., Wolff, J. A. & Van Hofe, F. H. (1960) Comparison of oral and intramuscular iron for prevention of the late anemia of premature infants. *Pediatrics*, **26**, 375.

Strauss, N. B. (1933) Anaemia of infancy from maternal iron deficiency in pregnancy. *J. Clin. Invest.*, **12**, 345.

Sturgeon, P. (1956) Iron metabolism. Review with special considerations of iron requirements during normal infancy. *Pediatrics*, **18**, 267.

Sutton, D. R., McLean Baird, I., Stewart, J. S. & Coghill, N. F. (1970) 'Free' iron loss in atrophic gastritis, post-gastrectomy states, and adult coeliac disease. *Lancet*, **ii**, 387.

Tunnessen, W. W., Smith, C. & Oski, F. A. (1969) Beeturia: A sign of iron deficiency. *Amer. J. Dis. Child.*, **117**, 424.

Webb, M. G. T., Taylor, M. R. H. & Gatenby, P. B. B. (1967) Iron absorption in coeliac disease of childhood and adolescence. *Brit. med. J.* **ii**, 151.

Wilson, J. F., Heiner, D. C. & Lahey, M. E. (1962) Studies on iron metabolism. I. Evidence of gastrointestinal dysfunction in infants with iron deficiency anemia. A preliminary report. *J. Pediat.*, **60**, 787.

Wilson, J. F., Lahey, M. E. & Heiner, D. C. (1974) Studies on iron metabolism. V. Further observations on cow's milk-induced gastrointestinal bleeding in infants with iron-deficiency anaemia. *J. Pediat.*, **84**, 335.

Woodruff, C. W. (1961) The utilization of iron administered orally. *Pediatrics*, **27**, 194.
Woodruff, C. W., Wright, S. W. & Wright, R. P. (1972) The role of fresh cow's milk in iron deficiency. II. Comparison of fresh cow's milk with a prepared formula. *Amer. J. Dis. Child.*, **124**, 26.
Zee, P., Walter, T. & Mitchell, C. (1970) A nutritional survey of preschool children from impoverished black families, Memphis. *J.A.M.A.*, **213**, 739.

2. Folate Metabolism and Deficiency

Biochemistry of folic acid and its derivatives, Dietary sources of folate, Absorption of folates | Determination of folate status, *Folate assays in blood, Figlu test, Haematological changes* | Folate balance in infancy and childhood, *Daily folate requirements, Folate status in the newborn* | Conditions associated with folate deficiency in childhood, *Prematurity, Infection, Malabsorption, Haemolysis, Nutritional deficiency, Anticonvulsants and other drugs associated with megaloblastic anaemia, Inborn errors related to folate metabolism, Conditions with increased folate loss* | Clinical features and treatment.

BIOCHEMISTRY OF FOLIC ACID AND ITS DERIVATIVES

Pteroylglutamic acid (Fig. 2.1) is the parent substance of the group of compounds included under the general term folic acid or folate (Commission on Biochemical Nomenclature, 1966).

coenzymes for some of the 1-carbon transfer reactions may be in this polyglutamyl conjugate form.

The 1-carbon groups involved in these transfer reactions can exist at three different levels of oxidation, equivalent to that of an alcohol, aldehyde or carboxylic acid:

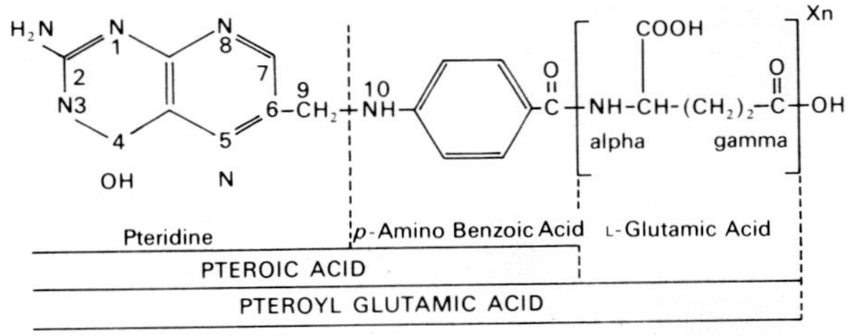

Fig. 2.1 Pteroylglutamic acid and its conjugates. Pteroylglutamic acid is a monoglutamate, n=1. In the tri- and heptaglutamyl conjugates n=3 and 7, respectively.

The compounds of biochemical importance in folate metabolism are derived from pteroylglutamic acid by:

1. Reduction to 7, 8-dihydro—and 5, 6, 7, 8-tetrahydrofolates.
2. Substitution of formyl or other 1-carbon group in place of H at position 5 or 10, or bridging 5 to 10.
3. Conjugation of the gamma-glutamyl carboxyl group with further molecules of L-glutamic acid to form tri- and heptaglutamyl derivatives.

It is only in the reduced form that folic acid is capable of fulfilling its metabolic role of accepting and donating methyl, formyl or other 1-carbon fragments. The polyglutamyl conjugates are of importance since the bulk of folate activity in animal tissues, including red cells, and in the diet is present in this form. Also the physiological

Compound		Oxidation level
5-methyl-tetrahydrofolate		methanol
5-10-methylene	,,	formaldehyde
5-formimino	,,	
5-10-methenyl	,,	formate
10-formyl*	,,	

*Folinic acid or (citrovorum factor) is 5-formyl-tetrahydrofolate. It does not itself occur *in vivo* but is probably converted to 10-formyl-tetrahydrofolate if administered therapeutically.

A series of dehydrogenases, reductases and deaminases can convert one folate derivative to another. The different levels of oxidation in these coenzymes determine the metabolic processes in which they participate (Fig. 2.2).

It is apparent that folate occupies a key position in many aspects of cell metabolism including aminoacid and nucleic acid synthesis particularly

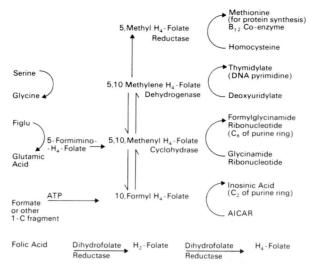

Fig. 2.2 The function of tetrahydrofolate (H_4-folate) derivatives in 1-carbon unit transfer. H_4-Folate, or its conjugates, is the universal acceptor of 1-carbon fragments from the reactions shown on the left, and is itself regenerated by the reactions shown on the right.

relevant to proliferating cells and growing tissues. The formylation of methionyl—sRNA, which is essential for the initiation of protein synthesis in microbiological systems, is also folate dependent. For more detailed reviews of folate metabolism reference should be made to Stokstad and Koch (1967) or Chanarin (1969).

In B_{12} deficiency 5-methyl-folate may accumulate at the expense of a depletion of tetrahydrofolate, thereby depriving the body of the main 1-carbon unit acceptor. This irreversible consumption of tetrahydrofolate has been termed the 'methyl folate trap hypothesis' (Herbert and Zalusky, 1962). It would provide a unifying metabolic concept to explain the similar cellular effects of B_{12} and folate deficiency, viz. tetrahydrofolate levels would become lowered in either folate or B_{12} deficiency. Recent evidence, however, casts doubt on the validity of this hypothesis (Chanarin, 1973; Cooperman, 1974).

DIETARY SOURCES OF FOLATE

Chanarin, Rothman, Perry and Stratfull (1968) have shown that only 25 per cent of dietary folate is in the 'free' monoglutamate form available to microbiological assay. Perry (1971) found an even lower figure of 10 per cent. The remainder is present as polyglutamate conjugates (mainly heptaglutamate) which require hydrolysis to the monoglutamate (or triglutamate) forms before they become available to microbiological assay. Conjugates which split off the polyglutamyl chains, are present in many animal and plant tissues, including the chick pancreas. Their physiological significance may vary from species to species. In the chick conjugated forms of folate are fully available for nutrition. In man the evidence is conflicting but suggests that approximately one third of conjugated folate is nutritionally available (Perry and Chanarin, 1968).

Over half of the folate, whether conjugated or free, is present as the 5-methyl tetrahydro derivatives detectable by *L. casei* but not by *strep. faecalis* assay. Not only is the bulk of dietary folate present as 5-methyl-tetrahydrofolate but this is also the form in which folates are absorbed into the portal blood (Perry and Chanarin, 1970). The *L. casei* assay is therefore probably the best single measure of nutritionally available food folate, although it may be a slight underestimate.

Table 2.1 shows the folate content of a number of foodstuffs relevant to childhood nutrition.

The figures are based upon *L. casei* assays performed without prior hydrolysis of the polyglutamates by conjugase treatment. The highest concentrations are found in green vegetables but chocolate is also a rich source. In the context of infant nutrition goat's milk is particularly low in folate. Some of the earliest reports of megaloblastic anaemia in infancy was caused by diets in which goat's milk was a major food source (Glanzmann, 1926; Zuelzer and Ogden, 1946). The introduction of mixed feeding at a relatively early age increases the folate intake above that obtainable from a diet of milk or milk products alone.

FOLATE METABOLISM AND DEFICIENCY   15

Table 2.1   *L. Casei* activity of food

Solid food	μg folate per 100 g moist weight
	Mean
Beef (steak)	9·2
Eggs (yolk)	12·9
Eggs (white)	0·6
Bread (white)	15·0
Cornflakes	5·5
Carrots	8·0
Lettuce	21·0
Brussel sprouts	49·9
Spinach	75·0
Ice-cream	4·0
Chocolates	99·0
Processed cheese	9·4–13·3
Data from Herbert (1963)	

Milk products	μg folate per litre	
	Mean	Range
Human milk (pooled)	52	31–81
Fresh cow's milk	55	37–72
Pasteurized cow's milk	51	40–65
Goat's milk	6	2–11
Reconstituted National dried milk		44–52
Reconstituted proprietary brands		20–71
Liquid proprietary brand (dil. 1 in 2)		6–19
Evaporated milks		40–60
Data from Ford and Scott (1968)		

Cooking of solid foods and terminal sterilization of milk cause serious loss of folate, greatly lowering these values.

The folate content of a number of dried milk preparations available in 7 European countries (given in micrograms per gram of dry powder) have recently been determined by Ford *et al.* (1974), *Archives of Disease in Childhood*, **49**, 874.

Preparation and treatment of the food is also important. Hurdle (1967) showed that 80 per cent of the folate in cabbage was destroyed by boiling for 8 minutes and 90 per cent of that in broccoli after steaming for 10 minutes. Ghitis (1966) showed that boiling, but not pasturization, of milk reduced its *L. casei* activity by approximately 50 per cent. Boiling of pasteurized milk, however, caused a more marked loss of between 70 and 90 per cent. It was suggested that preliminary pasteurization may destroy much of the ascorbic acid which normally protects the reduced forms of folate from oxidation during boiling, although Naiman and Oski (1964) were unable to show this. Terminal sterilization of infant milk feeds has been particularly incriminated as a cause of folate destruction (Ford and Scott, 1968). These considerations may explain the fact that artificially fed infants have a poorer state of folate nutrition than breast-fed infants in spite of cow's milk having a slightly

higher initial folate content (Matoth, Pinkas and Spoka, 1965).

Absorption of folates

Absorption of folates takes place largely in the proximal jejunum (Hepner, Booth, Cowan, Hoffbrand and Mollin, 1968) with an efficiency of 80 to 90 per cent for monoglutamates and perhaps 30 per cent for polyglutamates (Jandle and Lear, 1956; Perry and Chanarin, 1968). It is uncertain if the conjugase enzymes present in human intestinal juice are active at the prevailing pH and whether a proportion of the polyglutamates are absorbed without hydrolysis. Pteroylglutamic acid is absorbed by an active process, against a 30-fold concentration gradient, in the upper jejunum but possibly by diffusion only in the lower small intestine. It is the active absorption in the upper jejunum that is impaired in coeliac disease, rather than the slower distal absorption (Hepner et al., 1968). Recent work has shown that folinic acid is also well absorbed (Nixon and Bertino, 1972).

Much of the absorbed folate enters the portal circulation as the 5-methyl-tetrahydro derivative, presumably as a result of metabolism in the intestinal epithelium (Perry and Chanarin, 1970). Both this and parenterally administered folates reach the liver and other tissues where they equilibrate with existing folate stores and displace into the systemic circulation an equivalent amount of 5-methyl-tetrahydrofolate, the major component of serum folate activity (Whitehead and Cooper, 1967; Johns et al., 1961). Most of the hepatic folate is stored in the polyglutamate form (Whitehead, 1963). Various tests of folate absorption have been described based upon urinary excretion after oral v. parenteral administration (Doig and Girdwood, 1960), upon blood levels following 40 μg folate per kg body weight after folate saturation (Chanarin and Bennett, 1962), or upon the absorption of tritium-labelled folate (Anderson et al., 1960). They are not wholly suitable for routine use in paediatrics.

DETERMINATION OF FOLATE STATES

Folate assays in blood

Low serum folate levels indicate a state of negative folate balance; low red cell folate levels indicate depleted erythropoietic folate stores; increased FIGLU excretion indicates an interference with folate 1-carbon acceptor function; morphological criteria of megaloblastic changes and anaemia indicate a final stage of folate exhaustion sufficiently severe to impair haemopoiesis. Fig. 2.3 shows the sequence with which these biochemical and haematological changes developed during experimental deprivation in man (Herbert, 1962).

Determinations of serum and red cell folate levels are performed by microbiological assay using *Lactobacillus casei* since the major part of the activity is in the form of 5-methyl-tetrahydrofolate to which this organism is sensitive. The red cell folate, however, is in a conjugated form requiring hydrolysis before it is microbiologically available. Serum folate levels are labile, temporarily increasing after a meal, and should therefore be measured in the fasting state. Red cell folate levels are greater than the concentration in serum so that whole blood folate level depends almost entirely upon red cell folate and reflects this measurement if a correction is made based upon the packed cell volume:

$$\text{Red cell folate} \simeq \text{Whole blood folate} \times \frac{100}{\text{PCV}}$$

The red cell folate is less susceptible to transient fluctuations than is the serum folate and is thought to be the best single index of the folate status, in particular of the stores available for erythropoiesis (Hoffbrand, Newcombe and Mollin, 1966; Cooper and Lowenstein, 1966). A low red cell folate correlates more accurately with the presence of megaloblastic changes in the marrow than does a low serum folate. The red cell folate, is, however, slower to fall than the serum folate (Fig. 2.3) because of the duration of red cell survival (110 days) and the fact that the folate content of individual cells reflects the folate status at the time of their formation in the marrow (Streiff and Little, 1967). Blood transfusion invalidates the measurement because of the contribution from the healthy donor cells. A practical advantage in

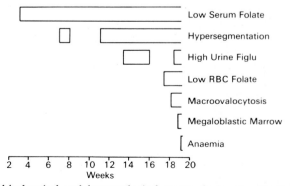

Fig. 2.3 The sequence of biochemical and haematological events during the development of folate deficiency. A low serum folate, only, indicates negative folate balance, and the RBC folate starts to fall. Only after the latter becomes subnormal do megaloblastic changes and anaemia develop. (Reproduced by permission of the author and the *Recorder of the Association of American Physicians*, from the paper by Herbert (1962)).

paediatrics is that the whole blood folate, and therefore the red cell folate by calculation, can be determined on as little as 0·05 ml of blood obtained by finger or heel-stab (Strelling et al., 1966). A theoretical disadvantage, of little consequence in paediatrics, is that the red cell folate, unlike that in serum, is low in B_{12} deficiency as well as in folate deficiency. The normal ranges are given in Table 2.2

formimino group for its further metabolism (Fig. 2.2). In folate deficiency or other metabolic block of this pathway there is an increased excretion of FIGLU after histidine loading (Fig. 2.4). Both histidine load and FIGLU excretion should be quantitated for accurate results. Luhby and Cooperman (1964) suggested an oral histidine dose of 0·12 g per lb body wt. (0·26 g/kg), but Vanier and Tyas (1966) showed that 0·1, 0·2 or 0·3 g/kg

Table 2.2 Normal ranges for folate assays and FIGLU test

L. casei activity expressed as ng/ml

	Range	Mean	Author
Serum folate			
Adults	6·0–18·6	9·7	Hoffbrand et al., 1966
Children 1 year	3·0–35	9·3	Vanier & Tyas, 1966
Children 1–6 years	4·1–21·2	11·4	Shojania & Gross, 1964
Children 1–10 years	6·5–16·5	10·3	Dormandy et al., 1963
Red cell folate			
Adults	160–640	316	Hoffbrand et al., 1966
Infants <1 year	74–995	277	Vanier & Tyas, 1966
Children 1–11 years	96–364	215	McNeish & Willoughby, 1969
Whole blood folate			
Adults	50–150	89	Izak et al., 1961
Adults	60–400	195	Vanier & Tyas, 1966
Infants <1 year	20–160	87	Kende et al., 1963
Infants 1 year	31–400	86	Vanier & Tyas, 1966
Infants 2–24 months	35–160	96*	Grossowicz et al., 1962
Children up to 11 years	52–164	97	McNeish & Willoughby, 1969

	Histidine load	Collection period	Total mg FIGLU	
FIGLU excretion				
Adults	15 G	0–8hrs	up to 17 mg	Chanarin & Bennett 1962
Infants	100–300 mg/kg	0–6 hrs	up to 6 mg	Vanier & Tyas, 1966
Children	0·12 G/lb	0–24 hrs	up to 30 mg	Luhby & Cooperman, 1964

Serum folate levels (fasting) below 3·0, red cell folate below 100 or whole blood folate below 60 can be regarded as abnormal. Normal values during the first year of life are shown in Fig. 2.6.
*Derived after correction for a PCV of 45 per cent.

FIGLU test

Formiminoglutamic acid (FIGLU) is a normal breakdown product of histidine but requires tetrahydrofolate as an acceptor for the 1-carbon

were equally satisfactory. Higher doses (0·5 g/kg) may produce pathological FIGLU excretion even in normal folate-sufficient infants or adults. By electrophoretic methods (Kohn, Mollin and Rosenbach, 1961) no FIGLU can be detected

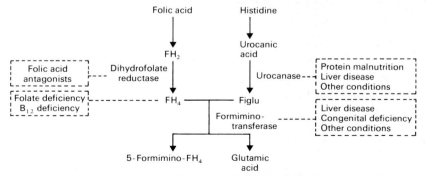

Fig. 2.4 Histidine metabolic pathway and sites of blockade. Tetrahydrofolate is a necessary acceptor of formimino groups resulting from histidine metabolism. In folate deficiency or metabolic blockade, unaltered FIGLU is excreted in the urine after a histidine load. (Reproduced from Today's Tests, *British Medical Journal* (1969), **2**, 100).

after a suitable histidine load in normal individuals, but by quantitative enzymatic methods, it is found that there is a small excretion of 1–17 mg (mean 9 mg) in normal adults (Chanarin and Bennett, 1962) and up to 6 mg in infants (Vanier and Tyas, 1966).

In megaloblastic anaemia due to folate deficiency the excretion is regularly increased many fold (Luhby and Cooperman, 1964; Kohn *et al.*, 1961; Chanarin, 1964). There is good correlation between low red cell folate, positive FIGLU test and megaloblastic anaemia. The sensitivity of the FIGLU test is closer to that of the red cell folate than to the serum folate (Fig. 2.3). It is, however, less specific than the red cell folate since it may be abnormal in liver disease, including children with infectious hepatitis (Gomirato-Sandrucci *et al.*, 1966), sarcoidosis (Kohn *et al.*, 1961), congenital formimino-transferase deficiency (Arakawa *et al.*, 1965) and in normal healthy infants in the first few months of life, possibly due to some degree of liver immaturity (Vanier and Tyas, 1966). Methotrexate therapy predictably increases FIGLU excretion (Acevedo and Mauer, 1965). B_{12} deficiency is frequently associated with a positive FIGLU test (Knowles and Prankerd, 1962), perhaps because of loss of tetra-hydrofolate to the 'methyl folate trap'. As in the case of red cell folate this diagnostic limitation is of less importance in paediatric than in adult medicine. To some extent a distinction between folate deficiency and conditions such as liver disease can be achieved by observing the effect of folate treatment upon the FIGLU test. In true folate deficiency FIGLU excretion diminishes after 24 hours of folate therapy. In B_{12} deficiency it diminishes after either B_{12} or folate therapy.

Urocanic acid is the immediate precursor of FIGLU in the breakdown of histidine (Fig. 2.4). Its conversion to FIGLU depends upon the hepatic enzyme urocanase. This is diminished in protein deprivation and may account for the increased urocanic acid excretion in infants with kwashiorkor (Whitehead and Arnstein, 1961) as well as in liver disease, malignant disease and infections. Urocanic acid excretion can also be increased in folate deficiency as a result of a 'feed-back' inhibition due to accumulation of FIGLU. These considerations assume importance when the enzymatic FIGLU assay of Chanarin and Bennett (1962) is used since this measures the combined FIGLU plus urocanic acid excretion (although duplicate tests with or without heat destruction of FIGLU permits independent measurement of both compounds).

Haematological changes

Megaloblastic changes are the penultimate, and anaemia the final consequence of folate deficiency (Fig. 2.3). Similar morphological changes develop in either folate or B_{12} deficiency. Careful examination of a well-spread and well-stained blood film is the most important step in the detection of a megaloblastic process (Chanarin, 1969, p. 345). Final confirmation is obtained by observing a reticulocyte response after 'physiological' doses of either folic acid or vitamin B_{12}.

PERIPHERAL BLOOD

In mild anaemia there is a uniform slight macrocytosis which can easily be overlooked unless examined under standardized conditions with a familiar microscope. The red cells have a normal degree of haemoglobinisation and some are oval. With more severe anaemia there is striking anisocytosis (viz. increased variation in cell size) due to the presence of poikilocytes as well as grossly enlarged macrocytes. It is probable that these red cell fragments arise from damage to the abnormally large macrocytes as they pass through capillaries, a situation analogous to the formation of fragmented burr cells in microangiopathic haemolytic anaemia (Chapter 9). This process could account for the haemolytic element sometimes seen in severe megaloblastic anaemia.

Hypersegmentation of the neutrophil polymorphs is an early change in the development of megaloblastic haemopoiesis. Normally not more than 5 per cent of the circulating polymorphs have more than 4 lobes (Herbert, 1967). In megaloblastic states this figure is often increased to over 10 per cent. Macropolycytes, abnormally large polymorphs with 8 or more lobes, may also be present in small numbers.

Examinations of films made from the 'buffy coat', obtained by centrifugation of blood, may show changes indicative of a megaloblastic state before it can readily be appreciated in ordinary blood films. In paediatric practice this technique can be adapted to capillary blood by using heparinized microhaematocrit tubes centrifuged at 750 r.p.m. for 5 minutes (Strelling *et al.*, 1966). Macrocytes, Howell-Jolly bodies and nucleated red cells with megaloblastic features are preferentially concentrated in this junctional zone between plasma and packed red cells. The finding of late megaloblasts in such films may on occasions make a marrow examination unnecessary.

MARROW

Marrow examination is the usual final arbiter in

determining the presence or absence of megaloblastic erythropoiesis. Well-fixed, well-stained and well-spread smears are again essential. 'Squash' or 'crush' preparations are unsatisfactory for purposes of detecting early megaloblastic changes (Chanarin, 1969, p. 350).

Erythroid precursors show the major changes but myeloid and megakaryocyte series are also affected. This is reflected in the leucopenia and thrombocytopenia that sometimes accompany severe megaloblastic anaemia.

Megaloblasts arise by a process of delayed nuclear maturation, dependent upon DNA synthesis for which tetrahydrofolate is required (Fig. 2.2). There is nucleo-cytoplasmic asynchronism with a relatively more mature cytoplasm for the stage of nuclear development, including the premature appearance of haemaglobin in the cytoplasm. Both nucleus and whole cell have increased diameters for the stage of maturation. The nuclear chromatin has a sieve-like appearance compared to the coarser chromatin clumping of normoblasts. Early megaloblasts and promegaloblasts have deep blue cytoplasm with Romanowsky stains (Leishman, May-Grunwald-Giemsa or Wrights stains); intermediate megaloblasts have purple to grey cytoplasm due to the presence of haemoglobin; late megaloblasts have orthochromatic, fully haemoglobinised cytoplasm, viz. the same colour as mature red cells. In a normoblastic marrow such orthochromatic erythroblasts are seldom seen (Dacie and White, 1959). In addition the megaloblast differs from the late normoblast in its size and the frequent presence of Howell-Jolly bodies, other nuclear fragments and sometimes bizarre mitoses. In severe megaloblastic anaemia all stages of megaloblasts are present, and the deeply basophilic pro- and early megaloblasts are prominent. In mild or early megaloblastic anaemia changes may be confined to a proportion of the late erythroblasts and perhaps the myeloid precursors. A practical point is that coincident iron deficiency or thalassaemia may partially obscure megaloblastic changes by virtue of impaired haem and globin synthesis respectively.

Although the whole myeloid series can be shown to have an increased average cell diameter in megaloblastic states it is the metamyelocyte that shows the most obvious enlargement compared to normal (Heinivaara and Kapainen, 1959). This late form of myelocyte has a kidney-shaped nucleus and a normal diameter of 11–15 μm (mean 13 μm). In megaloblastic states the majority exceed 14 μm, with some reaching 18 μm. The non-segmented 'band cells' are also larger (normal upper limit 13 μm to 16 μm); so-called giant band cells. It is probably unwise to diagnose megaloblastic anaemia from myeloid changes alone. The relationship between giant band cells in the marrow and hypersegmented polymorphs in the peripheral blood is not entirely clear. Both may simply reflect the same disordered myelopoiesis. It is not certain that the hypersegmented polymorph is derived from the giant band cell, and there is no evidence to support the traditional belief that a greater number of lobes implies increased age of the cell. Perhaps it is relevant that in the Pelger-Hüet anomaly, where most of the blood polymorphs are non-segmented, the marrow metamyelocytes are smaller than normal.

Megakaryocytes show a more open nuclear chromatin pattern than normal in severe megaloblastic anaemia. Even in the presence of thrombocytopenia they are usually normal in number and show platelet budding.

For a fuller morphological description of megaloblastic erythropoiesis the reader is referred to Whitby and Britton (1969) and Chanarin (1969).

FOLATE BALANCE IN INFANCY AND CHILDHOOD

Daily folate requirements

In adults this is probably between 50 and 100 μg per day. Estimates of the daily folate requirements in infants have ranged between 20 and 50 μg. That it is under 50 μg, is suggested by the investigation of Sullivan et al. (1966). They found that this dose produced a complete haematological response in 2 infants with megaloblastic anaemia caused by a diet of goat's milk contributing less than 12 μg per day. That the requirements lay in the region of 20–30 μg/day was suggested by the work of Velez et al. (1963). They found that 9 to 20 μg of folic acid per day caused remission in megaloblastic children with kwashiorkor or marasmus whose diet was contributing less than 10μg per day. This is consistent with the finding that folate deficiency occurred on a special diet for maple-syrup urine disease containing 9 to 11 μg/day (Levy et al., 1970). That the figure may vary from one patient to another was suggested by the observations of Ghitis and Tripathy (1970). Of two infants with nutritional megaloblastic anaemia one (9 months old and 5·6 kg) responded on two occasions to 35 μg but not to 15 or 25 μg; the other (12 months old and 5·4 kg) responded to the smaller dose of 15 μg/day on two separate occasions.

A different approach yields figures in the same range. Matoth et al. (1965) pointed out that the infant takes a daily intake of approximately 800 ml of breast milk per day. Based upon their estimate of a concentration of 24 μg/L. this volume would yield 20 μg/day, Based upon a more recent estimate of nearer 50 μg/l (Ford and Scott, 1968) the intake would be 40 μg/day.

By comparison with this figure of 40 μg/day, Vanier and Tyas (1966) showed that the total daily intake in two full-term infants on Cow and Gate full-cream milk was 29·7 and 26·6 μg per day. The same workers (1967) showed that the corresponding intake in a premature infant of 2 kg on half-cream Cow and Gate milk might be as low as 7 μg/day. Roberts et al. (1969) arrived at similarly low calculated intakes in premature infants fed on boiled pooled expressed breast milk.

Folate status in the newborn

Serum and red cell folate levels in the newborn are higher than the corresponding maternal values. This applies equally to premature or term infants (Figs 2.5 and 2.6). Even severe maternal folate deficiency with megaloblastic anaemia does not cause anaemia in the infant (Pritchard et al., 1970). There is conflicting evidence as to whether there is (Roberts et al., 1969) or is not (Vanier and Tyas, 1966) a relationship between maternal and foetal levels of red cell folate. The baby, however, appears to have a prior claim on available folate at the expense of the mother. It also seems highly probable that the widespread practice of folate supplementation of the mother during pregnancy improves the neonatal folate stores.

After birth there is a fall in both serum and red cell folate to subnormal values by adult standards (Figs 2.5 and 2.6). This fall is well-marked by 8 weeks (Matoth et al., 1964; Vanier and Tyas, 1966). Lower levels are found in infants from families of low economic status, and in artificially fed compared to breast-fed infants (Matoth et al., 1964). This is probably attributable to loss of folate during the preparation of artificial feeds as mentioned above. The conclusions of Vanier and Tyas (1966) are that the 'marginal folate stores during the first year are probably related to an intake that is barely adequate to meet the needs of rapid growth. This may result in the rapid development of overt deficiency during illness'. Also the dietary supply of folate is inadequate in the artificially fed infant. This is particularly true of the infant fed boiled, pasteurized or sterilized food (Matoth et al., 1965).

In *premature* infants the folate balance is even more precarious. The fall in serum and red cell folate is more marked than in term infants. Shojania and Gross (1964A) found that 9 out of 15 infants with birth weights under 1·7 kg had low serum folates at 1–2 months of age. Vanier and Tyas (1967) confirmed and extended these observations. They found that of 20 infants having birth weights between 1·1 and 2·0 kg (mean 1·4 kg) 13 developed low serum folate, 8 low red cell folate and 4 positive FIGLU tests at 2–3 months. (Normal infants do not show positive FIGLU tests at this age even although their folate assays may be low.) The striking fall in serum and red cell folate in a large series of premature babies (under 2·5 kg) is well illustrated by the results of Roberts et al. (1969) shown in Fig. 2.7. Even when the mothers have been taking prophylactic folic acid during pregnancy the premature infant's red cell folate falls below normal after the age of 3 months (Roberts et al., 1972).

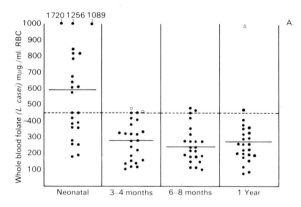

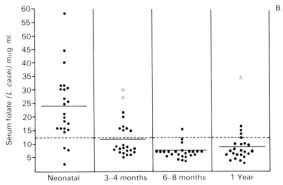

Fig. 2.5 RBC folate and serum folate changes in normal infants. A, whole blood folate during the first year of life. B, serum folate during the first year of life. ———, mean figure in each group; - - - -, normal adult mean; ○, breast-fed infants; △, infant receiving folate-fortified proprietary food. High levels at birth fall over the following months as shown by mean values, yet few individual values are below the lower limits of the normal adult range.

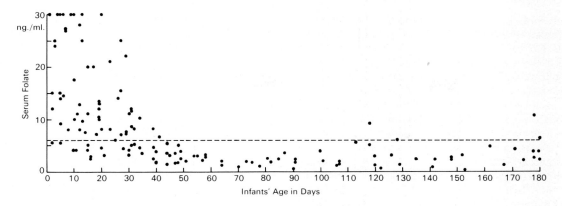
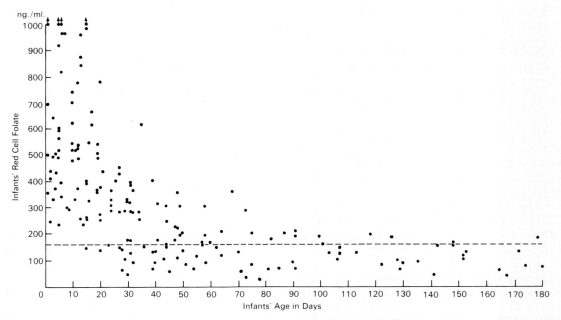

Fig. 2.6 Serum folate and RBC folate changes in premature infants. High levels at birth fall early in serum folate and later in RBC folate with many individual values well below the lower limit of normal adult range (- - - -). (Reproduced by permission of Dr Roberts and the Editor of the *Archives of Disease in Childhood*, from the paper by Roberts *et al.* (1969)).

CONDITIONS ASSOCIATED WITH FOLATE DEFICIENCY IN CHILDHOOD

Folate deficiency occurs mainly in four paediatric situations; prematurity, infection, malabsorption and haemolysis. Prematurity has been discussed above. In undeveloped countries primary deficiency, e.g. kwashiorkor, must be added to this list. Interference with folate metabolism can be caused by drugs such as methotrexate or anticonvulsants and by rare congenital enzyme deficiencies. For recent annotations on folate deficiency in childhood see Hoffbrand (1970) and *Lancet* (1973).

Prematurity

Overt megaloblastic anaemia may develop in premature infants during the second and third months of life, but is much less frequent than the low blood folate levels described above. Strelling *et al.* (1966) found megaloblastic changes between the ages of 5 and 11 weeks in 3 out of 18 with birth weights between 1·5 and 1·8 kg, and in all 6 with birth weights under 1·5 kg. Five of the 25 infants with megaloblastic anaemia originally described by Zuelzer and Ogden (1946) were premature. Three further examples of megaloblastic anaemia at 25, 33 and 50 days in infants with birth weights of 1·15 kg or less were described by Gray and Butler (1965). The Hb values had fallen to as low as 6·5 to 7·7 g/100 ml at the time of diagnosis. All showed a convincing reticulocyte response to folic acid. Three out of the 20 premature infants investigated by Vanier and Tyas (1967) developed anaemias with the Hb below 7 g/100 ml. Their birth weights were 1·2, 1·8 and 2·0 kg and the marrows showed giant metamyelocytes with or without partial megaloblastic changes when diagnosed at 2 months. Good reticulocyte and haemoglobin responses followed the administration of oral folic acid, 1·25 mg per day. The reticulocyte responses were accompanied by the appearance of large numbers of nucleated red cells in the peripheral blood.

Feeding difficulties, failure to gain weight, rhesus disease or the occurrence of infections, particularly gastroenteritis, have been associated with the development of megaloblastic anaemia in some but not all of the instances reported by the above authors. Indeed it appears from the literature that folate deficiency can occur in premature infants without any external factor such as infection, unlike the situation in full-term infants (Hoffbrand, 1970). This fact raises the question of the advisability of giving prophylactic folic acid to premature infants. A relevant finding is that the serum and red cell folate levels, although low at 2–3 months, return to normal by 6–8 months in the majority of infants (Vanier and Tyas, 1967). This is probably due to the introduction of mixed feeding at about this time. The premature infant is at risk therefore only over this relatively limited period. Burland et al. (1971) have shown that 14 I.M. doses of 100 μg of folic acid given during the first 5 weeks of life abolish the fall of serum and red cell folate seen in unsupplemented control premature infants under 1·8 kg birth weight. No instances of overt anaemia occurred in either group of infants but hypersegmentation of the polymorphs, which developed at 3 months in the control group, was prevented in the folic acid supplemented group. It was claimed that subclinical folate deficiency, present in the control infants, was prevented by the prophylactic dose of 1·4 mg folic acid. Mackintosh et al. (1969) had similarly found that 100 μg per day prevented the drop in whole blood folate seen at 12 weeks in control infants with birth weights under 2 kg. Hoffbrand (1970) has recommended prophylactic folic acid for all infants under 1·5 kg at birth and for all premature infants, and possibly all neonates, who suffer prolonged infections or other debilitating diseases impairing milk intake in the first few weeks of life. Vanier and Tyas (1967) came to similar conclusions regarding premature babies. Also it was recommended after exchange transfusion (since folate-rich foetal red cells are replaced by less well endowed adult cells) and when artificial diets low in folate are given as in phenylketonuria. The optimum dose and route of prophylactic folic administration is uncertain. An expert group of the W.H.O. has recommended 50 micrograms per day (Kendall et al., 1974). A double-blind trial, however, has shown no significant difference in weight gain, haemoglobin levels or incidence of infection in a group of infants with birth weights less than 2·5 kg (Kendall et al., 1974).

Infection

Many of the infants with megaloblastic anaemia reported in 1946 by Zuelzer and Ogden had suffered from a preceding infection, often of the upper respiratory tract. The Hb ranged from 2·7 to 6·6 g/100 ml at diagnosis. All were under 18 months of age, and most were between 7 and 12 months (this contrasts with the megaloblastic anaemia due to prematurity alone which occurs during the second and third months). All responded to folic acid, but not to ascorbic acid. Infection was also common in a similar series of infants with megaloblastic anaemia reported by Amato (1946). In 1953 Zuelzer and Rutsky described a further 27 infants with megaloblastic anaemia. All but 3 had a recent history of infection or diarrhoea. The three exceptions were premature infants. Not surprisingly the combination of infection and prematurity is particularly prone to cause megaloblastic anaemia, as in the three infants reported by Gray and Butler (1965). Zuelzer and Ogden rightly suggested that infections and nutritional deficiencies were significant causes, with prematurity, age and race (i.e. economic status) as contributory factors in the aetiology of megaloblastic anaemia of infancy. Line et al (1971) found evidence of folate deficiency in approximately half of a group of patients with tuberculous infection. There was a considerable improvement following 3 months anti-tuberculous chemotherapy.

Investigating the mechanism of these associations, Matoth et al. (1964B) showed that the whole blood folate (and therefore the red cell folate) was low in 80 per cent of infants with diarrhoea and in 75 per cent of those with infection. In a small group of infants with malnutrition without diarrhoea or evidence of infection the folate values were similarly low (Fig. 2.7). May et al. (1952) have shown that naturally occurring

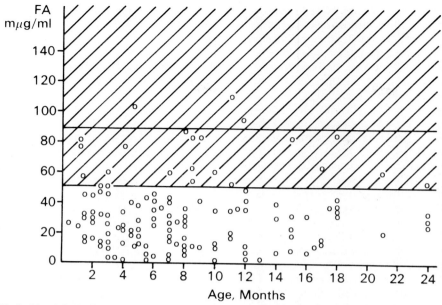

Fig. 2.7 Whole-blood folate in infants with infections, reflecting the RBC folate level, expressed per ml whole blood instead of per ml RBC. Many subnormal values occur in infants with infection irrespective of age. Shaded area, normal adult range; ———, adult mean. (Reproduced by permission of Professor Matoth and the Editor of *Pediatrics*, from the paper by Matoth et al. (1964B)).

infections or experimentally produced turpentine abscesses in monkeys caused a reduction in liver folate and led to megaloblastic anaemia. This could be prevented by folic acid but not by B_{12} or ascorbic acid. *In vitro* the reduction of folic acid to tetrahydrofolate by liver enzymes is inhibited by a rise in temperature to 39 °C (Panders, 1964). This may be relevant to the effect of infection in precipitating megaloblastic anaemia *in vivo*.

Malabsorption

If anaemia is present in childhood coeliac disease it is usually of the iron deficiency type with hypochromic red cells, whereas the anaemia in the adult form of the disease is more often macrocytic. Sheldon (1955) found overt megaloblastic anaemia in only 7 out of 74 children with coeliac disease. However, the FIGLU test is frequently positive e.g. in 39 out of 44 children (Visakorpi et al., 1967), and folate assays almost invariably low. Minor degrees of megaloblastic changes in the marrow are frequent. Thus Dormandy, Waters and Mollin (1963) found hypochromic red cells in 15 out of 19 childen with untreated coeliac disease and actual anaemia in 8, but a low serum folate and positive FIGLU test in all 19. Marrow examinations showed overt megaloblastic changes in 4, partial megaloblastic changes in a further 4 and giant metamyelocytes in a further 6. Similarly McNeish and Willoughby (1969) found a low whole blood and serum folate in all of a group of 30 children with untreated coeliac disease (Fig. 2.8), although only 15 had anaemia. In 11 of these

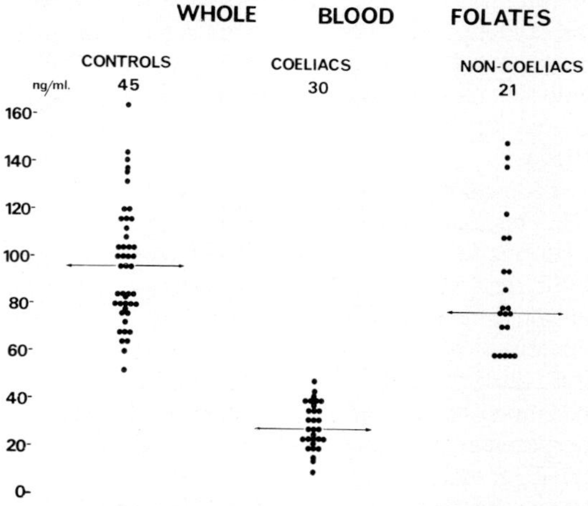

Fig. 2.8 Whole-blood folate in coeliac disease, associated with consistently low whole blood-folate levels at diagnosis. This is not so in other intestinal disorders. (Data from McNeish and Willoughby (1969), reproduced with permission of the Editor of *Lancet*).

the anaemia was hypochromic and in 4 macrocytic. The serum iron was low in 27 out of the 30 but the serum B_{12} normal in all.

By contrast the whole blood folate was normal in 20 children presenting with symptoms similar to coeliac disease but in whom the final diagnoses were of other disorders including post-infective malabsorption, cystic fibrosis, protein enteropathy and sucrose/iso-maltose deficiency (Fig. 2.8). It was suggested that this measurement was a useful screening test for coeliac disease (McNeish and Willoughby, 1969), but occasional mild cases of coeliac disease with normal folate status have since been reported (Cook et al., 1971).

After treatment with a gluten-free diet the serum folate and FIGLU excretion return to normal (Dormandy et al., 1963), in parallel with the return to normal of ³H-folate absorption (Kinnear et al., 1963) and of the mucosal pattern of the jejunum (Anderson, 1960). This is followed by a rise in red cell folate which reaches a normal level in approximately 20 weeks (Magnus, 1966). A follow-up study of 10 patients diagnosed as coeliac disease in childhood, but not treated with a gluten-free diet, showed a persistence of mucosal abnormalities into adult life together with low folate levels, abnormal red cell morphology and, in 3 patients, anaemia (Mortimer et al., 1968).

Studies in the adult form of the disease have similarly shown consistently lowered serum and red cell folate levels. Impaired folic acid absorption has been demonstrated in up to 100 per cent of such patients by a variety of different techniques including the uptake of tritium-labelled folate (Klipstein, 1963). The defect lies primarily in the duodenum and proximal jejunum. Xylose, glucose, fat and B_{12} are also poorly absorbed in decreasing order of frequency (Stewart et al., 1967).

Tropical sprue, usually a disease of adults, has also been reported in children (Santiago and Maldonado, 1968). All had megaloblastic changes. Folic acid therapy not only corrects the megaloblastic anaemia, but also improves the gastro-intestinal symptoms and malabsorption state in this disorder (Sheehy et al., 1962), raising the question as to whether folate deficiency can perpetuate the state of malabsorption and thus cause a vicious circle. Hoffbrand et al., (1969) showed a preferential defect of absorption for polyglutamates associated with a low jejunal content of conjugase in this disease.

Isolated congenital defects of folate absorption have also been described, presenting in the first few weeks or months with severe megaloblastic anaemia, diarrhoea and sore mouth (Lanzkowsky et al., 1969; Santiago-Borrero et al., 1973). Pharmacological doses of folate were, however, absorbed by passive diffusion. In Lanzkowsky's case there was also a failure of transport of folate from blood to CSF, with associated mental impairment and intracranial calcification. Luhby et al. (1961) also described mental retardation in association with a defect of folate absorption.

Haemolysis

Moderately low serum folate, abnormal FIGLU excretion and hypersegmentation of the polymorphs have been found in children with sickle cell disease, congenital spherocytosis, erythropoetic porphyria (Shojania and Gross, 1964B) and in thalassaemia (Luhby and Cooperman, 1961). These changes were corrected by folic acid administration, usually in large doses. All these patients, however, had a normoblastic marrow. Bearing in mind the sequence of changes in folate depletion (Fig. 2.3), these findings, as well as the rapid plasma clearance of injected folic acid in patients with chronic haemolytic anaemia (Chanarin et al., 1969), could indicate excessive folate utilization and increased requirement rather than true depletion to the stage where megaloblastic changes occur and erythropoiesis is impaired. A more recent investigation has shown a low serum folate in only 1 out of 16 children with compensated chronic haemolysis (Purugganan et al., 1971). These authors conclude that it is 'unlikely that folate deficiency in the usual sense exists in chronic haemolysis'. Nevertheless in 6 of these children undergoing an aplastic crisis serum folate was low in 3 and red cell folate low in 2.

When actual megaloblastic changes have been found in association with haemolysis there has usually been an additional factor of either infection or underlying malnutrition. For instance Chanarin et al. (1962) described a case of hereditary spherocytosis in a 10-year-old girl who developed a megaloblastic bone marrow arrest following fever and diarrhoea. Chatterjea (1959) found that 6 out of 27 patients with thalassaemia in India showed megaloblastic changes. The association of sickle cell disease and megaloblastic arrest in malnourished Jamaican children has been reported by McIver and Went (1960).

The possible role of folate deficiency in the precipitation of aplastic crises in haemolytic anaemia was raised by the observations of Pierce and Rath (1962). They found evidence of folate deficiency during aplastic crises in two patients with sickle-cell disease. This has not, however, been a consistent finding. Observations of Chanarin et al. (1962) in the 10-year-old girl with congenital spherocytosis with marrow arrest suggest that infection may induce megaloblastosis. The finding of a low red cell folate during aplastic crises may partly be due to the absence of reticulocytes, and other younger red cells, which have a higher folate content than older cells (Purugganan *et al.*, 1971; Hoffbrand *et al.*, 1966). Conversely the red cell folate may be misleadingly high in the presence of reticulocytosis making this an unsuitable investigation in haemolytic anaemia. Infection may precipitate megaloblastic arrest, as mentioned above (Kho *et al.*, 1961), perhaps due to a block in folate metabolism produced by the products of bacterial infection or by fever.

Nutritional deficiency

This has been mentioned already as a contributory factor in megaloblastic anaemia associated with haemolysis. Also the folate deficiency occurring in premature infants is nutritional insofar as it is caused by insufficient intake at a time when requirements are high. Primary nutritional deficiency must be a rare cause of megaloblastic anaemia in European children, although frequently encountered in underprivileged or coloured children. Kondi *et al.* (1963) found lower whole blood folate levels in normal infants from low income (Yemenite) parents than in infants from middle income parents. Matoth *et al.* (1964A) reported low blood folates in a group of infants from socially backward families in central Israel in whom no predisposing factors such as infection or diarrhoea were present. Jamaican children with marasmus due to severe malnutrition with or without infection were investigated by McIver and Black (1960). Fifty had megaloblastic anaemia which responded to folic acid. Similar instances of megaloblastic anaemia have been found in Djakarta, Indonesia (Lien-Keng and Odang, 1959), Durban (Walt *et al.*, 1956), Johannesburg (Spector and Metz, 1966), Kenya (Kondi *et al.*, 1963) South India (Pereira and Baker, 1966) and Columbia (Velez *et al.*, 1963). Most of these children, particularly those in Africa, were classified as having kwashiorkor. In many of the above series the serum folate was shown to be low, especially those without infection (Spector and Metz, 1966). The serum B_{12} was normal, or high in the presence of liver damage. The FIGLU excretion has been abnormal where measured and the anaemia responds to folic acid in doses as low as $20 \mu g$ per day (Velez *et al.*, 1963). A recent investigation by Khalil *et al.* (1973) in Egyptian infants has also confirmed that the megaloblastic anaemia associated with protein-calorie malnutrition is due to folate rather than B_{12} deficiency. Serum folate was low in 14 of 19 with kwashiorkor and 7 of 19 with marasmus.

Transient marrow aplasia, with all elements affected and peripheral pancytopenia, is a relatively frequent event in the course of kwashiorkor (Lien-Keng, 1961). It is probably precipitated by infection superimposed upon the state of folate deficiency. In underprivileged pre-school white children, from an economically depressed area of the USA, a low serum folate has been found in 17 per cent, with a low serum iron in a similar proportion (Sandstead *et al.*, 1971).

Unusual nutritional causes of megaloblastic anaemia in children from developed countries include the use of artificial diets for phenylketonuria (Hudson, 1961; Royston and Parry, 1962) and maple syrup urine disease (Levy *et al.*, 1970). In the latter condition the diet was found to supply only 9 to $11 \mu g$ per day. In homocystinuria folate deficiency has also been found (Carey *et al.*, 1968), but in this case increased folate consumption also occurs through excessive homocysteine methylation to methionine (Lancet, 1973). Paradoxically, treatment with pyridoxine in pyridoxine-responsive cases is followed by accentuation of the folate depletion and behaviour changes that are reversed by folate administration (Wilcken and Turner, 1973).

Goat's milk has been mentioned as a particularly poor source of folate ($5 \mu g/l$) and is a potent cause of megaloblastic anaemia in infants whose main source of nutrition is goat's milk. Cases of goat's milk anaemia have been reported from Germany (Glanzmann, 1926), America (Zuelzer and Ogden, 1946) and New Zealand (Becroft and Holland, 1966). Sullivan, Luhby and Streiff (1966) studied 3 further cases of megaloblastic anaemia due to this cause. These occurred at $6\frac{1}{2}$, 9 and 12 months, although other cases have been 18 to 20 weeks. The calculated folate intake from the diet of goat's milk was in the region of 1·5 to $12 \mu g$ per day. There was a response to $50 \mu g$ but not to $20 \mu g$ per day of oral folic acid. These observations are relevant to determination of the daily requirement in infants as referred to earlier.

Disturbances of folate metabolism secondary to deficiencies of ascorbic acid, vitamin E or iron have also been postulated. The problem is confused by the occurrence of multiple deficiencies in human malnutrition and infection, viz. a diet that is likely to cause scurvy is also likely to be folate deficient and probably iron deficient. The anaemia in scurvy is usually normochromic and responds to ascorbic acid alone (Cox *et al.*, 1962). In a proportion of cases, however, it is megaloblastic. The serum and whole blood folate levels are then low and the FIGLU test positive. Zalusky and Herbert (1961) showed that one such patient failed to respond to ascorbic acid while being kept on a folate-free diet, but that the addition of 50 μg per day of folic acid then produced a full haematological response. The implication is that the megaloblastic anaemia found in scurvy is in fact due to folate deficiency. Other observations, however, show that folic acid alone (in 250 μg doses) does not produce a full haematological response in such patients until ascorbic acid is also supplied (Jandle and Gabuzda, 1953). The probable explanation, as suggested from experimental work in monkeys (May *et al.*, 1952), is that folate requirements are increased in scurvy, and that treatment with ascorbic acid simply restores the folic requirement to normal. This amount would normally be supplied by a hospital diet. At physiological levels of intake, therefore, both ascorbic acid and folic acid are required for the full correction of the megaloblastic anaemia of scurvy.

It has also been questioned whether iron deficiency might predispose to folate deficiency both in children (Gross *et al.*, 1965; Vossough *et al.*, 1968) and in adults (Chanarin *et al.*, 1965). Recent investigations tend to exclude any causal relationship although a double deficiency could arise due to poor diet or malabsorption. In pure iron deficiency anaemia the red cell folate is normal or high (Purugganan *et al.*, 1971).

Vitamin E has similarly been incriminated. Majaj *et al.* (1963) have described megaloblastic anaemia in Jordanian infants and young children with deficiencies of vitamin E, folate and ascorbic acid who responded to vitamin E alone, with a return of folate and ascorbic levels to normal.

Anticonvulsants and other drugs associated with megaloblastic anaemia

It is now well established that megaloblastic anaemia can occur as a result of the administration of phenytoin (Dilantin, Epanutin) either alone or in combination with other anticonvulsant drugs; of primidone (Mysoline) alone or in combination with other drugs; and of barbiturates, of several types alone (Klipstein, 1964). It is more frequent in patients taking all three types of drug than in those taking two, e.g. phenobarbitone plus diphenylhydantoin or primidone. Malpas, Spray and Witts (1966) found macrocytosis in 11 per cent and low serum folate in 37 per cent of a

randomly selected group of such patients. Megaloblastic anaemia occurs in less than 0·75 per cent of patients. It is always due to folic acid deficiency and always responds to folic acid treatment (Reynolds, 1973).

Case 3. A 7-year-old boy (No. 134218) had been on primidone, 500 mg per day for 18 months for recurrent convulsions. These were successfully controlled. He became anorexic over a period of 2 months, followed by loss of weight and the development of pallor. On examination the spleen was palpable 2 cm below the costal margin and there was forearm pulsation, in addition to extreme pallor of the mucous membranes. There was no jaundice or oedema. The haemoglobin was 2·6 g/100 ml, WBC 1,400/mm^3 with 800 neutrophils/mm^3 and 128,000 platelets/mm^3. The blood film showed occasional macrocytes together with a marked degree of hypersegmentation of the polymorphs (48 per cent with 5 or more lobes). Small numbers of late megaloblasts could also be found in the blood film. Reticulocytes were 3 per cent, PCV 7 per cent and MCV 78 μm^3. Marrow examination showed marked megaloblastic changes and giant band cells. Serum folate was less than 2 ng/ml, B$_{12}$ 180 pg/ml.

Because of giddiness and dyspnoea on mild exertion, attributed to the severity of the anaemia, he was given a slow transfusion of one unit of packed red cell which raised his haemoglobin to 6·6 g/100 ml. This relieved the above symptoms without obscuring the subsequent reticulocyte response to therapy. He was given folic acid 5 mg, t.d.s., started prior to the transfusion, and continued on primidone 500 mg/day. A rapid reticulocyte response occurred; 12 per cent on the fourth day. Thereafter the haemoglobin rose slowly over to 9·0 g/100 ml, 4 weeks from start of folic acid. At this point the blood film suggested the development of superimposed iron deficiency, for which additional therapy was given. He did not develop fits while on the folic acid plus primidone.

In those patients with megaloblastic anaemia there is a low serum folate (Waters, 1963) and red cell folate (Case 3). The FIGLU excretion is often normal. The rate of clearance of injected folate is normal unless anaemia is present (Chanarin *et al.*, 1960). These findings have been interpreted as indicating a drug-induced, block in folate metabolism but not a true folate deficiency. Adequate diet may protect against the occurrence of macrocytosis (Malpas, Spray and Witts, 1966). In the presence of suboptimal folate intake, however, this block appears to induce a true megaloblastic anaemia. These changes are regularly reversed by administering folic acid, even in doses as small as 25 μg per day while continuing on diphenylhydantoin (Druskin *et al.*, 1962). Alternatively a haematological response occurs if the offending drug is stopped. Strangely the serum B$_{12}$ may also be low in the patients with megaloblastic anaemia. This is unlikely to indicate true deficiency since it, too, rises shortly after starting folic acid therapy.

The biochemical site of action of these anti-convulsant drugs is not known, but it may be significant that all three are substituted pyrimidines and that a pyridine ring is also present in the pteridine moiety of folic acid, as pointed out by Girdwood and Lenman (1956). There is some evidence that diphenylhydantoin inhibits *de novo* DNA synthesis and conflicting evidence as to whether it inhibits liberation of folate monogluta-mate from the heptaglutamate form (Baugh and Krumdieck, 1969). The anti-convulsants do not appear to inhibit the enzymes such as dihydrofolate reductase concerned with 1-carbon transfer re-actions (Fig. 2.2).

The CSF folate level is normally about three times the concentration in serum, and this re-lationship pertains in patients on anticonvulsants. The low CSF folate may be relevant to the mental state of children on long-term anticonvulsants (Reynolds *et al.*, 1969). Those on high doses may show progressive dementia, psychosis, depression, mental retardation and behaviour disorders. These symptoms can be improved by folic acid adminis-tration (Reynolds, 1967). Unfortunately this may result in an increased frequency of fits, but not, apparently, if B_{12} is given simultaneously. This has been confirmed by Neubauer (1970) who studied 50 epileptic children and showed that combined treatment with folic acid plus B_{12} can have a beneficial effect on their mental state without increasing the number or severity of fits. He used relatively large doses, viz. 10–15 mg of folic acid daily and 1,000 μg of B_{12} weekly until the serum levels were normal and then gave a reduced maintenance dose. Also it appears that the epi-leptogenic effects of folic acid only appear after 3–6

months administration of high doses (15 mg/day) (Reynolds, 1973).

Table 2.3 lists a number of other drugs that may cause megaloblastic anaemia. In most instances this complication is inconstant, but in the cases of methotrexate and pyrimethamine (Daraprin), which block dihydrofolate reductase, or cytosine arabinoside, which blocks DNA synthesis, a megaloblastic state is invariable.

Recent interest has focused upon the anti-bacterial combination co-trimoxazole. It appears to accentuate the severity of pre-existing megalo-blastic anaemias in normal doses and can produce megaloblastic changes in normal individuals if given in abnormally high doses (Lancet, 1973B). A precarious folate balance may be a prerequisite. A 10-day course in Ugandan children with severe protein-calorie malnutrition caused an increase in FIGLU excretion but no anaemia or macrocytosis (Poskitt and Parkin, 1972). It should not be given in pregnancy.

Inborn errors related to folate metabolism

One group of these disorders is characterized by a megaloblastic anaemia in which there is neither folate nor B_{12} deficiency. The other group is characterized by mental retardation with abnormally high serum folate with or without increased FIGLU excretion (Table 2.4). All these conditions are extremely rare, the reports mostly being of single patients or a single family.

Orotic aciduria has been reported a little more frequently than the other disorders, with four patients being described so far. They presented with megaloblastic anaemia in infancy at 2, 3, 3, and 7 months respectively. The serum folate levels were high and the serum B_{12} levels normal. There

Table 2.3   Drugs known to cause megaloblastosis

Anticonvulsants
  phenytoin (Dilantin, Epanutin)
  primidone (Mysoline)
  phenobarbitone
  amylobarbitone $\left.\right\}$ (Tuinal)
  quinalbarbitone
  phenyl methyl barbituric acid
Antimetabolites
  azathioprine
  6-mercaptopurine
  methotrexate
  pyrimethamine (Daraprim)
  homofolic acid
  5-fluorouracil
  vitamin B_{12} antagonists
  cytosine arabinoside
	Antituberculous drugs
	  para-amino salicylic acid
	  pyrazinamide
	  cycloserine
	Antibacterial drugs
	  nitrofurantoin
	  co-trimoxazole
	Other
	  cyclophosphamide
	  phenylbutazone
	  arsenic

was no response to therapy with folic acid, B_{12} or crude liver extract. Clinically the infants were retarded in growth and development. The urine contained abundant colourless crystals of orotic acid separating out in the cold (Huguley et al., 1959).

The biochemical block has been traced to a defect of the two enzymes immediately preceding the synthesis of uridine-5-phosphate. Very low levels of these enzymes, orotidylic pyrophosphorylase and orotidylic decarboxylase, have been found in erythrocytes, leucocytes and skin fibroblast cultures (Smith et al., 1966). A partial enzyme defect was found in many of the relatives in one family and it is thought that this indicated the

suggested that the block was a little later in the pyrimidine synthetic pathway than that found in orotic aciduria. But the conversion of deoxyuridine phosphate to thymidine phosphate, which is critically dependent upon folate coenzymes (Fig. 2.3) appeared to be intact.

Congenital deficiency of formimino transferase results in abnormal FIGLU excretion (Fig. 2.4) and hyperfolicacidaemia associated with mental retardation, but no megaloblastic anaemia (Arakawa et al., 1965). Since experimental iron deficiency in rats similarly results in reduction of this enzyme and consequent FIGLU excretion (Vitale et al., 1965) it has been suggested

Table 2.4   Rare congenital abnormalities of folate metabolism

	Megaloblastic anaemia	Mental deficiency	FIGLU excretion	Serum folate	Effective therapy	References
Orotic aciduria	+	—	—	↑	Uridine 1 g/day	Huguley et al., 1959
Folinic acid responsive anaemia	+	—	+	N not given	Folinic acid (100 μg)	Walters, 1967
Thiamine responsive anaemia	+	—	—		Thiamine 20 mg/day	Rodgers et al., 1969
Congenital familial megaloblastic anaemia	+	—	+	↑	High dose folic acid +B_{12}	Lampkin et al., 1969
N^5-methyltetrahydrofolate transferase deficiency	+	+	—	↑	—	Arakawa et al., 1967
Forminotransferase deficiency	—	+	+	↑	—	Arakawa et al., 1965
Cyclohydrase deficiency	—	+	—	↑	—	Arakawa et al., 1966

heterozygous carrier state (Fallon et al., 1963). As predicted by the site of the metabolic block, prior to uridylic acid, a complete haematological response and a restoration of normal growth occurred after treatment with uridine, 1 to 1·5 g per day (Becroft and Phillips, 1965). The output of orotic acid also is reduced by this therapy. In one older child, aged 5, there was a partial response to folic acid (Meimann et al., 1965).

Other examples of congenital or hereditary megaloblastic anaemia have been reported which respond to folinic acid (Hauran et al., 1960; Walters, 1967) or to thiamine (Rogers et al., 1969) but not to folic acid or B_{12}. Two sisters presenting with severe megaloblastic anaemia at 3 and 7 weeks but with normal serum folate and B_{12} levels responded to pharmacological doses of folic acid, 15 mg per day, plus B_{12}, 1,000 micrograms I.M. per week (Lampkin et al., 1971). There was no excretion of orotic acid nor response to folinic acid in these infants and the evidence

that this provides a possible explanation of how iron deficiency may cause a defect of folate metabolism.

Hyperfolicacidaemia without increased FIGLU excretion has been found in congenital cyclohydrase deficiency (Table 2.4). Again this was associated with mental retardation but no megaloblastic anaemia (Arakawa et al., 1966). These 3 congenital enzyme deficiencies in mentally defective Japanese infants have clinical and EEG features in common and have been reviewed by Arakawa (1970). Bearing in mind the association of mental impairment in congenital defects of folate absorption, with low serum folate levels, and the above syndromes with high serum folate this assay is clearly contributory to investigation of unexplained mental defects.

Conditions with increased folate loss

Patients with chronic renal disease appear to lose folate, but not B_{12}, during peritoneal (Sevitt and Hoffbrand, 1969) or haemodialysis (Hampers et al., 1967). Whereas the serum folate level was normal in 11 patients with chronic renal failure not requiring haemodialysis, it was low in 9 out of 10 having regular dialysis. On this basis Hampers et al. (1967) recommended folic acid supplementation in such patients.

Liver disease may also cause increased folate loss. Urinary excretion was increased from a normal mean of $9.5\,\mu g/day$ to 31.1 during active viral hepatitis and to 35.7 in congestive hepatomegaly due to cardiac failure (Retief and Huskisson, 1969). It was thought that this loss might be a significant factor in precipitating folic acid deficiency in chronic liver disease when the intake is poor. It might also explain the abnormal FIGLU tests found by Rook et al. (1973) in infants and children with heart disease.

Increased renal loss of folate has also been demonstrated in the newborn (Landon and Hey, 1974). This is thought to be due to poor tubular reabsorption. The average daily loss during the first 5 days of life was nearly eight times that in adult life and more than enough to account for the observed fall in plasma folate level over the same period. In the one preterm infant studied the renal losses remained high throughout the first month of life. The mean loss was $1.87\,\mu g/kg$ per day over the first five days which is of the same order as the daily folate intake from milk preparations of 2 to $10\,\mu g$ for a 3 kg baby (Roberts et al., 1969). These considerations could account for the precarious folate balance of the newborn.

CLINICAL FEATURES AND TREATMENT

The clinical picture in infants is characterized by anorexia, failure of continued weight gain and weakness with liability to infections and gastrointestinal disturbances. A sore tongue or mouth is seldom seen in temperate climates, although commoner in tropical sprue. These symptoms may be more striking than the anaemia. Haemorrhagic manifestations may occur secondary to thrombocytopenia, or infection, due to neutropenia.

Established folic acid deficiency may be adequately treated by giving 5 mg of folic acid orally per day. This dose of the pure monoglutamate is adequately absorbed even in the presence of an active malabsorption syndrome. The only practical indication for parental folic acid is the presence of vomiting or in the severely ill child where speed of action of the first dose might be vital. The I.M. route would be contra-indicated in the presence of thrombocytopenia.

If severe anaemia is present a small blood transfusion is indicated since no significant rise in haemoglobin can be expected in under a week. The transfusion should be given as slowly as possible for fear of precipitating cardiac failure and, in view of the general systematic effects of folate deficiency, the folic acid should be given even before the transfusion. In uncomplicated folate deficiency there will be a complete haematological response to 'physiological' doses of $200\,\mu g/day$. The serum iron falls to low levels between 24 and 48 hours, reticulocytosis appears at between 2 and 3 days, followed by circulating normoblasts and reaching a reticulocyte peak between 5 and 7 days. A rise in leucocytes and platelets may parallel the rise in reticulocytes. The Hb and red cell count rises appreciably during the second week and thereafter somewhat less rapidly. Hypersegmentation of the polymorphs disappears during the second week. A clinical improvement may be noticeable much sooner.

The possibility of multiple deficiencies should be considered; particularly iron, ascorbic acid and, in the malabsorption syndromes, vitamins A, D and K together with the B complex.

REFERENCES

Acevodo, G. & Mauer, A. M. (1965). The effect of large intravenous doses of methotrexate on urinary formiminoglutamic acid excretion. *J. Pediat.*, **66**, 753.

Anderson, B., Belcher, E. H., Chanarin, I. & Mollin, D. L. (1960) The urinary and faecal excretion of radioactivity after oral doses of 3H-folic acid. *Brit. J. Haemat.*, **6**, 439.

Anderson, C. M. (1960) Histological changes in the duodenal mucosa in coeliac disease. Reversibility during treatment with a wheat gluten free diet. *Arch. Dis. Child.*, **35**, 419.

Arakawa, T., Ohara, K., Takahashi, Y., Ogasawara, J., Hayashi, T., Chiba, R., Wada, Y., Tada, K., Mizuno, T., Okamura, T. & Yoshida, T. (1965) Forminotransferase-deficiency syndrome: A new inborn error of folic acid metabolism. *Ann. Paediat.*, **205**, 1.

Arakawa, T., Fujii, M., Chara, K., Watanabe, S., Karahashi, M., Kobayashi, M. & Hirono, H. (1966) Mental retardation with hyperfolic-acidemia not associated with formiminoglutamic-aciduria: cyclohydrase deficiency syndrome. *Tohoku J. Exp. Med.*, **88**, 341.

Arakawa, T., Narisawa, K., Tanno, K., Ohara, K., Higashi, O., Honda, Y. et al. (1967) Megaloblastic anemia and mental retardation associated with hyperfolic-acidemia, probably due to N_2-methyltetrahydrofolate transferase deficiency. *Tohoku J. Exp. Med.*, **93**, 1.

Arakawa, T. (1970) Congenital defects of folate utilization. *Am. J. Med.*, **48**, 594.

Bangh, C. M. & Krumdieck, C. L. (1969) Effects of phenytoin on folic-acid conjugases in man. *Lancet*. **2**, 519.

Becroft, D. M. O. & Phillips, L. I. (1965) Hereditary orotic aciduria and megaloblastic anaemia: A second case with a response to uridine. *Brit. med. J.* **1**, 547.

Becroft, D. M. O. & Holland, J. T. (1966) Goat's milk and megaloblastic anaemia of infancy. *N.Z. med. J.*, **65**, 303.

Burland, W. L., Simpson, K. & Lord, J. (1971) Response of low birthweight infants to treatment with folic acid. *Arch. Dis. Childh.*, **46**, 189.

Carey, M. C., Fennelly, J. J. & Fitzgerald, O. (1968) Homocystinuria II. Subnormal serum folate levels, increased folate clearance and effects of folic acid therapy. *Amer. J. Med.*, **45**, 26.

Chanarin, I., Dacie, J. V. & Mollin, D. L. (1959) Folic acid deficiency in haemolytic anaemia. *Brit. J. Haemat.*, **5**, 245.

Chanarin, I., Laidlaw, J., Loughbridge, L. W. & Mollin, D. L. (1960) Megaloblastic anaemia due to phenobarbitone. The convulsant action of therapeutic doses of folic acid. *Brit. med. J.* **1**, 1099.

Chanarin, I. & Bennett, M. C. (1962) The disposal of small doses of intravenously injected folic acid. *Brit. J. Haemat.*, **8**, 28.

Chanarin, I. & Bennett, M. C. (1962) A spectrophotometric method for estimating formimino-glutamic and urocanic acid. *Brit. med. J.*, **1**, 27.

Chanarin, I., Burman, D. & Bennett, M. (1962) Familial aplastic crisis in hereditary spherocytosis. Urocanic acid and FIGLU excretion studies in a case of megaloblastic anaemia. *Blood*, **20**, 33.

Chanarin, I. (1964) Studies on urinary formiminoglutamic acid excretion. *Proc. Roy. Soc. Med.*, **57**, 384.

Chanarin, I., Rothman, D. & Berry, V. (1965) Iron deficiency and its relation to folic acid status in pregnancy: Results of a clinical trial. *Brit. med. J.*, **1**, 480.

Chanarin, I., Rothman, D., Perry, J. & Stratfull, D. (1968) Normal dietary folate iron, and protein intake, with particular reference to pregnancy. *Brit. med. J.*, **2**, 394.

Chanarin, I. (1969) The megaloblastic anaemias, p. 233, p. 339, p. 345 and p. 350. Oxford and Edinburgh: Blackwell Scientific Publications.

Chanarin, I. (1973) Hypothesis: New light on pernicious anaemia. *Lancet*, **ii**, 538.

Chatterjea, J. B. (1959) *Section on haemoglobin in India*. Jonxix, J. H. P. and Delafresnaze, J. F. (eds.): Abnormal haemoglobins. Springfield, Illinois: Charles C. Thomas.

Commission on biochemical nomenclature (1966) Tentative rules. Nomenclature and symbols for folic acid and related compounds. *J. Biol. Chem.*, **241**, 2991.

Cook, D. M., Frans, N., Lloyd, A. & Stewart, J. S. (1971). Coeliac disease. Reappraisal of clinical diagnosis. *Arch. Dis. Childh.*, **46**, 705.

Cooper, B. A. & Lowenstein, L. (1966) Vitamin B_{12}-folate interrelationships in megaloblastic anaemia. *Brit. J. Haemat.*, **12**, 283.

Cooperman, J. M. (1974) Biochemical lesion in pernicious anaemia. *Lancet*, **ii**, 1144.

Cox, E. V., Meynell, M. J., Cooke, W. T. & Gaddie, R. (1960) Scurvy and anaemia. *Am. J. Med.*, **32**, 240.

Dacie, J. V. & White, J. C. (1949) Erythropoiesis with particular reference to its study by biopsy of human bone marrow: A review. *J. Clin. Path.*, **2**, 1.

Doig, A. & Girdwood, R. H. (1960) The absorption of folic acid and labelled cyanocobalamin in intestinal malabsorption. *Q. J. Med. n.s.*, **29**, 333.

Dormandy, K. M., Waters, A. H. & Mollin, D. L. (1963) Folic-acid deficiency in coeliac disease. *Lancet*, **1**, 632.

Druskin, M. S., Wallen, M. H. & Bonagura, L. (1962) Anticonvulsant-associated megaloblastic anaemia. *New Eng. J. Med.*, **267**, 483.

Fallon, H. J., Smith, L. H. J., Lctz, M. Graham, J. B. & Burnett, C. H. (1963) Hereditary orotic acidemia. *Trans. Ass. Am. Physns.*, **76**, 214.

Food and Agriculture Organization/World Health Organization (1970) *Requirements of ascorbic acid, vitamin D, vitamin B_{12}, folate and iron*. Geneva: W.H.O. Technical Report Series, No. 452, W.H.O.

Ford, J. E. & Scott, K. J. (1968) The folic acid activity of some milk foods for babies. *J. Dairy Research.*, **35**, 85.

Ghitis, J. (1966) The labile folate of milk. *Am. J. clin. Nutr.*, **18**, 452.

Ghitis, J. & Tripathy, K. (1970) Availability of milk folate: Studies with cow's milk in experimental folic acid deficiency. *Am. J. clin. Nutr.*, **23**, 141.

Girdwood, R. H. & Lenman, J. A. R. (1956) Megaloblastic anaemia occurring during primidone therapy. *Brit. med. J.*, **1**, 146.

Glanzmann, E. (1926) Klinische und experimentelle Studien über Ziegermilchanämie und Dystropie. *Jb. Kinderheilk. phys. Erzieh.*, **111**, 127.

Gomirato-Sandrucci, M., Nigro, N., Bonenti, G. & Benso, L. (1966). *L'escrezione urinaria dell 'acido formimino glutammico (Figlu) nell'epatite contagiosa dell'infanzia*. Congr. Intern. sulla. Rigenerazione epatica, Montecantini Terne.

Gray, O. P. & Butler, E. B. (1965) Megaloblastic anaemia in premature infants. *Arch. Dis. Childh.*, **40**, 53.

Gross, S., Keefer, V. & Newman, A. J. (1965) Folate metabolism and iron deficiency. *Lancet*, **2**, 744.

Grossowicz, N., Mandelbaum-Shavit, F., Davidoff, R. & Aronovitch, J. (1962) Microbiologic determination of folic acid derivatives in blood. *Brit. J. Haemat.*, **6**, 296.

Hampers, C. L., Streiff, R., Nathan, D. G., Snyder, D. & Merrill, J. P. (1967) Megaloblastic haematopoiesis in uremia and in patients on long-term haemodialysis. *New Eng. J. Med.*, **276**, 551.

Haurani, F. I., Wang, G. & Tocantins, L. M. (1960) Megaloblastic anaemia probably caused by defective utilization of folinic acid. *Blood*, **16**, 1546.

Heinivaara, O. & Kaipainen, W. J. (1959) Occurrence of large cells in myelopoiesis of megaloblastic anaemias. *Annls. Med. intern. Fenn.*, **48**, 177.

Hepner, G. W., Booth, C. C., Cowan, J., Hoffbrand, A. V. & Mollin, D. L. (1968) Absorption of crystalline folic acid in man. *Lancet*, **2**, 302.

Herbert, V. (1962) Experimental nutritional folate deficiency in man. *Tr. Assoc. Amer. Phys.*, **745**, 307.

Herbert, V. & Zalusky, R. (1962) Interrelations of vitamin B_{12} and folic acid metabolism: Folic acid clearance studies. *J. Clin. Invest.*, **41**, 1263.

Herbert, V. (1963) A palatable diet for producing experimental folate deficiency in man. *Am. J. clin. Nutr.*, **12**, 17.

Herbert, V. (1967) Biochemical and haematological lesions in folic acid deficiency. *Am. J. clin. Nutr.*, **20**, 562.

Hoffbrand, A. V., Newcombe, B. F. A. & Mollin, D. L. (1966) Method of assay of red-cell folate activity and the value of the assay as a test for folate deficiency. *J. clin. Path.*, **19**, 17.

Hoffbrand, A. V., Nechfles, J. N., Maldonado, N., Horta, E. & Santini, R. (1969) Malabsorption of folate polyglutamates in tropical sprue. *Brit. med. J.*, **2**, 543.

Hoffbrand, A. V. (1970) Folate deficiency in premature infants. *Arch. Dis. Childh.*, **45**, 441.

Hudson, F. P. (1961) Phenylketonuria. *Brit. med. J.*, **1**, 1105.

Huguley, C. M., Bain, J. A., Rivers, S. L. & Scoggins, R. B. (1959) Refractory megaloblastic anaemia associated with excretion of orotic acid. *Blood*, **14**, 615.

Hurdle, A. D. F. (1967) *The fotate content of a hospital diet.* University of London: M.D. thesis.

Izak, G., Rachmilewitz, M., Sadovsky, A. *et al.* (1961) Folic acid metabolites in whole blood and serum in anemia of pregnancy. *Am. J. clin. Nutr.*, **9**, 473.

Jandl, J. H. & Gabuzda, G. J. (1953) Potentiation of pteroylglutamic acid by ascorbic acid in anaemia of scurvy. *Proc. Soc. exp. Biol. Med.*, **84**, 452.

Jandl, J. H. & Lear, A. A. (1956) The metabolism of folic acid in cirrhosis. *Ann. intern Med.*, **45**, 1027.

Johns, D. G., Sperti, S. & Burgen, A. S. V. (1961) The metabolism of tritiated folic acid in man. *J. clin. Invest.*, **40**, 1684.

Kendall, A. C., Jones, E. E., Wilson, C. I. D., Shinton, N. K. & Elwood, P. C. (1974) Folic acid in low birthweight infants. *Arch. Dis. Childh.*, **49**, 736.

Kende, G., Ramot, B. & Grossowicz, N. (1963) Blood folic acid and vitamin B_{12} activities in healthy infants and in infants with nutritional anaemias. *Brit. J. Haemat.*, **9**, 328.

Khalil, M., Tanios, A., Moghazy, M., Aref, M. K., Mahmoud, S. & El Lozy, M. (1973) Serum and red cell folates, and serum B_{12} in protein calorie malnutrition. *Arch. Dis. Childh.*, **48**, 366.

Kho, L. K., Odang, O. & Markum, A. H. (1961) Acute erythroblastopenia (aplastic crisis) in children with megaloblastic anaemia. *Ann. Paediat.*, **196**, 379.

Kinnear, D. G., Johns, D. G., MacIntosh, P. C., Burgen, A. S. V. & Cameron, D. G. (1963) Intestinal absorption of tritium-labelled folic acid in idiopathic steatorrhoea: Effect of a gluten-free diet. *Can. med. Ass. J.*, **89**, 975.

Klipstein, F. A. (1963) The urinary excretion of orally administered tritium-labelled folic acid as a test of folic acid absorption. *Blood*, **21**, 626.

Klipstein, F. A. (1964) Subnormal serum folate and macrocytosis associated with anti-convulsant drug therapy. *Blood*, **23**, 68.

Knowles, J. P. & Prankerd, T. A. J. (1962) Abnormal folic acid metabolism in vitamin B_{12} deficiency. *Clin. Sci.*, **22**, 233.

Kohn, J., Mollin, D. L. & Rosenbach, L. M. (1961) Conventional voltage electrophoresis for formiminoglutamic-acid determination in folic acid deficiency. *J. clin. Path.*, **14**, 345.

Kondi, A., MacDoug ll, L., Foy, H., Mehta, S. & Mbaya, V. (1963) Anaemia of marasmus and kwashiorkor in Kenya. *Arch. Dis. Childh.*, **38**, 267.

Lampkin, B. C., Pyesmany, A., Hyman, C. B. & Hammond, D. (1971) Congenital familial megaloblastic anaemia. *Blood*, **37**, 615.

Lancet (1973A) Editorial: Folate deficiency in childhood. *Lancet*, **ii**, 813.

Lancet (1973B) Editorial: Co-Trimoxazole and blood. *Lancet*, **ii**, 950.

Landon, M. J. & Hey, E. N. (1974) Renal loss of folate in the newborn infant. *Arch. Dis. Childh.*, **49**, 292.

Lanzkowsky, P., Erlandson, M. E. & Bezan, A. I. (1969) Isolated defect of folic acid absorption associated with mental retardation and cerebral calcification. *Blood*, **34**, 452.

Levy, H. L., Truman, J. T., Ganz, R. N. & Littlefield, J. W. (1970) Folic acid deficiency secondary to a diet for maple syrup urine disease. *J. Pediat.*, **77**, 294.

Lien-Keng, K. & Odang, O. (1959) Megaloblastic anaemia in infancy and childhood in Djakarta. *Am. J. Dis. Child.*, **97**, 209.

Lien-Keng, K. (1961) Red-cell aplasia in marasmus and kwashiorkor. *Brit. med. J.*, **2**, 1086.

Line, D. H., Seitanidis, B., Morgan, J. O. & Hoffbrand, A. V. (1971) The effects of chemotherapy on iron, folate, and vitamin B_{12} metabolism in tuberculosis. *Quart. J. Med. n.s.*, **40**, 331.

Luhby, A. L. & Cooperman, J. M. (1961) Folic acid deficiency in thalassaemia major. *Lancet*, **2**, 490.

Luhby, A. L., Eagle, F. J., Roth, E. & Cooperman, J. M. (1961) Relapsing megaloblastic anemia and mental retardation associated with defect in gastrointestinal absorption of folic acid. *Amer. J. Dis. Child.*, **102**, 482.

Luhby, A. L. & Cooperman, J. M. (1964) Folic acid deficiency in man and its interrelationship with vitamin B_{12} metabolism. *Advanc. Metabolic Disorders*, **1**, 263.

MacIver, J. E. & Went, L. N. (1960) Sickle-cell anaemia complicated by megaloblastic anaemia of infancy. *Brit. med. J.*, **1**, 775.

Mackintosh, T. F. P., Strelling, M. K., Walker, C. H. M. & Goodall, H. B. (1969) Folic acid trends and prophylaxis in prevention of megaloblastic anaemia of infants of low birthweight. *Arch. Dis. Childh.*, **44**, 137.

McNeish, A. S. & Willoughby, M. L. N. (1969) Whole-blood folate as a screening test for coeliac disease in childhood. *Lancet*, **1**, 442.

Magnus, E. M. (1966) Low serum and red cell folate activity in adult coeliac disease. *Am. J. dig. Dis. n.s.*, **11**, 314

Majaj, A. S., Dinning, J. S., Assam, S. A. & Darby, W. J. (1963) Vitamin E responsive megaloblastic anaemia in infants with protein-calorie malnutrition. *Amer. J. clin. Nutr.*, **12**, 374.

Malpas, J. S., Spray, G. H. & Witts, L. J. (1966) Serum folic-acid and vitamin B_{12} levels in anticonvulsant therapy. *Brit. med. J.*, **1**, 955.

Matoth, Y., Pinkas, A., Zamie, R., Mccallem, F. & Grossowitcz, N. (1964A) Blood levels of folic and folinic acid in healthy infants. *Pediatrics*, **33**, 4.

Matoth, Y., Zamir, R., Bar-Shani, S. & Grossowitcz, N. (1964B) Studies on folic acid in infancy: II. Folic and folinic acid blood levels in infants with diarrhoea, malnutrition and infection. *Pediatrics*, **33**, 694.

Matoth, Y., Pinkas, A. & Spoka, C. (1965) Studies on folic dacid in infancy III. *Amer. J. clin. Nutr.*, **16**, 356.

May, C. D., Stewart, C. T., Hamilton, A. & Salmon, R. J. (1952A) Infection as a cause of folic acid deficiency and megaloblastic anaemia. *Am. J. Dis. Child.*, **84**, 718.

May, C. D., Hamilton, A. & Stewart, C. T. (1952B) Experimental megaloblastic anaemia and scurvy in the monkey. IV. Vitamin B_{12} and folic acid compounds in the diet, liver, urine and faeces and effects of therapy. *Blood*, **7**, 978.

Meimann, N., Nahean, Y., Scialom, C., Boulard, M., Pierson, M. & Bernard, J. (1965) Étude d'un case d'anémie megaloblastique de l'enfant avec excrétion anormale d'acide orotique. *Nouv. Revue fr. Hémat.*, **5**, 445.

Mortimer, P. E., Stewart, J. S., Norman, A. P. & Booth, C. C. (1968) Follow-up study of coeliac disease. *Brit. med. J.*, **3**, 7.

Naiman, J. L. & Oski, F. A. (1964) The folic acid content of milk: Revised figures based on an improved assay method. *Pediatrics*, **34**, 274.

Neubauer, C. (1970) Mental deterioration in epilepsy due to folate deficiency.

Nixon, P. F. & Bertino, J. R. (1972) Effective absorption and utilization of oral formyltetrahydrofolate in man. *New Eng. J. Med.*, **286**, 175.

Panders, J. T. (1964) *De invloed van temperatuer op enkele enzymen van de foliuminzuurstofwisseling*. Utrecht M. D. Thesis.

Pereira, S. M. & Baker, S. J. (1966) Hematologic studies in kwashiorkor. *Am. J. clin. Nutr.*, **18**, 413.

Perry, J. & Chanarin, I. (1968) Absorption and utilization of polyglutamyl forms of folate in man. *Brit. med. J.*, **4**, 546.

Perry, J. & Chanarin, I. (1970) Intestinal absorption of reduced folate compounds in man. *Brit. J. Haemat.*, **18**, 329.

Perry, J. (1971) Folate analogues in normal mixed diets. *Brit. J. Haemat.*, **21**, 435.

Pierce, L. B. & Rath, C. E. (1962) Evidence for folic acid deficiency in genesis of anaemic sickle cell crisis. *Blood*, **20**, 19.

Poskitt, E. M. E. & Parkin, J. M. (1972) Effect of trimethoprim-sulphamethoxazole combination on folate metabolism in malnourished children. *Arch. Dis. Childh.*, **47**, 626.

Pritchard, J. A., Scott, D. E., Whalley, P. J. & Haling, R. F. (1970) Infants of mothers with megaloblastic anaemia due to folate deficiency. *J.A.M.A.*, **211**, 1982.

Purugganan, G., Leikin, S. & Gantier, G. (1971) Folate metabolism in erythroid hyperplastic and hypoplastic states. *Amer. J. Dis. Child.*, **122**, 48.

Retief, F. P & Huskisson, Y. J. (1969) Serum and urinary folate in liver disease. *Brit. med. J.*, **ii**, 150.

Reynolds, E. H. (1967) Effects of folic acid on the mental state and fit-frequency of drug-treated epilectic patients. *Lancet*, **1**, 1086.

Reynolds, E. H., Preece, J. & Chanarin, I. (1969) Folic acid and anticonvulsants. *Lancet*, **1**, 1265.

Reynolds, E. H. (1973) Anticonvulsants, folic acid and epilepsy. *Lancet*, **i**, 1376.

Roberts, P. M., Arrowsmith, D. E., Rou, S. M. & Monk-Jones, M. E. (1969) Folate state of premature infants. *Arch. Dis. Childh.*, **44**, 637.

Roberts, P. M. M., Arrowsmith, D. E., Lloyd, A. V. C. & Monk-Jones, M. E. (1972) Effect of folic acid treatment on premature infants. *Arch. Dis. Childh.*, **47**, 631.

Rogers, L. E., Porter, F. S. & Sidbury, J. B. (1969) Thiamine-responsive megaloblastic anaemia. *J. Pediat.*, **74**, 494.

Rook, G. D., Lopez, R., Shimizu, N. & Cooperman, J. M. (1973) Folic acid deficiency in infants and children with heart disease. *Brit. Heart J.*, **35**, 87.

Royston, N. J. W. & Parry, T. E. (1962) Megaloblastic anaemia complicating dietary treatment of phenylketonuriam infancy. *Arch. Dis. Childh.*, **37**, 430.

Sandstead, H. H., Carter, J. P., House, F. R., McConnell, F., Horton, K. B. & Zwaag, R. V. (1971) Nutritional deficiencies in disadvantages pre-school children—Their relationship to mental development (economically depressed area of Nashville). *Amer. J. Dis. Child.*, **121**, 455.

Santiago, P. J. & Maldonado, N. (1968) *Tropical sprue in children*. New York: XII Congr. Intern. Soc. Hemat.

Santiago-Borrero, P. J., Santini, R., Pérez-Santiago, E. & Maldonado, N. (1973) Congenital isolated defect of folic acid absorption. *J. Pediat.*, **82**, 450.

Sevitt, L. H. & Hoffbrand, A. V. (1969) Serum folate and vitamin B_{12} levels in acute and chronic renal disease. Effect of peritoneal dialysis. *Brit. med. J.*, **ii**, 18.

Sheehy, T. W., Baggs, B., Perez-Santiago, E. & Floch, M. H. (1962) Prognosis of tropical sprue. *Ann. Intern. Med.*, **57**, 892.

Sheldon, W. (1955) Coeliac disease. *Lancet*, **2**, 1097.

Shojania, A. M. & Gross, S. (1964A) Folic acid deficiency and prematurity. *J. Pediat.*, **64**, 323.

Shojania, A. M. & Gross, S. (1964B) Hemolytic anaemias and colic acid deficiency in children. *Am. J. Dis. Child.*, **108**, 53.

Smith, L. H., Huguley, C. M. & Bain, J. A. (1966) *Hereditary orotic aciduria*. Stanbury, J. B., Wyngaarden, J. B. and Frederickson, D. S. (eds.); The metabolic basis of inherited disease, 2nd edn., p. 739. New York: McGraw-Hill.

Spector, I. & Metz, J. (1966) Giant myeloid cells in bone marrow of protein malnourished infants: Relationship to folate and vitamin B_{12} nutrition. *Brit. J. Haemat.*, **12**, 737.

Stewart, J. S., Pollock, D. J., Hoffbrand, A. V., Mollin, D. L. & Booth, C. C. (1967) A study of proximal and distal intestinal structure and absorptive function in idiopathic steatorrhoea. *Q. J. Med., n.s.*, **36**, 425.

Stokstad, E. L. R. & Koch, J. (1967) Folic acid metabolism. *Physiol. Rev.*, **47**, 83.

Streiff, R. R. & Little, A. B. (1967) Folic acid deficiency in pregnancy. *New Eng. J. Med.*, **276**, 776.

Strelling, M. K., Blackledge, G. D., Goodall, H. B. & Walker, C. H. M. (1966) Megaloblastic anaemia and whole-blood folate levels in premature infants. *Lancet*, **i**, 898.

Sullivan, L. W., Luhby, A. L. & Streiff, R. R. (1966) Studies of the daily requirement for folic acid in infants and the etiology of folate deficiency in goat's milk megaloblastic anaemia. *Amer. J. Clin. Nutr.*, **18**, 311.

Vanier, T. M. & Tyas, J. F. (1966) Folic acid status in normal infants during the first year of life. *Arch. Dis. Childh.*, **41**, 658.

Vanier, T. M. & Tyas, J. F. (1967) Folic acid status in premature infants. *Arch. Dis. Childh.*, **42**, 57.

Velez, H., Ghitis, J., Pradilla, A. & Vitale, J. J. (1963) Cali-Harvard nutrition project, I. Megaloblastic anaemia in kwashiorkor. *Am. J. Clin. Nutr.*, **12**, 54.

Visakorpi, J. K., Immonen, P. & Kuitunen, P. (1967) Malabsorption syndrome in childhood. *Arch. Paediat. Scand.*, **56**, 1.

Vitale, J.J., Streiff, R. R. & Hellerstein, E. E. (1965) Folate metabolism and iron deficiency. *Lancet*, **2**, 393.

Vossough, P., Leikin, S. & Purugganan, G. (1968) Evaluation of parameters of folic acid and vitamin B_{12} deficiency in patients with iron deficiency anaemia. *Pediat. Res.*, **2**, 179.

Walt, F., Holman, S. & Hendrickse, R. G. (1956) Megaloblastic anaemia of infancy in kwashiorkor and other diseases. *Brit. med. J.*, **i**, 1199.

Walters, T. R. (1967) Congenital megaloblastic anaemia responsive to N^5—formyl-tetrahydrofolic acid administration. *J. Pediat.*, **70**, 686.

Whitby, L. & Britton, C. J. C. (1969) *Disorders of the blood*. Edited by Britton, C. J. C. London: Churchill, J. & A.

Whitehead, R. G. & Arnstein, H. R. V. (1961) Imidazole acrylic acid excretion in kwashiorkor. *Nature, Lond.*, **190**, 1105.

Whitehead, V. M. & Cooper, B. A. (1967) Absorption of unaltered folic acid from the gastrointestinal tract in man. *Brit. J. Haemat.*, **13**, 679.

Whitehead, V. M. (1973) Polygammaglutamyl metabolites of folic acid in human liver. *Lancet*, **i**, 743.

Wilcken, B. & Turner, B. (1973) Homocystinuria. Reduced folate levels during pyridoxine treatment. *Arch. Dis. Childh.*, **48**, 58.

Zalusky, R. & Herbert, V. (1961) Megaloblastic anaemia in scurvy with response to 50 micrograms of folic acid daily. *New Eng. J. Med.*, **265**, 1033.

Zuelzer, W. W. & Ogden, F. N. (1946) Megaloblastic anaemia in infancy. *Am. J. Dis. Child* **71**, 211.

Zuelzer, W. W. & Rutzky, J. (1953) Megaloblastic anaemia of infancy. *Advances in Pediatrics*, **6**, 243.

3. Vitamin B₁₂ Metabolism and Deficiency

Biochemistry / Absorption and transport / Assessment of B_{12} status / B_{12} balance in infancy / Classification of B_{12} deficiency in infancy and childhood, *Intrinsic factor deficiency, Selective ileal malabsorption of B_{12}, Other causes of malabsorption, Nutritional B_{12} deficiency, Transcobalomin II deficiency.*

BIOCHEMISTRY

Vitamin B_{12} belongs chemically to the group of cobalamines. It is found in animal tissues but not in vegetable matter. That in animal tissues is ultimately derived from bacteria which are the only organisms capable of synthesizing vitamin B_{12} in nature. In animal tissues liver is a particularly rich source of B_{12} activity. The major portion of this activity is present in the coenzyme form, complexed with 5'-deoxyadenosine and bound to a specific protein. Substitution of hydroxyl, cyanide or methyl groups in place of the deoxyadenosyl radical results in hydroxo-, cyano- or methyl-cobalamines. These derivatives are found in small amounts in tissues and plasma, probably representing intermediary B_{12} metabolites. The hydroxo and cyanocobalamines are the forms used therapeutically. Rapid conversion of injected cyanocobalamine to the other forms occurs *in vivo*.

The main known biochemical reactions in which B_{12} participates in mammalian metabolism are (a) transfer of the methyl group from 5-methyl-tetrahydrofolate to homocysteine to form methionine, and (b) the intramolecular rearrangement of carbon atoms in methyl malonyl CoA to form succinyl CoA (Fig. 3.1).

The relationship of these B_{12}-dependent metabolic reactions to the development of megaloblastic changes in B_{12} deficiency is not clear. The 'folate trap' hypothesis (Chapter 2) can no longer explain all the facts (Chanarin, 1973). A rare hereditary disorder has been described in childhood where there is a defect of both the above B_{12}-coenzyme dependent reactions resulting in excessive excretion of both methyl-malonic acid and homocysteine (Fig. 3.1), but in spite of these metabolic blocks erythropoiesis is normal (Levy *et al.*, 1970; Goodman *et al.*, 1970). Some patients, however, have neurological involvement with mental retardation, increased tendon jerks and impaired proprioception, and Chanarin (1973) has suggested that the haemopoietic effects of B_{12} deficiency may have an entirely separate mechanism from that involved in neural tissue and the biochemical reactions in Figure 3.1. On the basis of folate uptake studies on lymphocytes (Das and Hoffbrand, 1970) and marrow cells (Tisman and Herbert, 1973) it has been suggested that B_{12} deficiency impairs transport of 5-methyl-tetrahydrofolate into haemic cells resulting in megaloblastic changes.

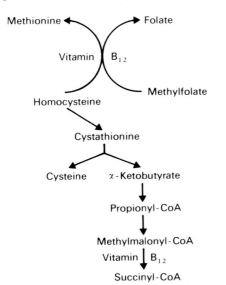

Fig. 3.1 Vitamin B_{12}-dependent metabolic pathways. (Reproduced with permission of the author and the Editor of *Lancet*, from the paper by Chanarin (1973)).

ABSORPTION AND TRANSPORT

Three stages in absorption can be defined (Mackenzie and Donaldson, 1969). Firstly there is interaction of dietary B_{12} with gastric intrinsic factor (IF) to form a macromolecular IF-B_{12} complex. Secondly this IF-B_{12} complex attaches to specific surface receptor sites on the ileal mucosal cells. Thirdly there is an active transport mechanism across the intestinal cells.

During transport in the portal blood B_{12} is thought to be attached to transcobalamin II rather than to IF (Cooper and White, 1968). Transcobalamin II (TC II) has the electrophoretic mobility of a beta globulin, is largely unsaturated in the circulating blood and readily binds B_{12} from oral or parenteral administration. The half-life of TC II-bound B_{12} is rapid and TC II enhances the uptake of B_{12} by a number of human cells including red cells (Retief et al., 1966). Another B_{12}-binding protein TC I, with electrophoretic mobility of an alpha globulin, is nearly fully saturated, has a half-life of 9 to 10 days and does not readily exchange with tissues (Finkler and Hall, 1967). These considerations suggest that TC II is the main transport protein of B_{12}, and that TC I forms a circulating B_{12} storage complex (Hakami et al., 1971). The clinical relevance is that congenital TC II deficiency causes megaloblastic anaemia and systemic manifestations within a few weeks of birth with a normal serum B_{12} level (Hakami et al., 1971), whereas congenital TC I deficiency causes a low serum B_{12} level without significant manifestations of deficiency (Carmel and Herbert 1969).

ASSESSMENT OF B_{12} STATUS

Microbiological assay of the serum B_{12} level using *Lactobacillus Leishmanii* or *Euglena gracilis* as the test organism is the key investigation. The normal adult range has been given as 140–900 picogrammes (pg) per ml, with values between 100 and 140 considered as 'borderline' (Mollin, 1960). Dormandy, Waters and Mollin (1963) similarly found a range of 220 to 770 in 12 children aged under 1 year, and of 150 to 1,180 in children between 1 and 10 years. In generalized malabsorption states such as coeliac disease 'borderline' results (e.g. 115) may be found even although folate is the prime deficiency. In true B_{12} deficiency states such as pernicious anaemia the serum B_{12} level is well below 100 pg/ml at presentation. In TC I deficiency the serum B_{12} level is low, but it is normal in TC II deficiency (*vide supra*).

The serum folate is normal or reciprocally elevated in isolated B_{12} deficiency but paradoxically the red cell folate is low in B_{12} deficiency as well as in folate deficiency (Waters and Mollin,

1961), perhaps because of the B_{12}-dependent entry of 5-methyl-tetrahydrofolate into cells mentioned above. This lack of discriminant value of a low red cell folate result can be resolved by follow-up serum B_{12} and (fasting) serum folate assays.

Methylmalonic acid excretion may also be used as an index of B_{12} deficiency (Fig. 3.1), as originally shown by Cox and White (1962). Valine loading increases the excretion and renders the test more sensitive (Gompertz, Hywell Jones and Knowles, 1967). Practical modifications making the test rapid and suitable for routine pathology laboratories have been described by Green and Pegrum (1968). Adults are given a 10 g valine load and methylmalonic acid excretion above 40 mg/24 hours is diagnostic of B_{12} deficiency. In general this test would only be used in paediatrics in metabolic study of special cases. In the rare disorder of methylmalonic aciduria described by Levy et al. (1970) and Goodman et al. (1970) the metabolic block occurs without associated haematological changes.

Absorption of B_{12} can best be studied by the Schilling test using labelled B_{12}, usually [57]Co, administered orally with and without added normal gastric juice or IF (Schilling, 1953). As this involves the administration of a radioactive isotope it is not, in general, a desirable test in young children, being reserved for special investigative problems. It does, however, allow definitive distinction between absence of IF or impaired absorption of the IF-B_{12} complex, e.g. in the selective B_{12} malabsorption defect of Immerslund's syndrome (Mackenzie et al., 1972). In this work the family had reached the ages of 15, 16 and 21 years before the Schilling test was performed.

Haematological consequences of B_{12} and folate deficiency are indistinguishable and include not only oval macrocytosis and megaloblastic anaemia (Plate A) but also neutropenia and thrombocytopenia in severe cases. Clinical features include pallor, soreness and smoothness of the tongue, with systemic effects such as 'failure to thrive' and poor weight gain in infants (e.g. Hakami et al., 1971) sometimes accompanied by diarrhoea and vomiting.

By the use of small, 'physiological' doses of folic acid and B_{12} in initial therapy distinction between the two types of deficiency can often be achieved (Marshall and Jandle, 1960; Hansen and Weinfeld, 1962). Adults with folic acid dependent anaemia respond fully to 0.2 mg I.M. of folic acid (1.3–7.0 μg/kg body weight) per day with optimum reticulocyte response and normoblastic marrow conversion after 8–10 days. Slight response can occur in some cases of B_{12} deficiency at doses of 0·3 to 0·4 mg per day, but a second and optimum response follows the subsequent administration of 3 μg I.M. B_{12} per day immediately following the folic acid course (Hansen and Weinfeld, 1962). In children a proportionately lower dose of I.M. B_{12} is effective, e.g. 0·1 μg/day will give a full haematological response in infants with B_{12} deficiency (Jadhav, Webb, Vaishnava and Baker, 1962).

B_{12} BALANCE IN INFANCY

The infant is born with a higher serum B_{12} level than its mother even when there is maternal deficiency (Baker et al., 1958) although there is a degree of correlation with maternal levels (Zachan-Christiensen et al., 1962). The hepatic stores are in the region of 20–25 μg in normal infants but have been found to be as low as 2–4 μg in infants born to mothers with B_{12} deficiency (Baker et al., 1962). Serial serum B_{12} levels followed in 10 premature infants showed a gradual fall from the initial normal or high values, with lowest levels reached at around 40 days. In 5 the serum B_{12} fell below 200 pg/ml and in 1 it reached 77 pg/ml. Subsequently the levels spontaneously returned to normal (Pathak and Godwin, 1972). These changes were thought to be due to low B_{12} intake at a time of increased demand.

Human milk contains a mean of 0·11 μg/100 ml supplying around 0·5 μg of B_{12} per day (Hansen, 1964) and cow's milk contains more than this. In maternal B_{12} deficiency the concentration in her milk is similar to that in her serum (Fig. 3.2), and the daily supply to the infant would be less than 1/10th of normal, i.e. less than 0·05 μg/day.

The requirement in adults is thought to be between 2 and 5 μg/day (Chanarin, 1969A) but the requirements in infancy are not known. McIntyre et al. (1965) suggested that it might be 0·04 μg/day for a 3 kg infant, but this figure was based upon simple weight proportion taking the daily requirement of a 70 kg adult as 1 μg. Baker et al. (1962) suggested 0·06 μg/day on similar reasoning. Because of probable increased requirements during rapid growth the figure of 0·04 μg is likely to be an underestimate. Since megaloblastic anaemia develops at 8 to 12 months in many of the infants with congenital intrinsic factor deficiency, in whom normal stores of 20–25 μg at birth would be expected, the average requirement during the first year of life may be nearer 0·1 μg/day. This is also the daily oral dose which is capable of giving a full haematological response in infancy (Fig. 3.3).

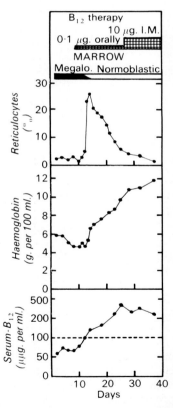

Fig. 3.3 Haematological response to vitamin B_{12} during deficiency. The infant (9 months) was given a daily oral supplement of vitamin B_{12} (0·1 μg) while remaining on B_{12}-deficient breast milk containing 32 pg/ml of B_{12}. (Reproduced by permission of Professor Baker and the Editor of Lancet, from the paper by Jadhav et al. (1962)).

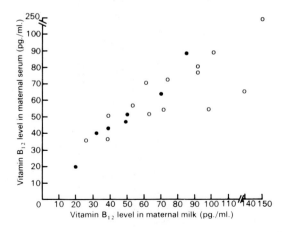

Fig. 3.2 Relationship between maternal serum and breast-milk vitamin B_{12} levels in B_{12} deficiency. ●, values taken from Baker et al. (1962). (Reproduced by permission of Dr Srikantia and the Editor, from the paper by Srikantia and Reddy (1967)).

CLASSIFICATION OF B_{12} DEFICIENCY IN INFANCY AND CHILDHOOD

Vitamin B_{12} deficiency is very rare in paediatric practice and could easily be missed unless a serum B_{12} assay is performed in all cases of megaloblastic anaemia. Systemic deficiency arises either from impaired absorption or from dietary deficiency as in breast fed infants of mothers with B_{12} deficiency. Tissue deficiency can arise by a rare defect of the transport mechanism viz. TC II deficiency (Table 3.1).

abnormalities. Thirdly, malabsorption of B_{12} in the presence of normal IF secretion, due either to a generalized malabsorption state, extensive intestinal surgery or pathology, or to a familial selective defect of ileal B_{12} absorption accompanied by benign proteinuria (Imerslund-Gräsbeck syndrome).

Whereas the patients with systemic deficiency due to malabsorption can be maintained in haematological remission by relatively small parenteral doses of B_{12} such as 100 μg per month, those with TC II deficiency require much larger and more

Table 3.1 Causes of B_{12} deficiency in infancy and childhood

IMPAIRED ABSORPTION	

Isolated congenital IF deficiency
  Normal gastric function. No antibodies to IF
  Autosomal recessive	

IF deficiency with gastric atrophy
  Achlorhydria. Antibodies to IF
  ±Endocrine abnormalities
  ?True juvenile Addisonian PA
	'Juvenile pernicious anaemia' (Arthur, 1972)

Familial selective B_{12} malabsorption (Imerslund)
  Normal IF. Normal ileal mucosa
  Associated benign proteinuria
  Autosomal recessive	

Generalized malabsorption e.g. tropical sprue, rarely in coeliac disease	

Abnormal intestinal flora
  Blind loops and anastamoses
  Intestinal scleroderma
	Not specifically juvenile or paediatric

Ileal lesion Extensive gut resection or pathology	
NUTRITIONAL	

Secondary to maternal deficiency
  Maternal PA, tropical sprue or strict
    vegetarianism + breast feeding
Dietary
  Strict vegetarianism, e.g. vegans	

TISSUE DEFICIENCY	
Hereditary transcobalamin II deficiency	

B_{12} malabsorption in the paediatric age group is of 3 types: Firstly isolated congenital absence of IF with otherwise normal gastric function, with megaloblastic anaemia usually appearing before the age of 2½ years. Secondly, pernicious anaemia, similar to the adult disease, with gastric atrophy and anti-IF antibodies in the serum, but occurring as early as the second decade. A proportion of children in the latter group have multiple endocrine

frequent doses, e.g. 1,000 μg twice-weekly (Hakam et al., 1971).

Intrinsic factor deficiency

Less than 50 cases have been reported in the literature. McIntyre et al. (1965) suggested that they fell into two types. The first of these, the majority, develop a megaloblastic anaemia before the age of $2\frac{1}{2}$ years (Case 4), and show an isolated deficiency of intrinsic factor with normal gastric histology and acid secretion without the development of serum antibodies to intrinsic factor. Arthur (1972) has described a girl of $3\frac{1}{2}$ in this category. The haemoglobin was $4\cdot8$ g/100 ml with a megaloblastic marrow, serum B_{12} of 60 pg/ml and serum folate of 17 μg/ml. The Schilling test showed impaired B_{12} absorption corrected by giving IF. Her gastric IF was absent but gastric biopsy was normal, with no gastritis or atrophy. Both height and weight were below the third percentile, but there was a remarkable growth spurt after instituting parenteral cyanocobalamine therapy.

There is a high familial incidence among siblings but probably no relation between this type of juvenile PA and the adult form of PA (Chanarin, 1969B).

Case 4. A full-term male infant (No. 96110) presented with pallor and listlessness at the age of 8 months, the general practitioner having found a haemoglobin of '40–50 per cent'. There had been weight loss over the previous 2 weeks. On examination there was fever (39 °C), but no lymphadenopathy or hepatosplenomegaly. The fever responded to ampicillin and cloxacillin. The peripheral blood showed a haemoglobin of $4\cdot3$ g/100 ml with macrocytes on the blood film. A marrow examination showed megaloblastic erythropoiesis with giant band cells. After a blood transfusion of 120 ml he was started on B_{12} 250 μg I.M. twice-weekly. Within two weeks his appetite was improving. The reticulocytes rose from 2 per cent before treatment to 22 per cent 6 days after injection of B_{12}.

He was maintained on 250 μg/month and the haemoglobin was kept at normal levels until default occurred. After 8 months off therapy he was again admitted with severe pallor and anaemia. The haemoglobin had fallen to $5\cdot1$ g/100 ml, serum B_{12} was 18 pg/ml, serum folate over 10 ng/ml, serum iron 188 μg/100 ml, and TIBC 270 μg/100 ml. Again the marrow was megaloblastic. One unit of packed cells was given and I.M. B_{12} restarted. Satisfactory maintenance has been achieved on monthly injections of 250 μg of B_{12}, the patient remaining in good health with a normal haemoglobin level (i.e. over 12 g/100 ml).

In this family there is no question of maternal malnutrition and a sibling is haematologically normal. The patient does not have a malabsorption state. The time of presentation, low serum B_{12} and response to low doses of B_{12} favour congenital deficiency of IF.
I am indebted to Dr. W. R. McAinsh of Law Hospital, Carluke, for details of this infant.

The second, smaller group described by McIntyre *et al.* (1965) have been older children, usually aged 10 years or over, and have shown in addition histamine-fast achlorhydria, gastric atrophy and antibodies to intrinsic factor. It was thought that these children were suffering from the same disease as adult pernicious anaemia but, although many features are in common, there are also slight differences. These include the high incidence of endocrine disorders in the children including idiopathic hypoparathyroidism, candidiasis, Addison's disease, hypothyroidism, polyendocrinopathy, juvenile cirrhosis, ovarian failure, agenesis of spleen and immunological abnormality in the patients and their family (Wuepper and Fudenberg, 1967; Blizzard and Gibbs, 1968). The basis of these associated abnormalities appears to be a genetically determined tendency to develop organ-specific antibodies. The abnormalities of gastric function are indistinguishable from those of adult Addisonian pernicious anaemia but the cause of the disease may be different (Chanarin, 1969B). Inheritance is probably recessive (Spinner *et al.*, 1968).

Selective ileal malabsorption of B_{12}

A quite distinct familial syndrome due to an isolated defect of intestinal B_{12} absorption with normal gastric acidity, histology and intrinsic factor but with associated persistent proteinuria has been described by Imerslund (1960) and Gräsbeck *et al.* (1960). Together with more recent reports (Mackenzie *et al.*, 1972) 37 children of both sexes and between the ages of 7 months and 14 years, but usually under 2 years, have been described. There appears to be an isolated defect of absorption of IF–B_{12} after this attaches to the surface of the ileal cell and before the B_{12} is bound to transcobalamin II (Mackenzie *et al.*, 1972). There are no other defects of intestinal absorption and the ileal mucosa is normal on light and electron microscopy. A familial tendency is apparent, three brothers showing the defect but both parents having normal absorption in Mackenzie's report. The megaloblastic anaemia but not the proteinuria respond to parenteral B_{12} therapy (100 μg per month). Also the proteinuria was recorded at 1 year in a patient developing the anaemia 10 years later.

Other causes of malabsorption

Surgical blind-loops, anastomes and fistulae may be associated with impaired B_{12} absorption attributed to change in the bacterial gut flora (Doig and Girdwood, 1960; Dellipiani and Girdwood, 1964). Treatment with tetracycline may result in a haematological remission (Siurala and Kaipainen, 1953). Intestinal scleroderma may also be associated with a megaloblastic anaemia due to impaired B_{12} absorption from a similar cause (Salen *et al.*,

1966). Extensive resection of the distal small intestine following gangrene due to volvulus at 20 days was followed by a megaloblastic anaemia with low serum B_{12} at 11 months (Clark and Booth, 1960). Dallman and Diamond (1960) described an infant who had total resection of the ileum at the age of 36 hours for intestinal atresia and who later developed B_{12} deficiency and megaloblastic anaemia at the age of 3 years and 4 months. As in the adult infestation with the fish tapeworm diphyllobothrium latum can cause B_{12} deficiency by competing with the host for the vitamin.

B_{12} deficiency as part of the coeliac syndrome is rare; only 1 out of 19 such children had a low serum B_{12} (Dormandy et al., 1963). Deficiency is probably more common in tropical sprue since there is more extensive gut involvement (Sheehy et al., 1961). Malabsorption of crystalline B_{12} but not of dietary, protein-bound B_{12} has been found in children with cystic fibrosis of the pancreas. Systemic B_{12} deficiency did not, however, occur (Deren et al., 1973).

Nutritional B_{12} deficiency

In the rare event of maternal B_{12} deficiency, either due to incipient pernicious anaemia (Lampkin et al., 1966), to strict vegetarianism or to tropical sprue (Jadhav et al., 1962; Srinkantia and Reddy, 1967), the infant may develop megaloblastic anaemia between 7 and 12 months if breast feeding is prolonged. Initial foetal B_{12} stores may have been suboptimal (Baker et al., 1962) and the B_{12} content of the breast milk is severely reduced as mentioned above (Fig. 3.2). The infants are not underweight but show pallor, apathy, developmental regression, skin pigmentation of axillae, groins, palms and dorsum of fingers, and characteristic involuntary movements with megaloblastic anaemia developing between 4 and 12 months. The serum B_{12} level is very low ranging from 25 to 64 pg/ml, and haemoglobin 3·6 to 8·5 g/100 ml. They can respond to as little as 0·1 μg of oral B_{12} per day (Fig. 3.3).

After infancy pure dietary deficiency of B_{12} is found only in strict vegetarians such as vegans in Western countries or certain Hindu sects among Indians. A case of subacute combined degeneration of the cord in a 15-year-old boy has been reported due to this cause (Badenoch, 1954).

Transcobalamin II deficiency

Early development of severe megaloblastic anaemia with neutropenia, thrombocytopenia, liability to infections, failure to thrive, diarrhoea, vomiting, red, inflamed tongue and oral ulceration has been reported in two siblings with deficiency of the B_{12} transport protein TC II. Presentation was at 3 and 5 weeks although the haemoglobin levels had been normal at birth. Complete clinical and haematological remission could only be obtained with large doses of parenteral B_{12} such as 1,000 μg twice-weekly or 500 μg every second day. There was no response to folic acid. Withdrawal of B_{12} therapy in one sibling led to relapse of megaloblastic anaemia in six weeks. The serum B_{12} levels were 267 and 855 pg/ml in the two infants and the serum folate 20 ng/ml in one. Decreased B_{12} absorption was demonstrated, which was uncorrected by IF suggesting that TC II plays a part in normal absorption of B_{12}. Both parents and several other members of the family had low levels of TC II, although haematologically normal, suggesting an autosomal recessive mode of inheritance (Hakami et al., 1971).

Identification of the different B_{12}-binding proteins is achieved by DEAE-cellulose ion exchange chromatography or polyacrylamide gel electrophoresis of serum after equilibration with ^{59}Co B_{12} (Fig. 3.4). When serum from these patients or normals is exposed to abnormally high concentrations of B_{12} then secondary binding 'peaks' appear. It is possible that these secondary binders come into play when large therapeutic doses of B_{12} are given and replace the normal TC II

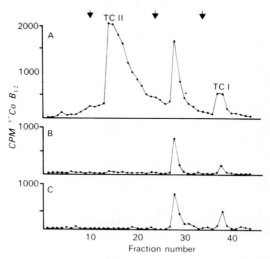

Fig. 3.4 Elution pattern of serum with ^{57}Co-B_{12} (2600 pg/ml) on DEAE-cellulose column. A, normal child; B, Case 1; C, Case 2. Arrows indicate change in buffer. A third vitamin B_{12}-binder is eluted with 0·1 M buffer at ph 5·8. (Reproduced by permission of Professor Hakami and the New England Journal of Medicine (1971), **285**, 1166).

protein in the function of delivering B_{12} to the tissues.

A further test that can be used to study this type of disorder is measurement of the serum unsaturated vitamin B_{12} binding capacity (Gottlieb et al., 1965) by adding ^{57}Co B_{12} to serum at room temperature and measuring the amount that can be removed by exposure to haemoglobin-coated charcoal. As expected the unsaturated binding capacity is reduced in TC II deficiency.

A further family with this disorder has recently been reported in Switzerland (Hitzig et al., 1974). The initial presenting features were predominantly those of increased liability to infection associated with agammaglobulinaemia and impaired antibody production (Hitzig and Kenny, in press).

REFERENCES

Arthur, L. J. H. (1972) Juvenile pernicious anaemia. Proc. Roy. Soc. Med., 65, 728.

Badenoch, J. (1954) The use of labelled vitamin B_{12} and gastric biopsy in the investigation of anaemia. Proc. Roy. Soc. Med., 47, 426.

Baker, H., Ziffer, H., Pasher, I. & Sobotka, H. (1958) A comparison of maternal and foetal folic acid and vitamin B_{12} at parturition. Brit. med. J., 1, 978.

Baker, S. J., Jacob, E., Rajan, K. T. & Swaminathan, S. P. (1962) Vitamin B_{12} deficiency in pregnancy and puerperium. Brit. med. J., 1, 1658.

Blizzard, R. M. & Gibbs, J. H. (1968) Candidiasis: Studies pertaining to its association with endocrinopathies and pernicious anemia. Pediatrics, 42, 231.

Carmel, R. & Herbert, V. (1969) Deficiency of vitamin B_{12}—binding alpha globulin in two brothers. Blood, 33, 1.

Chanarin, I. (1969A) The megaloblastic anaemias, p. 56. Oxford: Blackwell Scientific Publications.

Chanarin, I. (1969B) The megaloblastic anaemias, p. 733. Oxford: Blackwell Scientific Publications.

Chanarin, I. (1973) New light on pernicious anaemia. Lancet, ii, 538.

Clark, A. C. L. & Booth, C. C. (1960) Deficiency of vitamin B_{12} after extensive resection of the distal small intestine in an infant. Arch. Dis. Childh., 35, 595.

Cooper, B. A. & White, J. J. (1968) Absence of intrinsic factor from human portal plasma during ^{57}Co B_{12} absorption in man. Brit. J. Haemat., 14, 73.

Cox, E. V. & White, A. M. (1962) Methylmalonic acid excretion: an index of vitamin B_{12} deficiency. Lancet, 2, 853.

Dallman, P. R. & Diamond, L. K. (1960) Vitamin B_{12} deficiency associated with disease of the small intestine. Observations on an infant following extensive small bowel resection. J. Pediat., 57, 689.

Das, K. C. & Hoffbrand, A. V. (1970) Studies of folate uptake by phytohaemagglutinin stimulated lymphocytes. Brit. J. Haemat., 19, 203.

Dellipiai, A. W. & Girdwood, R. H. (1964) Bacterial changes in the small intestine in malabsorptive states and in pernicious anaemia. Clin. Sci., 26, 359.

Deren, J. J., Arora, B., Toskes, P. P., Hansell, J. & Sibinga, M. S. (1973) Malabsorption of crystalline vitamin B_{12} in cystic fibrosis. New Eng. J. Med., 288, 949.

Doig, A. & Girdwood, R. H. (1960) The absorption of folic acid and labelled cyanocobalamin in intestinal malabsorption. Q. J. Med. n.s., 29, 333.

Dormandy, K. M., Waters, A. H. & Mollin, D. L. (1963) Folic-acid deficiency in coeliac disease. Lancet, 1, 632.

Finkler, A. E. & Hall, C. A. (1967) Nature of the relationship between vitamin B_{12} binding and cell uptake. Arch. Biochem., 120, 79.

Gomperts, D., Hywel Jones, J. & Knowles, J. P. (1967) Metabolic precursors of methylmalonic acid in vitamin B_{12} deficiency. Clin. Chim. Acta, 18, 197.

Goodman, S. I., Moe, P. G., Hammond, K. B., Mudd, S. H. & Uhlendorf, B. W. (1970) Homocystinuria with methylmalonic aciduria: Two cases in a sibship. Biochem. Med., 4, 500.

Gottlieb, C., Lau, K. S., Wasserman, L. R. & Herbert, V. (1965) Rapid charcoal assay for intrinsic factor (IF), gastric juice unsaturated B_{12} binding capacity, antibody to IF, and serum unsaturated B_{12} binding capacity. Blood, 25, 875.

Gräsbeck, R., Gordin, R. Kantero, I. & Kuhlback, B. (1960) Selective vitamin B_{12} malabsorption and proteinuria in young people: a syndrome. Acta Med. Scand., 167, 289.

Green, A. E. & Pegrum, G. D. (1968) Value of estimating methylmalonic acid excretion in anaemia. Brit. med. J., 3, 591.

Hakami, N., Neiman, P. E., Canellos, G. P. & Lazerson, J. (1971) Neonatal megaloblastic anemia due to inherited transcobalamin II deficiency in two siblings. New Eng. J. Med., 285, 1163.

Hansen, H. A. & Weinfeld, A. (1962) Metabolic effects and diagnostic value of small doses of folic acid and B_{12} in megaloblastic anemias. Acta Med. Scand., 172, 427.

Hansen, H. A. (1964) On the diagnosis of folic acid deficiency. Goteburg: Almqvist and Wiksell.

Herbert, V., Streiff, R. R., & Sullivan, L. W. (1964) Notes on vitamin B_{12} absorption; autoimmunity and childhood pernicious anaemia; relation of intrinsic factor to blood group substance. Medicine, 43, 679.

Hitzig, W. H. Döhmann, U., Plüss, H. J. & Vischer, D. (1974) Hereditary transcobalamin II deficiency: Clinical findings in a new family. J. Pediatrics, 85, 622.

Hitzig, W. H. & Kenny, A. B. The role of vitamin B_{12} and its transport globulins in the production of antibodies. Clin. Exper. Immunology (in press).

Imerslund, O. (1960) Idiopathic chronic megaloblastic anaemia in children. Acta Paediat., 49, Suppl. 191.

Jadhav, M., Webb, J. K. G., Vaishnova, S. & Baker, S. J. (1962) Vitamin B_{12} deficiency in Indian infants. A clinical syndrome. *Lancet*, **2**, 903.

Lampkin, B. C., Shore, N. A. & Chadwick, D. (1966) Megaloblastic anemia of infancy secondary to maternal pernicious anemia. *New Eng. J. Med.*, **274**, 1168.

Levy, H. L., Mudd, S. H., Schulman, J. D., Dreyfus, P. M. & Abeles, R. H. (1970) A derangement in B_{12} metabolism associated with homocystinemia, cystathioninemia, hypomethioninemia and methylmalonic aciduria. *Am. J. Med.*, **48**, 390.

Marshall, R. A. & Jandl, J. H. (1960) Responses to 'physiologic' doses of folic acid in the megaloblastic anemias. *A. M. A. Arch. Int. Med.*, **105**, 352.

Mollin, D. L. (1960) The megaloblastic anemias. *Ann. Rev. Med.*, **11**, 333.

McIntyre, O. R., Sullivan, L. W., Jefries, G. H. & Silver, R. H. (1965) Pernicious anemia in childhood. *New Eng. J. Med.*, **272**, 981.

Mackenzie, I. L. & Donaldson, R. M. (1969) Vitamin B_{12} absorption and the intestinal cell surface. *Fed. Proc.*, **28**, 42.

Mackenzie, I. L., Donaldson, R. M., Trier, J. S. & Mathan, V. I. (1972) Ileal mucosa in familial selective vitamin B_{12} malabsorption. *New Eng. J. Med.*, **286**, 1021.

Pathak, A. & Godwin, H. A. (1972) Vitamin B_{12} and folic acid values in premature infants. *Pediatrics*, **50**, 584.

Retief, F. P., Gottlieb, C. W. & Herbert, V. (1966) Mechanism of vitamin B_{12} uptake by erythrocytes. *J. Clin. Invest.*, **45**, 1907.

Salen, G., Goldstein, I. & Wirts, C. W. (1966) Malabsorption in intestinal scleroderma, relation to bacterial flora and treatment with antibiotics. *Ann. intern. Med.*, **64**, 834.

Schilling, R. F. (1953) Intrinsic factor studies. II. The effect of gastric juice on the urinary excretion of radioactivity after the oral administration of radioactive B_{12}. *J. Lab. clin. Med.*, **42**, 860.

Sheehy, T. W., Perez-Santiago, E. & Rubini, M. E. (1961) Tropical sprue and vitamin B_{12}. *New Eng. J. Med.*, **265**, 1232.

Siurala, M. & Kaipainen, W. J. (1953) Intestinal megaloblastic anaemia treated with aureomycin and terramycin. *Acta Med. Scand.*, **147**, 197.

Spinner, M. W., Blizzard, R. M. & Childs, B. (1968) Clinical and genetic heterogeneity in idiopathic Addison's disease and hypoparathyroidism. *J. clin. Endocrinol.*, **28**, 795.

Srikantia, S. G. & Reddy, V. (1967) Megaloblastic anaemia of infancy and vitamin B_{12}. *Brit. J. Haemat.*, **13**, 949.

Tisman, G. & Herbert, V. (1973) B_{12} dependence of cell uptake of serum folate: An explanation for high serum folate depletion in B_{12} deficiency. *Blood*, **41**, 465.

Waters, A. H. & Mollin, D. L. (1961) Studies on the folic acid activity of human serum. *J. clin. Path.*, **14**, 335.

Wuepper, K. D. & Fudenberg, H. H. (1967) Moniliasis, 'autoimmune' polyendocrinopathy and immunologic family study. *Clin. exp. Immun.*, **2**, 71.

Zachan-Christiansen, B., Hoff-Jorgensen, E. & Kristensen, H. P. (1962) The relative haemoglobin, iron, vitamin B_{12} and folic acid values in the blood of mothers and their newborn infants. *Dan. Med. Bull.*, **9**, 157.

4. Aplastic Anaemia

Introduction, Classification / Constitutional aplastic anaemia, *Aetiology, Clinical features, Laboratory diagnosis, Treatment and prognosis* / Acquired aplastic anaemia, *Aetiology, Clinical features, Laboratory Diagnosis, Association of haemolysis, including PNH, Treatment* / Pure red-cell aplasia, *Aetiology, Clinical features, Laboratory diagnosis, Course of treatment.*

Introduction

Aplastic anaemia can be defined as a 'physiological and anatomical failure of the bone marrow with marked decrease or absence of blood-forming elements in the marrow, peripheral pancytopenia and no splenomegaly, hepatomegaly or lymphadenopathy' (Shahidi and Diamond, 1961).

Both deficiency anaemias and aplastic anaemias are characterized by reduced red cell production. Whereas haematinic deficiencies impair the function of erythroblasts at a biochemical level aplastic anaemias do so at a cellular level in that the erythroblasts themselves are absent or reduced in number. In most forms of aplastic anaemia the myeloid and megakaryocyte series are also affected resulting in a pancytopenia, i.e. neutropenia and thrombocytopenia, in addition to anaemia.

Pathologically the characteristic lesion is replacement of the haemopoietic marrow elements by hypocellular fatty tissue containing reticulum cells, lymphocytes, plasma cells and usually tissue mast cells (Fig. 4.1). In the pancytopenic forms there is an absence of megakarayocytes, myelocytes and normoblasts.

Knospe and Crosby (1971) have put forward the hypothesis that the primary cause of marrow depopulation is damage to the sinusoidal microcirculation of the marrow with secondary effects upon the haemopoietic stem cells. Such vascular lesions can be produced by large doses of localized X-irradiation in rats but may result from immunological damage in the human disease. In several types of aplastic anaemia, however, there is a hereditary basis with chromosomal instability probably affecting the haemopoietic stem cells (Swift and Hirschhorn, 1966; Bloom *et al.*, 1966). The good response to marrow transplant also

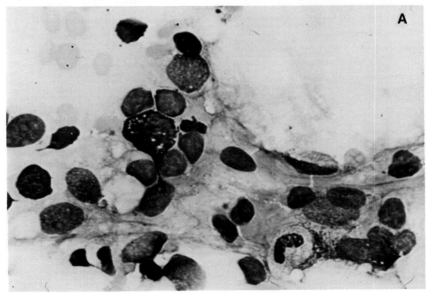

Fig. 4.1A *(caption on next page).*

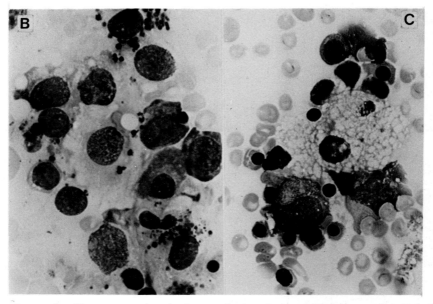

Fig. 4.1 Photomicrographs of bone marrow in aplastic anaemia. A, reticulum cells and mast cell (x 800); B, reticulum cells and plasma cell (x 800); C, phagocytic reticulum cell and erythroblasts (x 800). (Reproduced from Frisch and Lewis (1974) by permission of Dr S. M. Lewis the Editor of the *Journal of Clinical Pathology*, and the publishers the British Medical Association).

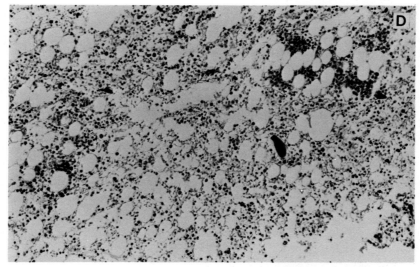

Fig. 4.1D, marrow fragment from patient shown in Fig. 4.3 (x 40).

suggests that aplastic anaemia is a disorder of marrow stem cells and that the primary insult which produces this failure is transient, although the damage sustained on the patient's stem cells is often continued (*Lancet*, 1975).

Classification

Essentially the aplastic states may be *constitutional,* as shown by a familial tendency or associated congenital defects, or *acquired*. If acquired there may be an identifiable cause, toxic or infective, or no such identifiable cause, when it is classified as being 'idiopathic'. Aplastic anaemia is usually a pancytopenic disorder with all three haemopoietic cell lines involved, but on rare occasions only one cell line is affected, e.g. granulocytes or platelets. Although described again under neutropenic and thrombocytopenic disorders respectively these isolated forms of aplastic

APLASTIC ANAEMIA   45

Table 4.1   Aplastic anaemia and related states

	Pancytopenic forms		Relevant author
Constitutional	*Type 1*	(a) With associated congenital defects	Fanconi (1927)
		(b) Familial but without associated congenital defects	Estren and Dameshek (1947)
		(c) Dyskeratosis congenita	Steier *et al.* (1972)
	Type 2	Preceded by neonatal thrombocytopenia	O'Gorman Hughes and Diamond (1964)
		No congenital defects. Males only	
Acquired		(a) Following drugs, toxic agents or infections	Wolff (1957)
		(b) Idiopathic, sometimes associated with PNH	Dacie and Lewis (1961)

	Isolated defects	
Pure Red cell aplasia	Congenital (erythrogenesis imperfecta)	Diamond and Blackfan (1938)
	Acquired, e.g. thymoma	Matras and Priesel (1928)
Infantile genetic agranulocytosis	Isolated familial agranulocytosis	Kostman (1956)
Reticular dysgenesis	Congenital aleucocytosis	De Vaal and Seynhaeve (1959)
Congenital amegakaryocytic thrombocytopenia	Associated with bilateral absence of radii	Bell *et al.* (1956)

marrow disease are included in the general classification of aplastic anaemia and related states shown in Table 4.1.

All these conditions are rare, the incidence of fatal aplastic anaemia being approximately 1·1 per million per year for children up to the age of 9 according to a recent survey in California (Wallerstein *et al.*, 1969), but the acquired forms of pancytopenia are several times more frequent than the constitutional forms. The Fanconi variety comprises the majority of the latter. Of the isolated defects only the pure red cell aplasia occurs with any frequency. The relative frequency of the different types of aplastic anaemia in childhood is indicated by the large combined series collected from 11 years at the Childrens' Hospital of Boston (Dr. Diamond) and 8 years at the Royal Alexandra Hospital for Children in Sydney (O'Gorman Hughes, 1966):

```
140 cases of aplastic anaemia in childhood
Constitutional        29
Acquired             104
   Toxic              70
      Chloramphenicol      40
      Anticonvulsants       4
      Chemicals            6
      Other               10
   Infection           16
   Idiopathic          28
Miscellaneous
   Associated with pancreatic insufficiency   1
      „        „    osteochondrodystrophy      1
   Preleukaemia                                5
```

CONSTITUTIONAL APLASTIC ANAEMIA

Aetiology

Three siblings were affected in the original description by Fanconi in 1927. The hereditary basis of the disease is shown by the fact that among 82 reported cases there is a familial background in 62, these occurring in 30 families, usually as siblings (Nilsson, 1960). In 5 families other members displayed the associated congenital anomalies without anaemia and in 3 families there were haematological disorders other than aplasia, e.g. acute leukaemia (Cowdell *et al.*, 1955). Consanguinity of the parents was present in 6 families and on rare occasions one or other parent showed neutropenia or mild pancytopenia. It is generally agreed that the inheritance is autosomal recessive (Beautyman, 1951; Reinhold *et al.*, 1952; Cowdell *et al.*, 1955). The slight excess of males compared to females reported in the literature is not greater than could occur by chance (Nilsson, 1960). There is no evidence of a sex-linked mode of inheritance, but in one family where a mother and child were similarly affected it was suggested that the inheritance was dominant (Imerslund, 1953). Congenital aplastic thrombocytopenia has also been described in siblings and may have a similar hereditary basis to Fanconi's anaemia (Shaw and Oliver, 1959).

Structural chromosome aberrations in cultured peripheral blood lymphocytes support the genetic basis of the disease and were first described in Fanconi's anaemia by Schroeder *et al.* (1964). The abnormalities include chromatid exchanges, chromatid breaks and endoreduplication (Fig. 4.2). The number of chromosomes remains normal (apart from endoreduplication). Similar morphological changes of the chromosomes have been found in infantile genetic agranulocytosis (Matsaniotis *et al.*, 1966), an aplastic disorder

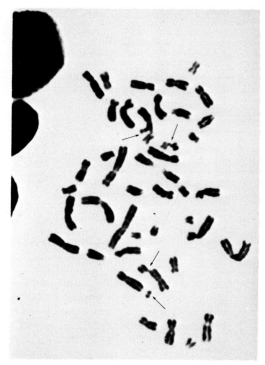

Fig. 4.2 Chromosome structural abnormalities in a child with Fanconi's aplastic anemia. Arrows indicate chromatid breaks and fragments. (Histological preparation and photograph prepared by Dr Elizabeth Boyd, Department of Genetics, Royal Hospital for Sick Children, Glasgow).

confined to the myeloid series, and in an infant with the skeletal anomalies of Fanconi's syndrome thought to be in the preanaemic state of this disease (Varela and Sternberg, 1967). Bloom, Warner, Gerald and Diamond (1966) found such chromosomal abnormalities in 10 out of 12 patients with Fanconi's anaemia (Type I) but not in 2 patients with Type II constitutional aplastic anaemia. Neither are they found in acquired forms of aplastic anaemia (Cobo et al., 1970). The chromosomal instability affects more than one tissue in Fanconi's anaemia, having been demonstrated in marrow cells and cultured skin fibroblasts, as well as lymphocytes (Swift and Hirshhorn 1966). Hirshhorn (1968) has suggested that it is possible to explain all the manifestations of Fanconi's anaemia on the basis of a hereditary susceptibility to chromosome breakage: 'Many of the cells with broken chromosomes would be lost during development, causing the developmental anomalies, and during haemopoiesis causing aplastic anaemia, but some of the remaining cells would be more susceptible to neoplastic transformation'. In support of this concept is the observation that fibroblast cultures from patients with Fanconi's anaemia, as well as from heterozygous carriers, are more easily transformed *in vitro* than normal cells by an oncogenic virus, SV^{40} (Todaro et al., 1966). Blood lymphocytes and skin fibroblast cultures from children with Fanconi's anaemia also show increased chromosome breakage after exposure to X-rays (Higurashi and Conen, 1971). It may also be relevant that the most frequently involved organ systems undergo embryonic differentiation at a similar time, the 25th to 34th day of foetal life (Althoff, 1953).

The chromosomal changes in Fanconi's anaemia resemble those found in acute leukaemia or following irradiation. It is of interest, therefore, that these patients and their families have an increased liability to acute leukaemia (Garriga and Crosby, 1959).

Among the 48 families in which the 66 reported cases of Fanconi's anaemia occurred there were 5 instances of leukaemia, usually acute. In one instance the leukaemia developed in a patient who had had aplasia for four years. Similar chromosomal changes are also seen in Bloom's syndrome (German et al., 1965), a hereditary immunological disorder with telangiectatic erythema of the face, molar hypoplasia, short stature as in Fanconi's anaemia, and likewise an increased liability to leukaemia (Sawitsky et al., 1966). Several patients with typical chromosomal changes and Fanconi's anaemia with growth retardation have recently been shown to have a deficiency of growth hormone (Pochedly et al., 1971; Zachmann et al., 1972; Gleadhill et al., 1975). Treatment with growth hormone for one year did not accelerate growth rate or improve the anaemia in the 8-year-old boy described by Gleadhill et al. Their endocrine studies suggested that the major defect of growth in this syndrome was due to end organ unresponsiveness.

Changes in the red cells characteristic of paroxysmal nocturnal haemoglobinuria (PNH) resulting in a haemolytic process have been recorded in Fanconi's anaemia (Dacie and Gilpin, 1944) and also in acquired aplastic anaemia. The association is rare, however, and the nature of the link between hypoplasia and the PNH defect remains a mystery (Dacie and Lewis, 1961).

Clinical features

In spite of the familial pattern and associated congenital abnormalities the pancytopenia does not usually appear until 4–7 years of age in boys and 6–10 years in girls. Very rare cases have

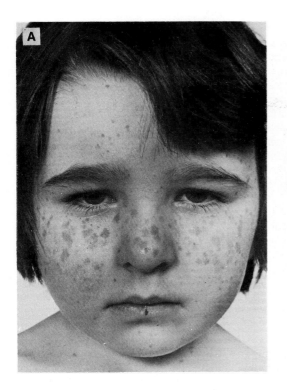
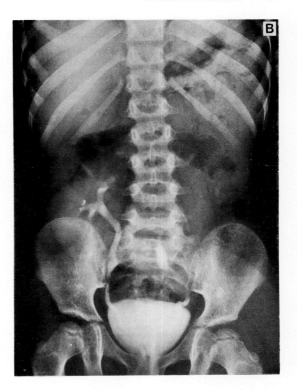
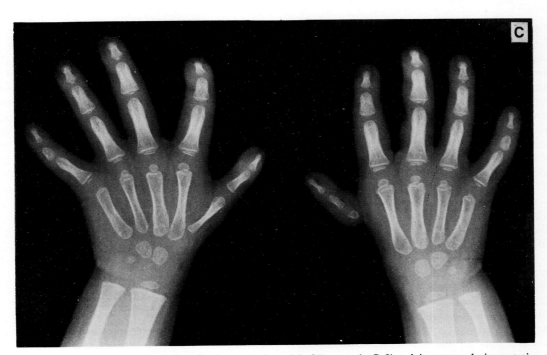

Fig. 4.3 Clinical features of Fanconi's aplastic anemia in a girl of 5 years. A, Café au lait spots and pigmentation of lip; B, renal abnormalities; C, thumb abnormalities; D, small stature.

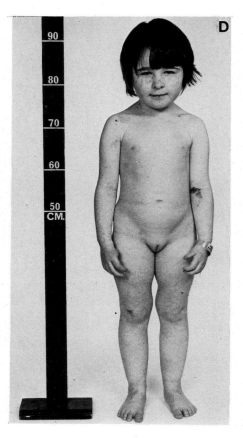

Fig. 4.3D

developed at the age of a few months or after the second decade. When recorded the birth weight has been lower than normal for the maturity. Anaemia is not present at birth or in the neonatal period but purpura may appear at this time in the rare Type II variety. When the anaemia develops, in later childhood, it is insidious in onset with pallor out of proportion to the degree of limitation of normal activity. Bruising, purpura and haemorrhage are often the presenting symptoms. There may be a simultaneous liability to infection. There is no hepatosplenomegaly or generalized lymphadenopathy although local, particularly cervical, glands may be moderately enlarged secondary to infection.

The characteristic associated abnormalities seen in the Fanconi syndrome (Fig. 4.3) include hyperpigmentation of the genitals, nipples and upper trunk, short stature, microcephaly, strabysmus, ptosis, nystagmus, increased tendon reflexes, mental retardation, abnormalities of the ears, deafness and skeletal deformities including anomalies of thumbs, radii, long bones, congenital dysplasia of the hip and syndactyly. Investigation may show abnormalities of the renal tract or congenital heart disease (Table 4.2). Siblings may show some of these abnormalities even if they have not inherited the anaemia. An excellent review of the clinical features is that of Nilsson (1960). In the closely related disorder dyskeratosis congenita cutaneous and mucosal abnormalities are more prominent than skeletal and renal changes, and include telangiectatic erythema, skin atrophy, mucosal leukoplakia, dental dysplasia and ridging of the nails. These features are illustrated in the paper of Steier, van Voolen and Selmanowitz (1972).

X-ray of the long bones, wrist and hand shows 2 to 4 years retardation of the bone age in most patients with the constitutional form but not in the acquired form (Shahidi and Diamond, 1961).

Laboratory diagnosis

The characteristic blood picture is one of pancytopenia with a haemoglobin level of 5 to 9 g/100 ml, neutropenia of 250 to 1,000 granulocytes per mm^3, less severe than in the acquired form, and a platelet count of 2,000 to 30,000 per mm^3. The red cells are well haemoglobinized and macrocytic. This macrocytosis could be a reflection of the high erythropoietin level in this disorder (Hillman and Finch, 1971). Rarely there are features of mild or intermittent haemolysis. Likewise the reticulocytes are usually low or absent, but occasionally elevated to around 3 per cent at an early stage of the disease since erythropoiesis appears to be preserved longer than the other marrow functions. Toxic granulations of the polymorphs are a constant finding but there are no other morphological abnormalities of the leucocytes. With the reduction of neutrophils, there is a relative lymphocytosis and monocytosis. Normoblasts, myelocytes and blast cells are absent. The ESR is extremely high and the serum iron normal or high. The bleeding time would be prolonged due to the thrombocytopenia but would be a superfluous investigation. There is no coagulation defect.

Although pancytopenia is the usual finding a minority of patients with Fanconi's anaemia present with isolated anaemia or leucopenia or combinations of anaemia plus leucopenia or anaemia plus thrombocytopenia, as in Fanconi's original Case 3. In addition, as indicated in Table 4.1, there are other hereditary aplastic states which are characterized by isolated neutropenia or thrombocytopenia.

In practice the main clinical and haematological distinction that has to be made in the usual

APLASTIC ANAEMIA 49

Table 4.2 Physical abnormalities in Fanconi's anaemia

Different abnormalities in 68 published cases		Different skeletal deformities in 40 cases of Fanconi's anaemia	
Abnormal pigmentation	51	Thumb deformities	28
Skeletal deformities	40	Reduced number of ossification centres in the wrist	17
Stunted growth	38	Aplasia of 1st metacarpal	7
Small head	29	Hypoplasia of 1st metacarpal	2
Renal anomalies	19	Aplasia of radius	7
Strabismus	18	Hypoplasia of radius	3
Microphthalmia	9	Absence of lower arm	1
Ptosis	2	Broad base in proximal phalanges	3
Epicanthus	2	Congenital dislocation of the hip	3
Nystagmus	2	Syndactylism	3
Deafness	7	Sprengel's deformity	1
Deformities of the ear	3	Scoliosis	1
Exaggerated reflexes	9	Cervical rib	1
Mental backwardness	14	Hip disease of Perthe's type	1
Hypogenitalism	15	Club foot	1
Cryptorchism	5	Increased impressiones digitatae in cranium	4
Hypospadias	3	Generalized osteoporosis	5
Transposition of penis and scrotum	1		
Adiposity	5		
Cardiac murmurs	19		
Congenital heart disease	4		

Various renal deformities in 19 cases of Fanconi's anaemia	
Renal aplasia	10
Double pelvis and/or ureters	5
Horseshoe kidney	3
Hydronephrosis	2
Abnormally low situation of kidney	2
Congenital renal cyst	1

Data from Nilsson (1960), *by permission of the author and publishers.*

pancytopenic form of aplastic anaemia is from aleukaemic leukaemia and idiopathic thrombocytopenic purpura (ITP). The critical investigation is examination of the bone marrow.

Aspiration is often more difficult than usual. Only a little fatty material may be aspirated among an excess of free blood. Typically the marrow smears and 'squashes' show a relative deficiency of haemopoietic cells, particularly myeloid precursors and total absence of megakaryocytes. Normoblasts are better preserved and may appear relatively increased. The remaining nucleated cells are lymphocytes, plasma cells, reticulum cells, tissue mast cells and sometimes small numbers of eosinophils (Fig. 4.1). The presence of darkly staining, almost opaque, tissue mast cells is very characteristic of the aplastic processes and is a helpful point in diagnosis although infrequently stressed in the literature. A proportion of the erythroid precursors show morphological abnormalities including megaloblastic changes, binuclear chromatin bridges, intercellular cytoplasmic connections and nuclear degenerative changes (Frisch and Lewis, 1974). The erythroid precursors often show megaloblastic features but

giant band cells are absent. Any myeloid precursors present are likely to be myeloblasts or promyelocytes. In spite of the megaloblastic changes the folate and B_{12} status is normal and there is no therapeutic response to either haematinic (Case 5). It should be emphasized that the marrow in constitutional aplastic anaemia is *hypoplastic*, in contrast to the finding in acquired forms where there is usually a more severe reduction of haemic cells justifying the term *aplastic* (Shahidi and Diamond, 1961). The distinction between active acute leukaemia, where the marrow is densely packed with a uniform type of blast cell, or ITP, where the marrow is of normal cellularity and composition with numerous megakaryocytes, is easy to make providing adequate marrow samples are obtained. Other differential diagnoses are considered in the section on acquired aplastic anaemia. The main practical difficulty that may arise in the interpretation of marrow smears is that there are sometimes islands of hyperactive haemopoiesis scattered amongst a predominantly inactive marrow. This problem can be resolved by histological examination of marrow fragments or a marrow trephine.

Case 5. A boy of 13 months (No. 138298) presented with bleeding from his gums, cough and low weight (7·9 kg). His haemoglobin fell from 9·2 g/100 ml to 5·3 g/100 ml over a period of weeks. Tests for malabsorption were normal. He was transfused as the anaemia did not respond to iron and folic acid. Thrombocytopenia was recorded on a number of occasions (e.g. 23,000/mm³).

At the age of 19 months he was referred to the Royal Hospital for Sick Children for investigation. Haemoglobin was 10·4 g/100 ml, WBC 4,000/mm³, polymorphs 2,300/mm³ and platelets 40,000/mm³, subsequently falling to 22,000/mm³. Marrow examination showed partial megaloblastic changes with 'maturation arrest' of the myeloid series, slight reduction of megakaryocytes and an increase in tissue mast cells. It was thought that these features suggested an early stage of marrow hypoplasia. Blood counts on parents and two siblings were normal. The patient did not have splenomegaly nor any skeletal or other physical abnormality. Mild neutropenia developed over the next few weeks (600–1,000/mm³), Foetal haemoglobin was 13 per cent, whole blood folate 120 ng/ml, serum folate 1·8 ng/ml and serum B_{12} 360 pg/ml. Duodenal intubation showed the presence of normal trypsin, lipase and amylase, excluding the syndrome of marrow dysfunction associated with pancreatic insufficiency. As the serum folate was low 5 mg of folic acid per day was given for a trial period to determine if the neutropenia and thrombocytopenia responded.

In fact, he deteriorated both clinically and haematologically while on folic acid, and was readmitted a month later with a severe napkin rash, bilateral blepharitis, stomatitis and the following blood count: Hb 8·4 g/100 ml, WBC 2,600/mm³, neutrophils 360/mm³, platelets 10,000/mm³. The red cells were macrocytic. This sequence of events was interpreted as indicating a progression from thrombocytopenia to pancytopenia in spite of haematinic therapy. Taken together with the marrow findings and elevated Hb.F he was thought to be an example of Diamond's Type II constitution aplastic anaemia, in which thrombocytopenia precedes pancytopenia. Oxymetholone 50 mg/day and prednisolone 10 mg/day were commenced and he was transfused.

Over the next 6 months his clinical and haematological state remained relatively static with several hospital admissions for infections, including pneumonia and stomatitis. The thrombocytopenia persisted. Oxymetholone was reduced to 10 mg b.d. and prednisolone to 5 mg on alternate days. After 6 months from initiating androgen and corticosteroid therapy the platelet count returned to around 100,000 and the Hb gradually rose to 13 g/100 ml with disappearance also of the neutropenia. These improvements persisted and steroids and oxymetholone were finally stopped 18 months from their institution. He has remained well with an entirely normal blood count since.

An ancillary aid to diagnosis, is measurement of the amount of circulating foetal haemoglobin. In children over 3 years of age normally less than 2 per cent of the haemoglobin is foetal. In either constitutional or acquired aplastic anaemia this is increased, usually to between 3 and 15 per cent (Shahidi *et al.*, 1962). It was also found in the sibling of a patient with constitutional aplastic anaemia. This finding is not specific for aplastic anaemia and probably represents a reversion to gamma chain synthesis by erythroblasts under stress. It is also seen for instance in pure red cell aplasia, juvenile chronic myelocytic leukaemia, hereditary spherocytosis and, of course, in thalassaemia and the haemoglobinopathies. In the case of acquired aplastic anaemias the absolute amount of foetal haemoglobin has been found to have prognostic significance (Bloom and Diamond, 1968). Seventeen out of 18 patients who died had less than 400 mg/100 ml, whereas 11 of 12 who survived and were doing well had more than 400 mg/100 ml at the initial examination. The concentration may also increase during corticosteroid-androgen induced reticulocytosis. The level of foetal haemoglobin returns to normal only after complete remission has occurred. The absolute concentration in mg/100 ml of blood is a more valid measurement than the percentage foetal haemoglobin since it is less affected by blood transfusion. By the Kleihauer film technique it is seen that the foetal haemoglobin is confined to a limited number of the patient's red cells probably indicating a clone of erythroblasts functioning under stress. The low values in patients with a bad prognosis may indicate a more complete inhibition of erythroblast function in their marrows. A similar foetal stigma is the persistence of the i-antigen on red cells (O'Gorman Hughes, 1966). Normally this is present at birth but has gone by 2 years of age (Giblett and Crookston, 1964).

A further unusual finding in patients with aplastic anaemia, including those with Fanconi's anaemia, is a decrease in tryptic activity of their duodenal juice (Desposito *et al.*, 1964; Ozsoylu and Argun, 1967). The nature of this association is unknown but the observation sprung from the reports of a syndrome consisting of pancreatic insufficiency, steatorrhoea and marrow dysfunction, predominantly affecting the myeloid series (Schwachman *et al.*, 1964; Burke *et al.*, 1967). In none of these disorders is there any evidence that the abnormal marrow function is caused by malabsorption. There is an increased concentration of urinary aminoacids, especially proline, in approximately half the patients with the constitutional form but not the acquired form of the disease.

Treatment and prognosis

Good reviews of the supportive therapy (Heyn *et al.*, 1969) and specific therapy (Diamond and

Shahidi, 1967) covering both the constitutional and acquired types of aplastic anaemia are available.

Initial blood transfusion is required in all cases of aplastic anaemia with haemoglobin levels less than 7·0 g/100 ml. This will need to be repeated at two to three week intervals, or more frequently in the presence of blood loss, until haemopoietic recovery or improvement occurs. For this reason particular care of the veins is necessary. Diagnostic venepunctures should be restricted to the minimum, every investigation being carried out on capillary blood so far as is possible. Regular antibody screening tests should be performed at the time of blood cross-matching so as to avoid shortened survival of transfused cells due to the immune antibodies that these patients are liable to develop after multiple transfusions. Antibodies to donor leucocytes may also develop in highly transfused-patients. The first clinical evidence of these is the occurrence of urticarial reactions or angioneurotic oedema after whole blood transfusions. The leucocyte antibodies can be identified by *in vitro* cytotoxicity tests and subsequent reactions can then be avoided by using saline-washed red cells, prepared in an aseptic closed system by the Blood Transfusion Service. Unfortunately platelet-rich plasma and platelet concentrates also contain sufficient white cells to cause similar reactions. Intravenous antihistamines plus hydrocortisone are of value in treating such reactions if they occur.

It is not necessarily wise to transfuse up to a haemoglobin level much above 9 g/100 ml since the stimulus to red cell production may thereby be impaired (Birkhill *et al.*, 1951; Emlinger *et al.*, 1952). Other supportive measures such as platelet transfusions, attempts to reduce oral and skin pathogenic flora (Chap. 20) are sometimes required in patients with severe thrombocytopenia and neutropenia. Local septic lesions require immediate and vigorous antibiotic (bactericidal) therapy, but avoiding intramuscular injections in the presence of thrombocytopenia. Pyrexia in excess of 38 °C is an indication for blood culture and the institution of combined antibiotic therapy before bacteriological results are available if there is a clinical likelihood of septicaemia. Intravenous Gentamicin 140 mg/M^2/day, given 6-hourly is a good initial blind choice since it is active against most gram negative infections, which constitute a major hazard. It may be combined with cloxacillin orally or parenterally.

Specific therapy with androgens plus corticosteroids was introduced by Shahidi and Diamond (1959, 1961) and has transformed the management and prognosis of both constitutional and acquired forms of aplastic anaemia, particularly the constitutional (Fanconi's) type. Prior to that time vitamins and haematinics had been used without benefit, corticosteroids had produced an improvement of haemostasis but without any effect upon the platelet count or producing any other haemopoietic response. Splenectomy had been tried with limited success in severe cases (Bernard *et al.*, 1958). Its benefit appeared to be confined to patients with relatively cellular marrows. Analysis of cases of aplastic anaemia admitted to the Children's Hospital in Boston over the preceding 20 years showed that only 2 out of 40 had a remission and one of these relapsed and died, giving an overall survival rate of 2·5 per cent (Shahidi and Diamond, 1959). Other series of aplastic anaemia in childhood gave similarly poor results. Out of nine children, Scott *et al.* (1959), had no survivors, out of 81 Wolff (1959) had 1, out of 20 Gasser (1961) had 2 survivors. The Fanconi's variety was uniformly fatal.

By contrast Shahidi and Diamond (1961) obtained a haematological remission with subsequent survival by the use of androgens in all of six patients with Fanconi's anaemia, and also in 9 out of 17 patients with acquired aplastic anaemia, although not in one patient with Type II constitutional aplastic anaemia (developing at the age of 5 following neonatal amegakaryocytic thrombocytopenia). The androgen was given in the form of testosterone proprionate or methyl testosterone as 10 mg sublingual tablets at a dose of 1 or 2 mg/kg/day. Alternatively a small number of patients were given fluoxymesterone or testosterone enanthate (I.M.) at a similar dosage. For the average child 15 mg per day was inadequate, 40 mg per day was optimal and higher doses than this produced no better response. The androgen was combined with corticosteroid, triamcinalone, at a dose of 8–12 mg/day.

The sequence of response in these patients was as follows: The reticulocytes rose to 8–20 per cent within a few months of treatment, accompanied or followed by a rise in haemoglobin and then of neutrophil polymorphs. The platelet count, by contrast, did not respond to the same extent, a modest rise occurring in one patient only. Hypochromia of the red cells tended to appear at the time of erythropoietic response, but this was accompanied by a normal or high serum iron level and may represent a block in haem synthesis. Those with the highest reticulocyte counts did not necessarily have the greatest rise in haemoglobin, and this discrepancy may be attributed to the presence of haemolysis in some patients. Sequential examination of the marrow showed the appearance of prominent foci of erythroid hyperplasia amongst marrow fragments at the time of reticulocytosis. Megaloblastic features tended to persist, however.

Desposito et al. (1964) similarly found that four out of four patients with constitutional aplastic anaemia responded to testosterone plus prednisone. After 1 to 3 months of this therapy a reticulocyte response occurred and this was followed by a rise in haemoglobin. Correction of neutropenia and thrombocytopenia was incomplete.

Cessation of androgen therapy in the constitutional form of aplastic anaemia uniformly results in a return of anaemia and neutropenia, but a second response occurs when the androgens are restarted. It is believed that patients with the constitutional disorder remain permanently androgen dependent, unlike those with the acquired form. It is possible, however, to achieve satisfactory maintenance with a lower dose than used to initiate the response, i.e. 10 mg methyl-testosterone plus 5 mg triamcinalone per day or a similar dose given twice weekly. The lowest effective maintenance dose is found by trial and error. The overall survival of children with constitutional aplastic anaemia is superior to those with the acquired disease (Fig. 4.7), with 40 to 50 per cent surviving 10 years (Li et al., 1972).

Growth rate improved (to 13 cm/year) in a boy of 8 given oxymetholone with low growth hormone levels who had previously shown no response to growth hormone therapy (Gleadhill et al., 1975).

Side effects of the androgen therapy include flushing, acne, hirsutism, sero-sanguinous discharge from the nipple and deepening of the voice. These changes regress within a month of stopping or reducing the drugs. Growth of pubic hair and enlargement of the genitalia also occur and regress to a lesser degree. These side effects are acceptable as the cost of survival and normal activity.

The possibility that so-called non-virilizing androgens would prove effective at maintaining an established remission remains *sub judice*. Oxymetholone (Anapolon) occupies an intermediate position, being approximately 1/5th as androgenic as the testosterone derivatives on a weight basis. This allows it to be given at a higher dosage of 4–5 mg/kg/day, compared to 1–2 mg/kg/day for testosterone derivatives. A response in reticulocytes, haemoglobin and neutrophils, but not in platelets, has been recorded with this drug in a boy of 5 with Fanconi's anaemia who was apparently refractory to testosterone proprionate (Allen et al., 1968) (Fig. 4.4). On stopping the drug he relapsed in two months, but had a further remission on restarting it at a dose of 5 mg/kg/day. Similarly McCredie (1969) has reported a response in haemoglobin after 2 months on oxymetholone (100 mg/day) and a slight response in white cells, but none in the platelets, in a girl of 14 with Fanconi's anaemia. She was also on prednisone at the time but had failed to respond to this drug alone. The haemoglobin appeared to be satisfactorily maintained on 25 mg oxymetholone per day or less. She had developed a deep husky voice on the higher dose, but this improved as the dose was reduced. A personally observed patient with Type II constitutional aplastic anaemia, preceded by neonatal thrombocytopenia, responded fully to oxymetholone and prednisolone (Case 5).

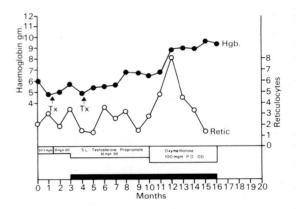

Fig. 4.4 Haemoglobin and reticulocyte response in Case 5 related to therapy with testosterone and prednisone followed by oxymetholone and prednisone. Relapse occurred as the oxymetholone dosage was lowered (not shown). (Reproduced from Allen et al. (1968), *Blood*, **32**, 83, by permission of the author and publishers).

Fears that androgen and steroid might interfere with subsequent growth have proved unfounded. Androgens accelerate the closure of epiphyses, corticosteroids delay closure. Long-term follow-up of children on the combined therapy revealed no significant discrepancy between linear growth and skeletal maturation. Subsequent endocrine investigation of two adolescent patients following this therapy revealed no abnormality. Testicular biopsy was also normal (Shahidi and Crigler, 1967). Liver dysfunction of the cholestatic type is a hazard of androgen therapy and has been reported in patients with refractory anaemia on oxymetholone in some series but not in other series (Allen et al., 1968). Rare instances of raised intracranial tension on the combined therapy have rapidly responded to chlorothiazide or diuretics.

The original rationale for androgen therapy in aplastic disorders sprung from the observation of erythropoietic stimulation in patients on this treatment for breast cancer (Kennedy and Nathanson, 1953), myeloid metaplasia (Pringle and Gardner, 1959) and in eunochoid men (McCullagh and Jones, 1942). A similar erythropoietic effect has been found in myelofibrosis (Kennedy, 1962). It had also been noted that spontaneous remissions occurred at the time of puberty in two boys with aplastic anaemia (Shahidi and Diamond, 1959).

The mechanism of this erythropoietic stimulation is not known. In mice there is a synergistic action between testosterone and erythropoietin (Gurney and Fried, 1965). It has been suggested that the action of androgens is at the bone marrow level but is dependent upon the presence of erythropoietin (Jepson and Lowenstein, 1967) rather than acting by stimulation of erythropoietin production. In aplastic anaemia the erythropoietin level is elevated (Lange et al., 1961) and this anaemia often responds to androgens. In the anaemia of chronic renal failure the erythropoietin level is reduced (Adamson et al., 1968) and there is no haemopoietic response to oxymetholone (McCredie, 1969). Ferrokinetic studies show that plasma iron clearances return to normal and red cell utilization rises to normal (Silink and Firkin, 1968), and red cell iron utilization rises to normal (McCredie, 1969) in aplastic anaemia following oxymetholone treatment. A recent and comprehensive review of the effect and mechanism of androgens upon erythropoiesis is that of Shahidi (1973). Androgens probably both increase the level of erythropoietin and also the pool of erythropoietin-responsive stem cells (Fig. 4.5).

ACQUIRED APLASTIC ANAEMIA

Aetiology

In this group of patients there is no familial tendency to anaemia, no associated congenital abnormality and the disorder is not present in the neonatal period. It may arise at any age in childhood or adult life, can sometimes be related to a specific toxic exposure or infection, but often not, when it is deemed 'idiopathic'.

Some drugs such as 6-mercaptopurine, methotrexate, cyclophosphamide or busulphan have a predictable dose-dependent marrow depressant effect which if allowed to continue will result in marrow aplasia, usually short-lived after the drug is stopped. The mechanism by which these drugs damage the normal marrow cells is similar to that by which they suppress leukaemic cell growth, the biochemical mechanisms being reasonably well understood (Chap. 20). Radiation damage to the marrow falls into the same category.

Other drugs such as quinacrine, chloramphenicol, phenylbutazone, or anti-convulsants used in normal therapeutic doses are unpredictably followed by severe marrow aplasia in a very small proportion of individuals, This is often irreversible, being fatal in approximately half the patients. Exposure to insecticides such as DDT and certain organic solvents fall into the same category. There is often some uncertainty in the individual patient as to whether a particular drug can be incriminated. Exposure within the past 6 months is a prerequisite. A list of drugs thought to cause occasional aplastic anaemia is given in table 4.3. The best known and most studied of these is chloramphenicol. This drug heads the list of known causative agents in the series of acquired aplastic anaemia reported by Scott et al. (1959), and in the similar paediatric series reported by Shahidi and Diamond (1961), Desposito et al. (1964), O'Gorman Hughes (1966) and Heyn et al. (1969). O'Gorman Hughes saw 16 cases attributed to chloramphenicol in 8 years in Sydney. The absolute incidence of fatal acquired aplastic

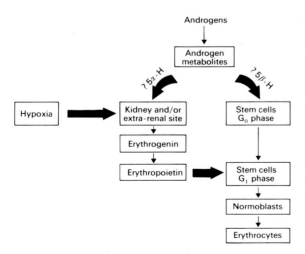

Fig. 4.5 Hypothetical scheme of the mechanism of action of androgens on erythropoiesis. (Reproduced by permission from the *New England Journal of Medicine* (1973), **289**, 78, and from Dr N. T. Shahidi.)

54 PAEDIATRIC HAEMATOLOGY

Table 4.3 Drugs frequently associated with aplastic anaemia

	Reports of aplastic anaemia in A.M.A. registry	
	All reports implicating drug	Reports where drug was given alone
	Number (1)	Number (3)
Group I. Toxic potentiality definite		
Chloramphenicol	312	163
Phenylbutazone	35	17
Mephenytoin (Mesantoin)	22	9
Gold compounds	10	8
Tolbutamide	11	6
Mepazine	5	4
Sulfamethoxypyridizine (Kynex)	14	3
Quinacrin (Atabrine)	5	3
Chlorpropamide (Diabinese)	4	2
Colchicine	5	2
Trimethadione	5	2
Carbutamide	2	1
Meprobamate	12	0
Organic Arsenicals	1	1
Group II. Toxic potentiality probable		
Potassium perchlorate	9	6
Acetazolamide (Diamox)	10	3
Chlorpromazine	20	3
Diphenyl-hydantoin (Dilantin)	21	3
Phenacetin	32	3
Sulfisoxazole (Gantrisin)	29	3
Thiacetazone (Thiosemicarbazone)	3	2
Pyrimethamine (Daraprim)	5	2
Chlordiaze/oxide (Librium)	7	2
Amodiaquine	2	2
Chlorpheniramine (Chlortrimeton)	17	2
Primidone (Mysoline)	11	2
Salicylamide	4	2
Sulfadimethoxine	6	2
Sulfathiazole	2	2
Tripelennamine (Pyribenzamine)	12	1
Streptomycin	27	0
Group III. Toxic potentiality minimal		
Penicillin	100	4
Acetylsalicylic acid	83	2
Tetracyclines	91	4

Reproduced from Bithell and Wintrobe (1967), Seminars in Haematology, 4, 194–221, by permission of Professor Wintrobe and the publishers, Grune and Stratton, Inc.

anaemia (a) in populations not known to be exposed to any particular drug hazard and (b) in those known to be exposed to various drugs including chloramphenicol are shown in table 4.4.

Treatment with chloramphenicol increases the chance of developing aplastic anaemia 13-fold but the small hazard involved is also apparent. For other drugs the hazard is still smaller. Nevertheless the British Committee on Safety of Drugs (1967) recommend that in conditions other than typhoid fever and haemophilus influenzal menin-

gitis it should only be used systemically after careful clinical, and usually laboratory assessment indicates that no other antibiotic will suffice. It should never be used systemically for trivial infections.

The mechanism by which chloramphenicol produces aplastic anaemia is not understood. It is not related to the dose or duration of exposure (Best, 1967). Nor is it related to defective excretion in susceptible individuals (Wagner and Smith, 1962). Inhibition of nucleic acid synthesis by normal marrow cells *in vitro* can be demonstrated,

Table 4.4 Incidence of fatal aplastic anaemia in various populations

Population	Incidental of fatal aplastic anaemia	Author
Unexposed		
US Armed Forces	1:500,000 ⎱ Good	Custer (1946)
California 1963–64	1:524,600 ⎰ agreement	Wallerstein et al. (1969)
Exposed		
To chloramphenicol		
California	1:36,118 ⎱ Good	Wallerstein et al. (1969)
UK	1:41,600 ⎰ agreement	Safety on drugs (1967)
	Increased incidence = ×13	
To quinacrine		
US Armed Forces	1:50,000	Custer (1946)
	Increased incidence = ×10	
To oxyphenylbutazone	1:124,000	Wallerstein et al. (1969)
	Increased incidence = ×4	

but only at a drug concentration in excess of that attained *in vivo* (Yunis and Harrington, 1960). The possibility that small amounts of chloramphenicol might be ingested in milk from cows treated for mastitis and that this might sensitize the marrow to later therapeutic doses has been suggested (Garrod, 1965), as has undiscovered synergism with a second drug, possibly innocuous when given alone (*B.M.J.*, 1966). In discussing the aetiology of pancytopenic fatal aplasia due to chloramphenicol it should be pointed out that an entirely different reversible dose-related marrow depression is seen in a high proportion of patients receiving this drug (Rosenbach et al., 1960). In 10 out of 22 patients receiving chloramphenicol multiple large vacuoles were found in the early erythroblasts of the marrow, often associated with a fall in red cell and reticulocyte counts (Saidi et al., 1961). These changes are reversed within one week of stopping the drug. Increased dosage, delayed plasma clearance (Fig. 4.6) (Suhrland and Weisberger, 1969), and accelerated erythropoiesis appeared to favour the development of these changes. Similar vacuoles are seen in phenylalanine or riboflavin deficiency (Sherman et al., 1964).

Regarding the aetiology of other drug-induced aplasias it has always been tempting to invoke immunological mechanisms (Osgood, 1953), perhaps of the drug-haptene type (see Sedormid purpura, Chap. 16). This, however, has never been demonstrated. In only one clinical situation, namely the graft versus host reaction in transfused immunologically incompetent infants, has aplastic anaemia been shown to have an immunological basis (Hathaway et al., 1965 and 1966). The occurrence of a severe anaphylactoid reaction following accidental re-exposure to DDT in a susceptible patient also suggests an immunological mechanism (Sánchez-Medal et al., 1963). Nieweg (1973) has suggested that there are three possible explanations of drug-induced aplasia: (a) Direct toxic action on the marrow cells, e.g. after chronic industrial exposure to benzene; (b) true allergy, with manifestations developing rapidly after exposure to only a small dose: (c) prolonged exposure to large doses, 'high-dose allergy'. This is the more usual pattern. He attributes this to cell membrane damage in the first place. Genetic susceptibility is also possible, and is suggested by the occurrence of blood dyscrasia following chloramphenicol exposure in identical twins (Best, 1967). Recent reviews on drug-induced aplastic anaemia are those of Nieweg (1973), Williams, Lynch and Cartwright (1973), and an annotation in the Lancet (1974).

The association of preceding virus infection

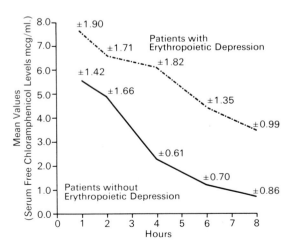

Fig. 4.6 Differences in the clearance rates of chloramphenicol in erythropoietic depressive and normal patients. (Reproduced from Suhrland and Weisberger (1969), *Blood*, **34**, 466, by permission of Professor L. G. Suhrland and the publishers).

with aplastic anaemia poses similar problems. This has been well-studied in the case of infectious hepatitis (Levy *et al.*, 1965). Aplastic anaemia followed the onset of hepatitis by 1 to 7 weeks in 5 patients aged 4 to 19 years. A number of similar cases have been reported including 3 by Schwartz, Baehner and Diamond (1966). These authors pointed out that transient depression of granulocytes, platelets and haemoglobin were common in infectious hepatitis, and that the progressive changes leading to marrow aplasia in a very small number of individuals might be an extension of this process, perhaps dependent upon genetic susceptibility. There is an analogy here with chloramphenicol toxicity. Pancytopenia with temporary marrow hypoplasia has also been seen in association with a number of RNA virus infections including rubella and the myxoviruses of influenza, parainfluenza, measles and mumps. Two experimental virus infections in mice, MVH-3 and the Trinidad strain of Venezuelan equine encephalitis (VEE) cause pancytopenia, and marrow hypoplasia, and the virus can be cultured from the marrow (Schwartz *et al.*, 1966). As in other causes of aplastic anaemia an autoimmune process has been suggested (Deller *et al.*, 1962).

In approximately half the cases of acquired aplastic anaemia no significant preceding infection or exposure to toxic agents can be determined. In the large series of 334 cases of acquired pancytopenia reported by Wolff (1957) 191 or 57·2 per cent were classified as idiopathic. In the series of O'Gorman Hughes (1966) the proportion was smaller, 28 out of 104 with acquired aplasia. Five out of 17 in Shahidi and Diamond's series (1961) and 5 out of 9 in that of Desposito *et al.* (1964) were idiopathic. Whether these cases are caused by infections with unidentified viruses remains uncertain. At least some of these idiopathic cases appear to be a different group which might be termed preleukaemia or leukaemia in an aplastic phase (O'Gorman Hughes, 1966). Melhorn *et al.* (1970) have described 6 children diagnosed upon firm, indisputable grounds as aplastic anaemia between the age of 1 year 11 months and 6 years but all of whom eventually developed acute lymphoblastic leukaemia 9 weeks to 20 months later. One common feature in these 6 patients was a more than usually rapid response of the aplastic anaemia to initial corticosteroid therapy. This had also been noted by O'Gorman Hughes (1966) and has been seen in one personally observed case who developed acute lymphoblastic leukaemia 3 months later. This rapid response of the pancytopenia to corticosteroids alone is in marked contrast to the usual lack of response in other cases of aplastic anaemia. It should be mentioned that a similar leukaemic transformation of aplastic anaemia caused by benzene (Erf and Rhoads, 1939) and chloramphenicol (Fraumeni, 1967) has been recorded.

Clinical features

The symptoms and signs of acquired aplastic anaemia are similar to those of the constitutional forms but pigmentation, short stature and congenital skeletal or visceral anomalies are absent. The age span is broader except perhaps in the case of chloramphenicol-induced aplasia where the peak age incidence is 3–7 years (Best, 1967). A history of exposure, sometimes repeated exposure, usually within the preceding six months, to drugs or chemicals known to predispose to aplastic anaemia was found in 43 and 67 per cent of patients with the acquired form of the disease in the two large collected series of Wolff (1957) and O'Gorman Hughes (1966) respectively.

Neiman *et al.* (1963) in a description of 14 children with idiopathic pancytopenia emphasized that in addition to the three main signs of anaemia, fever and purpura their negative features of importance including an absence of hepatosplenomegaly, lymphadenopathy, buccal ulceration or jaundice. There may, however, be purpura of the buccal mucosa and bleeding from the gums. On occasions there may be inflammatory lymphadenopathy related to local sepsis.

The occurrence of red urine should lead one to suspect the development of PNH (see following section).

Laboratory diagnosis

The peripheral blood picture is similar to that in the constitutional form but neutropenia is more severe, sometimes approaching agranulocytosis. Also the bone marrow is more markedly aplastic with little more than fat spaces devoid of haemic cells (Table 4.5). Megaloblastic changes, and other features indicative of 'dyserythropoiesis' are present in 5–90 per cent of the erythroid precursors present (Frisch and Lewis, 1974). In the case of dose-related, reversible marrow depression due to chloramphenicol vacuolation of the erythroid and myeloid precursors is found in the marrow, similar to those seen in phenylalanine deficiency (Sherman *et al.*, 1964). The foetal haemoglobin level may be elevated to a similar degree to that seen in constitutional forms (Shahidi *et al.*, 1962), but is less consistent in this respect.

Table 4.5 Comparison of features of constitutional and acquired aplastic anaemia

	Constitutional	Acquired
Age of onset	4–7 years in boys 6–10 years in girls	Any age
Sex ratio	61 per cent Male	Equal
Neutropenia	Less marked 250–950/mm^3	Severe
Marrow cellularity	Hypocellular	Aplastic
Erythropoiesis	Often megaloblastic	Virtually absent
Reticulocytes	Up to 3 per cent	Usually less than 1 per cent
Foetal haemoglobin	6–12 per cent	3–15 per cent
i-antigen	Usually present	Present in approx. half
Aminoaciduria	Present in $\frac{1}{2}$ patients	Absent
Retarded bone growth	Present	Absent
Response to androgens	Invariable	Approx 50 per cent
Effect of withdrawal of androgens	Rapid relapse	Transitory drop in Hb, but no relapse

Levels above 400 mg/100 ml (or 5 per cent) have been thought to indicate a better prognosis in the acquired disease (O'Gorman Hughes, 1966; Bloom and Diamond, 1968), but an analysis of more recent cases from the same institute has failed to confirm this finding, perhaps due to a change in technique (Li *et al.*, 1972).

There is no aminoaciduria as seen in approximately half of the patients with the constitutional form, nor retarded bone age (Shahidi and Diamond, 1961). The i-antigen is present in approximately half the patients (O'Gorman Hughes, 1966).

Lymphopenia and hypogammaglobulinaemia with subnormal IgG has been found in more than half the adult patients with this disease (Lewis, 1969). The association of similar changes with neutropenia are discussed later (Chap. 15).

Association of haemolysis, including PNH

Shortened red cell survival is seen in a proportion of patients with aplastic anaemia, indicating that the red cell defect is sometimes qualitative as well as quantitative (Lewis, 1969). Increased sequestration in the spleen may then be found. The expected reticulocytosis is, of course, usually precluded by the concomitant marrow aplasia. Haptoglobins are reduced in some cases. One cause of haemolysis in this disease is the strange syndrome of associated paroxysmal nocturnal haemoglobinuria (PNH) and aplastic anaemia (Dacie and Lewis, 1961). This should be suspected when an elevation of the bilirubin or spontaneous reticulocytosis occurs in an aplastic patient. It is confirmed by the acid serum haemolysis (HAM's) test for PNH and by testing for haemosiderinuria. In some cases the PHN abnormality is found only by testing the most sensitive erythrocyte population viz. the reticulocytes and young red cells obtained by carefully pipetting off the layer below the 'buffy coat' after centrifugation of 20–30 ml of blood at 500 G, (Gardner and Blum, 1967).

The usual sequence in this syndrome is that PNH is discovered during the course of aplastic anaemia, often some degree of erythropoietic recovery has occurred. In a few cases the reverse sequence has occurred with severe or fatal marrow failure developing during the course of PNH. By routinely testing all their patients with aplastic anaemia Lewis and Dacie (1967) found that 7 out of 46 (15 per cent) had the laboratory criteria of PNH. Two of these subsequently developed clinically typical PNH. Looked at from the other viewpoint they found that at least 15 of their 60 patients with PNH presented initially with evidence of aplasia. Normally PNH is a disease of adult males. However, the form which follows aplasia appears to have a younger age distribution and may actually affect children. The series of 11 such patients observed by Gardner included 6 under the age of 25, two being aged 7 years and 9 years. These two were male children who were considered to have aplastic anaemia for 2 and 5 years before the diagnosis of PNH (Gardner and Blun, 1967).

An interesting aspect of this associated syndrome is that the aplastic anaemia may be of the Fanconi type (Dacie and Gilpin, 1944), may be of the acquired type following exposure to chloramphenicol, tranquillizers, insecticides, weed killers or other drugs (Quagliana *et al.*, 1964) or may be of the idiopathic variety (Lewis and Dacie, 1967). Lewis and Dacie conclude that the essential link is between marrow aplasia and PNH, rather than between the aetiological factor responsible for the marrow damage and PNH. Both these authors and Gardner and Blum (1967) suggest that a somatic mutation occurs in the marrow stem cells during the period of aplasia which results in a second clone of abnormal PNH red cells being produced when marrow regeneration subsequently occurs. It should be added that, although the characteristic abnormality of PNH resides in the red cells, the granulocytes are also abnormal, having decreased phagocytic activity in the skin window technique (Frame et al., 1962) and low alkaline phosphatase activity (Beck and Valentine, 1951). This is in contrast to the usually increased alkaline phosphatase activity in granulocytes in uncomplicated aplastic anaemia.

Treatment

This is essentially the same as for constitutional aplastic anaemia, but there is the additional matter of ensuring that there is no further exposure to the offending drug or toxic agent where this can be identified. Re-exposure may induce a fatal relapse in patients who had recovered from the first episode of aplasia and may even provoke a fatal anaphylactic shock (Sánchez-Medal et al., 1963).

Supportive measures likewise include blood transfusion at times when the anaemia is severe enough to produce symptoms, usually this corresponds to a haemoglobin level of 4–6 g/100 ml. Packed red cells are used other than in the treatment of overt haemorrhage, and one aims to elevate the level to 8–9 g/100 ml. Higher haemoglobin levels produce a more severe depression of erythropoiesis (Diamond and Shahidi, 1967). Thrombocytopenic bleeding is treated by rapid infusions of platelet rich plasma, or platelet concentrates (4 units/m^2). Intramuscular injections are avoided, strict asepsis is observed in the performance of all procedures and infections are treated vigorously by bactericidal antibiotics. Because neutropenia tends to be particularly severe in the acquired forms of aplastic anaemia a neutropenia régime may be used during the neutropenic phase:

0·1 per cent Hibitane* mouth washes q.d.s. p.c.
Naseptin cream to anterior nares t.d.s.
Hibiscrub baths daily.
1·0 per cent Hibitane dental gel to gums b.d. (instead of using toothbrush) (Corsodyl, B.D.H.).

During periods of admission to hospital some form of isolation with reverse barrier nursing is advisable so as to lessen the chance of infection with hospital pathogens. Prophylactic systemic antibiotic therapy is strongly to be condemned since it increases the liability to fungal and antibiotic resistant infec-

*Made up from pure antiseptic, free of detergent or dye.

tions. Infection may first manifest itself by an increase in bleeding tendency. Not only does infection lower the platelet count but it also increases the bleeding tendency for a given platelet count (Vincent and DeGruchy, 1967).

ANDROGENS

Specific therapy with androgens plus corticosteroids is similar to that in constitutional forms viz. oral oxymetholone 4–5 mg/kg per day plus prednisolone 5 mg twice daily for children under 20 kg, 5 mg three times per day if 20–40 kg, and four times per day if over 40 kg. The difference lies in the lower proportion of patients responding in the acquired forms of aplasia, (Fig. 4.7) their slower response and the fact that those who

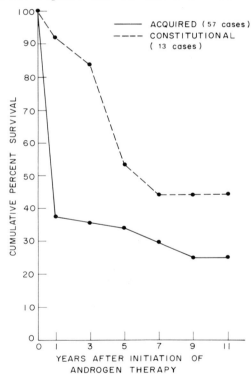

Fig. 4.7 Survival after initiation of androgen therapy in children with aplastic anemia. (Reproduced from Li, Alter and Nathan (1972), Blood, **40**, 153, by permission of the author and the publishers).

respond remain in remission after the androgen and corticosteroid therapy is stopped. In Fanconi's anaemia marrow failure promptly recurs on stopping this therapy. It has even been suggested that this can be used to distinguish between acquired and constitutional forms in difficult cases (Diamond and Shahidi, 1967).

Early results with the use of androgens and steroids gave impressive results. Out of 17 children with acquired aplastic anaemia (12 toxic and 5 idiopathic) 10 showed a sustained reticulocytosis reaching a peak of 5 to 15 per cent after 1 to 7 months of combined androgen and corticosteroid therapy (Shahidi and Diamond, 1961). Nine of these survived and showed a subsequent rise in haemoglobin. Three others showed a transient reticulocytosis but on other response. The discrepancy between the time of onset of reticulocytosis and the haemoglobin response has been attributed to haemolysis in these patients. Also the red cells formed during the early stage of this marrow regeneration are hypochromic, in the presence of normal serum iron levels and an increase in free protoporphyrin in the red cells (Shahidi, 1963), suggesting a cellular block in haemoglobin synthesis. The maximum rise in haemoglobin was found at $2\frac{1}{2}$ to 15 months from the beginning of androgen therapy. Serial marrow examination during the early stages of therapy showed groups of reticulum cells maturing into erythroid foci in those patients destined to respond. All those with a haemoglobin response also showed a rise in polymorphs to over 1,500/ mm^3, but the platelet response was less pronounced, reaching only 25,000 to 90,000 per mm^3. In general the polymorph rise was slower than the haemoglobin rise, and the platelet rise was slowest of all. The total duration of androgen therapy was $2\frac{1}{2}$ to 15 months in these patients and

logical improvement which was permanent. Two were idiopathic and 3 toxic in origin. (Of the non-responders 3 were idiopathic and 1 was toxic.) Similar time relationships were again seen. Signicant rises in the platelet count did not occur until 9 to 17 months on therapy, and even then this was only 50,000/mm^3 in one patient and 100,000/mm^3 in two others, at a time when haemoglobin and polymorphs were normal. Drugs were stopped after 7 to 11 months and this was followed by a transient fall in haemoglobin of 1 to 3 months duration in 4 out of the 5 patients. No relapse occurred during 1 to 3 years observation.

These two reports indicate that just over half these children responded, and that this occurred in both idiopathic and toxic forms of aplastic anaemia, with a questionably better response rate in the toxic group:

	Total no.	Survivors no.	Survivors per cent
Toxic	16	11	69
Idiopathic	10	4	40
Total	26	15	58

Data from Shahidi and Diamond (1961) and Desposito et. al (1964).

By contrast the results in children receiving corticosteroids or supportive therapy but no androgens are given below:)

Acquired aplastic anaemia		Total no. of children	Survivors no.	Survivors per cent
Scott et al.	(1959)	9	0	0
Wolff, J. A.	(1957)	81	1	1
Shahidi and Diamond	(1959)	40	1	5
Gasser	(1961)	20	2	10
Neiman et al.	(1963)	14	0	0
O'Gorman Hughes	(1966)*	48	9	19
Heyn et al.	(1969)	33	15	46
Total		245	28	11

*Including some of the patients in Shahidi and Diamond's series.

they remained in remission indefinitely after stopping therapy. Two of the responders had idiopathic aplasia and 8 toxic. Three of the non-responders had idiopathic and 4 toxic forms of aplasia. The suggestion that long-continued corticosteroids of high doses may actually impair marrow function by increasing the fat in the marrow was made by these authors.

Rather similar results were obtained with the use of androgens plus steroids by Desposito et al. (1964). Five out of nine children with acquired aplastic anaemia experienced a marked haemato-

Until the more recent of these reports it appeared that survival without androgen therapy seldom occurred. The improved survival occurring in the two most recent of these series can be attributed to advances in supportive therapy including antibiotics and platelet transfusions. In particular the series of Heyn et al. (1969) casts new light on the natural course of the disease and appears to be closing the gap between those treated with and without androgens. (Thirty of their 33 patients, however, were toxic rather than idiopathic in origin and this may have given a slightly more favourable prognosis.) O'Gorman Hughes (1966) in a review including 104 chidren with acquired aplastic anaemia from Boston and Sydney found a crude survival rate of 34 per cent for combined androgen plus corticosteroid therapy compared to 19 per cent for corticosteroid or supportive therapy alone.

More recent reports, including the current results from the same Boston children's hospital, have shown less satisfactory results with 70 to 80 per cent mortality in spite of androgen, corticoteroid and supportive therapy (Davis and Rubin, 1972; Li et al., 1972). There is a biphasic survival curve with many early deaths from infection and haemorrhage in the first 6 months (Fig. 4.7). The value of androgens in cases with severe acquired aplasia is now being questioned (Williams et al., 1973; Li et al., 1972).

PROGNOSTIC FEATURES

Prognostic features that have emerged from the review of O'Gorman Hughes (1966) are that this appears to be worse in aplastic anaemia following infection, particularly infectious hepatitis, or following a single short course of chloramphenicol. The prognosis appears to be better in idiopathic cases and in those attributable to anticonvulsants or to repeated courses of chloramphenicol. It was suggested that the bone marrow of a child who develops aplastic anaemia after a single short course is often more severely depressed than that of a child who requires repeated courses of the drug to induce pancytopenia. It is also well recognized that those with severely hypocellular marrows, greater than 85 per cent lymphocytes in the marrow (Li et al., 1972), less than 200 neutrophils/mm^3 or less than 20,000 platelets/mm^3 have an especially grave prognosis (Lancet, 1975). These considerations have led Camitta et al. (1974) to suggest that severe post-hepatic aplasia should be considered an indication for early marrow transplantation in view of the fact that only around 10 per cent in this category survive with supportive therapy plus androgens and steroids.

MARROW TRANSPLANTATION

The failure of androgens in severe acquired aplastic anaemia has encouraged exploration of the possibilities of marrow transplantation. Intravenous infusion of marrow from identical twins was followed by prompt recovery of marrow function in 5 out of 10 attempts (Pillow et al., 1966). When identical twin donors are unavailable the problems of graft rejection or, if the graft is accepted, graft versus host reaction present major

obstacles. Among ordinary siblings, however, there is a 1 in 4 chance of finding a histocompatible donor selected on the basis of HL-A typing and mixed lymphocyte (M.L.C.) testing to take account of other histocompatibility loci. These precautions lessen but do not entirely obviate the problems of graft incompatibility (Lancet, 1975). Additional immunosuppressive therapy such as high dose cyclophosphamide before the marrow transplant and a methotrexate course after the transplant are required to lessen or obviate the graft versus host reaction. Massive supportive therapy, including nursing in a sterile environment, leucocyte and platelet transfusions during the critical early days as well as considerable team expertise are needed before this therapeutic manoeuvre is attempted (Kay, 1974). The technique of marrow collection, processing and infusion is described by Thomas and Storb (1970). Twenty four patients (8 under 14 years) with severe aplastic anaemia (14 idiopathic, 4 post-hepatitis, 4 drug-induced, 1 PNH, 1 Fanconi) failing to respond to conventional therapy were given grafts from HL-A identical siblings (Storb et al., 1974). Twenty one showed prompt marrow regeneration in most instances confirmed by genetic markers to be due to donor cells. Four patients rejected the graft and died. Four died of graft versus host disease. Eleven are surviving with functioning grafts between 141 and 823 days. Ten have returned to normal activity. These results obtained by the Seattle group have encouraged others to apply the procedure. The result of the first British case, performed by the Royal Marsden Hospital Bone Marrow Transplant Team (Kay, 1974) is shown in Fig. 4.8. This may be the treatment of the future for selected cases with bad prognostic features at presentation (Camitta et al., 1974).

MISCELLANEOUS THERAPY

Splenectomy has been advocated in patients refractory to other therapy and possessing a cellular marrow (Bernard et al., 1958). The alleged benefit has not been confirmed by analysis of a large series of cases (Scott et al., 1959), and since the operation carries a considerable hazard in these thrombocytopenic patients it is not in general recommended (Diamond and Shahidi, 1967). A possible exception is in those patients where a haemolytic element is present and where there is demonstrable red cell sequestration in the spleen (Lewis and Dacie, 1967). Splenectomy has also been shown to increase platelet survival in aplastic patients who become refractory to platelet transfusion (Flatow and Freireich, 1966).

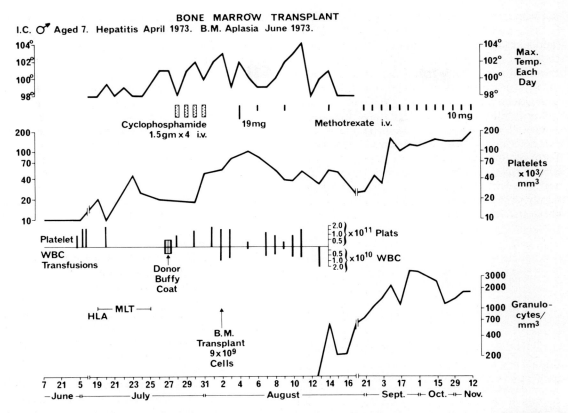

Fig. 4.8 Bone marrow transplantation in post-hepatitic marrow aplasia. Treatment and blood changes. (Reproduced from Kay (1974) and the Royal Marsden Hospital Bone Marrow Transplant Team, by permission of the author, the Editor and the publishers the British Medical Association).

Intravenous phytohaemagglutinin has been suggested in aplastic anaemia (Hunble, 1964), but present evidence does not support its use. Iron therapy is contraindicated as is cobalt therapy, which produces nausea and vomiting as well as thyroid enlargement. Folic acid and B_{12} are without effect, even in those patients with megaloblastic changes.

PURE RED-CELL APLASIA

This disorder has been described under many names of which the following are the most descriptive or most widely used: 'congenital hypoplastic anaemia' (Burgert et al., 1954; Pearson and Cone, 1957; Diamond et al., 1961), 'Pure red cell anaemia' (Smith, 1959), 'erythrogenesis imperfecta' (Cathie, 1950), 'primary red cell aplasia' (Donnely, 1953), and 'Blackfan-Diamond syndrome' the latter an acknowledgement to the definition of this disease and the description of five cases by Diamond and Blackfan in 1938. Two earlier cases had, however, been described by Josephs (1936). These descriptions indicate the essential nature of the disorder, namely that it is an isolated failure of red cell production in the marrow, with normal platelets and white cells, and is usually present from birth. In most cases there is a virtual absence of erythroblasts in the marrow which is why I favour the term 'pure red cell aplasia'. Actually the term 'erythrogenesis imperfecta' has been used for those cases showing a deficiency of effective red cell production in spite of adequate erythroblasts in the marrow; a state suggestive of ineffective erythropoiesis or refractory anaemia (Bomford and Rhoads, 1941), rather than aplasia. In two of Cathie's original cases the erythroblasts in the marrow were normal and in one they were increased.

Aetiology

The aetiology of this disease remains unknown. Its usual manifestation in the first few weeks of life and the fact that a proportion show anaemia at birth indicate that the cause is congenital, although not necessarily genetic. Favouring a genetic origin is the occurrence of affected siblings in the same family. Burgert et al. (1954) reported 2 affected brothers in their series of 12 children, and Diamond et al. (1961) found two affected siblings in five of their twenty eight families. Earlier generations were not affected. This pattern raised the possibility of a recessive form of inheritance. Förare (1963) made a significant contribution to this point by recording the anaemia in two children born to different mothers by the same father, plainly suggesting that it was carried by a 'dominant' gene. Mott et al. (1969) described a similar family (Fig. 4.9). In this instance it was possible to show that the father (4) had abnormal erythro-

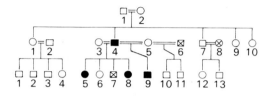

Fig. 4.9 Dominant transmission of pure red-cell aplasia from father to son and daughters of separate marriages. (Reproduced from Mott, Apley and Raper (1969) by permission of Dr Mott and the *Archives of Disease in Childhood*).

poiesis with persistence of foetal haemoglobin-containing red cells in spite of a normal haemoglobin level. His affected son (9) had a mild form of red cell hypoplasia which was brought to light only because of the previously affected daughters (5 and 8), and he never required transfusion therapy. This led the authors to suggest that the disease is transmitted as a dominant trait with modified expression in males, resulting a milder self-limiting anaemia, allowing survival into adult life and the perpetuation of the disease by transmission through these males. It was noticed by Diamond et al. (1961) that the chance of survival was greater in males although the incidence in the two sexes is similar. However, transmission from mother to daughter has also recently been reported (Hamilton, Dawson and Galloway, 1974), indicating that the mild form of the disease can sometimes occur in females.

The high incidence of associated congenital defects, in 7 out of 30 of Diamond's patients and 7 out of 8 of the series of O'Gorman Hughes (1961), further supports a congenital and possibly hereditary cause. The associated defects included dwarfism, skeletal anomalies, congenital heart defects, webbed neck and urinary tract malformations. The overall incidence of congenital anomalies is approximately 1 in 3 (Minagi and Steinback, 1966). A structural chromosome abnormality (on the short arm of one member of the A1 pair) was reported in one patient (Amarose et al., 1965), pericentric inversion of chromosome 1 in another patient (Heyn et al., 1974) but chromosome findings are in general normal. Likewise the associated biochemical findings of increased anthranilic acid excretion following an oral tryptophan load (Altman and Miller, 1953) has not proved constant (Pearson and Cone, 1957) in larger series. Rare association with hypocalcaemia (Tartaglia et al., 1966) and with hypogammaglobulinaemia (Brookfield and Singh, 1974) has been recorded.

Cathie (1950) showed in short term marrow cultures that the early erythoblasts matured normally into late erythroblasts but that there was a block in their further progress to reticulocytes. It was on this basis that he suggested an 'inborn error of development on the part of the late normoblast' and proposed the name 'erythrogenesis imperfecta'. This may explain the variable number of erythroblasts found in the marrow. There is no evidence that the disease is caused by a lack of erythropoietin (Hammond and Keighley, 1960). Recently Hammond has produced evidence that an inhibitor is present in the serum which most likely blocks erythropoietin-sensitive stem cell receptor sites (Ortega et al., 1975). Marrow from 9 anaemic patients responded sub-optimally to erythropoietin *in vitro*. Geller et al. (1975), however, found no serum inhibitors and suggest that it is premature to institute trials of immuno-suppression on presently available evidence.

An acquired form of pure red cell aplasia associated with thymoma (Dameshek et al., 1967) is well known in adults but virtually unknown in childhood. Acquired pure red cell anaemia with proerythroblast maturation arrest has, however, been reported in a boy of 5 without thymoma (Wranne et al., 1970). The response to prednisolone and azothioprine suggested an immunological cause in this patient.

Clinical features

Much of the following description is drawn from the review of 30 patients by Diamond, Allen and Magill in 1961. Pallor at the time of birth was present in 8 of these infants. If not present at birth it was usually first noted at 3 to 4 weeks. In 24 out of the 30 it was evident by 3 months and in only 4 did it develop after 1 year. Seven infants were small at birth and never achieved satisfactory growth levels for their age.

Apart from the possible non-specific congenital anomalies mentioned above the only clinical findings at diagnosis are those caused by anaemia. In particular there are no haemorrhagic manifestations nor liability to infection. Hepatomegaly and even splenomegaly may be present if there is congestive cardiac failure, but these gradually disappear following transfusion. A haemic cardiac murmur may also be present during periods of severe anaemia.

After 5 or more years of regular blood transfusion therapy (see below) all these patients develop skin pigmentation and other manifestations of transfusion haemosiderosis. Among 11 patients who had been transfused for 5 years or more 3 developed marked osteoporosis with vertebral compression fractures, 4 showed failure of secondary sexual maturation (4 out of the 6 who were 14 or over), 4 had hypersplenism, 6 had a bone age 3–4 years below normal and 8 showed growth retardation progressing from the 10th to the 3rd percentile as age advanced. It is possible that with the earlier use of chelating agents these complications will be less prominent in the future.

In the late stages of this disease liability to overwhelming infection seems to be a common mode of death, perhaps due to immunological deficiency secondary to involvement of the reticuloendothelial system by haemosiderosis or to the effects of hypersplenism. It has been particularly common in patients who have had splenectomy for this complication.

Laboratory diagnosis

The haemoglobin level may be as low as 9·4 g/100 ml at birth, and within the range of 2–8 g/100 ml at the more usual time of diagnosis of around one month. The red cells are normochromic and normocytic. Reticulocytes are usually less than 0·2 per cent or are totally absent. The blood picture is therefore in complete contrast to that seen in haemolysis or blood loss, where there would be reticulocytosis and circulating normoblasts as evidence of marrow overactivity. This point is of importance since one of the main clinical differential diagnoses is a late anaemia due to rhesus or ABO haemolytic disease. Although ABO incompatibility has been recorded on occasions (Smith, 1949) there is usually no evidence of maternal isoimmunization nor other evidence of haemolysis in the affected infant. Another differential diagnosis in these infants who are anaemic at birth would be acute or chronic foetomaternal haemorrhage. The former would be excluded by a Kleihauer test upon the mother's circulating blood (so as to detect circulating foetal RBCs); the latter would produce a hypochromic blood picture in the baby. At some point in time a reticulocytosis would be produced in the infant in both instances.

Cathie (1950) pointed out that not only were WBCs normal, but that both neutrophil leucocytosis and lymphocytosis occured normally in response to bacterial or viral infection. The platelet count is also normal at diagnosis.

The key investigation is a marrow examination. At the usual age of presentation this necessitates a tibial puncture since the posterior iliac crest is too small under 6 weeks of age. The cellularity of the marrow is normal and the myeloid and megakaryocyte series are normally represented but normoblasts are usually markedly reduced. Diamond et al. (1961) found the average number of erythroblasts was 4·3 per cent with a range of 0–13 per cent and an erythroid:myeloid ratio of 1:6 to 1:240 (normally 1:2 to 1:3). The red cell precursors that were present were mostly young proerythroblasts. No megaloblastic features were present. Other authors including Cathie (1950) and O'Gorman Hughes (1961) have reported otherwise typical cases where the proportion of erythroblasts was normal or even increased. These cases, however, showed defective maturation of normoblasts including multilobed and distorted nuclei, abnormal nuclear chromatin and defective haemoglobinisation. In Diamond's series 4 patients initially had normal numbers of erythroblasts in their marrows but over a period of months these disappeared. Hand in hand with the reduction in normoblasts there is often an increase in haematogones (Smith, 1959). These are similar to lymphocytes but a little larger and probably represent erythroid stem cells.

One case has been reported where a transition to a sideroblastic state with hypochromic red cells and erythroid hyperplasia occurred at 42 months (Boxer et al., 1971).

During the subsequent progress of the disease the haemoglobin level after transfusion falls at a steady rate corresponding to a red cell survival of approximately 110 days, unless there is a spontaneous or therapeutic remission of the disease. At this stage of the disease virtually all the circulating red cells are those of the donors. In spite of this foetal haemoglobin persists in some cases. Negative findings include an absence of biochemical evidence of haemolysis, absence of a haemoglobinopathy and no evidence of iron, folate, B_{12} or pyridoxine deficiency. Anthranilic acid excretion after tryptophan load has not proved a useful or constant diagnostic feature.

After some years of blood transfusion the serum iron and the percentage saturation of TIBC rises, the latter to close to 100 per cent. Progressive transfusion haemosiderosis leads to excessive iron deposition in the marrow reticulum cells and to hepatic cirrhosis. After 5 or more years a proportion of patients develop moderate thrombocytopenia and neutropenia and somewhat increased transfusion requirements due to hypersplenism secondary to portal hypertension. The myeloid and megakaryocyte series in the marrow are still normal at this stage.

Course and treatment

As indicated above many cases require repeated blood transfusion for survival. This inevitably leads to haemosiderosis which is the eventual 'killer' sometimes after 16 to 25 years. There is no erythropoietic response to any haematinic or marrow stimulant other than steroids.

Before the use of corticosteroids in this disease approximately 1 out of 3 cases experienced spontaneous remissions at some time between the ages of 1 to 13 years (Diamond et al., 1961). After the introduction of steroid therapy (Gasser, 1951) over half the patients had remissions, but a small maintenance dose is necessary thereafter in the majority (Allen and Diamond, 1961). Early institution of steroid therapy may be important since a response was obtained in 11 out of 13 infants where this was started as soon as the diagnosis had been established (3–9 months), but in only 1 out of 9 when there was a delay of a year or more before the institution of steroid therapy. The initial therapy should be prednisone 30 mg/day for 2 weeks, during which time a reticulocytosis usually occurs. Once the haemoglobin level has returned to normal the corticosteroid dose is reduced to the minimum level which will maintain the haemoglobin above 9–10 g/100 ml. A dose of 5.0 to 7.5 mg/day is usually adequate. Further reductions are subsequently made and intermittent therapy, for instance on alternate days or twice weekly, causes less retardation of growth than daily therapy (Pearson and Cone, 1957). Sjölin and Wranne (1970) found that 3 out of 6 patients responded well to prednisolone in a dose of 15–20

mg per day. Lower doses were ineffective and higher doses gave no better response. It has also been pointed out by Mauer (1969) that the addition of androgens should prevent the inhibition of growth produced by corticosteroids alone. There is the additional possibility that the androgen might further enhance the erythropoietic effect. Perhaps a quarter of those who respond may finally be weaned off all therapy without subsequent relapse.

It should be mentioned that other groups have had less success with steroids. Zuelzer et al. (1957) obtained a response in only 1 out of 5 patients, and subsequently in a larger series of 18 cases there were 4 spontaneous remissions and 7 corticosteroid induced remissions (quoted by Allen and Diamond, 1961). Both because of the steroid-resistant cases and because of patients surviving from the presteroid era the problem of the patient requiring regular transfusion and that of transfusion haemosiderosis are still with us. Mauer (1969) has pointed out that in a patient who is not forming red cells the transfusion requirement is similar if the haemoglobin level is kept above 9 g/100 ml as if a lower level is accepted. The patient is likely to remain fitter and growth performance may be better.★

For those patients requiring continuous transfusion therapy desferrioxamine is of value to reduce the degree of iron overload (Sephton Smith, 1962). One to 2 g can be given in 200 ml of saline before each blood transfusion. If this is supplemented by I.M. desferrioxamine (40 mg/kg) 3 times per week an iron excretion in the region of 5 mg per day can be expected in patients with 80 per cent or more saturation of their total iron binding capacity (TIBC) (11–40 mg of iron excreted per gram of desferrioxamine). This amount of iron loss is commensurate with the amount of iron derived from the transfused blood since 1 pint of blood contains approximately 200 mg of haemoglobin iron and may be required at approximately 40 day intervals. An alarming, but clinically insignificant finding, is a pink discoloration of the urine following desferrioxamine administration. It has also been shown that patients with transfusion siderosis may become deficient in ascorbic acid and that the amount of iron excreted after a given dose of desferrioxamine is increased by over 80 per cent by keeping them saturated with ascorbic acid, i.e. 1.5 g/day orally (Wapnick et al., 1969).†

★ In fact transfusion requirements are a little higher.

† An oral iron chelating agent, dihydroxybenzoic, acid, shows great promise for the future (Jones et al., 1975, Blood, **46**, 1027).

The development of irregular blood group antibodies (i.e. to blood group systems such as Kell or Duffy outside the Rh system) is a constant possibility necessitating careful X-matching in these patients so as to avoid transfusion reactions. Antileucocyte or antiplatelet antibodies may also develop producing allergic-type reactions during transfusion and necessitating the use of washed packed red cells on subsequent occasions. By the use of nitrogen stored red cells, washed free of plasma and leucocytes during their reconstitution, one not only avoids these reactions but also reduces the chance of transmitting serum hepatitis (Tullis et al., 1970).

Splenectomy does not appear to be effective in altering the course of the disease nor is it advisable at the late stage in the disease when hypersplenism develops. Of eight patients in Diamond's series who had splenectomy only 2 developed remissions and this occurred 4 and 14 months after the operation, These two patients and two others who had been splenectomized for hypersplenism died (of overwhelming infection in 3).

REFERENCES

Adamson, J. W., Eschbach, J. & Finch, C. A. (1968) The kidney and erythropoiesis *Amer. J. Med.*, **44**, 725.

Allen, D. M., & Diamond, L. K. (1961) Congenital (erythroid) hypoplastic anemia. *A.M.A. J. Dis. Child.*, **102**, 416.

Allen, D. M., Fine, M. H., Necheles, T. F. & Dameshek, W. (1968) Oxymetholone therapy in aplastic anemia. *Blood*, **32**, 83.

Althoff, H. (1953) Zur Panmyelopathie Fanconi als zustandsbild multipler Abartungen. *Ztschr. Kinderh.*, **72**, 267.

Altman, K. I. & Miller, G. (1953) A disturbance of tryptophan metabolism in congenital hypoplastic anaemia. *Nature, London*, **172**, 868.

Amarose, A. P., Tartaglia, A. P. & Propp, S. (1965) Cytogenic findings in Blackfan-Diamond syndrome. *Lancet*, **2**, 1020.

Beautyman, W. (1951) A case of Fanconi's anaemia. *Arch. Dis. Childh.*, **26**, 238.

Beck, W. S. & Valentine, W. N. (1951) Biochemical studies on leucocytes. II. Phosphatase activity in chronic lymphatic leucaemia, acute leucaemia and miscellaneous haematologic conditions. *J. Lab. Clin. Med.*, **38**, 245.

Bell, A. D., Mold, J. W., Oliver, R. A. & Shaw, S. (1956) Study of transfused platelets in a case of congenital hypoplastic thrombocytopenia. *Brit. med. J.*, **2**, 692.

Bernard, J., Mathé, G. & Najean, Y. (1958) Contribution a l'étude clinique et physiopathologique de la maladie de Fancon. *Rev. Franc. etude clin. et biol.*, **3**, 599.

Best, W. R. (1967) Chloramphenicol-associated blood dyscrasias: A review of cases submitted to the American Medical Association Registry. *J. Am. Med. Assoc.*, **201**, 181.

Birkhill, F. R., Maloney, M. A. & Levenson, S. M. (1951) Effect of transfusion polycythaemia upon bone marrow activity and erythrocyte survival in man. *Blood*, **6**, 1021.

Bithell, T. C. & Wintrobe, M. M. (1967) Drug-induced aplastic anemia. *Seminars in Hematology*, **4**, 194.

Bloom, G. E. & Diamond, L. K. (1968) Prognostic value of fetal hemoglobin levels in acquired aplastic anemia. *New Eng. J. Med.*, **278**, 304.

Bloom, G. E., Warner, S., Gerald, P. S. & Diamond, L. K. (1966) Chromosome abnormalities in constitutional aplastic anemia. *New Eng. J. Med.*, **274**, 8.

Bomford, R. R. & Rhoads, C. P. (1941) Refractory anemia. *Quart. J. Med.*, **10**, 175.

Boxer, L. A., Hussey, L. & Clarke, T. L. (1971) Sideroblastic anemia following congenital erythroid hypoplasia. *J. Pediat.*, **79**, 681.

B. M. J. (1966) Editorial: Mechanisms of aplastic anaemia. *Brit. med. J.*, **4**, 783.

Brookfield, E. G. & Singh, P. (1974) Congenital hypoplastic anemia associated with hypogammaglobulinemia. *J. Pediat.*, **85**, 529.

Burget, E. O., Kennedy, R. L. J. & Pease, G. L. (1954) Congenital hypoplastic anemia. *Pediatrics*, **13**, 218.

Burke, V., Colebatch, J. H., Anderson, C. M. & Simons, M. J. (1967) Association of pancreatic insufficiency and chronic neutropenia in childhood. *Arch. Dis. Childh.*, **42**, 147.

Camitta, B. M., Nathan, D. G., Forman, E. N., Parkman, R., Rappeport, J. M. & Orellana, T. D. (1974) Posthepatitic severe aplastic anemia—an indication for early bone marrow transplantation. *Blood*, **43**, 473.

Cathie, I. A. B. (1950) Erythrogenesis imperfecta. *Arch. Dis. Childh.*, **25**, 313.

Cobo, A., Lister, R., Cardova, M. S. & Pizzuto, J. (1970) Lack of chromosomal abnormalities in acquired aplastic anaemia (cf. Fanconi's). *Acta Haemat.*, **44**, 32.

Committee on Safety of Drugs (1967) Adverse reaction series No. 4., H.M.S.O., Jan. 1967.

Cowdell, R. H., Phizackerley, P. J. R. & Pyke, D. A. (1955) Constitutional anaemia (Fanconi's syndrome) and leukemia in two brothers. *Blood*, **10**, 788.

Custer, R. P. (1946) Aplastic anemia in soldiers treated with atabrine. *Amer. J. Med. Sci.*, **212**, 211.

Dacie, J. V. & Gilpin, A. (1944) Refractory anaemia (Fanconi type): Its incidence in three members of one family, with in one case a relationship to chronic haemolytic anaemia with nocturnal haemoglobinuria. *Arch. Dis. Childh.*, **19**, 155.

Dacie, J. V. & Lewis, S. M. (1961) Paroxysmal nocturnal haemoglobinuria: Variations in clinical severity and association with bone-marrow aplasia. *Brit. J. Haemat.*, **7**, 442.

Dameshek, W., Brown, S. M. & Rubin, A. D. (1967) Pure red cell anemia (erythroblastic hypoplasia) and thymoma. *Seminars in Hematology*, **4**, 222.

Davis, S. & Rubin, A. D. (1972) Treatment and prognosis in aplastic anaemia. *Lancet*, **i**, 871.

Deller, J. J., Cirksena, W. J. & Marcarelli, J. (1962) Fatal pancytopenia associated with viral hepatitis. *New Eng. J. Med.*, **266**, 297.

Desposito, F., Akatsuka, J., Thatcher, L. G. & Smith, N. J. (1964) Bone marrow failure in pediatric patients: I. cortisone and testosterone treatment. *J. Pediat.*, **64**, 683.

Diamond, L. K., Allen, D. M. & Magill, F. B. (1961) Congenital (erythroid) hypoplastic anemia. *A.M.A. J. Dis. Child.*, **102**, 403.

Diamond, L. K. & Blackfan, K. D. (1938) Hypoplastic anemia. *A.M.A. J. Dis. Child.*, **56**, 464.

Diamond, L. K. & Shahidi, N. T. (1967) Treatment of aplastic anemia in children. *Seminars in Hematology*, **4**, 273.

Djerassi, I., Farber, S. & Evans, A. E. (1963) Transfusions of fresh platelet concentrates to patients with secondary thrombocytopenia. *New Eng. J. Med.*, **268**, 221.

Donnely, M. (1953) A case of primary red cell aplasia. *Brit. med. J.*, **1**, 438.

Emlinger, P. J., Huff, R. L. & Oda, J. M. (1952) Depression of red cell iron turnover by transfusion. *Proc. Soc. Exp. Biol. Med.*, **79**, 16.

Erf, L. A. & Rhoads, C. P. (1939) The hematological effects of benzene (benzol) poisoning. *J. Indust. Hyg. Toxicol.*, **21**, 421.

Erslev, A. J. (1964) Drug-induced blood dyscrasias. I. aplastic anemia. *J. Am. Med. Assoc.*, **188**, 531.

Estren, S. & Dameshek, W. (1947) Familial hypoplastic anemia of childhood. Report of eight cases in two families with beneficial effect of splenectomy in one case. *A.M.A. J. Dis. Child.*, **73**, 671.

Fanconi, G. (1927) Familiare infantile pernizosaartige Anämie. *Jb. Kinderheilk.*, **117**, 257.

Flatow, F. A. & Freireich, E. J. (1966) Effect of splenectomy on the response to platelet transfusion in three patients with aplastic anemia. *New Eng. J. Med.*, **274**, 242.

Förare, S. A. (1963) Pure red cell anemia in step siblings. *Acta Pediat.*, **52**, 159.

Frame, B., Rebuck, J. & Riddle, J. M. (1962) Tissue leucocyte response in paroxysmal nocturnal hemoglobinuria. *Clin. Res.*, **10**, 199.

Fraumeni, J. F. (1967) Bone marrow depression induced by chloramphenicol or phenylbutazone. *J.A.M.A.*, **201**, 828.

Frisch, B. & Lewis, S. M. (1974) The bone marrow in aplastic anaemia: Diagnostic and prognostic features. *J. Clin. Path.*, **27**, 231.

Gardner, F. H. & Blum, S. F. (1967) Aplastic anemia in paroxysmal nocturnal hemoglobinuria. Mechanisms and therapy. *Seminars in Hematology*, **4**, 250.

Garriga, S. & Crosby, W. H. (1959) The incidence of leukemia in families of patients with hypoplasia of the marrow. *Blood*, **14**, 1008.

Garrod, L. P. (1965) Antibiotics in food. *Practitioner*, **195**, 36.

Gasser, C. (1951) Aplastische Anämie (chronische Erythroblastophtise und Cortison). *Schweiz. Med. Wschr.*, **81**, 1241.

Gasser, C. (1961) Panmyelopathien im kindesalter beitrag zur Fanconi-Anemie. *Helv. Paediat. acta*, **16**, 752.

Geller, G., Krivit, W., Zalusky, R. & Zanjani, E. D. (1975) Lack of erythropoietic inhibitory effect of serum from patients with congenital pure red cell aplasia. *J. Pediat.*, **86**, 198.

German, J., Archibald, R. & Bloom, D. (1965) Chromosome breakage in a rare and probably genetically determined syndrome in man. *Science*, **148**, 506.

Giblett, E. R. & Crookston, M. C. (1964) Agglutinability of red cells by anti-i in patients with thalassaemia minor and other haematological disorders. *Nature*, **201**, 1138.

Gleadhill, V., Bridges, J. M. & Hadden, D. R. (1975) Fanconi's aplastic anaemia with short stature—absence of response to human growth hormone. *Arch. Dis. Childh.* **50**, 318.

Gross, S., Melhorn, D. K. & Newmann, A. J. (1970) Acute childhood leukemia presenting as aplastic anemia: The response to corticosteroids. *J. Pediat.*, **77**, 647.

Gurney, C. W. & Fried, W. (1965) Further studies on the erythropoietic effect of androgens. *J. Lab. Clin. Med.*, **65**, 775.

Hamilton, P. J., Dawson, A. A. & Galloway, W. H. (1974) Congenital erythroid hypoplasic anaemia in mother and daughter. *Arch. Dis. Childh.*, **49**, 71.

Hammond, D. & Keighley, G. (1960) The erythrocyte-stimulating factor in serum and urine in congenital hyplastic anemia. *A.M.A. J. Dis. Child.*, **100**, 466.

Hathaway, W. E., Brangle, R. W., Nelson, T. L. & Roeckel, I. E. (1966) Aplastic anemia and alymphocytosis in an infant with hypogammaglobulinemia. *J. Pediat.*, **68**, 713.

Hathaway, W. E., Githens, J. H., Blackburn, W. R. Fulginiti, V. & Kempe, C. H. (1965) Aplastic anemia, hystiocytosis and erythrodermia in immunologically deficient children: Probable human runt disease. *New Eng. J. Med.*, **273**, 953.

Heyn, R. M., Ertel, I. J. & Tubergen, D. G. (1969) Course of acquired aplastic anemia in children treated with supportive care. *J.A.M.A.*, **208**, 1372.

Heyn, R., Kurczynski, E. & Schmickel, R. (1974) The association of Blackfan-Diamond syndrome, physical abnormalities and an abnormality of chromosome 1. *J. Pediat.*, **85**, 531.

Higurashi, M. & Conen, P. E. (1971) *In vitro* chromosomal radiosensitivity in Fanconi's anemia. *Blood*, **38**, 336.

Hillman, R. S. & Finch, C. A. (1971) Erythropoiesis. *New Eng. J. Med.*, **285**, 99.

Hirschhorn, K. (1968) Cytogenetic alterations in leukemia. In *Perspectives in Leukaemia*, p. 113. Edited by Dameshek, W., and Dutcher, R. M., New York: Grune and Stratton.

Huguley, C. M., Erslev, A. J. & Bergsagel, D. E. (1961) Drug-related blood dyscrasias. *J. Am. Med. Assoc.*, **177**, 23.

Humble, J. G. (1964) The treatment of aplastic anemia with phytohaemagglutinin. *Lancet*, **i**, 1345.

Imerslund, O. (1953) Hypoplastic anemia associated with multiple deformities. *Nord. Med.*, **50**, 1301.

Jepson, J. H. & Lowenstein, L. (1967) The effect of testosterone, adrenal steroids and prolactin on erythropoiesis. *Acta haemat.*, **38**, 292.

Josephs, H. W. (1936) Anemia of infancy and early childhood. *Medicine*, **15**, 401.

Kay, H. E. M. (1974) Bone marrow aplasia after infectious hepatitis treated by bone marrow transplantation. *Brit. med. J.*, **i**, 363.

Kennedy, B. J. (1962) Effect of androgenic hormone in myelofibrosis. *J.A.M.A.*, **182**, 116.

Kennedy, B. J. & Nathanson, I. T. (1953) Effects of intensive sex steroid hormone therapy in advanced breast cancer. *J.A.M.A.*, **152**, 1135.

Knospe, W. H. & Crosby, W. H. (1971) Aplastic anaemia: A disorder of the bone marrow sinusoidal microcirculation rather than stem cell failure?. *Lancet*, **1**, 20.

Kostman, R. (1956) Infantile genetic agranulocytosis. *Acta Paediat.*, **45**, 105.

Lancet (1974) Annotation: Drug-induced aplastic anaemia. *Lancet*, **i**, 251.

Lancet (1975) Editorial: Bone-marrow grafting for aplastic anaemia. *Lancet*, **i**, 22.

Lange, R. D., McCarthy, J. M. & Gallagher, N. I. (1961) Plasma and urinary erythropoietin in bone marrow failure. *Arch. Int. Med.*, **108**, 850.

Levy, R. N., Sawitsky, A., Florman, A. L. & Rubin, E. (1965) Fatal aplastic anemia after hepatitis—report of five cases. *New Eng. J. Med.*, **273**, 1118.

Lewis, S. M. (1969) Aplastic anaemia: Problems of diagnosis and of treatment. *J. Roy. Coll. Phycns., Lond.*, **3**, 253.

Lewis, S. M. (1969) Studies of the erythrocyte in aplastic anaemia and other dysterythropoietic diseases. *Nouv. Rev. Franç. Hemat.*, **9**, 49.

Lewis, S. M. & Dacie, J. V. (1967) The aplastic-anaemia—paroxysmal nocturnal haemoglobinuria syndrome. *Brit. J. Haemat.*, **13**, 236.

Li, F. P., Alter, B. P. & Nathan, D. G. (1972) The mortality of acquired aplastic anemia in children. *Blood*, **40**, 153.

Lukens, J. N. & Neuman, L. A. (1971) Excretion and distribution of iron during chronic desferoxamine therapy. *Blood*, **38**, 614.

McCredie, K. B. (1969) Oxymetholone in refractory anaemia. *Brit. J. Haemat.*, **17**, 265.

McCullagh, E. P. & Jones, R. (1942) Effect of androgens on blood count of man. *J. Clin. Endocr.*, **2**, 243.

Matras, A. & Priesel, A. (1928) Über einige gewächse des Thymus. *Beitr. Path. Anat.*, **80**, 270.

Matsaniotis, N., Kiossoglou, K. A., Karpauzas, J. & Anastaséa-Vlachou, K. (1966) Chromosomes in Kostmann's disease. *Lancet*, **2**, 104.

Mauer, A. M. (1969) *Pediatric Hematology*, p. 249. New York: McGraw-Hill.

Melhorn, D. K., Gross, S. & Newman, A. J. (1970) Acute childhood leukemia presenting as aplastic anemia: The response to corticosteroids. *J. Pediat.*, **77**, 647.

Minagi, H. & Steinback, H. L. (1966) Roentgen appearance of anomalies associated with hypoplastic anemias of childhood: Fanconi's anemia and congenital hypoplastic anemia (erythrogenesis imperfecta). *Am. J. Roentgenol.*, **47**, 100.

Mott, M. G., Apley, J. & Raper, A. B. (1969) Congenital (erythroid) hypoplastic anaemia: Modified expression in males. *Arch. Dis. Childn.*, **44**, 757.

Naiman, J. L. & Gerald, P. S. (1963) Fetal hemoglobin: Improved separation by a modified agar gel electrophoresis. *J. Lab. Clin. Med.*, **61**, 508.

Neiman, N., Pierson, M., Peters, A., Petit, J. & Bourges, M. (1963) Les pancytopénies idiopathic de l'enfant. *Sem. Hôp.*, **39**, 5.

Nieweg, H. O. (1973) Aplastic anemia (panmyelopathy). A review with special emphasis on the factors causing bone marrow damage. In *Blood Disorders due to Drugs and Other Agents*. Edited by R. H. Girdwood. Amsterdam: Exerpta Medica.

Nilsson, L. R. (1960) Chronic pancytopenia with multiple congenital abnormalities (Fanconi's anaemia). *Acta Paediat* **49**, 518.

O'Gorman-Hughes, D. W. (1961) Hypoplastic anaemia in infancy and childhood: Erythroid hypoplasia. *Arch. Dis. Childh.*, **36**, 349.

O'Gorman-Hughes, D. W. & Diamond, L. K. (1964) A new type of constitutional aplastic anemia without congenital anomalies presenting as thrombocytopenia in infancy. *J. Pediat.*, **65**, 1060.

O'Gorman-Hughes, D. W. (1966) Varied patterns of aplastic anemia in childhood. *Aust. Pediat. J.*, **2**, 228.

Ortega, J. A., Shore, N. A., Dukes, P. P. & Hammond, D. (1975) Congenital hypoplastic anemia inhibition of erythropoiesis by sera from patients with congenital hypoplastic anemia. *Blood*, **45**, 83.

Osgood, E. E. (1953) Drug induced hypoplastic anemias and related syndromes. *Ann. Int. Med.*, **39**, 1173.

Ozsoylu, S. & Argun, G. (1967) Tryptic activity of the duodenal juice in aplastic anemia. *J. Pediat.*, **70**, 60.

Pearson, H. A. & Cone, T. E. (1957) Congenital hypoplastic anemia. *Pediatrics*, **19**, 192.

Pillow, R. P., Epstein, R. B., Buckner, C. D., Giblett, E. R. & Thomas, E. D. (1966) Treatment of bone marrow failure by isogenic marrow infusion. *New Eng. J. Med.*, **275**, 94.

Pochedly, C., Collipp, P. J., Wolman, S. R., Suwansirikul, S. & Rezvani, I. (1971) Fanconi's anemia with growth hormone deficiency. *J. Pediatrics*, **79**, 93.

Pringle, T. C. & Gardner, F. H. (1959) Treatment of myeloid metaplasia with testosterone. *Clin. Res.*, **7**, 210.

Quagliana, J. M., Cartwright, G. E. & Wintrobe, M. M. (1964) Paroxysmal nocturnal haemoglobinuria following drug-induced aplastic anemia. *Annals Int. Med.*, **61**, 1045.

Reinhold, J. D. L., Neumark, E., Lightwood, R. & Carter, C. O. (1952) Familial hypoplastic anaemia with congenital abnormalities (Fanconi's syndrome). *Blood*, **7**, 915.

Rosenbach, L., Caviles, A. & Mitus, W. J. (1960) Chloramphenicol toxicity: Reversible vacuolization of erythroid cells. *New Eng. J. Med.*, **263**, 724.

Saidi, P., Wallerstein, R. O. & Aggeler, P. M. (1961) Effect of chloramphenicol on erythropoisesis. *J. Lab. Clin. Med.*, **57**, 247.

Sanchez-Medal, L., Castamedo, J. P. & Garciá-Rojas, F. (1963). Insecticides and aplastic anemia. *New Eng. J. Med.*, **269**, 1365.

Sawitsky, A., Bloom, D. & German, J. (1966) Chromosomal breakage and acute leukemia in congenital telangiectatic erythema and stunted growth. *Ann. Int. Med.*, **65**, 487.

Schiffer, L. M., Price, D. C. & Cronkite, E. P. (1965) Iron absorption and anemia. *J. Lab. Clin. Med.*, **65**, 316.

Schroeder, T. M., Anschütz, F. & Knopp, A. (1964) Spontane chromosomen Aberrationen bei familiarer Panmyelopathie. *Humangenetik*, **1**, 194.

Schwarz, E., Baehner, R. L. & Diamond, L. K. (1966) Aplastic anemia following hepatitis. *Pediatrics*, **37**, 681.

Scott, J. L., Cartwright, G. E. & Wintrobe, M. M. (1959) Acquired aplastic anaemia: An analysis of 39 cases and review of the pertinent literature. *Medicine*, **38**, 119.

Scott, J. L., Finegold, S. M., Belkin, G. A. & Lawrence, J. S. (1965) A controlled double blind study of the hematologic toxicity of chloramphenicol. *New Eng. J. Med.*, **272**, 1137.

Sephton Smith, R. (1962) Iron excretion in thalassaemia major after administration of chelating agents. *Brit. med. J.*, **4**, 1577.

Shahidi, N. T. & Diamond, L. K. (1959) Testosterone-induced remission in aplastic anemia. *A.M.A. J. Dis. Child.*, **98**, 293.

Shahidi, N. T. & Diamond, L. K. (1961) Testosterone-induced remission in aplastic anemia in both acquired and congenital types. Further observations in 24 cases. *New Eng. J. Med.*, **264**, 953.

Shahidi, N. T., Gerald, P. S. & Diamond, L. K. (1962 Alkali-resistant hemoglobin in aplastic anemia of both acquired and congenital types. *New Eng. J. Med.*, **266**, 117.

Shahidi, N. T. (1963) Morphologic and biochemical characteristics of erythrocytes in testosterone-induced remission in patients with acquired and constitutional aplastic anemia. *J. Lab. Clin. Med.*, **62**, 294.

Shahidi, N. T. & Crigler, J. F. (1967) Evaluation of growth and endocrine systems in testosterone-corticosteroid-treated patients with aplastic anemia. *J. Pediat.*, **70**, 233.

Shahidi, N. T. (1973) Androgens and erythropoiesis. *New Eng. J. Med.* **289**, 72.

Shaw, S. & Oliver, R. A. M. (1959) Congenital hypoplastic thrombocytopenia with skeletal deformities in siblings. *Blood*, **14**, 374.

Sherman, J. D., Greenfield, J. B. & Ingall, D. (1964) Reversible bone marrow vacuolizations in phenylketonuria. *New Eng. J. Med.*, **270**, 810.

Shwachman, H., Diamond, L. K., Oski, F. A. & Khaw, Kon-T. (1964) The syndrome of pancreatic insufficiency and bone marrow dysfunction. *J. Pediat.*, **65**, 645.

Silink, S. J. & Firkin, B. G. (1968) An analysis of hypoplastic anaemia with special reference to the use of oxymetholone in its therapy. *Aust. Ann. Med.*, **17**, 224.

Sjölin, S. & Wranne, L. (1970) Treatment of congenital hypoplastic anaemia with prednisone. *Scand. J. Haemat.*, **7**, 63.

Smith, C. H. (1949) Chronic congenital aregenerative anemia (pure red-cell anemia) associated with isoimmunization by the blood group factor 'A'. *Blood*, **4**, 697.

Steier, W., Van Voolen, G. A. & Selmanowitz, V. J. (1972) Dyskeratosis congenita: relationship to Fanconi's anemia. *Blood*, **39**, 510.

Smith, C. H. (1959) Pure red cell anemia. *J. Pediat.*, **54**, 609.

Storb, R., Thomas, E. D., Buckner, C. D., Clift, R. A., Johnson, F. L., Fefer, A., Glucksberg, E. R., Giblett, K. G., Lerner, K. G. & Neiman, P. (1974) Allogeneic marrow grafting for treatment of aplastic anemia. *Blood*, **43**, 147.

Suhrland, L. G. & Weisberger, A. S. (1969) Delayed clearance of chloramphenicol from serum in patients with hematologic toxicity. *Blood*, **34**, 466.

Swift, M. R. & Hirschhorn, K. (1966) Fanconi's anaemia: Inherited susceptibility to chromosome breakage in various tissues. *Ann. Intern. Med.*, **65**, 496.

Tartaglia, A. P., Propp, S., Amarose, A. P., Propp, R. P. & Hall, C. A. (1966) Chromosome abnormality and hypocalcemia in congenital erythroid hypoplasia. *Amer. J. Med.*, **41**, 990.

Thomas, E. D. & Storb, R. (1970) Technique for human marrow grafting. *Blood*, **36**, 507.

Todaro, G. J., Green, H. & Swift, M. R. (1966) Susceptibility of human diploid fibroblast strains to transformation by SV_{40} virus. *Science*, **153**, 1252.

Tullis, J. L., Hinman, J., Sproul, M. T. & Nickerson, R. J. (1970) Incidence of posttransfusion hepatitis in previously frozen blood. *J.A.M.A.*, **214**, 719.

Vaal, O. M. de, and Seynhaeve, V. (1959) Reticular dysgenesia. *Lancet*, **ii**, 1123.

Varela, M. A. & Sternberg, W. H. (1967) Preanaemic state in Fanconi's anaemia. *Lancet*, **2**, 566.

Vincent, P. C. & deGruchy, G. C. (1967) Complications and treatment of acquired aplastic anaemia. *Brit. J. Haemat.*, **13**, 977.

Wagner, H. P. & Smith, N. J. (1962) A study of detoxiflcation mechanisms in children with aplastic anemia. *Blood*, **19**, 676.

Wallerstein, R. O., Condit, P. K., Kasper, C. K., Brown, J. W. & Morrison, F. R. (1969) Statewise study of chloramphenicol therapy and fatal aplastic anemia. *J.A.M.A.*, **208**, 2045.

Wapnick, A. A., Lynch, S. R., Charlton, R. W., Seftel, H. C. & Bothwell, T. H. (1969) The effect of ascorbic acid deficiency on desferrioxamine-induced urinary iron excretion. *Brit. J. Haemat.*, **17**, 563.

Williams, D. M., Lynch, R. E. & Cartwright, G. E. (1973) Drug-induced aplastic anemia. *Sem. Hemat.*, **10**, 195.

Wolff, J. A. (1957) Anemias caused by infection and toxins: Idiopathic aplastic anaemia and anaemia caused by renal disease. *Pediat. Clin. N. Amer.*, **4P**, 469.

Wranne, L., Bonnevier, J. O., Killander, A. & Killander, J. (1970) Pure red cell anaemia with proerythroblast maturation arrest. *Scand. J. Haemat.*, **7**, 73.

Yunis, A. A. & Harrington, W. J. (1960) Patterns of inhibition by chloramphenicol of nucleic acid synthesis in human bone marrow and leukemic cells. *J. Lab. Clin. Med.*, **56**, 831.

Zachmann, M., Illig, R. & Prader, A. (1972) Fanconi's anemia with isolated growth hormone deficiency. *J. Pediat.* **80**, 159.

Zuelzer, W. W., Smith, C. H. & Sturgeon, P. (1957) Panels in therapy. XIII. Hypoplastic anemia of childhood. *Blood*, **12**, 303.

5. Haemolytic Anaemias: General Features

Red-cell changes, *Spherocytes, Red-cell fragmentation, Red-cell survival* | Compensatory marrow activity | Pigment metabolism.

The following features are common to many different types of haemolytic anaemia and are those which are likely to place an undiagnosed case of anaemia within this broad group of disorders. (The later sections describe the individual and distinguishing features of the specific varieties of haemolytic anaemia.) These general features of haemolysis can be grouped under red cell changes, marrow compensatory activity and changes in pigment metabolism. The clinical consequences of these are pallor, possible bone changes and, in particular, jaundice with dark stools and urine.

RED CELL CHANGES

Spherocytes

A spherocyte is a red cell which has lost its biconcave shape by becoming thicker and of smaller diameter, thereby approaching more closely the proportions of a sphere. This can be recognized in well-made blood films by the loss of the normal central area of pallor within the contours of the red cell. Together with the reduction in diameter this makes spherocytes appear as small, dark cells with a regular circular outline. To be significant several spherocytes must be detectable within each high-power field in the appropriately spread part of the film (Fig. 5.1).

Spherocytes are the characteristic morphological finding in hereditary spherocytosis (HS) but also occur in a wide variety of other haemolytic anaemias due to such diverse causes as burns, auto-immune disease, septicaemia, paroxysmal nocturnal haemoglobinuria (PNH), haemoglobin Köln disease, ABO incompatibility or drug-induced haemolysis.

Spherocytosis whether hereditary or acquired reflects an abnormality of the red cell membrane (Table 5.1) (Cooper and Shattil, 1971). The cause of this varies. In HS it may be the consequence of loss of membrane lipids (Jacob, 1968). In defects of the glycolytic pathway the cause is a failure of ATP generation (Weed *et al.*, 1969). Other causes include drug-induced oxidation of membrane sulphydryl groups (Jacob and Jandl, 1962), interaction of antibody-coated red cells with the

Table 5.1 Red cell defects in haemolytic anaemia

Mechanisms of hemolysis	Representative examples
Abnormalities of hemoglobin influencing flow:	
'Precrystalline state'	Hemoglobin C
Aggregation	Hemoglobin S
Precipitation	Oxidant drugs (G-6PD deficiency), unstable hemoglobins, and thalassemias
Exposure of red cells to inordinate physical trauma in the circulation:	
Impact extrinsic to the circulation	March hemoglobinuria
Turbulent flow	Faulty aortic-valve prosthesis
Cleavage by fibrin strands	Disseminated intravascular coagulation and thrombotic thrombocytopenic purpura
Abnormalities associated with the red cell membrane:	
Defects of shape, plasticity and permeability	HS and glycolytic defects
Decreased protein sulfhydryl reactivity	Oxidant drugs
Altered lipid composition	Spur cells
Interaction with immunoglobins or complement	Immunohemolytic anemias

Reprinted, by permission, from the New England Journal of Medicine (1971) **285**, 1515, *and by permission of Dr. R. A Cooper.*

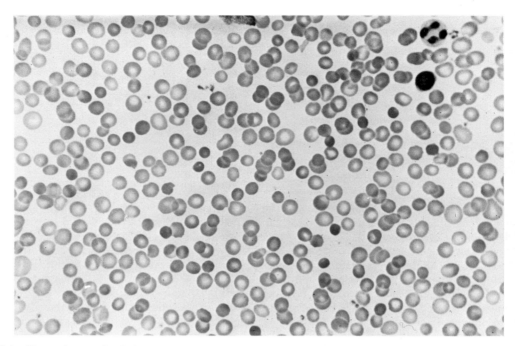

Fig. 5.1 Photomicrograph of blood film from a child with hereditary spherocytosis following a blood transfusion. The contrast between small, darkly staining spherocytes and normal red cells with central area of pallor is apparent (× 540).

reticuloendothelial system (LoBuglio et al., 1967), digestion of the membrane phospholipid by *Clostridium welchii* lecithinase (Dean et al., 1967) and the undue sensitivity of PNH red cell membrane to complement (Rosse and Dacie, 1966). Removal of insoluble intraerythrocytic inclusions such as Heinz bodies during the passage of red cells through the spleen (pitting) may simultaneously cause loss of surface membrane, also resulting in spherocyte formation (Jaffe, 1972).

Other types of red cell trauma such as impinging against intravascular fibrin in the microangiopathic states, against artificial valve prostheses or direct thermal injury in extensive burns or mechanical injury in march haemoglobinuria may similarly cause loss of membrane fragments (Cooper and Shattil, 1971).

Whatever the cause of spherocytosis the resulting cell suffers a loss of plasticity becoming less capable of surviving the changes in shape imposed upon it during its flow through the microcirculation, particularly when there is stagnation and a high haematocrit as in the spleen (Jandl and Aster, 1967). This is because the minimum surface area of a sphere for its enclosed volume does not permit any change in shape. *In vivo* this results in shortened red cell survival; *in vitro* it results in increased susceptibility to hypotonic lysis. Loss of plasticity may also occur in elliptocytosis, acanthocytosis, stomatocytosis and acquired spur cell anaemia (*vide infra*). In each case this can result in a reduced red cell survival *in vivo*.

One group of these disorders, viz. HS, hereditary elliptocytosis (HE) and stomatocytosis are characterized by an increased membrane permeability to cations. Jandl has referred to this state as 'leaky red cells' (1965). Compensation for the excessive influx of sodium ions can only be achieved by accelerated glycolysis and synthesis of ATP for the 'cation pump' concerned with sodium efflux (Jacob, 1968). Metabolic compensation may be possible in the systemic circulation but fails under the conditions of stagnation, glucose deprivation and acidosis existing in the splenic sinusoids (Young et al., 1951; Murphy, 1967). This is the explanation of the benefits from splenectomy in HS, HE and the partial benefit in stomatocytosis. By contrast when there is a block in glycolysis, as in some of the hereditary enzyme defects, the supply of glucose is not the limiting factor and splenectomy is not so beneficial.

Good recent reviews of the above topics are those of Dacie (1970), Cooper and Shattil (1971) and Jaffé (1972). The ionic factors concerned were well reviewed by Jandl (1965).

Red cell fragmentation

Fragmented red cells, 'burr' cells, pycnocytes, schistocytes, 'helmet' or 'pincered' cells are all irregularly distorted and contracted red cells which occur in a variety of acquired haemolytic states including the haemolytic-uraemic syndrome, other types of microangiopathic haemolytic anaemia, septicaemia, misplaced heart valve prostheses and some drug-induced haemolytic states. These cells can easily appear as artefacts, particularly in blood films allowed to dry slowly or made from anticoagulated blood which has been standing for some hours. A good practice is always to confirm their presence on more than one blood film freshly made from capillary blood. Different descriptive terms have been applied to the occurrence of these distorted cells in different clinical circumstances but it is doubtful if these represent separate entities or can usefully be distinguished in practice. Cells fitting the different descriptions can often be seen in one and the same blood film.

The genesis of these 'fragmented' or 'burr' cells is thought to be mechanical trauma usually associated with adhesion to microdeposits of fibrin (Brain et al., 1962; Bull et al., 1968). The latter may become temporarily adherent to the red cell membrane resulting in tearing of this envelope when shearing forces separate the two. This process is understandably associated with intravascular microcoagulation (consumptive coagulopathy) syndromes of diverse origin. In the case of acanthocytosis (hereditary abetalipoproteinaemia), 'spur' cell anaemia of severe hepatic failure and in lipid-deprived infants with acquired hypoproteinaemia increased membrane cholesterol appears to be the cause of the morphological abnormality. This results from stagnation of cholesterol on the red cell in the absence of a plasma lipoprotein carrier (McBride and Jacob, 1970). Strangely enough endogenous hyperlipaemia can also cause changes in red cell lipids and haemolysis (Bagade and Ways, 1968).

In the great majority of instances red cell fragmentation results in shortened red cell survival. This is probably due to loss of membrane plasticity, rendering the red cells less able to traverse the microcirculation, particularly that in the spleen (Cooper and Shattil, 1971).

Red cell survival

This can be measured directly by labelling a blood sample with ^{51}Cr, $DF^{32}P$ or ^3H–DFP and following the rate of decay of the label in the circulating blood. Details of the recommended methods for radioisotope red cell survival studies are given in the report of the International Committee for Standardization in Haematology (1971).

These techniques are seldom used in children since it is preferable to avoid the injection of radioactive material in childhood and also because the repeated venepunctures necessary in such investigations may present technical problems. The hazards of radioactivity may be overcome in future by methods using a non-radioactive compound for purposes of measurement by 'activation analysis' of the blood samples in vitro. This requires availability of a neutron source.

An advantage of conventional radiochromium labelling of the patient's blood in haemolytic anaemias is that subsequent surface counting can determine whether there is a preferential destruction of the red cells in the spleen or liver (Jandl et al., 1956). This information can be used to predict the value of splenectomy in certain cases of autoimmune haemolytic anaemia.

COMPENSATORY MARROW ACTIVITY

The healthy marrow is able to compensate for a 6–8 fold increase in the rate of red cell destruction before significant anaemia develops (Crosby and Akeroyd, 1952). This is especially so in the case of chronic haemolysis (Sànchez-Medal et al., 1969), since an increase in erythroid marrow, at the expense of fatty marrow, takes place. This is not possible, however, in infants since the marrow spaces are already filled with erythroid marrow. Compensation for haemolysis is then less efficient, being confined largely to extramedullary haemopoiesis. Other factors leading to impairment of marrow compensatory activity include folic acid deficiency, infection, toxic marrow depression or destruction of marrow erythroid precursors by the haemolytic agent.

The normal marrow response to haemolysis is by an increase of reticulocytes to above 2 per cent, often as high as 30 per cent, the appearance of normoblasts in the circulating blood and an increase in the number and proportion of the erythroid series in the bone marrow. The normal erythroid:myeloid ratio is about 1:5, but increases to 1:1 or more in response to haemolysis. Due to the accelerated erythroid turnover in the marrow some of the later divisions among the normoblasts series are 'skipped', resulting in macronormoblasts in the marrow and macrocytes in the peripheral blood.

These changes are due to erythropoietin stimulation, proportionate to the degree of anaemia, causing (a) an increase in erythroid precursor cells in the marrow, (b) an increase in haemoglobin complement per RBC and (c) a shift of marrow reticulocytes to the peripheral blood (Hillman and Finch, 1971). The 'shift' reticulocytes can be recognized in a blood film by their large diameter and marked basophilia. They also have an increased circulation time in the blood, for which a correction can be made if a quantitative assessment of erythropoiesis derived from the reticulocyte count is required (Hillman and Finch, 1969).

The increased erythroid activity results in increased folic acid utilization, which, if long-continued or occurring in a patient with low folate stores, may cause a lowering of the serum folate level and, at a later stage, overt megaloblastic anaemia (Chanarin et al., 1959). No such depletion of iron stores occurs since iron, being an indestructible element, is available for reutilization after haemolysis. The only exception to this is in the case of haemolytic anaemias accompanied by haemoglobinuria, e.g. PNH. Under these circumstances iron is lost to the body.

If the haemolysis is too rapid for adequate marrow compensation or if there is a failure of marrow erythropoiesis, as in an aplastic crisis, the haemoglobin falls progressively (Owren, 1948; Finch and Coleman, 1953).

Clinically the consequences of long-continued marrow hyperplasia may be bossing of the skull. Radiologically the radial striations produced by newly formed spicules of bone give the 'hair-on-end' appearance seen in severe thalassaemia after the age of 1 or 2 years (Fig. 5.2).

PIGMENT METABOLISM

The catabolism of 1 g of haemoglobin in the reticuloendothelial system results in the formation of approximately 35 mg of unconjugated bilirubin (Lemberg and Legge, 1949). Normally senescent red cells are entrapped and finally destroyed in the reticuloendothelial system of the bone marrow, liver or spleen and little free haemoglobin reaches the circulating blood during this process (Dacie, 1963A). In certain haemolytic anaemias, particularly those with acute episodes, intravascular haemolysis occurs with liberation of free haemoglobin into the circulating blood. Such haemoglobin is immediately bound to plasma haptoglobin, alpha-2 globulins synthesized in the liver. Their molecular size is too great for renal excretion so no haemoglobinuria occurs unless the haemolysis is sufficiently acute for free circulating haemoglobin to exceed the binding capacity of the plasma haptoglobins, normally equivalent to 125 mg Hb/100 ml (Smithies, 1955). The haemoglobin-haptoglobin complex is slowly removed from the

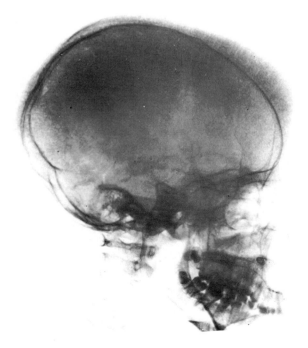

Fig. 5.2 'Hair-on-end' appearance on skull X-ray. Widening of diploic space and atrophy of outer table with radial striation giving characteristic appearance, in a case of chronic marrow hyperplasia due to haemoglobinopathy.
From (1973) *Textbook of Paediatrics*. Edinburgh: Churchill Livingstone, *Reproduced by permission of Dr. E. M. Sweet, Dr. P. Rawson and the editors.*

blood at a rate of approximately 13 mg/100 ml/hr (Laurell and Nyman, 1957) to the reticuloendothelial system (RES) where degradation of the haemoglobin to bilirubin then takes place. If the plasma haptoglobin level is determined at this stage, shortly after a period of haemolysis, it is found to be low or absent (Brus and Lewis, 1959). Although a good test for recent haemolysis it has to be remembered that haptoglobins are synthesized by the liver and low levels can occur with hepatocellular dysfunction. Also they are low or absent in the normal neonate (Allison and apRees, 1957).

If further haemoglobin is liberated into the plasma after the haptoglobins have been saturated or cleared by the RES the haem of haemoglobin becomes oxidized to haematin and combines with albumen to form methaemalbumen. This is detectable spectroscopically, absorbing at 630 mμ, or by the Schumms test in which an ammonium sulphide haemochromogen is formed which absorbs strongly at 558 mμ. If positive this test indicates intravascular haemolysis (Fairley, 1941). It is often accompanied by haemoglobinaemia (i.e. in excess of the normal upper level of 4 mg Hb/100 ml of plasma (Crosby and Dameshek, 1951) since the Hb-haptoglobin complex is fully saturated and only slowly cleared. Haemoglobinuria may also be present since the excess unbound haemoglobin passes into the glomerular filtrate. The excreted haemoglobin becomes oxidized to haematin and related products causing red to brown or black coloration of the urine, as in blackwater fever. Chronic haemoglobinuria of even slight amount produces excessive haemosiderin accumulation in the renal tubular cells resulting in ferrocyanide staining granules and casts in the urine (haemosiderinuria) a sensitive test for chronic or intermittent intravascular haemolysis (Crosby and Dameshek, 1951) such as PNH or cardiac valve prosthesis.

The bilirubin derived from haem groups from extravascular destruction of red cells, and from much of the intravascularly liberated haemoglobin, is normally conjugated and excreted by the liver. This process may be impaired in the newborn, and particularly in the premature baby because of low glucuronyl transferase activity (Brown and Zuelzer, 1958) and possibly also in the presence of severe anaemia which may reduce the excretory capacity of the liver. Chronic haemolytic anaemias can cause superaded biliary obstruction following the formation of pigment stones or 'sand' in the bile ducts or gall bladder. Mixed pigment stones are radio-opaque, pure pigment stones are not.

The normal hepatic excretion results in increased faecal stercobilin excretion which can be estimated quantitatively to assess the severity of the haemolytic process:

$$\text{Haemolytic Index} = \frac{\text{Av. daily output of faecal urobilinogen in mg} \times 100}{\text{Blood Hb (in g/100 ml)} \times \dfrac{\text{Total blood volume (in ml)}}{100}}$$

The normal range is 11–21 units (mg/day/100 g circulating haemoglobin).

A small portion of the stercobilin is reabsorbed into the circulation subsequently to be excreted in the urine as urobilinogen. This is a less certain test of haemolysis although of use in the side room (Miller *et al.*, 1942).

Black stools, due to stercobilin, and urine becoming darker on standing, due to urobilinogen changing to urobilin, are characteristic of haemolytic anaemias. Port wine or black urine, due to haemoglobinuria or methaemaglobinuria, suggest acute intravascular haemolysis.

REFERENCES

Allison, A. C. & apRees, W. (1957) The binding of haemoglobin by plasma proteins (haptoglobins). Its bearing on the 'renal threshold' for haemoglobin and the aetiology of haemoglobinuria. *Brit. med. J.*, **ii**, 1137.

Bagdade, J. D. & Ways, P. (1968) Lipemic hemolysis: Evidence for altered erythrocyte membrane composition and hemolytic anemia in hypertriglyceridemic states in man. *J. Clin. Invest.*, **47**, 4a.

Brain, M. C., Dacie, J. V. & Hourihane, D. O'B. (1962) Microangiopathic haemolytic anaemia: The possible role of vascular lesions in pathogenesis. *Brit. J. Haemat.*, **8**, 358.

Brown, A. K. & Zuelzer, W. W. (1958) Studies on the neonatal development of the glucuronide conjugating system. *J. Clin. Invest.*, **37**, 332.

Brus, I. & Lewis, S. M. (1959) Relationship between rates of haemolysis and disappearance of haptoglobins in haemolytic anaemia. Quoted by Dacie, J. V. (1963), in *Haemolytic Anaemias*, Part I, p. 13.

Bull, B. S., Rubenberg, M. L., Dacie, J. V. & Brain, M. C. (1968) Microangiopathic haemolytic anaemia: Mechanisms of red-cell fragmentation: *in vitro* studies. *Brit. J. Haemat.*, **14**, 643.

Chanarin, I., Dacie, J. V. & Mollin, D. L. (1959) Folic-acid deficiency in haemolytic anaemia. *Brit. J. Haemat.*, **5**, 245.

Cooper, R. A. & Shattil, S. J. (1971) Mechanisms of hemolysis—the minimal red-cell defect. *New Engl. J. Med.*, **285**, 1514.

Crosby, W. H. & Akeroyd, J. H. (1952) The limit of hemoglobin synthesis in hereditary hemolytic anemia. *Amer. J. Med.*, **13**, 273.

Crosby, W. H. & Dameshek, W. (1951) The significance of hemoglobinuria and associated hemosiderinuria, with particular reference to various types of hemolytic anemia. *J. Lab. Clin. Med.*, **38**, 829.

Dacie, J. V. (1963A) *The Haemolytic Anaemias—Congenital and Acquired.* Part I, p. 5. London: J. & A. Churchill Ltd.

Dacie, J. V. (1970) Autoimmune haemolytic anaemias. *Brit. med. J.*, **2**, 381.

Dean, H. M., Decker, C. L. & Baker, L. D. (1967) Temporary survival in clostridial hemolysis with absence of circulating red cells. *New Engl. J. Med.*, **277**, 700.

Fairley, N. H. (1941) Methaemalbumin. *Quart. J. Med. n.s.* **10, 95**, 115.

Finch, C. A. & Coleman, D. H. (1953) Patterns of erythropoiesis in hemolytic anemia. *J. Clin. Invest.*, **32**, 567.

Hillman, R. S. & Finch, C. A. (1969) The misused reticulocyte. *Brit. J. Haemat.*, **17**, 313.

Hillman, R. S. & Finch, C. A. (1971) Erythropoiesis. *New Engl. J. Med.*, **285**, 99.

International Committee for Standardization in Haematology (1971) Recommended methods for radioisotope red-cell survival studies. *Brit. J. Haemat.*, **21**, 241.

Jacob, H. S. (1968) Dysfunction of the red blood cell membrane in hereditary spherocytosis. *Brit. J. Haemat.*, **14**, 99.

Jacob, H. S. & Jandl, J. H. (1962) Effects of sulfhydryl inhibition on red blood cells. II. Studies *in vivo. J. Clin. Invest.*, **41**, 1514.

Jaffé, E. R. (1972) Oxidative hemolysis, or what made the red cell break? *New Engl. J. Med.*, **286**, 156.

Jandl, J. H., Greenberg, M. S., Yonemoto, R. H. & Castle, W. B. (1956) Clinical determination of the sites of red-cell sequestration in hemolytic anemias. *J. Clin. Invest.*, **35**, 842.

Jandl, J. H. (1965) Leaky red cells. *Blood*, **26**, 367.

Jandl, J. H. & Aster, R. H. (1967) Increased splenic pooling and the pathogenesis of hypersplenism. *Am. J. Med. Sci.*, **253**, 383.

Laurell, C. B. & Nyman, M. (1957) Studies on the serum haptoglobin level in hemoglobinemia and its influence on renal excretion of hemoglobin. *Blood*, **12**, 493.

Lemberg, R. & Legge, J. W. (1949) *Hematin Compounds and Bile Pigments.* New York: Interscience Publishers.

LoBuglio, A. F., Cotran, R. S. & Jandl, J. H. (1967) Red cells coated with immunoglobulin G: binding and sphering by mononuclear cells in man. *Science*, **158**, 1582.

McBride, J. A. & Jacob, H. S. (1970) Abnormal kinetics of red cell membrane cholesterol in acanthocytes: studies in genetic and experimental abetalipoproteinemia and in spur cell anemia. *Brit. J. Haemat.*, **18**, 383.

Miller, E. B., Singer, K. & Dameshek, W. (1942) The use of the daily fecal output of urobilinogen and the hemolytic index in the measurement of hemolysis. *Arch. Int. Med.*, **70**, 722.

Murphy, J. R. (1967) The influence of pH and temperature on some physical properties of normal erythrocytes and erythrocytes from patients with hereditary spherocytosis. *J. Lab. Clin. Med.*, **69**, 758.

Owren, P. A. (1948) Congenital hemolytic jaundice. The pathogenesis of the 'hemolytic crisis'. *Blood*, **3**, 231.

Rosse, W. F. & Dacie, J. V. (1966) Immune lysis of normal human and paroxysmal nocturnal hemoglobinuria (PNH) red blood cells. II. The role of complement components in the increased sensitivity of PNH red cells to immune lysis. *J. Clin. Invest.*, **45**, 749.

Sánchez-Medal, L., Pizzuto, J., Rodríguez-Moyado, H. & Espositó, L. (1969) Haemolysis and erythropoiesis. II. Reticulocytosis and rate of haemoglobin rise in haemolytic and deficiency anaemias. *Brit. J. Haemat.*, **17**, 343.

Smithies, O. (1955) Zone electrophoresis in starch gels: group variations in the serum proteins of normal human adults. *Biochem. J..*, **66**, 629.

Weed, R. I., LaCelle, P. L. & Merrill, E. W. (1969) Metabolic dependence of red cell deformity. *J. Clin. Invest.*, **48**, 795.

Young, L. E., Izzo, M. J. & Platzer, R. F. (1951) Hereditary spherocytosis. I. Clinical, hematologic and genetic features in 28 cases, with particular reference to the osmotic and mechanical fragility of incubated erythrocytes. *Blood*, **6**, 1073.

6. Hereditary Haemolytic Anaemias with Characteristic Red Cell Morphology

Hereditary spherocytosis (HS), *Aetiology and pathogenesis, Clinical features, Laboratory findings, Treatment* / Hereditary elliptocytosis (HE), *Aetiology, Clinical features, Laboratory findings, Treatment* / Stomatocytosis / Congenital haemolytic anaemia with dehydrated red cells / Acanthocytosis / Congenital dyserythropoietic anaemias (CDA).

Hereditary spherocytosis (HS) or acholuric jaundice was the first form of familial jaundice and anaemia to be defined, at the end of the last century. Many other forms of inherited haemolytic anaemia are now recognized and these are described in the succeeding sections under hereditary elliptocytosis, hereditary stomatocytosis, hereditary non-spherocytic haemolytic anaemia, thalassaemia and haemoglobinopathies. All these disorders have in common not only the fact that they are inherited but also that the haemolysis is due to an 'intrinsic' abnormality confined to the patient's red cells: viz. transfused normal red cells survive normally in these patients (Dacie and Mollison, 1943). This is in contradistinction to many acquired haemolytic anaemias, when the abnormality is often 'extrinsic' to the red cells, e.g. autoimmune haemolytic anaemia or microangiopathic haemolytic anaemia.

The hereditary or genetically determined haemolytic states may usefully be classified (Table 6.1) according to whether the defect affects (a) the cell wall (and therefore the red cell morphology), (b)

the metabolic processes leading to the synthesis of ATP (from glycolysis) or the maintenance of an adequate intracellular reduction potential (via pentose shunt and glutathione metabolism) and (c) the globin structure or synthesis (Van Eys, 1970). Although the haemoglobinopathies are rightly classified as haemolytic states it should be added that many are asymptomatic. Only a minority of the known aminoacid substitutions result in a functionally abnormal haemoglobin. In some instances the abnormal haemoglobin results in polycythaemia rather than haemolysis. In the sickling diseases the main clinical consequence is vascular occlusion rather than haemolysis. In the case of unstable haemoglobins there is a liability to haemolysis but methaemoglobinaemia may sometimes be the more prominent clinical feature. The thalassaemia syndromes show a haemolytic element but the anaemia is also to a large extent due to a failure of haemoglobin synthesis.

In those conditions where there is a severe metabolic or structural defect of the red cells haemolysis is present continuously, while in the

Table 6.1   Classification of genetically determined haemolytic anaemias

Defects in cell wall function
  Hereditary spherocytosis
  Hereditary elliptocytosis
  Various less well defined or rarer syndromes
Defects in metabolism
  Enzyme deficiencies in the shunt pathway and glutathione
    reduction or synthesis
  Glycolytic enzyme deficiencies
Defects of haemoglobin structure or synthesis
  Porphyrin synthesis abnormalities
  Haemoglobin protein structure
    Structural changes resulting in haemoglobin aggregation
    Structural changes resulting in haemoglobin instability
    Structural changes resulting in abnormal haemoglobin function
  Haemoglobin protein synthesis – the thalassaemia syndromes

Based upon Table 1 from Van Eys (1968) reproduced by permission of the author and Paediatric Clinics of North America, (Vol. 17, p. 449).

less severe defects this is only precipitated at times of metabolic stress such as in the neonatal period or exposure to drugs or the presence of infection.

HEREDITARY SPHEROCYTOSIS (HS)

Together with hereditary elliptocytosis, stomatocytosis and acanthocytosis the red cells in this disorder have *characteristic morphological abnormalities*. This is in contradistinction to the 'non-spherocytic haemolytic anaemias' or enzyme defects, and the haemoglobinopathies in which only *non-specific morphological abnormalities* of the red cells are present.

Aetiology and pathogenesis

Males and females are equally affected. The mode of inheritance is dominant but with variable degrees of expression which results in occasional apparent 'skipping' of a generation and also variable degrees of severity of the disease within the same family. Out of a total of 54 affected families, documented in two large series, there were 9 families where both parents of the propositus were apparently normal (Race, 1942; Young, 1955). It is not confined to any particular races but it is more common in Northern Europeans. The incidence in Wisconsin is 220 per million population (MacKinney, 1965).

The fundamental defect is thought to be an abnormality of the red cell membrane which permits excessive sodium ion entry into the cell (Fig. 6.1). This can be compensated for only by

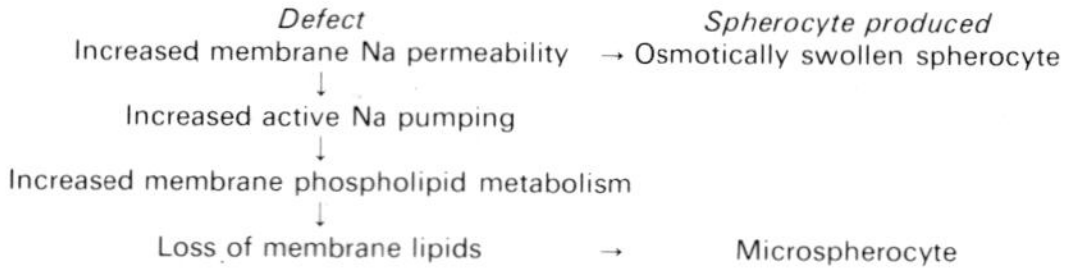

Defect
Increased membrane Na permeability → *Spherocyte produced* Osmotically swollen spherocyte
↓
Increased active Na pumping
↓
Increased membrane phospholipid metabolism
↓
Loss of membrane lipids → Microspherocyte

Fig. 6.1 Scheme relating increased membrane sodium permeability to spherocyte formation. (Reproduced from Jacob (1966), *American Journal of Medicine*, **41**, 734, by permission of the author and publishers).

overwork of the ATP-dependent cation pump, working in an opposite direction. This causes excessive demands for glucose metabolism. During splenic stagnation this demand may not be met, resulting in loss of cell viability (Jacob and Jandl, 1964; Mohler, 1965; Jacob, 1968). Loss of lipid from the red cell membrane during incubation (Prankherd, 1960) is thought to be a consequence of the increased cation transport. This loss seems to represent loss of whole fragments of cell membrane

(Weed and Bowdler, 1966). Since the smallest surface area for a given volume is a perfect sphere this loss of surface leads to the formation of spherocytes. The characteristic increased susceptibility to hypotonic lysis is the consequence of lack of distensibility of a sphere.

Clinical features

There is a wide variety in the severity of jaundice and anaemia in different patients and the course of the disease is usually episodal. About half manifest themselves in the neonatal period, mimicking haemolytic disease of the newborn. Rarely it may be discovered fortuitously in old age. Most commonly it is first diagnosed in children of school age. The manifestations are jaundice, anaemia, splenomegaly and less often gall stones or leg ulcers.

JAUNDICE

Neonatal jaundice occurred in 23 out of 43 patients in one series. Exchange transfusions were required in 4 of these patients (Stamey and Diamond, 1957). Signs of kernicterus have developed in a severely jaundiced baby not exchange transfused (Roddy, 1954). The jaundice in later childhood or adolescence is slight and intermittent. It may be precipitated by a coincident infection.

ANAEMIA

As mentioned above this is very variable. It is commonly of only moderate degree giving rise to slight pallor, but during 'crises' the anaemia becomes rapidly severe accompanied by dyspnoea, nausea, vomiting, abdominal pain, extreme lassitude and fever. These crises are more often 'aplastic' than 'haemolytic'. Jaundice increases in the haemolytic but not in the aplastic crises. They may be precipitated by an infection and perhaps by concomitant folic acid deficiency (Delamore *et al.*, 1961). Chronic anaemia may be accompanied by impaired growth and mental retardation.

SPLENOMEGALY

This is probably a constant feature but not necessarily to a degree where it is clinically palpable. In approximately 1/6th of patients the spleen cannot be felt. It is usually firm and not tender, but may become tender after splenic infarction or haemolytic crisis.

Gall stones and leg ulcer are uncommon in children but become more frequent with advancing age. Radiological evidence of bone changes in the skull are less frequent than in thalassaemia. Ectopic bony tumours, particularly in the thorax, have been described and these contain active erythropoietic tissue (Hanford et al., 1960).

Laboratory findings

The characteristic finding is the presence of spherocytosis, seen in blood films (Fig. 5.1), or demonstrated by increased osmotic fragility. (Fig. 6.2). In mild cases the spherocytes may be

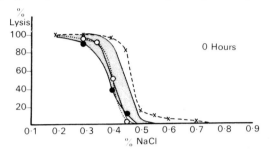

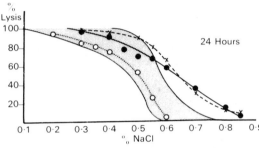

Fig. 6.2 Erythrocyte osmotic fragility curves from fresh blood (0 h) and blood incubated for 24 h at 37°. Patients suffered from hereditary spherocytosis, (x - - - - - x); hereditary non-spherocytic haemolytic anemia (Type I), (o . . . . o); and hereditary non-spherocytic haemolytic anemia (Type II), (● ———— ●). The shaded areas represent the normal range. (Reproduced from Dacie (1963), *The Haemolytic Anaemias, Part I*, p. 41, by permission of the author).

less obvious and the osmotic fragility so close to normal as to be inconclusive. In these cases the fragility curve performed after sterile incubation of the whole blood may prove more conclusive as this procedure accentuates the defects in hereditary spherocytosis (Young et al., 1951). Although sensitive this test is not entirely specific for hereditary spherocytosis, being abnormal whenever autohaemolysis is increased as in some of the non-spherocytic haemolytic anaemias. Figure 6.2 shows comparative fragility curves in fresh and incubated blood from a case of HS as well as from a case of Type II congenital non-spherocytic haemolytic anaemia in which autohaemolysis is characteristically increased.

Autohaemolysis at 24 and 48 hrs is increased in HS, and is corrected by the addition of glucose (or ATP) (Selwyn and Dacie, 1954). In some atypical cases of HS autohaemolysis may be diagnostic when the osmotic fragility is inconslusive (Zail et al., 1967).

Accompanying the spherocytosis there is usually a mild to moderate degree of anaemia together with polychromasia, circulating normoblasts and a reticulocytosis as evidence of increased erythropoiesis. If the haemolytic process is fully compensated there may be no anaemia but a chronically elevated reticulocyte count. The marrow shows normoblastic hyperplasia. Stainable iron tends to be increased.

An aplastic crisis is accompanied by a total change in the blood picture. Spherocytosis appears more marked. This may be due to a failure of RBC production leading to an ageing population (Dacie, 1963B). Reticulocytes are low or absent and no polychromasia or normoblasts are found on the blood film. The serum bilirubin falls. There is frequently thrombocytopenia and neutropenia, never found at other times in this disease (Owren, 1948; Gasser, 1950). The marrow shows transient hypoplasia with giant proerythroblasts but few normoblasts and a maturation arrest of the myeloid series (Dameshek and Bloom, 1948). The marrow arrest may persist for 7–14 days. Increased excretion of urocanic acid after a histidine load has been reported (Chanarin et al., 1962) in one megaloblastic case but it does not appear that folic acid deficiency is the usual cause of these crises. The simultaneous development among several members of the same family suggests an infective agent (Marson et al., 1950).

The pigment metabolism is similar to that in other haemolytic anaemias with the reservations mentioned regarding possible periods of superadded obstructive or hepatocellular jaundice. Indirect bilirubin is elevated in approximately 70 per cent of cases (MacKinney et al., 1962), usually to between 1 and 4 mg/100 ml. During aplastic crises there may be a reduction in bilirubin production and during haemolytic crises an increase.

Red cell survival studies are not required for purposes of routine diagnosis but have shown a rate of cell destruction 6–8 times that of normal (Motulsky et al., 1955). Surface counting shows sequestration in the spleen rather than the liver (Hughes Jones and Szur, 1957). Transfused cells survive normally.

Following splenectomy the anaemia, reticulocytosis, pigment excretion and red cell survival return to normal or near normal, but the spherocytosis and abnormal osmotic fragility persist indefinitely. Autohaemolysis tends to decrease after splenectomy (Selwyn and Dacie, 1954).

Concomitant iron deficiency in children may temporarily mask the spherocytosis due to the increase in thin, flat red cells at the expense of spherocytes. This does not alleviate the haemolytic process, however (Crosby and Conrad, 1960).

Distinction between other varieties of spherocytic haemolytic anaemia may be made by the negative Coombs test, negative Heinz body test, negative Ham's test and normal haemoglobin analysis. The latter point is mentioned since at least one type of haemoglobinopathy, haemoglobin Köln, is accompanied by spherocytosis. Foetal haemoglobin, however, is slightly elevated in a proportion of patients with hereditary spherocytosis. On rare occasions the direct Coombs test has been positive in association with infections. Unusual variants of the disease have been reported with associated thrombocytopenia in infants (Zetterström and Strindberg, 1958).

In the neonatal period the distinction between ABO haemolytic disease, which commonly shows spherocytosis, is made by a consideration of the foeto-maternal blood groups and the absence of a maternal alpha or beta haemolysin or other immune antibodies. The incubation fragility test in neonatal HS is sometimes clearly abnormal when the osmotic fragility would pass for normal by adult standards (Trucco and Brown, 1967). The autohaemolysis test in HS is corrected by glucose but there is no correction in ABO haemolytic disease (Kostinas et al., 1967).

Examination of the blood from both parents may disclose a mild or compensated spherocytic haemolytic anaemia in one or other, considerably simplifying the problems of diagnosis, as does a known family history of the disease. MacKinney et al. (1962) showed that haemoglobin, film, reticulocyte count and bilirubin estimation detected the great majority of carriers.

Treatment

Splenectomy is indicated in all patients with definite hereditary spherocytosis except perhaps the rare case of those with an entirely compensated haemolytic anaemia and no history of aplastic crisis or evidence of gall stones (Dacie, 1963C). It is advisable to defer this operation, however, until at least the age of 3–4 years (Glenn et al., 1954) because of possible liability to serious infections in young children following splenectomy. Eraklis

et al. (1967) found 2 deaths out of a series of 140 children having splenectomy for HS. In both these fatal cases splenectomy had been performed before the age of 2 years because of the severity of haemolysis. The liability to infection may have been related either to the age or the severity of the disease. The clinical results of splenectomy are excellent and it is doubtful if any true case of hereditary spherocytosis has failed to respond. The rare late recurrence of haemolytic anaemia is likely to be due to growth of an accessory spleen (MacKenzie et al., 1962).

The anaemia is cured, the reticulocytosis virtually disappears, the bilirubin excretion falls to the upper limit of normal and red cell survival returns to normal or to a value which can easily be compensated. In one of the larger reported series Welch and Dameshek (1950) obtained complete clinical remissions in all of their 38 patients. This is typical of other series.

Transfusion is needed as supportive therapy in the early months of life, at times of severe anaemia or aplastic crisis; and exchange transfusion if the bilirubin level approaches 20 mg/100 ml in the neonatal period.

Steroids have no place in treatment. Folic acid supplementation is advisable if there is any factor predisposing to deficiency such as poor diet or malabsorption.

HEREDITARY ELLIPTOCYTOSIS (HE)

This term is used synonymously with 'ovalocytosis' (Dacie, 1963D). The disease appears to be world wide and the incidence in one American series was 1 in 2,500 (Wyandt et al., 1941).

Aetiology

The inheritance is dominant and the genes for HE appear to be located on the same chromosome as those carrying the Rh blood groups (Goodall et al., 1953). There is a variable degree of expression and only a proportion of affected individuals show evidence of a haemolytic anaemia (Ozer and Mills, 1964). Rare probable homozygotes have been described who had a severe haemolytic anaemia (Prior and Pitney, 1967). The shortened red cell survival sometimes present in this disorder may not be due to the abnormal cell shape per se but to an increased membrane permeability to sodium, similar to that in HS (Peters et al., 1966). This is consistent with the excessive decrease in ATP levels during incubation of HE cells (De Gruchy et al., 1962).

Clinical features

Many patients are entirely symptom free but a small proportion, about 12 per cent, have a clinical syndrome indistinguishable from HS (Penfold and Lipscomb, 1943), including jaundice, splenomegaly, and occasionally gall stones and leg ulcers. In the more severe forms of HE anaemia and jaundice may occur in the neonatal period (Cutting et al., 1965; Lipton, 1955). At other times the anaemia may be precipitated by a recent infection.

Laboratory findings

The elliptocytes are seen in blood films as elongated or oval cells (Fig. 6.3). They constitute 25 to 90 per cent of the red cells and have to be distinguished from the small proportion, up to be present (Cutting et al., 1965). It is these patients with increased haemolysis and a tendency to spherocytosis that show increased osmotic fragility and autohaemolysis (De Gruchy et al., 1962; Weiss, 1963). No abnormal Hb is present, and usually there is no abnormal persistence of foetal haemoglobin (White et al., 1959).

The red cell survival is shortened in those cases with active haemolysis and preferential sequestration in the spleen can be demonstrated (Dacie, 1963E). The morphological abnormality persists after splenectomy and is then accompanied by an increased number of fragmented cells, but the red cell survival returns to normal.

Treatment

Transfusion is effective in so far as the transfused blood survives normally in the patient's

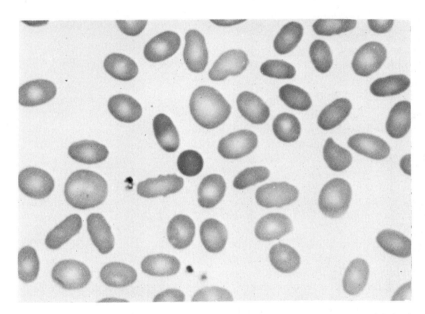

Fig. 6.3 Elliptocytosis with haemolysis. Both elliptocytes and spherocytes are present. This is the typical picture in the minority of elliptocytosis patients who have haemolysis. Blood film (x 5,000).

10 to 15 per cent of oval cells seen in normal blood or elongated cells in iron deficiency (Wyandt et al., 1941). The morphological abnormality may be absent at birth, developing at about 4–6 months (Helz and Menten, 1944). The MCHC is normal. Otherwise the blood picture may show no anaemia, a compensated haemolytic anaemia or an overt haemolytic anaemia. In those cases with marked haemolysis the cells are more oval than elliptic and oval spherocytes plus fragmented cells may also circulation. Splenectomy benefits those with active haemolysis (Lipton, 1955).

STOMATOCYTOSIS

A rare morphological abnormality in which 10–30 per cent of the red cells showed a linear instead of circular central area of pallor on a stained blood film (Fig. 6.4) was first described by Lock, Sephton Smith and Hardisty (1961). This

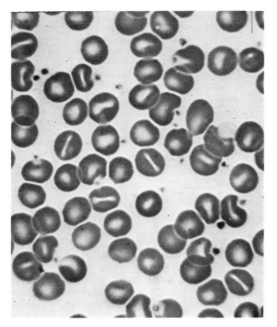

Fig. 6.4 Stomatocytes. In this rare congenital haemolytic anemia the central area of pallor of the red cells appears as a slit or mouth (x 1000).

appearance suggested a mouth-like orifice in the cell, leading to the term 'stomatocyte'. When suspended in plasma the cells assumed a bowl-shaped form. It was associated with a chronic haemolytic anaemia which was accentuated after infections and which persisted after splenectomy in a girl of 5 years and her mother. The same morphological changes were seen in an older patient with a less severe haemolytic anaemia, again improved but not cured by splenectomy (Miller et al., 1965). In this case the parents and a sibling were unaffected. Another single case with normal family studies, was described by Meadow (1967). Two other reports of stomatocytosis in a single case (Zarkowsky et al., 1968), and in a young boy, his father and grandfather (Oski et al., 1969) have drawn attention to the high sodium and low potassium content of the red cells. The anaemia was severe and improved but not cured by splenectomy in the first, and was mild in the second of these reports.

Presentation in these cases included mild jaundice at birth (Oski et al., 1969), splenomegaly at 6 months (Lock et al., 1961), and as a rather consistent feature, pallor and jaundice associated with infections. Fairly gross splenomegaly by the age of 3–4 years was also a consistent finding. There was a considerable liability for the patients to be diagnosed initially as HS and for splenectomy to be performed. The persistence of haemolysis after splenectomy led to a reinvestigation and the correct diagnosis (Meadow, 1967).

This condition mimics HS both in its mode of inheritance and by virtue of the increased osmotic fragility, incubation fragility and autohaemolysis. The autohaemolysis was as high as 61–65 per cent in Lock's patients after 48 hr at 37 °C with partial correction by added glucose.

In the report by Miller et al. (1965), but not in others, the autohaemolysis was particularly enhanced at 4 °C compared to 37 °C. An unusual feature noted by both Lock et al. (1961) and Oski et al. (1969) was that the older red cells in these patients became progressively lighter with age, which is opposite to the normal trend. Centrifugation studies showed that the older cells, at the top of the column of blood, showed more marked morphological changes and osmotic fragility than the younger cells. Osmometric studies suggest that there is inelasticity of the red cell membrane (Lock et al., 1961). Together with the demonstration of an increased membrane permeability to cations (Zarkowsky et al., 1968; Oski et al., 1969) it now appears that stomatocytosis falls within the same group of disorders as HS and HE. To confuse the issue, however, a similar defect of sodium transport has been found in a Negro family without evidence of haemolysis (Balfe et al., 1968). Red cell survival studies show that the spleen is the main site of removal when labelled stomatocytes are injected into normal recipients. The fact that they are also removed by the liver may explain the incomplete benefit from splenectomy.

Minor differences in the red cell metabolism have been observed in the reported cases, including decreased G-6-PD activity in one family and decreased glutathione content in another patient. It has been suggested, therefore, that stomatocytosis may be a heterogenous group of red cell disorders that share certain osmotic similarities (Oski et al., 1969). This suggestion has been supported by the description of a further variant of stomatocytosis with normal osmotic fragility (Miller et al., 1972).

CONGENITAL HAEMOLYTIC ANAEMIA WITH DEHYDRATED RED CELLS

A 21-year-old woman of French and Irish descent with a life-long history of anaemia, jaundice and hepatosplenomegaly, and with a similarly affected 3-year-old son has recently been described by Glader et al. (1974). The red cells appeared crenated and dehydrated on blood films and there was marked osmotic resistance. Red cell sodium was increased and potassium and water content reduced. The basic defect appeared to be increased membrane permeability to cations; this being greater for potassium than for sodium. Potassium loss exceeded sodium gain and total cation content was decreased. Haemolysis persisted after splenectomy in the mother.

ACANTHOCYTOSIS

A bizarre morphological abnormality in which 70–80 per cent of the red cells showed multiple spikes around their periphery (*Akantha* =

(Simon and Ways, 1964). It has been suggested syndrome is related to coincident vitamin E (tocopherol) deficiency, related to malabsorption or immaturity (Kayden and Silber, 1965; Dodge *et al.*, 1967). Other workers have emphasized the altered phospholipid composition of the red cell membrane (Weed and Reed, 1966) or the accumulation of membrane cholesterol and the effect of this on cell plasticity as the cause of haemolysis (McBride and Jacob, 1970). In the neonatal period this disorder may have to be distinguished from the benign non-hereditary disorder infantile pycnocytosis (Chap. 12). Also a closely related disorder consisting of haemolytic anaemia,

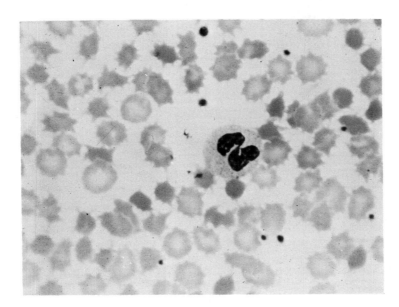

Fig. 6.5 Acanthocytosis. Blood film (x 2,700).

thorn in Greek) was first described in a consanguinous Jewish family by Singer, Fisher and Perlstein (1952). Inheritance was thought to be recessive and the abnormality was associated with atypical retinitis pigmentosa, coeliac syndrome and neurological manifestations. This patient showed no evidence of haemolysis nor other haematological abnormality. The defect is accompanied by abetalipoproteinaemia and low plasma cholesterol. Mild or intermittent haemolysis has been present in other cases (Farquar and Ways, 1966). *In vivo* red cell life span is slightly shortened. The degree of cell deformation increases with cell age. There is normal red cell glycolysis, ATP formation and methaemoglobin reduction but autohaemolysis is markedly increased both at 37 °C and 4 °C even in the presence of EDTA

dwarfism, and mental retardation associated with that the variable haemolytic element in this decreased lecithin content of red cells has been described in Japan. There were no other affected members of the family (Arakawa *et al.*, 1966).

CONGENITAL DYSERYTHROPOIETIC ANAEMIAS (CDA)

These rare congenital and hereditary anaemias differ from those described earlier in this chapter in that the characteristic morphological abnormalities are to be found in the marrow rather than the peripheral blood, although non-specific abnormalities are also present in the morphology of the circulating red cells. They also differ from the other forms of haemolytic anaemia described in this chapter in that much of the 'haemolysis' takes place at the level of marrow erythroblasts and is more accurately described as *ineffective erythropoiesis* (*Lancet*, 1974). Heimpel (1970) has defined CDA as a therapy-refractory anaemia with ineffective erythropoiesis which manifests itself in the first 15 years of life, often in the neonatal period. Clinically there is chronic mild anaemia seldom requiring regular transfusion, with chronic or intermittent mild hyperbilirubinaemia closely simulating Gilbert's syndrome (hereditary defect in uptake of conjugated bilirubin into the liver cells). Shortened red cell survival is present in some patients. Progressive iron overload occurs, irrespective of blood transfusion, leading eventually to haemosiderosis and hepatic cirrhosis. Granulopoiesis and thrombopoiesis remain normal. Most patients have been of European stock.

teristic serological reactions (Verwilghen *et al.*, 1973).

Recent detailed reports of CDA Type I (Lewis, Nelson and Pitcher, 1972) and CDA Type III (Goudsmit *et al.*, 1972) are also available. Photomicrographs in these reports show the most marked erythroblastic multinuclearity ('gigantoblasts') in Type III and the less bizarre binucleated normoblastic hyperplasia, including internuclear bridges, in Type I. Studies of DNA synthesis in the different types have suggested that in Type I the block is at the level of basophilic normoblast (Lewis, Nelson and Pitcher, 1972), in Type II at the polychromatic to orthocromatic level (Queisser *et al.*, 1970), while in Type III there is a departure from the normal diploid DNA content per normoblast nucleus, raising the possibility of amitotic divisions (Goudsmit *et al.*, 1972).

In HEMPAS (Type II) the most comprehensive

Table 6.2 Classification of CDA

	Marrow		Blood	Inheritance
Type I	Megaloblastic Internuclear chromatin bridges		Macrocytic	Autosomal recessive
Type II ('HEMPAS')	Bi-and multinuclearity. Pluripolar mitoses		Normocytic	Autosomal recessive
Type III	Giant multinuclearity with up to 12 nuclei		Macrocytic	Autosomal dominant

Data predominantly from Heimpel and Wendt (1968).

Heimpel and Wendt (1968) originally classified CDA into 3 types (Table 6.2) on the basis of miscellaneous case reports collected from the literature plus 2 cases of their own. Type II seems, from subsequent reports, to be the most common of these rare disorders with 39 cases collected in a recent review (Verwilghen *et al.*, 1973), and has acquired the acronyn HEMPAS by virtue of the distinguishing feature that the red cells are susceptible to lysis in acidified normal serum (hereditary erythroblastic multi-nuclearity associated with a positive acidified-serum test). The red cells in HEMPAS are strongly agglutinated by anti-i, unlike normal postnatal red cells, and lysed by anti-i and anti-I. Agglutination by an alloantibody present in normal serum, but not in the patient's serum, occurs (Crookston *et al.*, 1969). Electron microscopy demonstrates a double red cell membrane, 40 to 60 nm within the normal membrane, in some of the erythroblasts and red cells in HEMPAS and it is suggested that this abnormality is the cause of the defective cell division, the failure of the multinucleated erythroblasts to expel their nuclei, and the charac-

review by Verwilghen *et al.* (1973) showed anaemia and jaundice in 35 of 39 patients, with less than a quarter needing repeated transfusion. Splenomegaly was present in 25 of 34, hepatomegaly in 15 of 34, cirrhosis and/or hepatic haemosiderosis in 7 and gall stones in 8. Mental retardation was present in 5, and bilateral cataracts in 1 patient. Osmotic fragility was increased in 10 of 20 and autohaemolysis slightly increased in 5 of 20. Peripheral blood films showed irregularly contracted RBCs, with hypochromic cells, 'teardrop' poikilocytes, basophilic stippling and occasional circulating normoblasts. Marrow examination showed erythroblastic hyperplasia with many binucleated normoblasts together with the surprising finding of Gaucher-like cells, containing birefringent inclusions, in 15 out of 17 patients.

Splenectomy was performed in 11 patients, including the most severely affected, and resulted in moderate to marked improvement. Iron therapy is strongly contraindicated, and desferrioxamine had little effect on the iron overload. In a recent paediatric report of a Type II case vitamin E administration apparently improved the RBC survival and haemoglobin level with reduction in serum bilirubin and reticulocyte count. Red cell lipid pattern was restored to normal but morphological abnormalities increased (O'Regan *et al.*, 1974).

REFERENCES

Arakawa, T., Katsushima, N. & Fujiwara, T. (1966) A hemolytic anemia with abnormality of erythrocyte lipids and dwarfism—probably a new syndrome. *TOKOKU J. Exptl. Med.*, **88**, 35.

Balfe, J. W., Cole, C., Smith, E. K. M., Graham, J. B. & Welt, L. G. (1968) Hereditary sodium transport defect in human red cells. *J. Clin. Invest.*, **47**, 4a.

Chanarin, I., Burman, D. & Bennett, M. C. (1962) The familial aplastic crisis in hereditary spherocytosis. Urocanic acid and formiminoglutamic acid excretion in a case with megaloblastic arrest. *Blood*, **20**, 33.

Crookston, J. H., Crookston, M. C., Burnie, K. L., Francombe, W. H., Dacie, J. V., Davis, J. A. & Lewis, S. M. (1969) Hereditary erythroblastic multinuclearity associated with a positive acidified—serum test: A type of congenital dysterythropoietic anaemia. *Brit. J. Haemat.*, **17**, 11.

Crosby, W. H. & Conrad, M. E. (1960) Hereditary spherocytosis: Observations on hemolytic mechanisms and iron metabolism. *Blood*, **15**, 662.

Cutting, H. O., McHugh, W. J., Conrad, F. G. & Marlow, A. A. (1965) Autosomal dominant hemolytic anemia characterized by ovalocytosis. A family study of seven involved members. *Amer. J. Med.*, **39**, 21.

Dacie, J. V. (1963B) *The Haemolytic Anaemias*—Part I. p. 112. London: Churchill.

Dacie, J. V. (1963C) *The Haemolytic Anaemias*—Part I. p. 117. London: Churchill.

Dacie, J. V. (1963D) *The Haemolytic Anaemias*—Part I. p. 151. London: Churchill.

Dacie, J. V. (1963E) *The Haemolytic Anaemias*—Part I. p. 162. London: Churchill.

Dacie, J. V. & Mollison, P. L. (1943) Survival of normal erythrocytes after transfusion to patients with familial haemolytic anaemia (acholuric jaundice). *Lancet*, **1**, 550.

Dameshek, W. & Bloom, M. L. (1948) The events in the hemolytic crisis of hereditary spherocytosis, with particular reference to the reticulocytopenia, pancytopenia and abnormal splenic mechanism. *Blood*, **3**, 1381.

DeGruchy, G. C., Loder, P. B. & Hennessy, I. V. (1962) Haemolysis and glycolytic metabolism in hereditary elliptocytosis. *Brit. J. Haemat.*, **8**, 168.

Delamore, I. W., Richmond, J. & Davies, S. H. (1961) Megaloblastic anaemia in congenital spherocytosis. *Brit. med. J.*, **1**, 543.

Dodge, J. T., Cohen, G., Kayden, H. J. & Phillips, G. B. (1967) Peroxidative hemolysis of the red blood cells from patients with abetalipoproteinemia (acanthocytosis). *J. Clin. Invest.*, **46**, 357.

Eraklis, A. J., Kevy, S. V., Diamond, L. K. & Gross, R. E. (1967) Hazard of overwhelming infection after splenectomy in childhood. *New Engl. J. Med.*, **276**, 1225.

Eys, J. Van (1970) Recent progress in genetic hemolytic disorders: a practical approach. *Pediat. Clin. N. America*, **17**, 449.

Farquhar, J. W. & Ways, P. (1966) Abetalipoproteinemia. In *The Metabolic Basis of Inherited Disease*, 2nd edn. Edited by Stanbury, J. B., Wyngaarden, J. B. and Fredrickson, D. S. New York: McGraw-Hill Book Co.

Gasser, C. (1950) Erythroblastopénie aiguè dans les anémies hémolytiques. *Sang*, **21**, 237.

Glader, B. E., Fortier, N., Albala, M. M. & Nathan, D. G. (1974) Hemolytic anemia associated with RBC dehydration and potassium loss. *New Eng. J. Med.*, **291**, 491.

Glenn, F., Cornell, G. N., Smith, C. H. & Schulman, I. (1954) Splenectomy in children with idiopathic thrombocytopenic purpura, hereditary spherocytosis and mediterranean anaemia. *Surg. Gynec. Obstet.*, **99**, 689.

Goudsmit, R., Beckers, D., de Bruijore, J. I., Engelfriet, C. P., James, J., Morselt, A. F. W. & Reynierse, E. (1972) Congenital dyserythropoietic anaemia, type III. *Brit. J. Haema.*, **23**, 97.

Hanford, R. B., Schneider, G. R. & MacCarthy, J. D. (1960) Massive thoracic extramedullary hemopoiesis. *New Engl. J. Med.*, **263**, 120.

Goodall, H. B., Hendry, D. W. W., Lawler, S. W. & Stephen, S. A. (1953) Data on linkage in man: elliptocytosis and blood groups. II. Family 3. *Ann. Eugen. (London)*, **17**, 272.

Heimpel, H. & Wendt, F. (1968) Congenital dyserythropoietic anaemia with karyorrhexis and multinuclearity of erythroblasts. *Helv. Medica Acta*, **34**, 103.

Helz, M. K. & Menten, M. L. (1944) Elliptocytosis, a report of two cases. *J. Lab. Clin. Med.*, **29**, 185.

Heimpel, H. (1970) *Kongenital dyserythropoietische Anaemie n in Blut und Blutkrankheiten II*. Berlin: Springer.

Hughes Jones, N. C. & Szur, L. (1957) Determination of sites of red cell destruction using 51 Cr-labelled cells. *Brit. J. Haemat.*, **3**, 320.

Jacob, H. S. (1968) Dysfunction of the red blood cell membrane in hereditary spherocytosis. *Brit. J. Haemat.*, **14**, 99.

Jacob, H. S. & Jandl, J. H. (1964) Increased cell membrane permeability in the pathogenesis of hereditary spherocytosis. *J. Clin. Invest.*, **43**, 1704.

Kayden, H. J. & Silber, R. (1965) The role of vitamin E deficiency in the abnormal autohemolysis of acanthocytosis. *Trans. Assoc. Am. Physicians*, **78**, 334.

Kostinas, J. E., Cantow, E. F. & Wetzel, R. A. (1967) Autohemolysis of cord blood in congenital spherocytosis and ABO incompatibility. *J. Pediat.*, **70**, 273.

Lancet (1974) Editorial : Ineffective erythropoiesis. *Lancet*, **i**, 1164.

Lipton, E. L. (1955) Elliptocytosis with hemolytic anemia: The effects of splenectomy. *Pediatrics*, **15**, 67.

Lewis, S. M., Nelson, D. A. & Pitcher, C. S. (1972) Clinical and ultrastructural aspects of congenital dyserythropoietic anaemia Type I. *Brit. J. Haemat.*, **23**, 113.

Lock, S. P., Smith, R. S. & Hardisty, R. M. (1961) Stomatocytosis: A hereditary red cell anomaly associated with haemolytic anaemia. *Brit. J. Haemat.*, **7**, 303.

McBride, J. A. & Jacob, H. S. (1970) Abnormal kinetics of red cell membrane cholesterol in acanthocytes: Studies in genetic and experimental abetalipoproteinaemia and in spur cell anaemia. *Brit. J. Haemat.*, **18**, 383.

Mackenzie, F. A. F., Eastcott, H. H. G., Barkhan, P., Elliot, D. H., Hughes Jones, N. C. & Mollison, P. L. (1962) Relapse in hereditary spherocytosis with proven splenunculus. *Lancet*, **1**, 1102.

MacKinney, A. A. (1965) Hereditary spherocytosis. Clinical family studies. *Arch. Intern. Med. (Chicago)*, **116**, 257.

MacKinney, A. A., Morton, N. E., Kosower, M. S. & Schilling, R. F. (1962) Ascertaining genetic carriers of hereditary spherocytosis by statistical analyses of multiple laboratory tests. *J. Clin. Invest.*, **41**, 554.

Marson, F. G., Meynell, M. J. & Tabbush, H. (1950) Familial crisis in acholuric jaundice. *Brit. med. J.*, **2**, 760.

Meadow, S. R. (1967) Stomatocytosis. *Proc. Roy. Soc. Med.*, **60**, 13.

Miller, G., Townes, P. L. & MacWhinney, J. B. (1965) A new congenital hemolytic anemia with deformed erythrocytes (?Stomatocytes) and remarkable susceptibility of erythrocytes to cold hemolysis *in vitro*. *Pediatrics*, **35**, 906.

Miller, D. R., Rickles, F. R., Lichtman, M. A., LaCelle, P. L., Bates, J. & Weed, R. I. (1972) A new variant of hereditary hemolytic anemia with stomatocytosis and erythrocyte cation abnormality. *Blood*, **38**, 184.

Mohler, D. M. (1965) Adenosine triphosphate metabolism in hereditary spherocytosis. *J. Clin. Invest.*, **44**, 1417.

Motulsky, A. G., Giblett, E., Coleman, D., Gabrio, B. & Finch, C. A. (1955) Life-span, glucose metabolism and osmotic fragility of erythrocytes in hereditary spherocytosis. *J. IClin. Invest.*, **34**, 911.

O'Regan, S., Melhorn, D. K., Newman, A. J. & Graham, R. C. (1974) Erythrocyte lipids and vitamin E in type II congenital dyserythropoietic anemia. *J. Pediat.*, **84**, 355.

Owren, P. A. (1948) Congenital hemolytic jaundice. The pathogenesis of the 'hemolytic crisis'. *Blood*, **3**, 231.

Oski, F. A., Naiman, J. L., Blum, S. F., Zerkowsky, H. S., Whaun, J., Shohet, S. B., Green, A. & Nathan, D.G. (1969) Congenital hemolytic anemia with high sodium low potassium red cells. Studies of three generations of a family with a new variant. *New Engl. J. Med.*, **280**, 910.

Ozer, L. & Mills, G. C. (1964) Elliptocytosis with haemolytic anaemia. *Brit. J. Haemat.*, **10**, 468.

Penfold, J. B. & Lipscomb, J. M. (1943) Elliptocytosis in man, associated with hereditary haemorrhagic telangiectasia. *Quart. J. Med.*, **12**, 157.

Peters, J. C., Rowland, M., Israels, L. G. *et al.* (1966) Erythrocyte sodium transport in hereditary elliptocytosis. *Can. J. Physiol. Pharmacol.*, **44**, 817,

Prankherd, T. A. J. (1960) Studies on the pathogenesis of haemolysis in hereditary spherocytosis. *Quart. J. Med. n.s.*, **29**, 199.

Prior, D. S. & Pitney, W. R. (1967) Elliptocytosis: A report of two families from New Guinea. *Brit. J. Haemat.*, **13**, 126.

Queisser, W., Spiertz, E., Jost, E. & Heimpel, H. (1970) Proliferation disturbance of erythroblasts in congenital dyserythroblastic anaemia (CDA) Type I and II. In *Proc. XIII Congr. Int. Soc. Haematol.*, p. 236. New York: Springer Verlage.

Race, R. R. (1942) On the inheritance and linkage relations of acholuric jaundice. *Ann. Eugen. (Lond.)*, **11**, 365.

Roddy, R. (1954) Clinical conferences at St. Christopher's Hospital for Children: Two cases of hereditary spherocytosis manifest in the newborn period. *J. Pediat.*, **44**, 213.

Selwyn, J. G. & Dacie, J. V. (1954) Autohemolysis and other changes resulting from the incubation *in vitro* of red cells from patients with congenital hemolytic anemia. *Blood*, **9**, 414.

Simon, E. R. & Ways, P. (1964) Incubation hemolysis and red cell metabolism in acanthocytosis. *J. Clin. Invest.*, **43**, 1311.

Singer, K., Fisher, B. & Perlstein, M. A. (1952) Acanthocytosis: A genetic erythrocytic malformation. *Blood*, **7**, 577.

Stamey, C. C. & Diamond, L. K. (1957) Congenital hemolytic anemia in the newborn: Relationship to kernicterus. *Am. J. Dis. Child.*, **94**, 616.

Trucco, J. I. & Brown, A. K. (1967) Neonatal manifestations of hereditary spherocytosis. *Am. J. Dis. Child.*, **113**, 263.

Verwilghen, R. L., Lewis, S. M., Dacie, J. V., Crookston, J. H. & Crookston, M. C. (1973) HEMPAS: Congenital dyserythropoietic anaemia (Type II). *Quarterly Journal of Medicine*, **42**, 257.

Weed, R. I. & Bowdler, A. J. (1966) Metabolic dependence of the critical hemolytic volume of human erythrocytes: Relationship to osmotic fragility and autohemolysis in hereditary spherocytosis and normal red cells. *J. Clin. Invest.*, **45**, 1137.

Weed, R. I. & Reed, C. F. (1966) Membrane alterations leading to red cell destruction. *Am. J. Med.*, **41**, 681.

Weiss, H. J. (1963) Hereditary elliptocytosis with hemolytic anemia. *Amer. J. Med.*, **35**, 455.

Welch, C. S. & Dameshek, W. (1950) Splenectomy in blood dyscrasias. *New Engl. J. Med.*, **242**, 601.

White, J. C., Beaven, G. H. & Ellis, M. (1959) Unpublished observations, quoted by Dacie, J. V. (1963) *The Haemolytic Anaemias*, Part I. London: Churchill.

Wyandt, H., Bancroft, P. M. & Winship, T. O. (1941) Elliptic erythrocytes in man. *Arch. Intern. Med. (Chicago)*, **68**, 1043.

Young, L. E., Platzer, R. F., Ervin, D. M. & Izzo, M. J. (1951) Hereditary spherocytosis. II. Observations on the role of the spleen. *Blood*, **6**, 1099.

Young, L. E. (1955) Observations on inheritance and heterogeneity of chronic spherocytosis. *Trans. Ass. Amer. Phycns.*, **68**, 141.

Zail, S. S., Krawitz, P., Viljoen, E., Kramer, S. & Metz, J. (1967) Atypical hereditary spherocytosis: Biochemical studies and sites of erythrocyte destruction. *Brit. J. Haemat.*, **13**, 323.

Zarkowsky, H. S., Oski, F. A., Sha'afi, R., Shohet, S. B. & Nathan, D. G. (1968) Congenital hemolytic anemia with high sodium, low potassium red cells. I. Studies of membrane permeability. *New Engl. J. Med.*, **278**, 573.

Zetterström, R. & Strindberg, B. (1958) Sporadic congenital spherocytosis associated with congenital hypoplastic thrombocytopenia and malformations. *Acta Paediat.*, **47**, 14.

7. Hereditary Non-Spherocytic Haemolytic Anaemias (Enzyme Deficiencies)

Introduction / Biochemical considerations / Disorders of the hexose monophosphate shunt / Glucose-6-phosphate dehydrogenase (G-6-PD), *Clinical manifestations of G-6-PD* / Other defects affecting availability of reduced glutathione (GSH), *6-Phosphogluconate dehydrogenase (6-PGD)*, *Glutathione reductase (GSSG-R)*, *Glutathione peroxidase (GSH-Px)*, *Defects of glutathione (GSH) synthesis* / Disorders of the glycolytic pathway (Embden-Meyerhof), *Pyruvate kinase (PK)*, *Hexokinase (HK)*, *Phosphohexose isomerase (PHI)*, *Phosphofructokinase (PFK)*, *Triosephosphate isomerase (TPI)*, *Glyceraldehyde-3-phosphate dehydrogenase (G-3-PD)*, *Phosphoglycerate kinase (PGK)*, *2,3-Diphosphoglyceromutase (2,3-DPGase)*, *Adenosine triphosphatase (ATP-ase)*.

INTRODUCTION

The previous chapter described the hereditary anaemias characterized by specific abnormalities of red cell morphology, including spherocytosis (HS), elliptocytosis (HE) and stomatocytosis. The present chapter is concerned with a heterogenous group of red cell disorders, most of which are associated with chronic or intermittent haemolysis, in which there are only *non-specific* changes in red cell morphology, e.g. anisocytosis, macrocytosis, red cell fragmentation, polychromasia, basophilic stippling and sometimes small numbers of spherocytes or target cells. This group of disorders is characterized by (a) normal osmotic fragility in unincubated blood, (b) increased autohaemolysis of sterile blood incubated at 37°C and (C) defective red cell metabolism. The metabolic defects are due to deficiency or molecular abnormality of enzymes, or to unstable variants of haemoglobin. Jaffé and Gottfreid (1968) have also described a family with hereditary non-spherocytic haemolytic anaemia in which the only detectable abnormality was altered phospholipid composition of the red cell membrane. Further generalizations are that the mode of inheritance is usually recessive, whereas it is dominant in HS, HE and stomatocytosis, and that the benefit from splenectomy in the non-spherocytic haemolytic anaemias is less clear cut than is the case in HS or HE.

Historically the autohaemolysis test of Selwyn and Dacie (1954) played a major part in defining and subdividing this group of non-spherocytic haemolytic anaemias. Sterile defibrinated blood was incubated at 37°C and the percentage haemolysis measured at 48 hours, with normal results

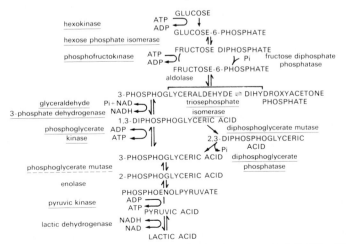

Fig. 7.1 Glycolytic pathway (Embden-Meyerhof). (Reproduced from Van Eys (1970), *Pediatric Clinics of North America*, **17**, 449, by permission of the author and the publishers.)

giving 0.4 to 4.5 per cent lysis, or approximately up to 5 per cent (Prager, 1967). A more recent modification of the autohaemolysis test, employing continuous rotation during incubation had given a lower normal range of 0–0.6 per cent lysis at 48 hours (Grimes *et al.*, 1968). This test demonstrated an intrinsic red cell abnormality in cases of haemolytic anaemia having a normal osmotic fragility curve and only non-specific changes in red cell morphology. Patients were classified tentatively as having Type I or Type II disorders on the basis of the autohaemolysis results. Type I cases gave autohaemolysis results either within or just outside the normal range, which, in either event, were reduced by the presence of added glucose, although less so than with normal blood. Type II results showed much more marked haemolysis, i.e. up to 40 per cent, well outside the normal range, and this was unaffected or even accentuated by added glucose. Subsequently this test has been used by many investigators. In 1960 de Gruchy *et al.*, added ATP as an alternative to glucose and found that this caused a marked reduction in autohaemolysis in both Type I and Type II cases. Since the

II patients. This enzyme catalyses the transfer of a high energy phosphate group from phosphoenol pyruvate to ADP with the formation of ATP plus pyruvate. Certain other enzyme deficiencies of this glycolytic pathway are now known to be associated with Type I or Type II autohaemolysis patterns (Table 7.1). The neat logic that led to the discovery of PK deficiency now appears fortuitous since it is probable that added ATP never enters the red cells under test, but exerts its retarding effect on haemolysis by virtue of lowering the pH of the medium (Grimes *et al.*, 1968).

BIOCHEMICAL CONSIDERATIONS

Mature red cells exist under distinct metabolic disadvantages. Unlike the normoblast or reticulocyte they lack the enzymatic machinery for oxidative phosphorylation, Krebs tricarboxylic acid cycle, protein synthesis, and lipid synthesis. Anaerobic glycolysis is their only source of energy (Fig. 7.1). This is because they lack nucleus and ribosomes and mitochondria on which the enzymes necessary for these missing functions are normally carried.

Table 7.1   Red-cell enzyme deficiencies associated with Types I or II autohaemolysis patterns

Abnormality	Type	Remarks
Hereditary spherocytosis	I, occ. II	Added glucose usually effects a marked reduction in lysis; following splenectomy lysis without additives is reduced
Hereditary elliptocytosis	Normal or I	Results do not correlate with degree of haemolytic anaemia
G6PD deficiency		
(a) without haemolysis	Normal	
(b) with congenital haemolytic anaemia	I	The degree of lysis without additives is smaller than in most cases of HS
PK deficiency	II	Splenectomy has no effect on the Type II classification
Diaphorase deficiency	Normal	
GSSG–R deficiency	II	
Hexokinase deficiency	I	
TPI deficiency	I	
Unstable haemoglobinopathy	I	Established for Köln and Hammersmith but Hb.H may give I or II
2,3–DPGase deficiency	I	
GPI deficiency	I	
Paroxysmal nocturnal haemoglobinuria	II	
Gamma glutamyl cysteine synthetase	II	

Reproduced, by permission of the author and publishers, from Grimes, British Journal of Haematology (1969) **17,** *129.*
(Gamma-glutamyl cysteine synthetase added to original table).

red cell content of ATP was known to be abnormally low in Type II cases Robinson, Loder and de Gruchy (1961) postulated that there was a block in ATP generation from the later steps of the Embden-Meyerhof glycolytic pathway (Fig. 7.1). Shortly thereafter Valentine, Tanaka and Miwa (1961) demonstrated a severe defect of pyruvate kinase (PK) activity in the red cells of three Type

Since the red cell cannot synthesize proteins or lipids beyond its first few days in the circulation it is particularly important that it is capable of protecting these elements of its structure throughout its circulating life span. The proteins in question are not only haemoglobin, but also the numerous enzymes necessary for glycolysis, the red cell's only source of energy. The lipids are the phospholipids present as lipoprotein complexes which constitute the red cell membrane.

Haemoglobin, sulphydryl-containing enzymes and phospholipids are constantly exposed to oxidative injury from small amounts of H_2O_2, peroxyhaemoglobin or equivalent free radicals formed during normal metabolism, and on occasions also from oxidative drugs, (e.g. naphthoquinones) or active drug metabolites (Beutler, 1971). In the case of haemoglobin the iron must remain in the divalent ferrous form for the pigment to function in oxygen transport. Yet, in the presence of high concentrations of oxygen the haemoglobin iron is constantly susceptible to oxidation to the trivalent ferric form, with the production of methaemoglobin (Met. Hb). Normally there is a continuous process of reduction of formed Met. Hb but this is both energy consuming and requires a constant supply of NAD.H, i.e. reduced nicotinamide adenine dinucleotide (DNP.H), plus the enzyme methaemoglobin reductase (or 'diaphorase'). In the absence of this enzyme there is a steady accumulation of Met. Hb at the rate of up to 3 per cent per day (Grimes, 1969). The necessary protection can be achieved in the normal red cell even with the limited metabolic machinery at its disposal. This is possible from the energy and NAD.H generated during the metabolism of glucose via the Embden-Meyerhof pathway (Fig. 7.1). If there is either a deficiency of Met. Hb reductase or if there is a structural abnormality of the haemoglobin molecule rendering the iron unusually susceptible to oxidation (haemoglobinopathy M and unstable haemoglobins) then methaemaglobinaemia occurs, particularly if the blood is incubated *in vitro*. Methaemoglobin formation compromises oxygen transport but is not necessarily associated with haemolysis. It is only in one form of Hb.M (Saskatoon) and in the unstable haemoglobin disorders that haemolysis occurs.

A second type of oxidative injury against which the red cell must protect itself is oxidation of sulphydryl groups. Haemoglobin has two particularly vulnerable SH-groups, viz. β 93 cystein, but similar groups are present in both the intracellular enzymes and the membrane lipoproteins. Protection of these SH- groups is normally achieved by a high level of reduced glutathione (GSH), maintained by a constant source of NADP.H (TPN.H) generated from the hexosemonophosphate shunt (Fig. 7.3). This is the alternative pathway through which glucose can be metabolized (aerobically). The bulk, however, (90–95 per cent) is metabolized via the anaerobic, Embden-Meyerhof, pathway. In particular, H_2O_2 in low concentration is destroyed

by glutathione peroxidase with concomitant oxidation of the glutathione (high concentrations of H_2O_2 are destroyed by catalase). Reduced glutathione (GSH) is normally present at a concentration of 160–380 μ moles per 100 ml of packed cells or one molecule for every two of haemoglobin. This concentration is reduced if there is a metabolic block in the generation of NADP.H, as in G-6-PD deficiency, especially if there is an oxidative challenge from a drug or its metabolite, or if there is continued oxidative stress from an unstable haemoglobin requiring constant reparative reduction. When most of the red cell glutathione is in the oxidized form (G-SS-G) protection of vulnerable SH groups no longer occurs and in fact there is evidence that mixed disulfides are formed between glutathione and the β 93 cysteine of haemoglobin:

$$G\text{-}SS\text{-}G + HS\text{-}Hb = GSH + G\text{-}SS\text{-}Hb.$$

Similar mixed disulfides with membrane sulphydryl groups may also be formed. Inactivation of these groups reduces red cell survival (Jacob and Jandle, 1962). This is thought to be the first step in a sequence of oxidative damage to Hb later leading to loss of the haem moiety, unfolding of polypeptide chains and the precipitation of Heinz body red cell inclusions characteristic of toxic haemolytic processes. These topics have recently been reviewed by Beutler (1971). Heinz bodies are rigid and probably impede the passage of red cells through small interstices of the reticuloendothelial system, especially of the spleen. Removal or 'pitting' of the red cell inclusions may result in loss of fragments of membrane, formation of microspherocytes and eventually total destruction of the red cells (Jaffé, 1972). This author emphasized that lipid peroxidation and membrane destruction may also be a consequence of this breakdown in the maintenance of an adequate level of reduced glutathione (GSH). Exposure of enzyme deficient cells to primaquine and related drugs increases their permeability for cations (Weed, 1961) probably as a consequence of membrane damage (George *et al.*, 1966). Deficiencies of any of the enzymes of the hexosemonophosphate shunt or of glutathione synthesis or metabolism (Fig. 7.3, Table 7.1) may be associated with 'oxidant drug' haemolysis *or* spontaneous haemolysis *or* haemolysis in association with bacterial infections, viral infections or acidosis. Imperfections in the current concepts include the fact that deficiencies of two of the enzymes on this pathway (G-SS-G reductase and 6-PGD) are less clearly related to spontaneous or drug induced haemolysis (Jaffé, 1972).

A third factor that is relevant to the survival of red cells in the circulation is the need for a constant supply of high energy phosphate bonds via ATP. In particular, this source of energy is required to maintain the cation pump which pumps potassium into the cell and sodium out of the cell so as to maintain the gradient of low intracellular sodium and high potassium. Energy may also be required for maintenance of the structural integrity of the cell membrane. Enzyme deficiencies of the later stages of the Embden-Meyerhof pathway, e.g. PK deficiency, cause such a defect. The consequences of such a block are more serious for the red cell than for other cells of the body since the red cell lacks alternative metabolic pathways capable of generating ATP. The nature of the metabolic lesion makes the red cell particularly susceptible to low glucose concentrations, such as in the splenic sinuses, and haemolysis may preferentially take place in that organ. On the other hand, haemolysis is not specifically related to oxidative injury from drugs in this type of metabolic defect. The phosphate ester present in the highest concentration within the red cell (15μ moles/g of Hb, equivalent to a 1:1 molar ratio) is 2,3 diphosphoglycerate (2,3 DPG). It is generated via the 2,3 DPG shunt (Rapoport and Luebering, 1952), and provides the red cell with a means of regulating the oxygen affinity of its Hb. The 2,3-DPG interacts with the beta chains of de-oxy Hb thereby stabilizing this reduced form and decreasing its affinity for oxygen. Increased concentrations of this ester may therefore favour oxygen release to tissues at low oxygen tensions (Benesch and Benesch, 1969). Since more 2,3-DPG is especially formed during glycolysis in the anoxic red cell, this provides a self-regulatory mechanism whereby there is greater oxygen release than would otherwise occur at the low oxygen tensions pertaining in the tissues (Bunn and Jandl, 1970; Hamasaki et al., 1970). The formation of 2,3-DPG is achieved at the expense of ATP synthesis since an energy yielding step, the dephosphorylation of 1:3 diphosphoglycerate is by-passed

by the shunt (Figs. 7.1 and 2). The existence of the shunt therefore provides the red cell with a means of regulating its supply of ATP relative to 2,3-DPG. Other ligands that similarly increase 0_2 release from Hb 0_2 are carbon dioxide and hydrogen ions (Finch and Lenfant, 1972).

Without the ability (a) to reduce Met. Hb, (b) to protect sulfhydryl groups from oxidation and (c) to maintain a supply of ATP the red cell would 'be a useless package of haemoglobin', and would 'quickly become sodium-logged, sphered and brown, and be removed from the circulation', (Beutler, 1969A).

DISORDERS OF THE HEXOSE MONOPHOSPHATE SHUNT

As described above these lead to a limited capacity of the mature red cell to produce NADP.H for the maintenance of glutathione in the reduced state (GSH), and thus render the red cell more susceptible to oxidative injury. Haemolysis occurs when the red cells are stressed, e.g. by drugs or in the neonatal period. If chronic haemolysis exists it is increased by these stresses (Beutler, 1969). This is in contradistinction to deficiencies of anaerobic glycolysis pathway which do not result in drug sensitivity, but are manifest by a non-spherocytic haemolytic anaemia.

The metabolic pathways involved in the maintenance of reduced glutathione are shown in Fig. 7.3. They include the synthesis of the tripeptide itself, the pathway leading to its reduction via NADP.H and the reoxidation of glutathione during its interaction with H_20_2.

GLUCOSE-6-PHOSPHATE DEHYDROGENASE (G-6-PD)

Over 50 variants of this red cell enzyme are known to exist among the different racial and ethnic groups of the world. These can be distinguished by their electrophoretic, kinetic or physio-

Summary of metabolic functions of mature red cell

Key metabolite	Source	Function
ATP production	Latter part of Embden-Meyerhof anaerobic glycolytic pathway	Maintaining cation pump and membrane stability
NAD.H production	Anaerobic glycolysis	Reduction of Met. Hb
NADP.H production	Hexosemonophosphate shunt	Maintenance of reduced glutathione, for protection of SH groups in Hb enzymes and membrane
2,3–DPG production	Rapoport Luebering cycle	Increasing 0_2 release by Hb at low PO_2 values

chemical properties (Kirkman *et al.*, 1968). 'Finger-print' analysis of highly purified enzymes has shown that the difference between normal G-6-PD and one common variant lies in a single substitution of asparagine for aspartic acid (Yoshida, 1968). This is analagous to the situation among the haemoglobinopathies. The normal enzyme is designated the B form. Among black American males there is a high incidence of two electrophoretically faster forms. One of these has essentially normal activity (A+ form) and is without clinical significance. The other (A— form) appears to have normal catalytic activity but has an increased degradation during red cell ageing, resulting in a rapid decay of activity during the life of the red cell. Mature red cells with this variant have approximately 10 per cent of the normal enzyme activity, but reticulocytes and young red cells have a nearly normal activity (Marks and Gross, 1959). This A- type of enzyme is now known to be associated with drug-induced haemolytic anaemia in the black American. Historically it was the observation of haemolysis in

sensitive black males following administration of the antimalarial drugs pamoquin (Earl *et al.*, 1948) and primaquin (Hockwald *et al.*, 1952; Dern *et al.*, 1954) that led to the discovery of G-6-PD deficiency by Carson *et al.*, in 1956. This was the first haemolytic anaemia shown to be caused by a defect of a red cell enzyme and the discovery led to the search for other examples of enzyme deficiency among the group of hereditary non-spherocytic haemolytic anaemias.

Mediterranean (Caucasian) and Oriental (Mongolian) variants of the enzyme also exist, and these are associated with a much lower level of activity (approx. 1 per cent of normal) in both mature and young red cells. Clinically there is a liability to neonatal haemolysis as well as a marked sensitivity to certain drugs, and to fava beans (favism) in the Mediterranean variant. An even more severe deficiency is seen with 'Chicago' and Northern European variants of G-6-PD, associated with almost complete absence of the enzyme, resulting in a chronic non-spherocytic haemolytic anaemia, further accentuated by drugs, infection and in the

Table 7.2   Some agents reported to produce haemolysis in patients with G–6–PD deficiency

Antimalarials
   Primaquine
   Pamaquine
   Pentaquine
   Plasmoquine
   Quinocide
   Quinacrine (Atabrine)
   Quinine (*C*)

Sulfonamides
   Sulfanilamide
   N² Acetylsulfanilamide
   Sulfacetamide (Sulamyd)
   Sulfamethoxypyridazine (Kynex, Midicel)
   Salicylazosulfapyridine (Azulfidine)
   Sulfisoxazole (Gantrisin)
   Sulfapyridine

Nitrofurans
   Nitrofurantoin (Furadantin)
   Furazolidone (Furoxone)
   Furaltadone (Altafur)
   Nitrofurazone (Furacin)

Antipyretics and Analgesics
   Acetylsalicylic acid (in large doses)
   Acetanilide
   Acetophenetidin (Phenacetin)
   Antipyrine (*C*)
   Aminopyrine (*C*)
   p-Aminosalicylic acid

Sulfones

Others
   Dimercaprol (BAL)
   Methylene blue
   Naphthalene
   Phenylhydrazine
   Acetylphenhydrazine
   Probenecid
   Vitamin K (large doses of water
     soluble analogues)
   Chloramphenicol (*C*)
   Quinidine (*C*)
   Fava beans (*C*)
   Chloroquine
   Nalidixic acid (Negram)
   Orinase

Infections
   Respiratory viruses
   Infectious hepatitis
   Infectious mononucleosis
   Bacterial pneumonias

Diabetic Acidosis

(*C*), to date, only Caucasians

Reproduced, by permission of the authors and publisher, from Oski and Naiman (1972).

neonatal period. A complete list of G-6-PD variants are given in Table 2 of the review by Beutler (1969B). It is only a small proportion of the total known variants that are subactive, i.e. associated with enzyme deficiency and liability to haemolysis.

The genetic locus for G-6-PD variants is on the X-chromosome and inheritance therefore follows the sex-linked recessive pattern. The locus is close to that for colour blindness (Adam, 1961), haemophilia and Christmas disease, but no linkage with the locus for Xg^a has been found (Siniscalco et al., 1966). It is typically the hemizygous male ($\bar{X}Y$) who is affected, as in other X-linked disorders, as well as the very rare homozygous female ($\bar{X}\bar{X}$). The more common heterozygous female carrier ($\bar{X}X$) shows a variable degree of clinical disorder since in effect she has a mosaic distribution of G-6-PD deficient and G-6-PD sufficient red cells circulating in her blood (Beutler and Baluda, 1964). The proportion of these two cell populations and the resulting overall enzyme level varies greatly among heterozygotes with parallel clinical consequences. Some women shown by pedigree analysis to be heterozygotes have normal red cell G-6-PD proportion of normal and abnormal cells in the X heterozygote. It was the study of G-6-PD deficiency that led Beutler et al. (1962) to make a similar suggestion. Another point of broad biological interest is that since G-6-PD deficiency gives some degree of protection against infection by falciparum infection its high incidence in malarious areas may represent a form of 'balanced polymorphism' accounting for persistence of the gene (Motulsky, 1964).

Clinical manifestations of G-6-PD

It has been estimated that 100 million individuals in the world suffer from one or other type of G-6-PD. It is by far the commonest enzyme deficiency known.

DRUG-INDUCED HAEMOLYSIS

This is the manifestation seen typically in black Americans, but also occurs in other groups. As mentioned above, it was the occurrence of haemolysis in sensitive black males after administration of antimalarial drugs which led to the discovery of this G-6-PD deficiency. A large number of drugs are now known to cause haemolysis in such patients

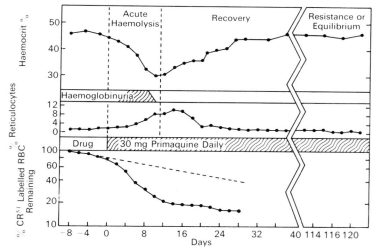

Fig. 7.2 Sequence of haematological events after primaquine administration to patients with genetic defects in glucose-6-phosphate dehydrogenase expression. The haemolysis is self-limiting even though primaquine (30 mg) administration is continued daily, since it stimulates erythropoiesis by the bone marrow. Reticulocytes and younger erythrocytes are more resistant to haemolysis by the oxidized degradation products of primaquine than are the older cells. Excess primaquine results in chronic haemolytic anemia. (Reproduced from Alving et al. (1960), Bulletin of the World Health Organization, 22, 621, by permission).

activity, while others have as severe a degree of deficiency as affected male hemizygotes (Beutler, 1970). The double population of red cells is explained by the *Lyon hypothesis* (1961), whereby only one X chromosome is genetically active in any cell during interphase, resulting in a fortuitous whether of Negro, Caucasian or Mongoloid stock (Table 7.2). Certain of the less active drugs only produce haemolysis in Caucasians since the enzyme deficiency is more severe in this variant, as indicated in the table. A full list of known active drugs, together with a discussion of the types of evidence by which the drugs have been incriminated, is given by Beutler (1969B). Individual differences in drug metabolism account for variations in sensitivity in some instances. Certain drugs appear to precipitate haemolysis only when an additional stress such as infection or the neonatal state exist. Such drugs are: aspirin, phenacetin, ascorbic acid, methylene blue, atabrine, chloramphenicol, dimercaprol, vitamin K and its analogues (Van Eys, 1970). Bacterial infection (Burka *et al.*, 1966), viral infection, especially hepatitis, (Salen *et al.*, 1966) and diabetic acidosis (Grant and Winks, 1961) may all mimic drug ingestion in precipitating haemolysis in sensitive patients. The clinical effect of drug ingestion is the appearance of dark urine, pallor and sometimes jaundice. The sequence of haematological events after ingestion of a standard dose of primaquine is shown in Fig. 7.2. The haemoglobin falls within 2–4 days. At this stage there may be Heinz bodies demonstrable in the circulating red

reaching a maximum response by 10–20 days. As the cohort of newly formed red cells replaces the older cells which are being destroyed the average enzyme level rises to nearly normal since in the A-variant reticulocytes have a high enzyme level. At this point a phase of relative resistance develops and even although the drug may be continued the haemolysis is self-limiting or greatly reduced. This resistance does not similarly develop in the Caucasian variants since even the reticulocytes have a low enzyme level in these more severe deficiencies.

Between episodes of drug or infection-induced haemolysis the affected black male is entirely symptom free with normal haemoglobin and reticulocyte levels in spite of a chronic slight reduction in red cell survival to 18–24.5 days half life compared to 25.5–31 days in normals (Brewer *et al.*, 1961). The haemolytic process is completely compensated even in the neonatal period.

Table 7.3 The sensitivity of tests for G–6–PD deficiency

| Method | % Giving Abnormal Test Results* Population Surveys For | | Artificial Mixtures† (Authors' Data) | |
	Affected Male	Carrier (Heterozygote)	Lowest % Abnormal Cells Consistently Giving Abnormal Test Results	Highest % Abnormal Cells Consistently Giving Normal Test Results
Brilliant cresyl blue	100	20–48	80	20
Methemoglobin reduction (nonquantitative)	100	75	60	10
Spot test	100	20	60	20
Fluorescence test	100	No data	60	10
Ascorbate test	100	No data	20	5
Spectrophotometric assay	100	76	60	20
6-Hour methemoglobin reduction	100	No data	40	10
Methemoglobin elution	100	76–100	5	0
G6PD-tetrazolium cytochemical method	100	80–100	5	0

* In the many field surveys made for determining the frequency of G6PD deficiency in various ethnic groups, it has been assumed that the screening tests detect all hemizygotes (males). It is, however, not certain that this assumption is correct, for some G6PD variants are expressed as mild (40%–60%) deficiency in the hemizygote and quite possibly some of these will be missed. There seems to be, at present, insufficient information as to the sensitivity of these tests for detection of mild deficiency variants. Data given here are based on previously published studies (see reference column) except for the spot test and the G6PD-tetrazolium test, which represent the authors' experience.

† Artificial mixtures were obtained by mixing known numbers of compatible normal and G6PD-deficient erythrocytes. See text for details. Fairbanks & Fernandez (1969).

Reproduced, from Fairbanks and Fernandez (1969), by permission of the authors and J.A.M.A.

cells and a blood film may show spherocytes and fragmented cells indicative of active haemolysis. The haemoglobin level continues to fall until 8–12 days but a reticulocytosis appears at 4–5 days,

Details of the various screening tests for detection of G-6-PD deficiency are described by Grimes (1969) and their relative sensitivity, especially with regard to heterozygotes, is shown in

Table 7.3 from Fairbanks and Fernandez (1969).

FAVISM

Acute, life-endangering haemolysis caused by ingestion of fava (broad) beans occurs in Mediterranean and Oriental forms of the disease but not in the Negro type. Although G-6-PD deficiency is a prerequisite for sensitivity to the fava bean it appears that some other, second factor is necessary for an individual to be affected by favism. For instance, it has been found that favism is more common in some G-6-PD deficient families than in others (Stamatoyannopoulos et al., 1966), and that when a whole G-6-PD deficient family has a meal of fava beans only some of the members are adversely affected.

Fava beans are uniquely rich in the amino acid L-dopa. Dopaquinone, the oxidation product of L-dopa, can catalyse GSH oxidation in G-6-PD deficient red cells (Beutler, 1970). This author has therefore suggested that perhaps excessive tyrosinase activity or unusually slow removal of dopaquinone might be the second metabolic abnormality, in addition to G-6-PD deficiency, necessary to produce favism.

The clinical and haematological features of an attack of favism are similar to those described for drug-induced haemolysis but much more severe, often leading to acute renal failure. Blood transfusion is lifesaving, whereas it is not required in the self-limiting drug-induced haemolytic episodes of the Negro type of deficiency.

NEONATAL JAUNDICE AND KERNICTERUS

This is particularly associated with the Mediterranean and Oriental types of G-6-PD deficiency, although also occurring in the much rarer chronic haemolytic form of the disease (Newton and Bass, 1958; Shahidi and Diamond, 1959). Typically, it does not occur in Blacks, although exceptions to this have recently been reported (Lopez and Cooperman, 1971). Strangely enough, the incidence of neonatal jaundice in the Mediterranean type of G-6-PD varies greatly in different populations. For instance the incidence is 5 per cent in infants born in Athens but 34 per cent in those born in Lesbos (Doxiadis et al., 1964). This has suggested that a second hereditary factor predisposing to this complication exists, rather analagous to the situation in favism.

Clinically, the infant will present with pallor, jaundice and dark urine. The jaundice seldom appears within the first 24 hours of life, but more often develops on the second day of life (Doxiadis and Valaes, 1964). One third of exchange trans-

fusions are for G-6-PD deficiency in Greece and the sex ratio of affected infants is approximately 3 males to 1 female. Often there is no exposure to an offending agent (Table 7.2). Another group of cases is seen where the jaundice develops much later. In these there has often been exposure to moth balls (naphthalene), aniline dye marking ink, or a drug (Zinkham and Childs, 1958). Kernicterus may develop due to jaundice as late as the second week in this disease (Naiman and Kosoy, 1964). Hepatosplenomegaly is usually absent, and if present should raise suspicion of an additional factor such as isoimmunization, or infection (Oski and Naiman, 1972).

The haemoglobin level may be near to normal in infants who have not been exposed to a toxic agent, reflecting the fact that very little haemolysis is needed to produce detectable jaundice in the newborn. In other infants there is distinct anaemia with reticulocytosis and an increase in normoblasts on the blood film. The red cells show fragmentation and some spherocytosis. Heinz bodies are present at early stages of haemolytic process. Diagnosis can be confirmed by relatively simple screening tests for G-6-PD deficiency (Grimes, 1969). The low levels (approx. 1 per cent) are not obscured in the types of deficiency associated with neonatal jaundice (i.e. Mediterranean or Oriental) since the young red cells and reticulocytes also have a low enzyme content (Kirkman et al., 1960).

Treatment may involve exchange transfusion if the serum bilirubin level approaches 20 mg/100 ml. It also involves avoidance of the toxic agents listed in Table 7.2 both in the baby and in the mother if she is breast feeding, and in any other affected members of the family. Ingestion of fava beans by the mother has resulted in haemolytic anaemia in her breast fed infant (Emanuel and Schoenfield, 1961). The effective application of these principles involves routine screening of neonates from high frequency ethnic groups and of siblings of affected patients.

Although the synthetic water soluble analogues of vitamin K (i.e. Synkavite and Hykinone) given in large doses (e.g. 5 to 10 mg) have been incriminated as causing Heinz body haemolytic anaemias in premature babies (Gasser, 1953; Meyer and Angus, 1956) doses of 1 mg do not produce jaundice or haemolysis in black infants with G-6-PD deficiency (Zinkham, 1963). Even larger doses of the naturally occurring vitamin K_1 (Aquamephyton, Konakion) are safe in such black infants. It is not known for certain what doses of these vitamin K preparations are safe in Mediterranean or other infants with G-6-PD deficiency. The advice of the American

Academy of Pediatrics (1961) is to restrict the dose to 1 mg of K_1 I.M.

The particular liability to haemolysis during the neonatal period may be due to additional factors rendering the red cell more susceptible to oxidative injury at this period including low vitamin E levels (Gordon et al., 1955), low methaemoglobin reductase levels (Ross, 1963) and, in a proportion of infants, low glutathione peroxidase levels (Whaun and Oski, 1970). The anaemia does not persist after the neonatal period in the usual Mediterranean or Oriental type of disease; only recurring in later life at times of drug exposure, infection or acidosis.

CHRONIC NON-SPHEROCYTIC HAEMOLYTIC ANAEMIA

This is the least common manifestation of G-6-PD deficiency and occurs chiefly in Northern European stock and only on rare occasions, in Blacks (Grossman et al., 1966). It is confined to males. The G-6-PD activity is lower than in the above mentioned types of deficiency, and differs qualitatively from other Caucasian variants. One of the associated variants is 'Chicago I' (Kirkman et al., 1964). The continuous haemolysis present in this disease may be related to an additional defect of ATP metabolism absent in the other forms (Mohler and Crockett, 1964). Biochemical characteristics of 22 different enzyme variants associated with chronic haemolysis are given by Rattazzi et al. (1971).

Anaemia and sometimes slight icterus persists throughout life even in the absence of drug exposure or other predisposing cause and is accompanied by mild splenomegaly. The haematological picture is that of a chronic non-spherocytic haemolytic anaemia, with reticulocytosis, shortened red cell survival and increased autohaemolysis of the Type I pattern, viz. slightly increased with only partial correction by glucose. It is of interest that the forms of G-6-PD deficiency without chronic haemolysis show normal autohaemolysis. The red cell morphology may be nearly normal or may show a small number of fragmented red cells plus polychromasia and anisocytosis. Heinz bodies are absent from circulating red cells except at times of a haemolytic crisis. Tests dependent upon the G-6-PD level show a gross enzyme deficiency or a total absence. The bilirubin may chronically be as high as 5 mg/100 ml.

In addition to the persisting haemolytic anaemia there are superimposed episodes of acute haemolysis precipitated by infections or drug exposure as well as the liability to neonatal jaundice mentioned above. Associated features of optic atrophy plus bilateral cortical atrophy (Escobar et al., 1964) and cataracts plus seizures (Westring and Pisciotta, 1966) have been reported on rare occasions.

Splenectomy is not usually beneficial in this disorder (Bowdler and Prankerd, 1964), although improvement has been reported in one patient with severe anaemia. Avoidance of all drugs known to be injurious in G-6-PD deficiency (Table 7.2) is the most important element of management.

OTHER DEFECTS AFFECTING AVAILABILITY OF REDUCED GLUTATHIONE (GSH)

The metabolic reactions involved are shown in Fig. 7.3.

6-Phosphogluconate dehydrogenase (6-PGD)

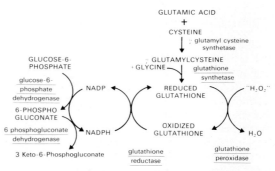

Fig. 7.3 Glutathione synthesis and reduction via the pentose shunt. (Reproduced from Van Eys (1970), Pediatric Clinics of North America, 17, 449, by permission of the author and publishers).

As in the case of G-6-PD there are also a large number of electrophoretic variants of this enzyme but only few are associated with deficient activity (Parr and Fitch, 1967). The 'Whitechapel' variant results in deficiency by virtue of enzyme instability. In another variant there is little or no enzyme present. Partial deficiency occurs in heterozygotes and severe deficiency only in homozygotes. This is not sex linked. There are only about 20 reported cases of 6-PGD deficiency. The incidence of deficiency in one survey was 0.3 per cent in black Americans and 0.7 per cent in Caucasians (Dern et al., 1966).

Deficiency of this enzyme would be expected to cause a similar but less severe block in glutathione reduction as occurs in the case of G-6-PD. Less severe since it is involved only in the generation of the second of the two molecuets of NADP.H resulting from glucose metabolism, whereas

G-6-PD deficiency will block both (Fig. 7.4). This is somewhat borne out by clinical observations. In some instances there are no clinical manifestations of deficiency (Brewer and Dern, 1964), in another report drug challenge with primaquine in a heterozygote resulted in questionable mild haemolysis (Dern et al., 1966). while in another instance, an infant with 6-PGD deficiency, there was sufficient haemolysis to necessitate an exchange transfusion in the neonatal period (Lausecker et al., 1965). Haemolysis persisted in this infant. At the age of two months the haemoglobin level was 6.4 g/100 ml and the reticulocytes 21.6 per cent. This is the most severe example of haemolysis so far reported in 6-PGD deficiency.

There are no simple screening tests for detecting 6-PGD deficiency but NADP-linked enzyme assays exist and their references are given by Grimes (1969).

Glutathione reductase (GSSG-R)

This deficiency came to light while investigating patients who had drug-induced haemolytic anaemia but who had normal G-6-PD levels. Desforges et al. (1959) described a patient who developed haemolysis and methaemoglobinaemia induced by Sulfoxone but in whom both G-6-PD and 6-PGD levels were normal, while the red cell GSSG-R was 60 per cent of normal. They found that susceptibility to haemolysis was related to red cell age; only after 50 days did the red cells become sensitive. Presumably the defective enzyme is unstable in vivo. Carson et al. (1961) similarly described a Caucasian man of German ancestry whose red cells were sensitive to a number of drugs including primaquine. The G-6-PD level was normal but the GSSG-R was 57 per cent of normal. Later Carson and Frischer (1966) reported a further case, a female of German extraction who developed a mild episode of haemolysis following Gantrisin, with a GSSG-R level of 38 per cent. This review referred to two other patients also from Germany with lower enzyme levels. The largest number of cases have been reported by Waller et al. (1965) from Germany. Individuals from four families showed relatively severe haemolysis, the pattern of inheritance being autosomal dominant. There are now more than 60 reported cases of this deficiency.

The particular point that emerges from the work of Waller is that a range of haematological disorders seem to be associated with GSSG-R deficiency including not only drug-induced haemolytic anaemia but also non-spherocytic haemolytic anaemia, thrombocytopenia, pancytopenia and neurological disorders including mental deficiency, spasticity and an abnormal EEG. The enzyme deficiency affects platelets and leucocytes as well as red cells. Also almost all known patients seem to be German or of German ancestry. The range of drugs to which these patients are sensitive are included in the review by Waller (1968).

Flavine adenine dinucleotide (FAD) is the co-enzyme of GSSG-R and it has been shown that addition of FAD to haemolysates in vitro increases the amount of active enzyme as does the administration of riboflavin in vivo (Beutler, 1969). It appears that only a fraction of the enzyme is fully active under normal conditions, and the relevance of this fact to the pathogenesis and perhaps treatment of the enzyme deficiency states is not understood at present. The situation is further complicated by the existence of different electrophoretic variants of the enzyme (Blume et al., 1968).

The biochemical effects of a deficiency of this GSSG-R would be expected to result in a failure to maintain adequate levels of GSH (Fig. 7.3) as in G-6-PD or 6-PGD deficiencies. As in these there is glutathione instability (Beutler, 1957) with increased Heinz body formation during incubation with acetyl phenylhydrazine (Beutler et al., 1955). Autohaemolysis is increased, showing the Type II pattern (Grimes, 1969). A screening test for GSSG-R deficiency has been devised based on UV fluorescence of NADP.H (Beutler, 1966).

Glutathione peroxidase (GSH-Px)

This is the final enzyme in a series of reactions catalysing the reduction of H_2O_2 (Fig. 7.3), and therefore important in the protection of red cell membrane, enzymes and haemoglobin from the deleterious effects of oxidizing agents (Cohen and Hochstein, 1963). Deficiency of GSH-Px would be expected to render the red cells unduly sensitive to drug-induced haemolysis (as in G-6-PD A-deficiency) and perhaps to haemolysis in the neonatal period (as in G-6-PD, Mediterranean).

GSH-Px is one of the more recently discovered enzyme deficiencies of the red cell. Low levels are found in two circumstances: (a) in normal full term and premature infants (Gross et al., 1967), and (b) as a life-long autosomally inherited defect recognizable as either a heterozygous (Necheles et al., 1968) or homozygous state (Necheles et al., 1969). The levels are lower in premature infants than in term infants. Transient deficiency is therefore common, and permanent, hereditary deficiency rare. Then the homozygous individual has a level equivalent to the lowest range of normal premature infants and the heterozygous individual has a level nearer that of normal term infants (Fig. 7.4).

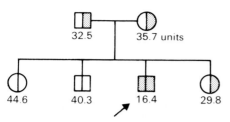

Fig. 7.4 Family study in erythrocyte glutathione peroxidase deficiency; activity expressed in units/g Hb. (Reproduced from Necheles et al. (1969), Blood, **33**, 164, by permission of Dr Necheles and the publisher).

The neonatal GSH-Px deficiency occurring in normal infants was shown by Gross et al. (1967) to render the red cells unduly susceptible to low concentrations of H_2O_2 in vitro, resulting in increased formation of Heinz bodies and methaemoglobin. The clinical effect of this neonatal deficiency was investigated by Whaun and Oski (1970). GSH-Px deficiency alone did not appear to result in hyperbilirubinaemia, but their findings suggested that infants with low GSH-Px levels had an increased chance of developing severe degrees of jaundice. As with G-6-PD all deficient infants are at potential risk, but only some become jaundiced, possibly as a result of an added factor such as vitamin E deficiency or drug exposure. This type of GSH-Px deficiency may account for some instances of otherwise unexplained neonatal jaundice.

Necheles, Boles and Allen (1968) first described the genetically determined form of GSH-Px deficiency in 4 young children. Three had significant hyperbilirubinaemia during the first week of life, one severe enough to require exchange transfusion. One had anaemia, all had reticulocytosis. By the age of 6 months all evidence of haemolysis had disappeared but the GSH-Px levels were still low (unlike the more common neonatal deficiency). The enzyme deficiency was only partial and it was thought that these patients were heterozygotes of an autosomal trait of significance mainly in the neonatal period. A sibling, however, later developed a moderate haemolytic anaemia while on sulfisoxazole (Gantrisin). Nitrofuradantin and acetyl salicylic acid have precipitated haemolysis in other similar cases (Necheles et al., 1970) suggesting that some of these patients are permanently susceptible to drug-induced haemolysis. But heterozygotes do not suffer from a persistent haemolytic anaemia. About 20 such patients have so far been reported. Most are Caucasians but one Puerto Rican family and one black American have also been affected

One certain homozygote (Necheles et al., 1969) and another probable homozygote, both with very low GSH-Px levels, showed chronic reticulocyte counts of 3 and 6 per cent suggesting that they had a well-compensated non-spherocytic haemolytic anaemia (Necheles et al., 1970).

Haematological features include the occurrence of circulating Heinz bodies during active haemolysis, increased Heinz body formation after incubation but normal GSH stability in vitro (Boivin et al., 1969). There is no spot-test available but an assay based upon the oxidation of GSH by H_2O_2 is discussed in the recent review by Necheles et al. (1970).

Defects of glutathione (GSH) synthesis

Two enzymatic steps are involved in the synthesis of GSH. The first of these is gammaglutamyl cysteine synthetase (gamma-GC synthetase) and the second is glutathione synthetase (GSH synthetase) (Fig. 7.3). The result of a block at either point is deficiency of glutathione and therefore of reduced glutathione (GSH), with consequences to the red cell similar to those of G-6-PD deficiency. Hereditary deficiency of the second enzyme was first described in a Dutch family by Oort, Loos and Prins in 1961, while deficiency of the first enzyme has only recently been described by Konrad et al. (1972) in a man and his sister of German descent.

Prins et al. (1966) reported a comprehensive study of GSH synthetase deficiency in a large Dutch family with 5 affected members. The defect was observed in both sexes but only in the offspring of consanguinous marriages, consistent with an autosomal recessive type of inheritance. The GSH level was less than 10 per cent of normal and this was associated with a chronic non-spherocytic haemolytic anaemia which was fairly well compensated. Red cell life span was reduced to $\frac{1}{3}$ to $\frac{1}{4}$ of normal. In addition, there appeared to be increased susceptibility to drug-induced haemolysis since the rate of red cell destruction was increased by administration of 30 mg primaquine per day, while another patient passed 'cola-coloured' urine after eating fava beans. Similar German (Löhr et al., 1963) and French cases (Boivin et al., 1966) have been described. A further more recent report confirms the autosomal recessive pattern of inheritance (Mohler et al., 1970). A 32-year-old male with a well-compensated haemolytic anaemia had no GSH-synthetase activity in his red cells, whereas cells from both his parents and his 4 children had levels that were half those of normals. In all the above reports there were no haematological abnormalities in the heterozygote carriers. Also it has been shown in several investigations that the defect resides solely in the second of GSH-synthetase enzymes, there being no other metabolic defect.

In homozygotes the haemoglobin has been 11.6 to 14.4 g/100 ml, reticulocytes 2.4 to 8.5 per cent and osmotic fragility normal. No striking abnormality of red cell morphology has been present. In the Heinz body formation test (Beutler *et al.*, 1955) during incubation with acetyl phenyl hydrazine there is a much greater number of relatively small Heinz bodies formed by comparison with G-6-PD deficiency (Prins *et al.*, 1966). The critical test is the determination of red cell GSH levels. This is readily measured colourimetrically on a metaphosphoric acid filtrate prepared from whole blood, using dithiobis-2-nitrobenzoic acid (Beutler *et al.*, 1963).

Gamma-glutamyl-cysteine synthetase deficiency is the most recently described red cell enzyme defect (Konrad *et al.*, 1972). A brother and sister of German descent with less than 5 per cent of the normal level of GSH in their red cells had suffered from mild anaemia and intermittent jaundice from birth. The spleens were palpable 3 cm below the costal margin. There was no mention of neonatal jaundice or drug sensitivity.

The haemolytic anaemia was non-spherocytic, with normal osmotic fragility, and usually adequately compensated with reticulocytes between 4 and 21.4 per cent. The autohaemolysis was increased up to 9.3 per cent and was not corrected by added glucose or adenosine. Biochemical investigations showed that the second enzyme, GSH synthetase, was normally present. The inheritance was probably autosomal recessive since the probands' male children as well as the probands' mother had intermediate levels of gamma-GC synthetase activity and no haematological abnormality. A neurological disorder was present in both affected patients but it is not known if this is related to the enzyme defect.

DISORDERS OF THE GLYCOLYTIC PATHWAY (EMBDEN-MEYERHOF)

This is the pathway (Fig. 7.1) through which over 90 per cent of glucose is metabolized in red cells. It is the sole source of ATP in the mature red cell. Defects of this pathway cause a chronic non-spherocytic haemolytic anaemia rather than the drug-induced haemolysis characteristic of defects affecting availability of GSH (Table 7.4). This is because the cation pump is impaired in the absence of adequate ATP and cell integrity compromised. The generation of NADP.H and GSH, required for protection from drug-induced haemolysis, remains unimpaired.

Table 7.4 Major clinical features of different red cell enzyme deficencies

	Clinical Features			Simple, Specific Diagnostic Test Available
Enzyme Affected	No Anemia	CNSHA*	Drug-Induced Hemolysis	
G6PD				Yes
Mediterranean variant	+		+	
African variant A–	+		+	
Rare variants	+	+	+	
Glutathione peroxidase	+	+	+	No
Glutathione reductase	+		+	Yes
Pyruvate kinase		+		Yes
Triose phosphate isomerase		+		Yes
6-Phosphogluconate dehydrogenase		+†	+	No
Hexokinase		+		No
2, 3-Diphosphoglycerate mutase		+		No
Glutathione synthetase		+	+	No
Glucose phosphate isomerase		+		No
Phosphoglycerate kinase		+		No
Adenosine triphosphatase		+		No

* Congenital nonspherocytic hemolytic anemia.
† Data from Waller, H. D., and Löhr, G.W.[2]

Reproduced, by permission of the authors and publishers, from Fairbanks and Fernandez (1969).

These defects of ATP formation tend to result in increased autohaemolysis but not in Heinz body formation or glutathione instability (Table 7.1).

Pyruvate kinase (PK)

Since the original description by Valentine, Tanaka and Miwa in 1961 first linking this deficiency with a form of congenital non-spherocytic anaemia there have been many subsequent reports, including those of Tanaka et al. (1962), Oski and Diamond (1963), Brunetti et al. (1963), Bowman and Procopio (1963), Bowdler and Prankerd (1964) and Necheles et al. (1966). After G-6-PD it is probably the second commonest defect causing haemolysis, with approximately 100 known cases. The majority of these patients are of Northern European descent but Mexican, Italian, Japanese, black American and Syrian individuals have also been affected.

Inheritance is of the autosomal recessive pattern with heterozygotes showing an intermediate level of enzyme in their red cells, but no evidence of haemolysis. In the homozygotes there is great variation in clinical severity. Oski et al. (1964) described one of the more severely affected patients, a boy of 5 whose haemoglobin ranged between 5.8 and 8.5 g per 100 ml, reticulocytes between 34 and 94 per cent and circulating normoblasts usually between 5 and 10 per 100 WBC. During his early life he required monthly transfusion (before splenectomy). The usual history includes neonatal jaundice, sometimes requiring exchange transfusion, followed by a life-long tendency to moderate anaemia and mild jaundice. These features are exacerbated by infections, but not by drug exposure. Milder cases show only intermittent anaemia or jaundice. On examination splenomegaly is a constant finding.

Haematologically the picture is of a non-spherocytic haemolytic anaemia with macrocytes, including some oval forms, polychromasia, anisocytosis and only occasional spherocytes. In addition, there is in PK deficiency a variable proportion of contracted red cells with multiple projecting spicules, rather like acanthocytes or pycnocytes. In the severe case described by Oski et al. (1964), 80 per cent of the red cells were of this form, but in other reports the proportion is much lower. Heinz bodies are only present after splenectomy. Osmotic fragility on unincubated blood is normal or decreased, although increased if performed after incubation. The most characteristic feature of PK deficiency is a markedly increased rate of autohaemolysis. This is of the Type II pattern showing no correction with glucose or adenosine, although usually with ATP, ADP, or AMP (Tanaka et al., 1962). When this association was first found it was thought for a while that all Type II cases were due to PK deficiency, but it is now known that the same pattern is found in GSSG-R, gamma-GC synthetase and sometimes in 2, 3 DPGM deficiencies. Biochemical investigations in the severe case mentioned above showed an absence of glucose consumption by the red cells except in the presence of an oxidant drug such as primaquine, which stimulates the hexose monophosphate shunt. As a result of defective ATP generation the red cells leak K^+ outwards and are unable to sustain a compensated overaction of the ATP dependent cation pump (Fig. 7.5). This defect

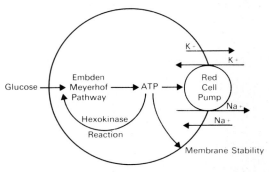

Fig. 7.5 Schematic model of the economy of ATP in the normal human RBC. (Reproduced from Nathan (1965), New England Journal of Medicine, 272, 118, by permission of the Editors and Dr D. G. Nathan).

is thought to lead to premature senescence and death of the red cell (Nathan et al., 1965). It explains the low ATP content of fresh red cells and the more rapid fall in ATP on incubation characteristic of non-spherocytic haemolytic anaemia with Type II autohaemolysis originally found by Robinson et al. (1961).

Specific diagnosis is made by quantitative assay of the enzyme as described by Valentine et al. (1961) or by a spot test devised by Beutler (1966) based on an NAD.H-linked reaction (Table 7.5). It is important that the red cell lysate is uncontaminated by leucocytes since these contain a different PK enzyme unaffected by red cell PK deficiency. The red cells of homozygotes have 10–20 per cent of normal PK activity while heterozygotes have 50 per cent or more activity.

The severity of the haemolysis is not directly related to the level of PK activity (Necheles et al., 1966), although proportional to the degree of autohaemolysis (Oski and Diamond, 1963). This

102   PAEDIATRIC HAEMATOLOGY

Table 7.5   Fluorescent tests for red cell enzyme deficiencies

Test			Results With	
			Normal Blood	Enzyme-Deficient Blood
For G6PD				
Glucose-6-phosphate + NADP	$\xrightarrow{\text{(G6PD)}}$	NADPH + 6-phosphogluconate	Fluorescence develops	No fluorescence
For Pyruvate Kinase (PK)				
Phosphoenol pyruvate + ADP	$\xrightarrow{\text{(PK)}}$	pyruvate + ATP	Fluorescence decreases	Fluorescence persists
Pyruvate + NADH	$\xrightarrow{\text{(lactic dehydrogenase)}}$	lactate + NAD		
For Glutathione Reductase (GSSG-R)				
Oxidized glutathione (GSSG) + 2 NADPH	$\xrightarrow{\text{(GSSG-R)}}$	2 GSH + 2 NADP	Fluorescence decreases	Fluorescence persists
For Triose Phosphate Isomerase (TPI)				
Glyceraldehyde-3-phosphate	$\xrightarrow{\text{(TPI)}}$	dihydroxy acetone phosphate	Fluorescence decreases	Fluorescence persists
Dihydroxy acetone phosphate + NADH	$\xrightarrow{\text{(n-glycerophosphate dehydrogenase)}}$	n-glycerophosphate + NAD		

Reproduced, by permission of the authors and publisher, from Fairbanks and Fernandez (1969).

may be because, at least in some cases, there is a kinetically abnormal PK which can be shown to be ineffective at the low substrate concentrations pertaining *in vivo*, although the defect is less apparen⁺ when tested at higher *in vitro* substrate concentrations (Boivin and Galand, 1967; Paglia *et al.*, 1968). Genetically determined isoenzymes may therefore exist for PK as in the case of G-6-PD and the severity of the clinical disorder could depend upon the particular variant inherited.

Preferential splenic sequestration of PK deficient cells can be demonstrated and these cells may be particularly sensitive to the glucose deprivation that occurs in the splenic sinuses (Necheles *et al.*, 1966). Splenectomy has been found to reduce transfusion requirements in severely affected patients (Oski *et al.*, 1964). It should probably be reserved for such cases since there is only partial benefit.

Hexokinase (HK)

This is the first enzyme on the glycolytic pathway (Fig. 7.1) and is thought to be the rate-limiting step in the process. A deficiency of HK is one of the rarer causes of hereditary non-spherocytic haemolytic anaemia, only 6 cases being known. The patient described by Valentine *et al.* (1967) was a girl of English and Polish extraction who had suffered from chronic anaemia and mild icterus since birth, required exchange transfusions in the neonatal period and a further blood transfusion at 6 weeks. She developed hepatosplenomegaly by 5 months and splenectomy was performed. After this she did not require further transfusions but a chronic anaemia with haemoglobin levels between 7.5 and 9.8 g/100 ml and reticulocytes of 7.4–24 per cent persisted. There was an episode of haemoglobinuria during an upper respiratory infection but no evidence of drug-induced haemolysis. The blood film showed a proportion of small densely staining red cells with spickle-like surface projections similar to those described in PK deficiency. Also there were target cells, normoblasts and rare spherocytes.

The enzyme deficiency is confined to the red cells. In the asymptomatic parents and siblings a partial deficiency is present suggesting an autosomal recessive pattern of inheritance. Since this is one of the enzymes where there is a much greater concentration in very young cells compared to older cells, due to rapid fall-off with cell age, the result has to be related to the reticulocyte count, in order to deduce the true degree of deficiency. Other investigations show a slight increase in autohaemolysis corrected by glucose and adenosine (Type I), normal GSH stability and normal enzyme kinetics.

A rather different disorder associated with HK deficiency had been described by Löhr et al. in 1965. This was a familial pancytopenia of the Fanconi type affecting 3 boys. There was a shortened red cell survival as well as decreased production. The enzyme deficiency affected the platelets and leucocytes as well as the red cells in these patients.

Recent investigations by Necheles et al. (1968) and Keitt (1969) have disclosed the presence of HK variants associated with haemolytic anaemia in which electrophoretic and kinetic abnormalities exist, resulting in decreased enzyme activity at low substrate concentrations. In the report by Keitt the product of the HK reaction, glucose-6-phosphate, was markedly decreased in the red cells of two anaemic patients and was partially reduced in four non-anaemic relatives.

Phosphohexose isomerase (PHI)

This is the second enzyme in the glycolytic pathway. To some extent a block at this point can be circumvented by glucose metabolism via the hexose monophosphate shunt (Fig. 7.3). Deficiency of PHI is a rare cause of chronic non-spherocytic haemolytic anaemia, 12 cases being so far reported. Baughan et al. (1968) described a boy of French and Irish descent with this deficiency. Anaemia was severe in the first seven months (Hb 4.7 to 6.8 g/100 ml). Splenomegaly developed and splenectomy was performed at 9 months, after which transfusion requirements ceased other than at times of infections. Chronic haemolysis continued, however, with a haemoglobin level of around 10 g/100 ml and reticulocytes of 28 per cent. The same group of workers (Paglia et al., 1969) subsequently reported 3 siblings with PHI deficiency who were Anglo-Saxon and unrelated to the first case. The anaemia was more severe, but again ameliorated by splenectomy. Although the anaemia has been accentuated by infections it does not appear to be drug-induced. Neonatal jaundice was mentioned in one patient. No leucocyte, platelet or neurological defects have been recorded.

The blood film in these patients showed the usual non-specific changes of a haemolytic anaemia together with the presence of a small proportion of darkly staining spiculated microspherocytes as in the two preceding enzyme deficiencies. Osmotic fragility was normal in unincubated blood but increased after incubation. Autohaemolysis is of the Type I pattern. Glutathione stability and the Heinz body formation test are normal. Detailed study of the enzyme has shown normal kinetics but electrophoretic heterogeneity (Detter et al., 1968).

Specific enzyme assay has shown levels of 14–30 per cent of normal in presumptive homozygotes with haemolysis, and intermediate values of around 50 per cent in assymptomatic heterozygous carriers. The pattern of inheritance is autosomal recessive. Interpretation of enzyme levels in patients with reticulocytosis is complicated by the higher enzyme levels in younger cells as in HK. The leucocytes also show PHI deficiency in affected individuals, but this appears to be without clinical significance. A screening test based upon the formation of fluorescent TPNH via an enzyme-linked reaction has recently been developed (Blume & Beutler, 1972).

Combined deficiency of PHI (homozygous) and G-6-PD (hemizygous) has been reported in a German boy (Schröter et al., 1971). He suffered from a moderate chronic non-spherocytic haemolytic anaemia since early childhood with haemolytic crises during infections and after the ingestion of haemolytic drugs.

Phosphofructokinase (PFK)

This is the third enzyme on the glycolytic pathway. PFK catalyses the conversion of fructose-6-phosphate to fructose-1, 6-diphosphate. ATP is a cosubstrate for PFK function, but in excess is an inhibitor of the reaction. This dual role of ATP in the PFK reaction leads to its function as one of the rate limiting steps in glycolysis. Frenkel and Waterbury (1972) have described the only patient so far known with PFK deficiency confined to the red cells and associated with haemolysis. Both the enzyme deficiency (60 per cent of normal) and the degree of haemolysis (9 per cent reticulocytes) were mild. A similar enzyme level was found in the mothers' and maternal grandmothers' red cells and it is possible that inheritance is linked to the X-chromosome. The enzyme showed abnormal lability *in vitro* and also increased inhibition by ATP.

The haemolysis was well compensated, the $T\frac{1}{2}$ by the ^{51}Cr method being 12–14 days (normal 28–32 days). Red cell morphology and osmotic fragility were normal, but autohaemolysis slightly increased and corrected by glucose.

This isolated defect of red cells has to be distinguished from Type VII glycogen storage disease with myoglobinuria occurring in Japanese and Jewish families. In this disorder there is a severe deficiency of muscle PFK and a mild deficiency of red cell PFK, to 50 per cent of normal, again with a mild compensated haemolytic anaemia (Tarui *et al.*, 1970).

Triosephosphate isomerase (TPI)

This enzyme is used to convert one half of each molecule of glucose metabolized from dihydroxyacetone phosphate to glyceraldehyde-3-phosphate (Fig. 7.1). Deficiency of TPI has been found to occur not only in red cells but also in leucocytes, skeletal muscle, serum and CSF in affected patients. In its absence there is an accumulation of dihydroxyacetone phosphate and this may be toxic to red cells and possibly to other tissues as well (Jaffé, 1970).

Schneider *et al.* (1964; 1965) reported the first family with this deficiency. A young girl of French and Negro extraction with TPI deficiency of red cells and leucocytes suffered from a chronic non-spherocytic haemolytic anaemia, recurrent infections and a progressive neurological disease with generalized spasticity. There was neither neonatal jaundice nor drug sensitivity. A sibling and a cousin, however, had died of neonatal haemolytic anaemia. The family history was consistent with an autosomal recessive type of inheritance. TPI deficiency has since been described in patients of Anglo-Saxon extraction. At least nine affected individuals are known and all but one have died before the age of six with a progressive neuromuscular disorder (Jaffé, 1970). The nature of this is imperfectly understood, but may be related to the widespread tissue deficiency of this enzyme in affected individuals.

The blood film shows slight macrocytosis, small numbers of target cells and occasional small, densely contracted red cells. Osmotic fragility is normal on fresh blood; increased after incubation. Autohaemolysis is increased to between 6.9 and 10.6 per cent but was fully corrected by glucose, adenosine or ATP (Schneider *et al.*, 1965). The enzyme activity is approximately 6 per cent of normal in homozygotes and 50 per cent in heterozygotes. A spot-test has been developed which may be useful for screening patients with neurological disease (Kaplan *et al.*, 1968A). Electrophoretic abnormality of the enzyme as well as deficient activity has also been found (Kaplan *et al.*, 1968B).

Glyceraldehyde-3-phosphate dehydrogenase (G-3-PD)

A father and son of English ancestry, both with a compensated haemolytic anaemia and 20–30 per cent the normal G-3-PD level, were described by Harkness (1966). Their serum showed slight hyperbilirubinaemia and there was a chronic reticulocytosis of 10–15 per cent. GSH stability was normal, osmotic fragility normal and autohaemolysis increased but corrected by glucose or ATP. The blood film showed the non-specific changes seen in the other glycolytic enzyme deficiencies together with small numbers of fragmented cells. A further report of G-3-PD deficiency associated with haemolysis has been made by Oski and Whaun (1969). The enzyme kinetics were normal, haemolysis was aggravated by oxidant compounds and the inheritance was possibly autosomal recessive.

Phosphoglycerate kinase (PGK)

This enzyme catalyses one of the ATP-productive steps in glycolysis. Deficiency would be expected to impose a severe metabolic handicap upon mature red cells. Even although a metabolic by-pass is possible via 2, 3-diphosphoglyceric acid (the Rapoport-Leubering shunt), this would not compensate for ATP production since none is generated in this shunt (Fig. 7.1).

Moderate deficiency of PGK, especially in the older red cells, was associated with a relatively well compensated non-spherocytic haemolytic anaemia in a 63-year-old Caucasian woman reported by Kraus *et al.* (1968). As no relatives were alive the pattern of inheritance could not be investigated. Valentine *et al.* (1969) described a Chinese family in which two male children were severely affected, and in which five male relatives in the maternal portion of the pedigree died in early childhood and may have had the same disorder. Female carriers had milder haemolysis and a moderate decrease in red cell PGK activity (Fig. 7.6). It appeared that PGK deficiency was X-chromosome linked, with intermediate expression in female heterozygotes compared to male hemizygotes.

The blood film was similar to that seen in other defects of the glycolytic system described above. Autohaemolysis was increased, and not reduced by glucose or ATP (Type II). The ATP concentration was low when related to the reticulocyte count. The 2,3-DPG concentration was elevated as

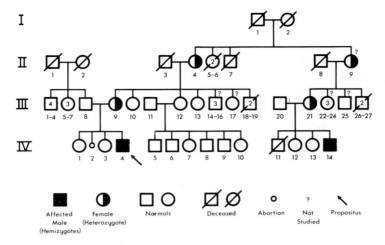

Fig. 7.6 Family study in phosphoglycerate kinase deficiency. (Reproduced from Valentine (1969), *New England Journal of Medicine*, **280**, 528, by permission of the Editors and Dr W. N. Valentine).

expected from metabolic considerations. Leukocytes as well as red cells are deficient in the enzyme but with no known adverse consequence.

Both the severely affected males in the later report suffered from moderate neurological abnormalities including convulsive seizures, mental retardation and emotional instability. There is a suspicion that the deficiency in PGK activity may directly or indirectly account for the mental defect (Valentine *et al.*, 1969).

There is no 'spot' test for PGK deficiency but Valentine *et al.* (1969) describe an enzyme linked assay. There is some evidence that the enzyme was different in the patient of Kraus *et al.* (1968) and that genetic polymorphism may exist as with certain other red cell enzymes.

2, 3-Diphosphoglyceromutase (2, 3-DPGase)

Deficiency of this enzyme is not quite so uncommon since there are 12 known cases; of German, French and British extraction (Lohr and Waller, 1963; Bowdler and Prankerd, 1964; Schröter, 1965; Syllm-Rapoport *et al.*, 1965).

Schröter's patient was a young infant with severe anaemia who survived only 3 months with transfusions. The parents were first cousins and their red cells contained approximately 50 per cent of the normal enzyme activity. They were considered to be asymptomatic heterozygotes, the inheritance being autosomal recessive. The occurrence of haemolysis in both son and father in the report of Bowdler and Prankerd (1964), however, suggests that it may be autosomal dominant.

Chronic haemolytic anaemia with mild splenomegaly and the haematological stigmata of non-spherocytic haemolytic anaemia have been found. Autohaemolysis is increased and corrected by glucose, adenosine or ATP. The ATP content is only slightly decreased and, unlike PGK deficiency, 2, 3-DPG, is decreased since 2, 3-DPGase is necessary for its formation (Fig. 7.1).

Splenectomy improves the anaemia without fully correcting the haemolysis (Bowdler and Prankerd, 1964), as is the case with many of the anaemias due to defects of the glycolytic pathway.

Adenosine triphosphatase (ATP-ase)

Harvald *et al.* (1964) described three Danish patients with this deficiency, and subsequently a French patient has been reported (Cotte *et al.*, 1968). It was suggested by Harvald *et al.* that the inheritance was 'dominant' with approximately 50 per cent ATP-ase activity in heterozygotes. The severity of anaemia is variable and accompanied by splenomegaly and intermittent jaundice. Haematological data are scanty but there is spherocytosis and the osmotic fragility was *decreased* in the French patient, which is the opposite to that expected if this is the same ATP-ase that is involved in the 'cation pump'. One of Harvald's patients benefited from splenectomy.

An excellent recent review of the diagnosis and management of red cell enzyme deficiencies in the context of haemolysis in the newborn is that by Gilman (1974). Another authoritative review of these disorders is that by Jaffé (1970). A useful annotation on laboratory diagnosis is that of Grimes (1969).

REFERENCES

Adam, A. (1961) Linkage between deficiency of glucose-6-phosphate dehydrogenase and colour blindness. *Nature (Lond.)*, **189**, 686.

Baughan, M. A., Valentine, W. N., Paglia, D. E., Ways, P. O., Simons, E. R. & de Marsh, Q. B. (1968) Hereditary hemolytic anemia associated with glucose-phosphate isomerase (GPI) deficiency—a new enzyme defect of human erythrocytes. *Blood*, **32**, 236.

Benesch, R. & Benesch, R. E. (1969) Intracellular organic phosphates as regulators of oxygen release by haemoglobin. *Nature (Lond.)*, **221**, 618.

Beutler, E. (1957) The glutathione instability of drug-sensitive red cells: A new method for the *in vitro* detection of drug sensitivity. *J. Lab. Clin. Med.*, **49**, 84.

Beutler, E. (1966) A series of new screening procedures for pyruvate kinase deficiency, glucose-6-phosphate dehydrogenase deficiency, and glutathione reductase deficiency. *Blood*, **28**, 553.

Beutler, E. (1969) Effect of flavin compounds on glutathione reductase activity: *in vivo* and *in vitro* studies. *J. Clin. Invest.*, **48**, 1957.

Beutler, E. (1969A) Genetic disorders of red cell metabolism. *Medical Clinics of North America*, **53**, 813.

Beutler, E. (1969B) Drug-induced hemolytic anemia. *Pharmacological Reviews*, **21**, 73.

Beutler, E. (1970) Annotation: Glucose-6-phosphate dehydrogenase deficiency. *Brit. J. Haemat.*, **18**, 117.

Beutler, E. (1971) Abnormalities of the hexose monophosphate shunt. *Semin. Hematol.*, **8**, 311.

Beutler, E., Dern, R. J. & Alving, A. S. (1955) The hemolytic effect of primaquine. *VI*. An *in vitro* test for sensitivity to erythrocytes to primaquine. *J. Lab. Clin. Med.*, **45**, 40.

Beutler, E., Yeh, M. & Fairbanks, V. F. (1962) The normal human female as a mosaic of X-chromosome activity: Studies using the gene for G–6–PD deficiency as a marker. *Proc. Nat. Acad. Sci.*, **48**, 9.

Beutler, E., Duron, O. & Kelly, B. M. (1963) Improved method for the determination of blood glutathione. *J. Lab. Clin. Med.*, **61**, 882.

Beutler, E. & Baluda, M. C. (1964) The separation of glucose–6–phosphate dehydrogenase-deficient erythrocytes from the blood of heterozygotes for glucose–6–phosphate dehydrogenase deficiency. *Lancet*, **i**, 189.

Blume, K. G., Rüdiger, H. W. & Lohr, G. W. (1968) Electrophoresis of glutathione reductase from human blood cells. *Biochim. Biphys. Acta.*, **151**, 686.

Blume, K. G. & Beutler, E. (1972) Detection of glucose phosphate isomerase deficiency by a screening procedure. *Blood*, **39**, 685.

Boivan, P., Galand, C., André, R. & Debray, J. (1966) Anémies hémolytiques congénitales avec déficit isolé en glutathione réduit par déficit en glutathione synthétase. *Nouv. Rev. Franc. Hemat.*, **6**, 859.

Boivan, P. & Galand, C. (1967) Constante de michaelis anormale pour le phospho-enol-pyruvate au cours d'un déficit en pyruvate-kinase erythrocytaire. *Rev. Franc. Etud. Clin. Biol.*, **12**, 372.

Boivan, P., Galand, C., Hakim, J., Roge, J. & Guéroult, N. (1969) Anémie hémolytique avec déficit en glutathione-peroxydase chez un adulte. *Enzym. Biol. Clin.*, **10**, 68.

Bowdler, A. J. & Prankerd, T. A. L. (1964) Studies in congenital non-spherocytic haemolytic anaemias with specific enzyme defects. *Acta Haemat.*, **31**, 65.

Bowman, H. S. & Procopio, F. (1963) Hereditary non-spherocytic hemolytic anemia of pyruvate-kinase deficient type. *Ann. Int. Med.*, **58**, 567.

Brewer, G. J., Tarlov, A. R. & Kellermeyer, R. W. (1961) The hemolytic effect of primaquine: *XII*. Shortened erythrocyte life span in primaquine sensitive male Negroes in the absence of drug administration. *J. Lab. Clin. Med.*, **58**, 217.

Brewer, G. J. & Dern, R. J. (1964) A new inherited enzymatic deficiency of human erythrocytes: 6-phosphogluconate dehydrogenase deficiency. *Am. J. Human Genet.*, **16**, 472.

Brunetti, P., Puxeddu, A., Nenci, G. & Migliorini, E. (1963) Haemolytic anaemia due to pyruvate-kinase deficiency. *Lancet*, **2**, 169.

Bunn, H. F., & Jandl, J. H. (1970) Control of hemoglobin function within the red cell. *New Eng. J. Med.*, **282**, 1414.

Burka, E. R., Weaver, Z. & Marks, P. A. (1966) Clinical spectrum of hemolytic anemia associated with glucose–6–phosphate dehydrogenase deficiency. *Ann. Intern. Med.*, **64**, 817.

Busch, D. & Heimpel, H. (1969) Hereditäre nicht sphrozytäre hämolytische Anämie mit hohen Erythrocyten—ATP. *Blut.*, **19**, 293.

Carson, P. E., Flanagan, C. L., Ickes, C. E. & Alving, A. S. (1956) Enzymatic deficiency in primaquine-sensitive erythrocytes. *Science*, **124**, 484.

Carson, P. E., Brewer, G. J. & Ickes, C. (1961) Decreased glutathione reductase with susceptibility to hemolysis. *J. Lab. Clin. Med.*, **58**, 804.

Carson, P. E. & Frischer, H. (1966) Glucose–6–phosphate dehydrogenase deficiency and related disorders of the pentose phosphate pathway. *Amer. J. Med.*, **41**, 744.

Cohen, G. & Hochstein, P. (1963) Glutathione peroxidase: The primary agent for elimination of hydrogen peroxide in erythrocytes. *Biochemistry*, **2**, 1420.

Committee on Nutrition (1961) Vitamin K compounds and the water-soluble analogues. Use in therapy and prophylaxis. *Pediatrics*, **28**, 501.

Cotte, J., Kissin, C., Mathieu, M., Poncet, J., Monnet, P., Salle, B. & Germain, D. (1968) Observation d'un cas de déficit partiel en ATPase intraérythrocytaire. *Rev. Franc. Etudes Clin. Biol.*, **13**, 284.

DeGruchy, G. C., Santamaria, J. N., Parsons, I. C. & Crawford, H. (1960) Non-spherocytic congenital hemolytic anemia. *Blood*, **16**, 1371.

Dern, R. J., Weinstein, I. M., LeRoy, G. V., Talmage, D. W. & Alving, A. S. (1954) The hemolytic effect of primaquine: I. The localization of the drug induced hemolytic defect in primaquine sensitive individuals. *J. Lab. Clin. Med.*, **43**, 303.

Dern, R. J., Brewer, G. J., Tashian, R. E. & Shows, T. B. (1966) Hereditary variation of erythrocytic 6-phosphogluconate dehydrogenase. *J. Lab. Clin. Med.*, **67**, 255.

Desforges, J. F., Thayer, W. W. & Dawson, J. P. (1959) Hemolytic anemia induced by sulfoxone therapy, with investigations into the mechanisms of its production. *Amer. J. Med.*, **27**, 132.

Detter, J. C., Ways, P. O., Giblett, E. R., Baughan, M. A., Hopkinson, D. A., Povey, S. & Harris, H. (1968) Inherited variations in human phosphohexose isomerase. *Ann. Human Genet.*, **31**, 329.

Doxiadis, S. A. & Valaes, T. (1964) The clinical picture of glucose–6–phosphate dehydrogenase deficiency in early infancy. *Arch. Dis. Childh.*, **39**, 545.

Doxiadis, S. A., Valaes, T., Karaklis, A. & Stavrakakis, D. (1964) Risk of severe jaundice in glucose 6-phosphate-dehydrogenase deficiency of the newborn. *Lancet*, **ii**, 1210.

Earle, D. P., Bigelow, F. S., Zubrod, C. G. & Kane, C. A. (1948) Studies on the chemotherapy of the human malarias. IX. Effect of pamaquine on the blood cells of man. *J. Clin. Invest.*, **27**, 121.

Emanuel, B. & Schoenfield, A. (1961) Favism in a nursing infant. *J. Pediat.*, **58**, 263.

Escobar, M. A., Heller, P. & Trobaugh, F. E. (1964) Complete erythrocyte glucose–6–phosphate dehydrogenase deficiency, non-spherocytic hemolytic anemia in a Caucasian adult associated with neurological abnormalities. *Arch. Intern. Med.*, **113**, 428.

Eys, J. Van (1970) Recent progress in genetic hemolytic disorders: A practical approach. *Pediat. Clinics of N. America*, **17**, 449.

Fairbanks, V. F. & Fernandez, M. N. (1969) The identification of metabolic errors associated with hemolytic anemia. *J.A.M.A.*, **208**, 316.

Finch, C. A. & Lenfant, C. (1972) Oxygen transport in man. *New Eng. J. Med.*, **286**, 407.

Frenkel, E. P. & Waterbury, L. (1972) Hereditary non-spherocytic hemolysis with erythrocyte phosphofructokinase deficiency. *Blood*, **39**, 415.

Gasser, C. (1953) Die hämolytische Frühgeburtenanamie mit spontaner Innenkörporbildung. Ein venes Syndrom, beobachtet an 14 Fallen. *Helv. Paediat. Acta.*, **8**, 491.

George, J. N., O'Brien, R. L., Pollack, S. & Crosby, W. H. (1966) Studies of *in vitro* primaquine hemolysis: substrate requirement for erythrocyte membrane damage. *J. Clin. Invest.*, **45**, 1280.

Gilman, P. A. (1974) Hemolysis in the newborn infant resulting from deficiencies of red blood cell enzymes: Diagnosis and management. *J. Pediat.*, **84**, 625.

Gordon, H. H., Nitowsky, H. M. & Cornblath, M. (1955) Studies of tocopherol deficiency in infants and childhood. *Amer. J. Dis. Child.*, **90**, 669.

Gordon-Smith, E. C. & White, J. M. (1974) Annotation: Oxidative haemolysis and Heinz body haemolytic anaemia. *Brit. J. Haemat.*, **26**, 513.

Grant, F. L. & Winks, G. F. (1961) Primaquine sensitive hemolytic anemia complicating diabetic acidosis. *Clin. Res.*, **9**, 27.

Grimes, A. J., Leets, I. & Dacie, J. V. (1968) The autohaemolysis test: appraisal of the method for the diagnosis of pyruvate kinase deficiency and the effect of pH and additives. *Brit. J. Haemat.*, **14**, 309.

Grimes, A. J. (1969) Annotation: The laboratory diagnosis of enzyme defects in the red cell. *Brit. J. Haemat.*, **17**, 129.

Gross, R. T., Bracci, R., Rudolph, N., Schroeder, E. & Kochen, J. A. (1967) Hydrogen peroxide toxity and detoxification in the erythrocytes of newborn infants. *Blood*, **29**, 481.

Grossman, A., Ramathan, K., Justice, P., Gordon, J., Shahidi, N. T. & Hsai, D. (1966) Congenital non-spherocytic hemolytic anemia associated with erythrocyte glucose–6–phosphate dehydrogenase deficiency in a Negro family. *Pediat.*, **37**, 624.

Hamasaki, N., Asakura, T. & Minakami, S. (1970) Effect of oxygen tension on glycolysis in human erythrocytes. *J. Biochem. (Tokyo)*, **68**, 157.

Harkness, D. R. (1966) A new erythrocytic enzyme defect with hemolytic anemia. Glyceraldehyde–3–phosphate dehydrogenase deficiency. *J. Lab. Clin. Med.*, **68**, 879.

Harvald, B., Hanel, K. V., Squires, R. & Trap-Jensen, J. (1964) Adenosine-triphosphatase deficiency in patients with non-spherocytic hemolytic anemia. *Lancet*, **2**, 18.

Hockwald, R. S., Arnold, J., Clayman, C. B. & Alving, A. S. (1952) Toxicity of primaquine in Negroes. *J. Am. Med. Assoc.*, **149**, 1568.

Jacob, H. S. & Jandl, J. H. (1962) Effects of sulphydryl inhibition on red blood cells. I. Mechanism of hemolysis. *J. Clin. Invest.*, **41**, 779.

Jaffé, E. R. (1970) Clinical profile: Hereditary hemolytic disorders and enzymatic deficiencies of human erythrocytes. *Blood*, **35**, 116.

Jaffé, E. R. (1972) Oxidative hemolysis, or What made the red cell break? *New Eng. J. Med.*, **286**, 156.

Jaffé, E. R. & Gottfried, E. D. (1968) Hereditary non-spherocytic hemolytic disease associated with an altered phospholipid composition of the erythrocytes. *J. Clin. Invest.*, **47**, 1375.

Kaplan, J. C., Shore, N. & Beutler, E. (1968A) The rapid detection of triosephosphate isomerase deficiency. *Amer. J. Clin. Path.*, **50**, 656.

Kaplan, J. C., Teeple, L., Shore, N. & Beutler, E. (1968B) Electrophoretic abnormality in triosephosphate isomerase deficiency. *Biochem. Biophys. Res. Commun.*, **31**, 768.

108 PAEDIATRIC HAEMATOLOGY

Keitt, A. S. (1969) Hemolytic anemia with impaired hexokinase activity. *J. Clin. Invest.*, **48**, 1997.

Kirkman, H. N., Riley, H. D. & Crowell, B. B. (1960) Different enzymic expressions of mutants of human glucose–6–phosphate dehydrogenase. *Proc. Natl. Acad. Sci.*, **46**, 938.

Kirkman, H. N., Rosenthal, I. M., Simon, E. R., Carson, P. E. & Brinson, A. G. (1964) Chicago I variant of glucose–6-phosphate dehydrogenase in congenital hemolytic disease. *J. Lab. Clin. Med.*, **63**, 715.

Kirkman, H. N., Kidson, C. & Kennedy, M. (1968) Variants of human glucose–6–phosphate dehydrogenase. Studies of samples from New Guinea. In *Hereditary Disorders of Erythrocyte Metabolism. City of Hope Symposium Series*, Vol. 1, p. 126. Ed. by E. Beutler. Grune and Stratton. New York.

Konrad, P. N. Richads, F., Valentine, W. N. & Paglia, D. E. (1972) Gamma-glutamyl-cysteine synthetase deficiency —a cause of hereditary hemolytic anemia. *New. Eng. Med., ed.*, **286**, 557.

Lausecker, C., Heidt, P., Fisher, D., Hartleyb, H. & Löhr, G. W. (1965) Anémie hémolytique constitutionnelle avec déficit en 6–phospho-gluconate-déshydrogénase. *Arch. Franc. Pediat.*, **21**, 789.

Löhr, G. W., Baum, P. & Kamm, G. (1963) Toxische hämolytische Anämien. *Med. Klin.*, **58**, 2111.

Löhr, G. W. & Waller, H. D. (1963) Zur Biochemie einiger angeboremer hämolytischer Anämien. *Folia Haematol.*, **8**, 377.

Löhr, G. W., Waller, H. D., Anschütz, F. & Knopp, A. (1965) Biochemische Defekte in den Blutzellen bei familiärer Pamyelopathie (Typ Fanconi). *Humangenetik*, **1**, 383.

Lopez, R. & Cooperman, J. M. (1971) Glucose–6–phosphate dehydrogenase deficiency and hyperbilirubinemia in the newborn. *Amer. J. Dis. Child.*, **122**, 66.

Lyon, M. F. (1961) Gene action in the X-chromosome of the mouse (*mus musculinus L.*). *Nature*, **190**, 372.

Marks, P. A. & Cross, R. T. (1959) Erythrocyte glucose–6–phosphate dehydrogenase deficiency: Evidence of differences between Negroes and Caucasians with respect to this genetically determined trait. *J. Clin. Invest.*, **38**, 2253.

Meyer, T. C. & Angus, J. (1956) The effect of large doses of Synkavit in the newborn. *Arch. Dis. Childh.*, **31**, 212.

Mohler, D. N. & Crockett, C. L. (1964) Hereditary hemolytic disease secondary to glucose–6–phosphate dehydrogenase deficiency: Report of three cases with special emphasis on ATP metabolism. *Blood*, **23**, 427.

Mohler, D. N., Majerus, P. W., Minnich, V., Hess, C. E. & Garrick, M. D. (1970) Glutathione synthetase deficiency as a cause of hereditary hemolytic disease. *New Eng. J. Med.*, **283**, 1253.

Motulsky, A. G. (1964) Pharmacogenetics. In *Progress in Medical Genetics*, **3**, 49. Ed. Steinberg, A. G. and Bearn, A. G. New York: Grune and Stratton.

Naiman, J. L. & Kosoy, M. H. (1964) Red cell glucose–6–phosphate dehydrogenase deficiency—a newly recognised cause of neonatal jaundice and kernicterus in Canada. *Canad. M.A.J.*, **91**, 1243.

Nathan, D. G., Oski, F. A., Sidel, V. W. & Diamond, L. K. (1965) Extreme hemolysis and red cell distortion in erythrocyte pryuvate kinase deficiency: II. Measurements of erythrocyte glucose consumption, potassium flux and adenosine triphosphate stability. *New. Eng. J. Med.*, **272**, 118.

Necheles, T. F., Finkel, H. E., Sheehan, R. G. & Allen, D. M. (1966) Red cell pyruvate kinase deficiency. The effect of splenectomy. *Arch. Intern. Med.*, **118**, 75.

Necheles, T. F., Boles, T. A. & Allen, D. M. (1968) Erythrocyte glutathione peroxidase deficiency and hemolytic disease of the newborn infant. *J. Pediat.*, **72**, 319.

Necheles, T. F., Rai, U. S. & Allen, D. M. (1968) A hexokinase variant associated with congenital non-spherocytic hemolytic disease. *Clin. Res.*, **16**, 540.

Necheles, T. F., Maldonado, N., Barquet-Chediak, A. & Allen, D. M. (1969) Homozygous erythrocyte glutathione-deficiency: Clinical and biochemical studies. *Blood*, **33**, 164.

Necheles, T. F., Steinberg, M. H. & Cameron, D. (1970) Erythrocyte glutathione-peroxidase deficiency. *Brit. J. Haemat.*, **19**, 605.

Newton, W. A. & Bass, J. C. (1958) Glutathione-sensitive chronic non-spherocytic hemolytic anemia. *Am. J. Dis. Child.*, **95**, 501.

Oort, M., Loos, J. A. & Prins, H. K. (1961) Hereditary absence of reduced glutathione in the erythrocytes—a new clinical and biochemical entity? *Vox Sanguinis*, **6**, 370.

Oski, F. A. & Diamond, L. K. (1963) Erythrocyte pyruvate kinase deficiency: report of three cases. *New Eng. J. Med.*, **269**, 763.

Oski, F. A., Nathan, D. G., Sidel, V. W. & Diamond, L. K. (1964) Extreme hemolysis and red cell distortion in erythrocyte pyruvate kinase deficiency. I. Morphology, erythrokinetics and family enzyme studies. *New. Eng. J. Med.*, **270**, 1023.

Oski, F. A. & Whaun, J. (1969) Hemolytic anemia and red cell glyceraldehyde–3–phosphate dehydrogenase (G–3–PD) deficiency. *Clin. Res.*, **17**, 601.

Oski, F. A. & Naiman, J. L. (1972) *Hematologic Problems in the Newborn*. Philadelphia: W. B. Saunders.

Paglia, D. E., Valentine, W. N., Baughan, M. A., Miller, D. R., Reed, C. F. & McIntyre, O. R. (1968) An inherited molecular lesion of erythrocyte pyruvate kinase. Identification of a kinetically aberrant isoenzyme associated with premature hemolysis. *J. Clin. Invest.*, **47**, 1929.

Paglia, D. E., Holland, P., Baughan, M. A. & Valentine, W. N. (1969) Occurrence of defective hexosemonophosphate isomerization in human erythrocytes and leukocytes. *New Eng. J. Med.*, **280**, 66.

Parr, C. W. & Fitch, L. I. (1967) Inherited quantitative variations of human phosphogluconate dehydrogenase. *Ann. Hum. Genet.*, **30**, 339.

Prager, D. (1967) The autohemolysis test. *J.A.M.A.*, **201**, 189.

Prins, H. K., Oort, M., Loos, J. A., Zürcher, C. & Beckers, T. (1966) Congenital non-spherocytic hemolytic anemia, associated with glutathione deficiency of the erythrocytes. Hematologic, biochemical and genetic studies. *Blood*, **27**, 145.

HEREDITARY NON-SPHEROCYTIC HAEMOLYTIC ANAEMIAS (ENZYME DEFICIENCIES) 109

Rapoport, S. & Luebering, J. (1952) The 2, 3–diphosphoglycerate cycle in human erythrocytes. *J. Biol. Chem.*, **196**, 583.

Ratazzi, M. C., Corash, L. M. van Zanen, G. E., Jaffé, E. R. & Piomelli, S. (1971) G–6–PD deficiency and chronic hemolysis: Four new mutants—relationships between clinical syndrome and enzyme kinetics. *Blood*, **38**, 205.

Robinson, M. A., Loder, P. B. & deGruchy, G. C. (1961) Red-cell metabolism in nonspherocytic congenital haemolytic anaemia. *Brit. J. Haemat.*, **7**, 327.

Ross, J. D. (1963) Deficient activity of DPNH-dependent methaemoglobin diaphorase in cord blood erythrocytes. *Blood*, **21**, 51.

Salen, G., Goldstein, F., Haurani, F. & Wirts, C. W. (1966) Acute hemolytic anemia complicating viral hepatitis in patients with glucose–6–phosphate dehydrogenase deficiency. *Ann. Internal Med.*, **65**, 1210.

Schneider, A. S., Valentine, W. N., Hattori, M. & Heins, H. L. (1964) A new erythrocyte enzyme defect with hemolytic anemia—triosephosphate isomerase (TPI) deficiency. *Blood*, **24**, 855.

Schneider, A. S., Valentine, W. N., Hattori, M. & Heins, H. L. (1965) Hereditary hemolytic anemia with triosephosphate isomerase deficiency. *New Eng. J. Med.*, **272**, 229.

Schröter, W. (1965) Kongenital nichtsphärocytare hämolytische Anämie bei, 2,–3–diphospho-glyceratmutase-mangel der Erythrocyten im frühen Säuglingsalter. *Klin. WSCHR.*, **43**, 1147.

Schröter, W., Brittinger, G., Zimmerschmitt, E., König, E. & Schrader, D. (1971) Combined glucosephosphate isomerase and glucose–6–phosphate dehydrogenase deficiency of the erythrocytes: A new haemolytic syndrome. *Brit. J. Haemat.*, **20**, 249.

Selwyn, J. G. & Dacie, J. V. (1954) Autohemolysis and other changes resulting from the incubation *in vitro* of red cells from patients with congenital hemolytic anemia. *Blood*, **9**, 414.

Shahidi, N. T. & Diamond, L. K. (1959) Enzyme deficiency in erythrocytes in congenital nonspherocytic hemolytic anemia. *Pediat.*, **24**, 245.

Siniscalco, M., Filippi, G., Latte, B., Piomelli, S., Ratazzi, M., Gavin, J., Sanger, R. & Race, R. R. (1966) Failure to detect linkage beteen Xg and other X-borne loci in Sardinians. *Ann. Hum. Genet.*, **29**, 231.

Stamatoyannopoulos, G., Fraser, G. R., Motulsky, A. G., Fessas, Ph., Akrivakis, A. & Papayannopoulou, Th. (1966) On the familial predisposition to favism. *Amer. J. Hum. Genet.*, **18**, 253.

Syllm-Rapoport, I., Jacobasch, G., Roigas, H. & Rapoport, S. (1965) 2, 3–PGase mangel als mögliche ursache erhöten ATP-gehaltes. *Folia Haemat.*, **83**, 363.

Tanaka, K. R., Valentine, W. N. & Miwa, S. (1962) Pyruvate kinase (PK) deficiency hereditary non-spherocytic hemolytic anemia. *Blood*, **19**, 267.

Tarui, S., Kono, N., Nasu, T. & Nishikawa, M. (1970) Enzymatic basis for the co-existence of a myopathy and hemolytic disease in inherited muscle phosphofructokinase deficiency. *Biochem. Biophys. Res. Commun.*, **34**, 77.

Valentine, W. N., Tanaka, K. R. & Miwa, S. (1961) Specific erythrocyte glycolytic enzyme defect (pyruvate kinase) in three subjects with congenital non-spherocytic hemolytic anemia. *Tr. A. Am. Physicians*, **74**, 100.

Valentine, W. N., Oski, F. A., Paglia, D. E., Baughan, M. A., Schneider, A. S. & Naiman, J. L. (1967) Hereditary hemolytic anemia with hexokinase deficiency. Role of hexokinase in erythrocyte ageing. *New Eng. J. Med.*, **276**, 1.

Valentine, W. N., Hsieh, H. S., Paglia, D. E., Anderson, H. M., Baughan, M. A., Jaffé, E. R. & Garson, O. M. (1969) Hereditary hemolytic anemia associated with phosphoglycerate kinase deficiency in erythrocytes and leukocytes: A probable X-chromosome linked syndrome. *New Eng. J. Med.*, **280**, 528.

Valentine, W. N., Anderson, H. M., Paglia, D. E., Jaffé, E. R., Konrad, P. N. & Harris, S. R. (1972) Studies on human erythrocyte nucleotide metabolism. II. Non-spherocytic hemolytic anemia, high red cell ATP, and ribosphosphate pyrophosphokinase deficiency. *Blood*, **39**, 674.

Waller, H. D., Löhr, G. W., Zysno, E., Gerok, W., Voss, D. & Strauss, G. (1965) Glutathion-reduktasemangel mit hämatologischen und neurologischen Störungen (Autosomal dominant vererbliche Bildung eines pathologischen Enzymes). *Klin. Wochschr.*, **43**, 413.

Waller, H. D. (1968) Glutathione reductase deficiency. In *Hereditary Disorders of Erythrocyte Metabolism*. Ed. Beutler, E. New York: Grune and Stratton.

Weed, R. I. (1961) Effects of primaquine on the red blood cell membrane. II. K^+ permeability in glucose–6–phosphate dehydrogenase deficient erythrocytes. *J. Clin. Invest.*, **40**, 140.

Westring, D. W. & Pisciotta, A. V. (1966) Anemia, cataracts and seizures in a patient with glucose–6–phosphate dehydrogenase deficiency. *Arch. Intern. Med.*, **118**, 385.

Whaun, J. M. & Oski, F. A. (1970) Relation of red blood cell glutathione peroxidase to neonatal jaundice. *J. Pediat.*, **76**, 555.

Yoshida, A. (1968) The structure of normal and variant human glucose–6–phosphate dehydrogenase in genetically determined abnormalities of red cell metabolism. *City of Hope Symposium Series*, **i**, 126. Ed. by E. Beutler.

Zinkham, W. H. (1963) Peripheral blood and bilirubin values in normal full-term primaquine sensitive Negro infants: effect of vitamin K. *Pediatrics*, **21**, 983.

Zinkham, W. H. & Childs, B. (1958) A defect of glutathione metabolism in erythrocytes from patients with naphthalene-induced hemolytic anemia. *Pediatrics*, **22**, 461.

8. Abnormalities of Haemoglobin Synthesis

Basic considerations, *Chemical structure of haemoglobin, Normal variants of haemoglobin, Haemoglobins present at birth, Detection of foetal haemoglobin, Physiological significance of foetal haemoglobin, Postnatal changes in Hb F concentration* / Genetically determined abnormalities of haemoglobin structure / The haemoglobinopathies, *Inheritance, Geographic distribution and incidence, Sickling states, Unstable haemoglobins, M-Haemoglobinopathies and other causes of methaemoglobinaemia, Thalassaemia syndromes.*

These include the haemoglobinopathies, thalassaemia syndromes, defects of porphyrin synthesis and defects of iron incorporation into haem (sideroblastic anaemias). They can cause haemolysis, impairment of haemoglobin production or both.

BASIC CONSIDERATIONS

Haemoglobinopathies result from a genetically determined amino acid substitution in one of the polypeptide chains of the globin portion of the molecule, causing synthesis of a pathological form of haemoglobin, e.g. Hb S, Hb C, etc. Thalassaemias result from a genetically determined impairment of production of one of the polypeptide chains (usually alpha or beta chains) of the molecule. No abnormally constituted polypeptide chains nor pathological haemoglobin are formed (Weatherall, 1968) but there is unbalanced overproduction of alternative polypeptide chains and consequently of certain forms of haemoglobin which are normally present in only trace amounts, e.g. Hb F and Hb A_2. Defects of porphyrin synthesis or of iron incorporation into haem do not result in abnormal or unbalanced haemoglobin formation.

Chemical structure of haemoglobin

Haemoglobin consists of four polypeptide chains to each of which is attached an identical haem group

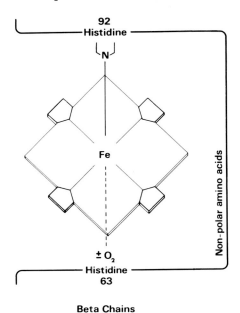
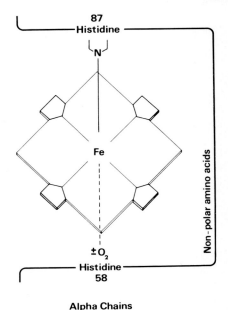

Fig. 8.1 Attachment of the haem plate within pockets of alpha and beta chains.

partially enclosed within a pocket of the chain. In normal adult haemoglobin (Hb A) there are two alpha chains of 141 amino acids and two beta chains of 146 amino acids. Many of the amino acid sequences are common to alpha and beta chains and they share a common three-dimensional structure. The conventional designation of Hb A is $\propto_2^A \beta_2^A$; indicating the presence of two alpha and two beta chains; the superscription 'A' indicating that these alpha and beta chains are of the normal type as found in Hb A. The four chains are arranged in such a way that there is close contact between the alpha and beta chains, but less contact between like chains (Huehens and Bellingham, 1969).

Furthermore the alpha 1 = beta 1 contact is firmer than the alpha 1 — beta 2 contact (Rosemeyer and Huehns, 1967). Movement takes place at the latter contact during reversible interaction between Hb and 0_2. The beta chains move 5 Å farther apart during reduction of oxyhaemoglobin (Perutz et al., 1968). This point is relevant to an understanding of the sickling process (vide infra) and of the behaviour of amino acid substitutions in the regions of alpha 1 = beta 1 or alpha 1 — beta 2 contacts (Huehens and Bellingham, 1969).

Haem groups are bound through their central iron to the imidazole groups of 'proximal' histidine units at position 92 of the beta chains and position 87 of the alpha chains respectively. The sixth co-ordination position of the haem iron, the site of reversible oxygenation, is oriented towards another 'distal' histidine unit at position 63 of the beta chain and position 58 of the alpha chain, which occupy analagous positions on their respective chains (Fig. 8.1). Amino acid substitutions in the

haemoglobin (Jacob et al., 1968; Carrell and Lehmann, 1969).

Normal variants of haemoglobin

After the neonatal period there are normally three types of haemoglobin in the blood; Hb A is the predominant form, and HB F and Hb A_2 are both present in much smaller amounts. Identical alpha chains of 141 amino acids are common to these three haemoglobins (Huehens and Shooter, 1961). It is the non-alpha chains of 146 amino acids which distinguish Hb A, F and A_2 (Table 8.1). During foetal life two further 'embryonic' haemoglobins are transiently present; Gower I and II. These contain epsilon chains present only in early foetal life (Table 8.1). The earliest form (Gower I) is a tetramer of epsilon chains; the later form (Gower II) consists of alpha chains plus epsilon chains (Huehens and Shooter, 1965).

Ingram (1961) has suggested that the different chains arose one from another by a process of gene duplication. Of the non-alpha chains gamma may have been the oldest (Hb F), from which beta chains evolved (Hb A), with 71 per cent of amino acid sequences identical. Finally, delta chains (Hb A_2) may have evolved from beta, with 96 per cent of amino acids identical (Lehmann et al., 1966).

Recently it has been found that there are two types of gamma chain; one (G gamma) with glycine at position 136, the other (A gamma) with alanine at this position (Schroeder et al., 1968). The ratio of G gamma to A gamma is 3.1 in the Hb F present at birth but 2.3 in the Hb F present after the neonatal period and in later life (Huisman et al.,

Table 8.1 Normal haemoglobins

	Proportion after age of 3	Constitution
Hb A	95–98 per cent	alpha$_2$ beta$_2$
Hb F	0–2 per cent	alpha$_2$ gamma$_2$
Hb A_2	1–3 per cent	alpha$_2$ delta$_2$
	Embryonic haemoglobins	
Gower I ⎫	Present only in first 3	epsilon$_4$
Gower II ⎭	months of foetal life	alpha$_2$ epsilon$_2$

proximity of the haem plate invariably produce a haematological disorder either by rendering the haem more susceptible to oxidation (M-haemoglobins, unstable haemoglobins) or by increasing (Hb Chesapeake) or decreasing (Hb Hammersmith) the oxygen affinity of the

1970). A further subdivision of HbF is that there is a minor component (F_1), constituting approximately 20 per cent of the Hb F in cord blood, which differs from the normal (F_{11}) form in that one of its two alpha chains is acetylated at the N-terminal amino group (Schroeder et al., 1962).

ABNORMALITIES OF HAEMOGLOBIN SYNTHESIS 113

Table 8.2 Types of haemoglobin present at birth

	Percentage of total	Composition
HbA	15–40	alpha$_2$ beta$_2$
HbF	50–85	alpha$_2$ gamma$_2$
HbA$_2$	< 0·3	alpha$_2$ delta$_2$
Hb Bart's	Trace, < 0·5	gamma$_4$

Haemoglobins present at birth

At birth Hb F is present in much higher concentrations than in later life (Table 8.2).

Not only is there a preferential synthesis of gamma chains during late foetal life resulting in the preponderance of Hb F, but there also appears to be a slight excess of gamma chains over alpha chains (Weatherall, 1963). These excess gamma chains combine to form the tetramer gamma$_4$, Hb Bart's, normally present in only trace amounts (<1 per cent). It is termed a 'fast' haemoglobin by virtue of its electrophoretic mobility. Examination of a blood film by the Kleihauer technique shows that virtually all red cells at birth contain some Hb F but that there is graduation in intensity of staining suggesting that there is a variable ratio of Hb F to Hb A among the different foetal red cells (Fraser and Raper, 1962; Shepherd et al., 1962). It is not the case that Hb F is synthesized in extramedullary sites and Hb A in the bone marrow during foetal life (Thomas et al., 1960; Zilliacus and Ottelin, 1967): Individual normoblasts in the marrow produce different proportions of Hb F and Hb A.

Hb A$_2$ is virtually absent at birth but reaches adult concentrations of 1–3 per cent at about 6 months (Erdem and Aksoy, 1969).

Detection of foetal haemoglobin

Detection and estimation of Hb F is facilitated by the fact that it is resistant to denaturation by acids and alkalis (this is not a unique property since embryonic haemoglobins are even more resistant). Resistance to denaturation during a one-minute exposure to 0.083 N NaOH at 30 °C is the basis of the Singer's alkali denaturation test (Singer et al., 1951). Agar gel electrophoretic (Robinson et al., 1957), spectrophotometric (Beaven et al., 1960), column chromatographic (Kirschbaum, 1962) and immunological (Heller et al., 1962) methods for its detection also exist. One of the most useful advances has been the application of acid elution to blood films (Kleihauer et al., 1957). Freshly fixed films are immersed in an acid-citrate buffer at pH 3.3 for 5 minutes at 37° C, after which they are counterstained. Red cells containing only Hb A appear as unstained 'ghosts'; those containing any Hb F stand out as well-stained haemoglobin-containing red cells (Fig 8.2). By this technique it is possible to detect a foetomaternal haemorrhage as small as 0.2 ml, which is an immunizing dose in the genesis of rhesus disease. It is also a useful rapid test for detecting foetal haemoglobin in the circulation in such varied conditions as aplastic anaemia, thalassaemia or haemoglobinopathy. It does not give the same quantitative result as a chemical estimation of Hb F in whole blood (e.g. the Singer's test) since the Kleihauer film shows all cells with even a small content of Hb F.

Physiological significance of foetal haemoglobin

For many years it has been assumed that Hb F confers an advantage to the foetus by increasing the transfer of O_2 from the maternal circulation. Foetal red cells have a greater affinity for oxygen than adult cells. A conventional plot of the oxygen dissociation curve shows a 'shift to the left' by comparison with adult blood (e.g. Fig. 8.3). Although increased affinity can be shown with intact foetal red cells no such difference can be found when pure solutions of Hb F and Hb A are compared (Allen et al., 1953). It was suspected therefore that the 'shift to the left' was due to some environmental factor operating within the foetal red cell. Generation of 2,3-DPG and other phosphate esters in the anoxic red cell has now been shown to be responsible. Whereas 2,3-DPG enhances the release of O_2 from Hb AO_2 (Benesch et al., 1968) its effect on oxy-Hb F is much less (Bauer et al., 1968). The esters interact with beta chains but these are absent in Hb F. At low PO$_2$ levels there is therefore a preferential transfer of oxygen from adult cells to foetal cells. Oski and Naiman (1972A) have pointed out that although this increased O_2 affinity of foetal cells may be of advantage in utero it may be a disadvantage after birth since it will impair O_2 release to the tissues

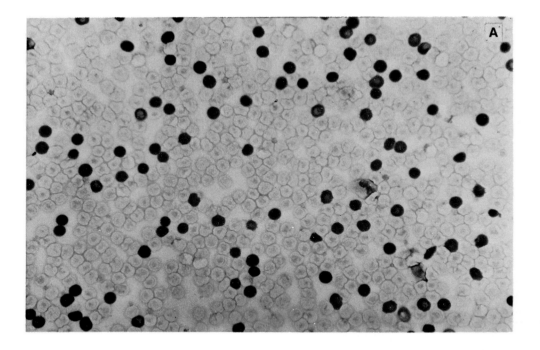

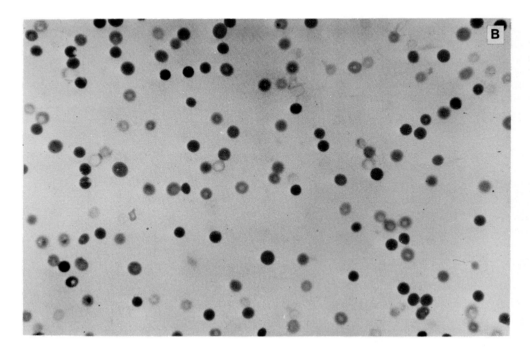

Fig. 8.2 Photomicrographs of Kleihauer film (× 540). A, foetal RBCs stain darkly due to persisting Hb F; adult RBCs stain as ghosts due to denatured and eluted Hb A. Figure B shows the appearance in Fanconis aplastic anemia, with graduations between strongly positive and negative-staining cells.

ABNORMALITIES OF HAEMOGLOBIN SYNTHESIS 115

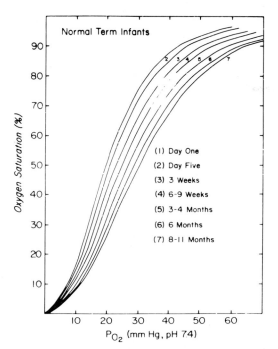

Fig. 8.3 Oxygen dissociation curves of blood from full-term infants at different post-natal ages. Normal P_{50} values are reached at approx. 11 months. (Reproduced with permission from Oski and Naiman (1972), *Hematologic Problems in the Newborn*, Philadelphia: Saunders).

under conditions of hypoxia. These authors further make the point that exchange transfusion with fresh adult blood is worthy of critical evaluation in situations of severe neonatal anoxia.

Premature babies show a further 'shift to the left' of the curve, the abnormality being more marked in those of lowest birth weight.

Postnatal changes in Hb F concentration

After birth there is a progressive reduction in the proportion of Hb F in the circulating blood, reaching 10–15 per cent by four months (Fig. 8.4B) and less than 2 per cent by three years (Singer *et al.*, 1951). These changes represent a continuation of the downward trend which commences at 34–36 weeks gestation when the proportion of Hb F is as high as 90 per cent. From then on an increased proportion of Hb A is synthesized (Brody and Nilsson, 1960) so that at birth the relative rate of Hb F synthesis has fallen to 50–65 per cent, and by three months to approximately 5 per cent. Fall in rate of synthesis precedes the fall in percentage of circulating Hb F because of the factor of cell survival (Garby *et al.*, 1962). In rhesus disease the rapid and random red cell destruction negates this factor, bringing the percentage of circulating Hb F closer to the percentage of Hb F synthesis and resulting in a higher proportion of Hb A in the cord blood compared to normal infants (Oppé and Fraser, 1961).

Figs. 8.4A and B also show the percentage of red cells staining as 'foetal', 'adult' and 'intermediate' at progressive stages of gestation and postnatal life

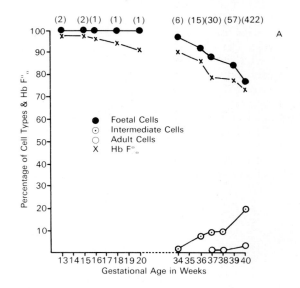

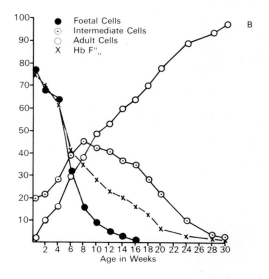

Fig. 8.4 Proportions of foetal, intermediate and adult RBCs present before (A) and after (B) birth. Number of observations are indicated in parenthesis. (Reproduced from Fraser and Raper (1962), *Archives of Disease in Childhood*, **37**, 289, by permission of the author and publishers).

as seen in Kleihauer films. These cells contain wholly Hb F, wholly Hb A or varying proportions of Hb F and A (Fraser and Raper, 1962). The postnatal decline in Hb F causes a progressive return of the oxygen dissociation curve to normal (Fig. 8.3). The position of this curve is dependent not only on the proportions of Hb F and Hb A but also on the concentration of red cell 2, 3-DPG (Delivoria-Papadopoulos et al., 1971; Orzalesi and Hay, 1971). Cells containing wholly foetal Hb are probably not produced after birth but small numbers can normally be found in the blood until about 16 weeks. Cells containing intermediate proportions of Hb F are probably produced up to about 16 weeks and occasional such cells persist until about 30 weeks. Progressively smaller proportions of Hb F are incorporated into successive generations of these intermediate cells (Fraser and Raper, 1962).

Disturbances in the pattern of transition from foetal to adult haemoglobin synthesis occur in association with a number of foetal and maternal conditions. These are shown in Table 8.3. Rhesus disease has already been mentioned. Prematurity appears to delay the normal transition in proportion to the gestational age (Fraser and Raper, 1962).

opathies. Abnormality of structure results from one or occasionally two amino acid substitutions in the polypeptide chains of the globin part of the molecule. It should be stressed that most of these variants do not cause any clinical disorder (Huehns and Bellingham, 1969).

Substitutions in the beta chain account for the better known haemoglobinopathies (Hb S,C,D,E) and are not normally demonstrable at birth since there has been very little beta chain synthesis by that time. Substitutions in the alpha chain are detectable both at birth and in later life, although mostly asymptomatic. Substitutions in the gamma chains are *only* detectable in the neonatal period, while those of the delta chain cannot be found until five or six months when Hb A_2 normally first appears. Haemoglobinopathies affecting the non-beta chains are rare and largely of academic interest, not resulting in anaemia, jaundice or other clinical manifestations (Oski and Naiman, 1972B).

Since the discovery of the genetic code it has been found that all the known amino acid substitutions in Hb can be accounted for by replacement of only one of the three bases coding for the

Table 8.3   Conditions affecting transition from foetal haemopioesis

Maternal		Authors
Chronic intra-uterine anoxia	Hb F % ↑	Bromberg et al., 1956
Diabetes	Hb F % ↓	Gerbie et al., 1959
Foetal		
'Small for gestation' babies	Hb F % ↑	Bard et al., 1970
Trisomy 13 (D_1)	Hb F % ↑	Walzer et al., 1966
Trisomy 13 (D_1)	+ Hb Gowers 2 + Bart's	Huehens et al., 1964
Trisomy 21 (G)	Hb F % ↓	Wilson et al., 1968
Erythroblastosis	Hb F % ↓	Oppé and Fraser, 1961
Hereditary		
Persistence of high Hb F	2–30 % throughout life	Conley et al., 1963
Fanconi's aplastic anaemia	3–15 % throughout life	Shahidi et al., 1962
Erythrogenesis imperfecta (?)	Hb F (trace)	Mott et al., 1969
Beta haemoglobinopathies and beta thalassaemia	Hb F ↑	Itano et al., 1956
Gamma thalassaemia	Hb F ↓	Kan et al., 1972B

Chronic anoxia after birth, e.g. cyanotic heart disease does not affect the post-natal decline of Hb F (Farrar and Bloomfield, 1963).

GENETICALLY DETERMINED ABNORMALITIES OF HAEMOGLOBIN STRUCTURE: THE HAEMOGLOBINOPATHIES

As in most defects of protein synthesis the abnormality may be quantitative affecting the rate of synthesis, in the thalassaemias, or qualitative due to an abnormality in structure, in the haemoglobin-

appropriate position (Beale and Lehmann, 1965). Such single base changes are the result of point mutations (Lehmann and Carrell, 1969).

The clinical consequence of the mutation depends upon the position on the polypeptide chain at which substitution occurs and on the change in polarity or electrostatic charge resulting from the substitution (Heller, 1965). For example replacement of the hydrophilic *glutamyl* residue at

Haemoglobinopathy	Hb S	Hb C and E	Hb Zurich
Amino acid substitution	Glu ⟶ Val	Glu ⟶ Lys	His ⟶ Arg
Change in m-RNA coding	GAG ⟶ GUG	GAG ⟶ AAG	CAU ⟶ CGU

See Lehmann et al., (1966) for full list.

the 6 position of the beta chain by the hydrophobic *valyl* leads to severe conformational change in the molecule resulting in sickling (Murayama, 1964). A hydrophilic but basic *lysyl* substitution in the same position causes the less severe Hb C disease with haemolysis but without sickling. But a *lysyl* in place of *glutamyl* at the neighbouring 7 position in Hb C Georgetown causes a sickling disorder. Tyrosine in place of histidine at position 63 forms a bond with the haem iron rendering it unsuitable for reversible oxygenation (Hb M Saskatoon) whereas arginine in the same position (Hb Zürich) increases the susceptibility of the molecule to oxidant denaturation by drugs (Gerald and Efron, 1961; Frick et al., 1962).

Inheritance

Separate pairs of alleles control the structure of the alpha, beta, gamma and delta chains. These may be multiple in the case of gamma chains (Schroeder et al., 1968) and alpha chains (Lehmann and Carrell, 1968). Point mutations in the genetic code mentioned above appear to be inherited on a pair of allelomorphic somatic genes (Ingram, 1959). Each haemoglobinopathy may exist as a heterozygous state or a homozygous state (Neel, 1951; Terry et al., 1954). For instance Hb S totally replaces Hb A in the homozygous sickle cell disease (S/S) but only partially replaces it in the heterozygous sickle cell trait (S/A). This parallel behaviour of molecular proportions and genetic status first led to the recognition of 'molecular diseases' (Pauling et al., 1949). The heterozygote shows a degree of abnormality intermediate between that of the homozygote and normal. Since different haemoglobinopathy genes for the same chain are allelomorphic mixed haemoglobinopathies such as Hb S/C can occur.

Thalassaemia genes (alpha thal and beta thal) are similarly inherited resulting in homozygous or heterozygous states for either alpha chain or beta chain thalassaemia. There are, however, genes of varying severity (e.g. alpha thal$_1$ and alpha thal$_2$) or possibly four rather than two genes controlling alpha chain synthesis (Lehmann et al., 1964). Since the beta thal genes are also allelomorphic with the beta haemoglobinopathy genes mixed haemoglob-inopathy/thalassaemia syndromes can occur, e.g. Hb E/beta thal.

Interaction occurs between the different haemoglobinopathy and thalassaemia genes, increasing the clinical severity in the double heterozygote if the same (e.g. beta) chain is affected, but not if different chains are affected. None of the normal chain can be synthesized if both allelomorphic genes for that chain are abnormal.

Geographic distribution and incidence

The main reservoir of sickle cell disease is Tropical Africa and Madagascar (Fig. 8.5). In

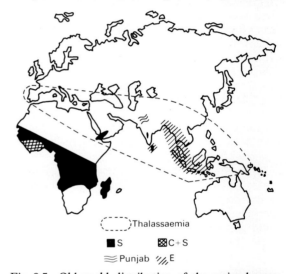

Fig. 8.5 Old-world distribution of the major haemoglobin abnormalities. (Reproduced from Lehmann and Huntsman (1975), *Association of Clinical Pathologists*, Broadsheet 33, revised 1975).

some areas the incidence of carriers of Hb S is as high as 40 per cent. It is also relatively frequent in Turkey, Greece and other Mediterranean countries including North Africa. The occurrence in Veddoid Indian hill tribes has given rise to the suggestion that a primitive Veddoid race in Arabia in neolithic times spread both into Africa and India carrying the Hb S gene with them. The incidence of 8–9 per cent in the black American population is merely a reflection of their importation from West Africa in the 17th century.

The distribution of the haemoglobin S gene in the old world is very similar to that of malignant tertian malaria. Since the heterozygote with sickle cell trait is relatively protected from the lethal complication of cerebral malaria this is likely to more than compensate for the death rate from homozygous sickle cell disease; and to be operative in causing a persistence of the gene. This phenomenon has been termed 'balanced polymorphism' (Allison, 1954). In A/S heterozygotes the parasitized cells are more prone to sickling than the non-parasitized cells and this may lead to rapid removal of parasites from the circulating blood (Luzzatto et al., 1970). There is also evidence that the heterozygote for HbS has increased fertility.

The main occurrence of Hb C is in West Africa, of Hb D in Western India and of Hb E in Burma and Thailand.

Beta thalassaemia (Mediterranean anaemia, Cooley's anaemia) occurs characteristically among races bordering on the Mediterranean (thalas = Greek for sea). In Turkey and Greece the incidence reaches 20 per cent, in Sicily and the Po delta 10 per cent, in Southern Italy 4 per cent. It is really, however, more widespread than its synonym would suggest. There is a high incidence in Burma and Thailand, with a lower incidence in China, India and Central Africa. Balanced polymorphism may also occur since the heterozygotes are thought to have a reduced susceptibility to malaria and increased fertility.

Alpha thalassaemia has the reverse distribution compared with the beta form since its main occurrence is in the Far East and in Negroes, with a very low incidence in Mediterranean stock.

Geographical distribution is further reviewed by Dacie (1963) and Lehmann et al. (1966).

Sickling states

It is not only in homozygous carriers of Hb S that sickling occurs, but also in double heterozygotes with sickle cell trait plus a second condition, as well as in carriers of certain variants of Hb C (Pierce et al., 1963; Ranney, 1970) (Table 8.4). The latter are not strictly confined to black populations (Rwylin and Benson, 1961; Thompson et al., 1965).

PATHOGENESIS OF SICKLING PHENOMENA AND RELATED HAEMOLYSIS

At the molecular level Murayama (1962, 1964) has produced evidence that a hydrophobic bond is formed between two valyl radicals at positions 1 and 6 on the surface of the beta chain, the latter

being the substituted amino acid characteristic of Hb S. This results in the formation of a ring in the beta chain of one molecule which can be regarded as a 'key' which fits into the 'lock' formed by a complementary portion of the alpha chain of a second Hb molecule. In the deoxygenated state the two beta chains are 7 Å closer together (Muirhead and Perutz, 1963) and the hypothesis is that it is only in this molecular configuration that the 'key' and 'lock' can come into apposition. It is thought that the 'Murayama hypothesis' satisfactorily explains the tactoid formation of deoxygenated Hb S by causing stacking of the molecules in linear array. The evidence is clearly discussed by Heller (1965) as well as the modifications necessary to explain sickling of Hb C Georgetown and crystal formation of Hb C, both of which have amino acid substitutions in the same area of the molecule. In Hb S Memphis an additional alpha chain abnormality modifies the severity of sickling by interfering with the above-mentioned alpha beta inter-action hybrid molecular species containing one beta chain of Hb A and one of Hb S, such as occur in S/A heterozygotes, would also inhibit the extended stacking of deoxygenated Hb S (Huehns and Bellingham, 1969; Jensen and Lessin, 1970). Recently the 'Murayama hypothesis' has been modified to the extent of postulating direct inter-action between the hydrophobic valyl residue of the beta chain with the alpha chain of a second molecule (Nalbandian et al., 1970). Six molecules of deoxy Hb S form a ring which, when stacked, gives a tubular spiral structure much firmer than any that can be formed by deoxy Hb A (Finch et al., 1973).

At the cellular level there is electron microscopy evidence of parallel rods within sickled cells (Bertles and Döbler, 1969). These become entwined to form rigid fibres which produce gross shape changes of the red cell and are visible as linear 'wrinkles' on the cell surface. As sickling proceeds the fibres become organized into parallel bundles in the long axis of the body or spicule of the sickled cell (Jensen and Lessin, 1970). The extreme distortion during sickling results in apposition of portions of the inner surface of the cell membrane, followed by compartmentalisation of the cell contents and subsequent loss of fragments of membrane and cell contents during unsickling. This is the origin of the 'freakish poikilocytes' characteristic of the disease (Jensen, 1969), which are irreversibly sickled cells with decreased surface area and shortened life span (Serjeant et al., 1969). These cells also have greatly reduced plasticity and deformability

ABNORMALITIES OF HAEMOGLOBIN SYNTHESIS   119

Table 8.4   Sickle cell diseases and allied disorders

Hemoglobin Phenotype	Mobility of the abnormal hemoglobin relative to hemoglobins A, C, S, or F	Morbidity	Splenomegaly	
Sickle cell disorders				
Homozygous sickle cell disease	S	Severe crises, anemia	Rare after 7 years of age	
Sickle cell trait	S and A	Rare, mild crises, hematuria	Frequent	
S–C disease	S and C	Generally milder than SS; crises do occur	Yes	
S–D disease	S and D	Mild to moderate	In about 30% of cases	
S–E disease	S and close to C	Mild to moderate, as trait	Yes	
S–E (Pittsburgh) disease	S and close to C	Severe, like homozygous SS	—	
S–G disease	S and between A and S	As sickle trait	—	
SS–Hgb Memphis	S and close to S	Milder than SS disease alone	—	
S–β thalassemia	S and A	Very mild	—	
S–β thalassemia	S, F, and a small amount of A	Moderately severe crises	Yes	
S–Hgb Lepore	S, F, and A	Moderately severe crises	Yes	a
S–persistent high F	S and F	Milder than SS but occasional crises	—	
Sickle cell anemia with hereditary spherocytosis	S (and A when trait)	Hereditary spherocytosis predominates	Yes, if trait	
Sickle cell anemia with hereditary ovalocytsosis	Presumably S and A	Mild	—	
Hemoglobin variants resulting in positive sickle cell preparations				
Hemoglobin C-Harlem	as C	—	—	
Hemoglobin C-Georgetown	as C	—	—	
Hemoglobin I	Faster than A	Essentially asymptomatic		
Hemoglobin variants resulting in morbidity mimicking mild sickle cell disease, but not resulting in positive sickle cell preparations				
Hemoglobin C disease	C	Very mild hemolytic anemia, occasional mild crises	Often	
Hemoglobin C–E(Pittsburgh) disease	C and close to C	As CC disease	—	

Reproduced, by permission, from Van Eys (1970) Pediat. Clin. N. Amer., 17, 449.

(Bertles and Milner, 1968) further decreasing the survival in the circulation.

Closely related to the molecular polymerization that occurs with Hb S is a less extensive molecular aggregation which occurs with deoxygenerated Hb C, resulting in the formation of intraerythrocytic crystals due to decreased solubility (Charache *et al.*, 1967). This is again due to an alteration of polarity on the surface of the beta chains apparently causing interaction with the alpha chains of the next molecule, this being accentuated in the deoxygenated configuration. The presence of crystals of precipitated Hb C within red cells results in the removal of the cells by the spleen (Diggs *et al.*, 1954). Membrane loss due to removal of microcrystals in the spleen is likely, as with Heinz bodies. Increased cell viscosity and reduced plasticity also occur. The target cells in Hb C disease may contain a centrally located haemoglobin crystal (Jensen and Lessin, 1970).

In vivo consequences of these cellular changes are haemolysis, vascular stasis and thrombotic crises in the sickling haemoglobinopathies shown in Table 8.4, but haemolysis alone in Hb C disease. Red cell survival in these disorders has been reported by McCurdy (1969). Mean red cell life span was 12–24 days (average 17.2 days) in 9 S/S patients, 16 and 20 days in S/C, 35 and 38 days in C/C, 53 and 96 days in S/beta thal and over 90 days (i.e. normal) in A/S heterozygotes. In general the cell destruction was exponential, i.e. random rather than age dependent. The capacity of the marrow to compensate for this haemolysis appeared to be slightly reduced either because of associated defective erythropoiesis in these disorders or because of a shift in the oxygen dissociation curve making O_2 more freely available to the tissues and consequently lessening the stimulus for erythropoietin release (Bellingham and Huehns, 1968). Decreased oxygen affinity has been shown for S/S, S/C, S/D and S/beta thal cells (Cawein *et al.*, 1969). In the case of Hb C a further series has confirmed decreased red cell survival in patients with only the trait (A/C) (Pringle and McCurdy, 1970).

Relevant to events precipitating *in vivo* sickling and vascular obstruction the percentage of sickled cells in arterial and venous blood is related to the percentage of Hb S in the blood, the type of the other Hb present and to the PO_2. A greater than expected degree of sickling, however, occurs in the presence of infection (Cawein *et al.*, 1969). Fever and acidosis also enhance sickling (Harris, 1959). It is clear that the presence of sickle cells increases blood viscosity and slows its rate of flow, predisposing to capillary stasis (Diggs, 1956). In low pressure vascular areas where the blood flow is normally at its slowest, further slowing and eventually stasis is precipitated by a process of 'log-jamming'. More oxygen is given up by the red cells to meet tissue requirements, the sickling is enhanced and a vicious circle established (Bird, 1972). Increased blood viscosity is the cause of many of the clinical features including chronic skin ulceration in older patients. In a study of pulmonary lesions in sickle cell anaemia Diggs (1969) described pulmonary artery emboli consisting of entangled mats of sickled red cells and fragments of intravascular clots preformed in systemic veins. Included in the emboli were globules of fat, bits of cellular marrow and trabecular bone from areas of ischaemic infarction of bone. There was no evidence of primary thrombi in pulmonary arteries.

Intravascular fibrin formation may, however, contribute to the capillary plugging and infarction of sickle crises in other tissues, justifying therapeutic trials with anticoagulants or defibrination with Ancrod (Mann *et al.*, 1972). Stuart, Stockman and Oski (1974) have adduced evidence of probable ADP release from red cells or platelets during vaso-occlusive sickle cell crises. Surviving platelets show a 'refractory state' with concomitant decrease in platelet adhesiveness, presumably a biological advantage.

HAEMATOLOGICAL DIAGNOSIS

A normochromic, normocytic anaemia of some severity is present, with Hb levels sometimes as low as 6 g/100 ml. There is no hypochromia as seen in the thalassaemia syndromes, but target cells, polychromasia and sometimes normoblasts. In Hb C target cells are particularly numerous. In homozygous sickle cell disease small numbers of sickled cells may be seen on the blood film (Fig. 8.6). Moderate reticulocytosis is present except at times of aplastic crisis. There is a neutrophil leucocytosis with a normal or high platelet count, again except at times of aplastic crisis. The osmotic fragility curve shows increased resistance (as discussed under thalassaemia). The bone marrow shows erythroid hyperplasia and increased stainable iron in reticulum cells and normoblasts. Megaloblastic changes can occur in the presence of folic acid depletion, and erythroid hypoplasia secondary to infection.

Rapid confirmation of the presence of Hb S, in either the homozygous or heterozygous state, can be made either by the traditional sickling test in which one drop of fresh blood is mixed on a slide with three drops of freshly prepared 2 per cent sodium metabisulphite, $Na_2S_2O_5$, and sealed under a cover slip with vaseline round the edges. The preparation is examined microscopically after $\frac{1}{2}$–2 hr incubation at 37°C. The presence of Hb S is indicated by the formation of grossly distorted, filamentous sickled cells. A normal control is advisable.

Because this test is unsuitable for rapid screening of large numbers of patients new methods have been developed based upon the relative insolubility of deoxygenated Hb S in solution (Binder and Jones, 1970; Loh, 1971). 'Sickledex' is a commercially available form of this screening test (Canning and Huntsman, 1970). Positive results should be confirmed initially by the sickling test and then by haemoglobin electrophoresis to distinguish homozygotes, heterozygotes and mixed haemoglobinopathies (Fig. 8.7).

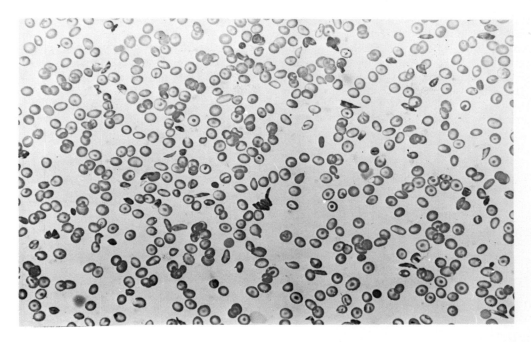

Fig. 8.6 Blood film from a child with sickle-cell anemia (S/S) (× 540). In this case actual sickle cells are present on the blood film.

Starch gel electrophoresis (discussed again under thalassaemia diagnosis) allows demonstration of the individual haemoglobins present and distinguishes, for instance, the sickle cell trait (with Hb S + A) from the sickle cell Hb C double heterozygote (with Hb S and C but no Hb A). Homozygous sickle cell disease has no Hb A present, showing predominantly Hb S (approx. 80 per cent) with the remainder Hb F. The technical details and points of interpretation are fully described by Hutchison (1967). Electrophoretic separation of haemoglobins can also be made on cellulose acetate using a smaller amount of material and a shorter run (Kohn, 1969). This has recently been used in a paediatric screening programme by Barnes et al. (1972) employing only a capillary sample of blood for the purpose. The newer methods of detecting Hb S are discussed also in an annotation (B.M.J., 1972).

Antenatal diagnosis based on an even smaller sample of foetal blood obtained by placental puncture may even be possible using the techniques of isotopic measurement of beta chain synthesis being developed by Hollenberg et al. (1971). This technique is discussed more fully under thalassaemia diagnosis. The possibility of obtaining foetal blood for the purpose by using either aspiration of placenta after ultrasonic localization or better, under direct vision from the foetus using fibre optics is currently being considered (Kan et al., 1972A).

CLINICAL MANIFESTATIONS OF SICKLING DISEASES

Clinical symptoms are rare before 3 months, but are present in half of S/S infants by one year and in ¾ by two years (Haggard and Schneider, 1961). Oski and Naiman (1972B) collected a total of only 7 infants where the onset of symptoms had occurred in the first month of life. This data was collected from 5 different reports representing a

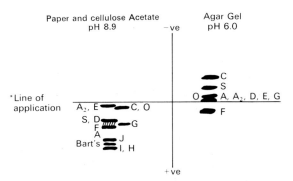

Fig. 8.7 Mobilities of common haemoglobins on cellulose acetate and agar gel. (Reproduced from *Association of Clinical Pathologists*, Broadsheet 33, revised 1975 by Lehmann and Huntsman, with permission from the author and publisher).

considerable pool of clinical experience over many years. Jaundice and haemolytic anaemia were present in 6, and this appeared to be triggered by infection in 2. Hepatosplenomegaly was present in 3. A difficulty in diagnosis is that the concentration of Hb S at this age may be too low for the sickling test to be positive. A negative test in the mother excludes the diagnosis, however.

Anaemia can be detected at the age of one month and pain most often in the back or abdomen, or of a bone or joint. Cerebral infarction can produce a wide variety of neurological pictures. A particularly characteristic presentation in infants under 2 years is sudden onset of pain and swelling of the short bones of the hands and feet with radiological findings similar to typhoid osteitis. This has been described as the 'hand–foot syndrome' (Watson et al., 1963) (Fig. 8.8).

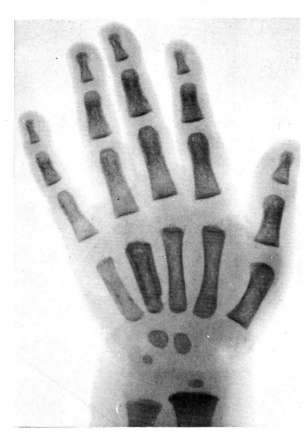

Fig. 8.8 X-ray of hand in a child with the hand-foot syndrome due to homozygous sickle-cell anemia. Dactylitis of the fourth metacarpal is present with extensive sub-periosteal new bone formation widening shaft–infarction with or without infection. (Reproduced with the permission of Dr P. Rawson, Consultant Radiologist, Royal Hospital for Sick Children, Glasgow. This plate also appears in *Textbook of Paediatrics* (1973), p. 2033, and is reproduced by permission of Professor J. O. Forfar).

in S/S infants but not in S/A infants. By 3 months the haemoglobin is often between 8–9 g/100 ml, but can exceptionally be as low as 6 g/100 ml (Van Baelen et al., 1969).

Beyond infancy the clinical course is one of extended periods of normality with perhaps only slight anaemia, punctuated by intermittent crises usually precipitated by respiratory or other infection (Wright and Gardner, 1959). Particular liability to both pneumococcal and salmonella infection exist to which these patients seem unduly prone (Lukens, 1972). The crises are commonly 'thrombotic', producing infarction rather than anaemia, or 'aplastic'. The thrombotic crises lasting from several days to a week, produce vomiting, anorexia, fever

Acute pulmonary disorders in these patients are often misdiagnosed as pneumonia when in fact they are pulmonary infarction. Distinguishing features include the tendency to recurrence in sickle cell infarction and a longer duration of fever than usually seen in pneumonia (Petch and Serjeant, 1970).

Aplastic crises are characterized by the sudden onset of severe pallor and anaemia rather than painful episodes. The anaemia may be of sufficient severity to precipitate congestive cardiac failure. They are commonly precipitated by quite trivial infection, when they are characterized by reticulocytopenia (Charney and Miller, 1964) but on occasions appear to be caused by folic acid deficiency consequent upon the greater utilization in chronic haemolytic states. Sequestration crises, due to sludging in the liver and spleen, are characteristic of the young patient before 'autosplenectomy' occurs and also require transfusion as a matter of urgency (Huntsman and Lehmann, 1974). Mann et al. (1975) investigated 16 episodes of sudden anaemia requiring blood transfusion in 13 S/S children. In 5 out of 7 episodes there was evidence of increased haemolysis, while in 10 out of 16 episodes reticulocytopenia indicated marrow depression. Cold agglutinins active at room temperature were present in 13 episodes, with anti-I specificity in 11. Warmed blood was used for transfusion in these cases without complication. An infective agent, possibly mycoplasmal, appeared often to be responsible for the anaemia.

Manifestations common to other chronic haemolytic anaemias include gall stone formation and chronic leg ulcers in older patients. Splenomegaly is frequently present in young children but tends to shrink after repeated infarctions in older children (autosplenectomy). Skeletal manifestations secondary to haemolysis include widening of the skull diploë with outward displacement and thinning of the outer table resulting in the radiological hair-on-end appearance, osteoporosis of the vertebrae and compression deformities (fish vertebrae). Recently it has been found that the more florid radiological changes are no longer being seen, presumably because of improved nutrition and lower rate of parasitic infection (Goldring, 1969). It is being recognized that the disease does not necessarily carry such a hopeless prognosis as previously thought (Gray, 1969).

A lesion of particular interest is that affecting the renal function resulting in hyposthenuria. Initially this lesion is reversible by transfusion of normal blood but later becomes irreversible (Keitel et al., 1956). Perillie and Epstein (1963) have suggested that sickling occurs in the hypoxic renal medulla restricting blood flow and limiting the production of the hypertonic environment necessary for osmotic resorption of water.

An excellent and fuller account of the clinical manifestations of sickle cell anaemia is given by Mauer (1969), and of these and their management by Pearson and Diamond (1971).

Patients with heterozygous S/A trait show none of these symptoms or signs except occasional episodes of benign haematuria and a liability to minor thrombotic crises if they become anoxic during anaesthesia or in high-flying aircraft. Mixed Hb S syndromes with other haemoglobinopathies or thalassaemia result in intermediate disability as indicated in Table 8.4. Homozygous Hb C disease causes mild chronic haemolysis but no thrombotic incidents (Spaet et al., 1953). Rare homozygotes of Hb E and D result in even milder chronic haemolysis, but this is more marked in the double heterozygote, e.g. E/β thal, (Bird and Lehmann, 1956; Lehmann et al., 1956). Rare variants of Hb C, viz. Hb C Harlem, Hb C Georgetown and Hb C^c are capable of sickling in vivo or in vitro (Van Eys, 1970).

TREATMENT OF SICKLING DISORDERS

Treatment of the thrombotic crises includes bed rest, analgesics, oral or parenteral hydration and antibiotics in the presence of infections. If anaemia is present blood transfusion achieves not only correction but also dilution of the sickling-prone cells, which reduces the pathological blood viscosity (Anderson et al., 1963). Correction of the decreased plasma volume and metabolic acidosis found in crises (Diggs, 1965) should also be attempted. No clear advantage has been found in using low molecular weight Dextran (Barnes et al., 1965). Hyperbaric oxygen at 2 atmospheric pressures reduces the percentage of circulating sickle cells but has not in general relieved the symptoms of painful crises (Desforges and Wang, 1966; Laszlo et al., 1969). Reynolds, (1971), however, reported successful response on 3 occasions in one patient.

There have been recent enthusiastic reports on the use of I.V. urea in sucrose for the relief of painful sickling crises (Nalbandian et al., 1971; McCurdy and Mahmood, 1971) since in high concentration urea can disrupt hydrophobic bonds (Bruning and Holtzer, 1961) and reverse sickling in vitro (Nalbandian et al., 1970). Sucrose is added to the I.V. urea to prevent haemolysis which would occur with urea alone. The most notable side-effect from this therapy is a 'Niagra-like' diuresis which may actually increase the risk of serious sickling through accentuation of the dehydration often already present (Desforges, 1971; Lancet, 1974). Recent controlled trials (Urea Co-operative Trials Group) have shown no response or shortening of crises with urea in high (15 per cent) or low (10 per cent) concentrations (Kraus et al., 1974; McCurdy et al., 1974) nor with alkali (M/6 lactate) (Rhodes et al., 1974) compared to controls treated with 10 per cent sucrose or N/4 saline in 5 per cent dextrose. Neither has prophylactic oral administration of urea to 11 children with sickle cell anaemia reduced the incidence of painful crises or the number of hospital admissions per year (Lubin and Oski, 1973). The subject has recently been discussed in an annotation in the *Lancet* (1974).

The suggestion had been made that any benefit from urea therapy could be due to the formation of trace amounts of cyanate ion (Cerami and Manning 1971), since this increases the *in vivo* survival of sickle cells (Cerami, 1972). May *et al.* (1972) have shown that this effect of cyanate is not due to direct inhibition of the sickling process but to the fact that it acts by increasing the red cell affinity for oxygen, decreasing the proportion of deoxy Hb present at any particular PO_2 level. A clinical trial in 31 patients with sickle cell disease, aged 7 to 49 years, has suggested that administration of sodium cyanate (10 to 35 mg/kg/day) for 6–18 months reduced the incidence of 'idiopathic' crises, but not of crises due to identifiable infection (Gillette *et al.*, 1974). Further, controlled trials are clearly indicated. At present neither urae or cyanate can be recommended (Huntsman and Lehmann, 1974).

Hyperbaric oxygen (Reynolds, 1971) and the defibrinating anticoagulant 'ancrod' (Mann *et al.*, 1972) have been found ineffective in the treatment of crises.

Prompt treatment of any infection and fever is probably the single most important point to emphasize in long-term management, since infection is the most frequent precipitating factor which 'triggers' a thrombotic crisis as well as potentially inducing an aplastic crisis due to inhibition of marrow function. Special arrangements should be made to expedite admission to hospital in the event of infection. A good standard of nutrition should be encouraged, including routinely administered oral folic acid, 5 mg/day, to all S/S patients to compensate for the increased folate requirements of a hyperactive marrow. Transfusions are seldom needed except during or following aplastic or thrombotic crises. Life-long hazards of anaesthesia and air travel should be remembered. Splenectomy is only rarely indicated when there is clear evidence of hypersplenism. 'Autosplenectomy' tends to occur with advancing age due to repeated splenic infarcts leading to fibrosis (Diggs, 1935), and splenomegaly becomes progressively less frequent after the age of 10 (Watson *et al.*, 1956).

General management includes testing other siblings to detect S/A carriers or even other S/S cases among the more recently born. Advice should be given regarding the risks of splenic infarction or other crisis due to altitude (over 7,000 feet) or anoxia during anaesthesia (Conn, 1954). Patients with sickle cell trait (S/A) are at hazard only in unpressurized aircraft; S/S patients seem to be able to fly in pressurized aircraft without hazard (? due to autosplenectomy), while by contrast S/C patients are the most prone to the effects of low pressure, and flying should be prohibited in this group (Green, Huntsman and Serjeant, 1971). In other respects the double heterozygotes such as S/β thal, S/C etc., have a disease of intermediate severity.

An associated deficiency of G-6-PD is worth detecting since it may increase the frequency of sickle cell crisis in S/S patients (Smits *et al.*, 1969).

Little specific therapy is needed in homozygous Hb C, D or E diseases, in which there is chronic mild haemolysis but no reduction in life expectancy (Tanaka and Clifford, 1958). Symptomatic management of recurrent periarticular and abdominal pain found in this disease (Smith and Krevans, 1959) may be required.

W.H.O. recommendations for the treatment of haemoglobinopathies and allied disorders are available (1972), as well as an excellent recent review by Huntsman and Lehmann (1974). Genetic engineering or transplantation may be used in future.

Unstable haemoglobins

Unlike the amino acid substitutions in Hb S and Hb C which affect the polarity of the *external surface* of the haemoglobin molecule resulting in polymerization (Hb S) or crystallization (Hb C), the substitutions in unstable haemoglobins occur *within the haem cavity or pocket* of the alpha or beta polypeptide chains (Figs. 8.1 and 8.9). Substitution in this region of haem attachment causes gross molecular instability resulting in a chronic non-spherocytic haemolytic anaemia characterized by an enhanced tendency to Heinz body formation, discoloration of the urine due to dypyrrolic pigment excretion and, in some instances, drug-induced haemolysis closely mimicking that seen in G-6-PD deficiency. The syndrome associated with this type of haemoglobinopathy has been described as 'unstable haemoglobin haemolytic anaemia (UHHA)' by Carrell and Lehmann, (1969) and as 'congenital Heinz body haemolytic anaemia (CHBHA)' by Jacob (1970) and others. Recent reinvestigation of the original case of idiopathic Heinz body anaemia reported by Cathie in 1952 has shown that the disease was due to an abnormal unstable haemoglobin (Steadman *et al.*, 1970). Since the disorders are fully manifest in heterozygotes the inheritance is, in effect, dominant. It is believed that the homozygous state is incompatible with life.

Closely related to the unstable haemoglobins are the M-haemoglobins discussed in the subsequent section. The substitution is in the region of haem attachment in these disorders also but results in increased susceptibility of oxidation of haem Fe^{++} to Fe^{+++} with consequent methaemoglobin accumulation and cyanosis, rather than haemolysis. There is some overlap among these disorders insofar as there is an increase in methaemoglobin formation in most types of UHHA (Table 8.5).

Changes in the oxygen affinity have also been found in some of the unstable haemoglobins (Bellingham and Huehns, 1968) and some of the M-haemoglobins (Ranney et al., 1968). An increase in O_2 affinity results in greater tissue anoxia and greater erythropoietin stimulation for a given level of anaemia. This can cause a better haemopoietic response to haemolysis but may also accentuate the symptoms of anaemia (Jacob, 1970). In at least one haemoglobinopathy, Hb Chesapeake, the only clinical manifestation is mild polycythaemia (Charache et al., 1966).

Table 8.5 Findings in the unstable haemoglobin diseases

Disease	Hb (g/100 ml)	Abnormal Hb%	Retics%	Methaemoglobin (Fresh blood)	Inclusion bodies Post-splenectomy	Inclusion bodies On incubation in vitro	Spleno-megaly	Dipyr-roluria	Electrophoretic abnormality Alkaline H, starch gel.†
Zürich	11–15	25	3–8	nil	—	+	+	+	Clear slow band
Köln	9–13	10–15	5–15	3–4	+	+	+	+	Diffuse slow band
Genova	—	25	—	—	—	+	—	—	No abnormality
Sydney	12–13	36	4–10	—	+	+	+	No	Slow band
Hammersmith	6–8	30	20–70	1·2	—	+	+	?+	Minor changes
Gun Hill	13*	30	4–10	—	+	+	+	No	Slow band
Bibba	6·5–7·5	11	6–16	12·3	—	—	—	—	No abnormality
Torino	—	8	—	4·7	—	—	—	—	Slow band
Santa Ana	7–9	15	15–20	—	+	+	+	+	Slow band
Riverdale-Bronx	11–12	30	10	—	—	+	+	—	Slow band

(The absence of information is represented by —).

*This figure is near 16 if a correction is made for the lower haem content of Hb Gun Hill

†Most of the β chain unstable haemoglobins also show an α chain band on starch gel electrophoresis (behind Hb A_2).

Reproduced, by permission, from Carrell and Lehmann (1969) *Seminars in Hematology*, **6**, 116–132.

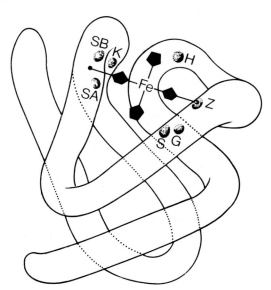

K = Köln; β^{98} *Valine → Methionine*
H = Hammersmith; β^{42} *Phenylalanine → Serine*
Z = Zurich; β^{63} *Histidine → Arginine*
G = Genova; β^{28} *Leucine → Proline*
S = Sydney; β^{67} *Valine → Alanine*
SA = Santa Ana; β^{88} *Leucine → Proline*
SB = Sabine; β^{91} *Leucine — Proline*

Fig. 8.9 Structural alterations in Heinz body-forming haemoglobins. The β-chain of haemoglobin, after Perutz, is depicted, emphasizing that the amino-acid substitutions in several CHBHA haemoglobins closely neighbour the β-chain haem group (portrayed as Fe-tetrapyrrole). (Reproduced from Jacob (1970), *Seminars in Hematology*, **7**, 341, with permission).

PATHOGENESIS OF ANAEMIA IN UHHA

The molecular abnormality in these disorders is more subtle than in the Hb S, C, D and E haemoglobinopathies. There is no change in electrophoretic mobility since the amino acid substitutions do not involve a change in polarity or charge (Carrell and Lehmann, 1969). It is thought that if such a gross change occurred adjacent to the haem contact the result would be incompatible with life. Only minor derangements in such a sensitive region of the molecule are consistent with survival. The first evidence of an abnormality of haemoglobin structure in these disorders was its increased tendency to precipitate on mild heating (50°C) associated with the presence of Heinz bodies, raised methaemoglobin levels and dipyrroluria (Dacie et al., 1964). Subsequent detailed peptide analysis has disclosed the common structural feature of substitution in the region of haem attachment (Fig. 8.9).

Haem attachment is jeopardized by these amino acid substitutions resulting in accelerated loss of haem (Jacob et al., 1968). Haem is an important structural component contributing to the stability of globin and its loss predisposes to denaturation of globin in vitro (as in the heat test) and in vivo (Fanelli et al., 1958). In particular the haem depleted beta chains tend to split off, undergo denaturation and precipitation to form Heinz bodies. These react with the cell GSH and the membrane thiols affecting cell permeability and plasticity (Jacob, 1970). Removal of the Heinz bodies from the red cells as they circulate through the splenic sinusoids takes place by a process of 'pitting' (Crosby, 1959; Rifkind, 1965). This results in loss of red cell membrane with subsequent sphering and haemolysis. Attachment of the Heinz bodies to the red cell membrane increases the mechanical fragility and the disulphide bonds with the membrane may account for the increased cation permeability and osmotic fragility seen, for instance, with Hb Köln (Jacob et al., 1968; Jensen and Lessin, 1970). It appears that the formation of intraerythrocytic precipitate or crystals is a common factor in the genesis of haemolysis not only in the Heinz body haemolytic anaemias (due to pentose shunt defects as well as haemoglobinopathy), but also in Hb C disease and in the thalassaemias, where it is free alpha, beta or gamma chains and their tetramers which are precipitated e.g. haemoglobin H (beta$_4$), haemoglobin Bart's (gamma$_4$), and the subsequent mechanism of haemolysis may be similar in all.

The free haem groups lost to the unstable haemoglobins are probably metabolized to dipyrroles rather than to bilirubin (Hutchison et al., 1964; Kreimer-Birnbaum et al., 1966A), accounting for the associated dark, pigmented urine. Similar pigments are excreted when solubilized Heinz bodies, presumably containing loosely associated haem, are fed to rats (Goldstein et al., 1968).

Elevated methaemoglobin, in both fresh and incubated blood, probably reflect the fact that the first step in Heinz body formation involves oxidation of the haem iron, as is the case when normal blood is incubated with phenylhydrazine (Jacob et al., 1968; Carrell and Lehmann, 1969).

CLINICAL AND HAEMATOLOGICAL FEATURES OF THE UNSTABLE HAEMOGLOBINOPATHIES

The unstable haemoglobinopathies are one cause of 'hereditary non-spherocytic haemolytic anaemia' similar in many respects to those caused by red cell enzyme defects. The anaemia may first appear in infancy. Its severity is very variable among the different haemoglobin variants and even within one family. There is often a history of crises induced by ingestion of drugs or by infection. The drugs are similar to those causing haemolysis in G-6-PD deficiency and are listed by Beutler (1969). Splenomegaly is usually present, with variable pallor and sometimes jaundice.

The majority of families are of European stock, several of German origin. A single Japanese family has also been recorded, probably representing a separate mutation.

Haematological features of Hb Köln disease, which is the best documented form of UHHA, are a normochromic or slightly hypochromic anaemia with a few irregularly contracted cells and microspherocytes, plus punctate basophilia and reticulocytosis. Thrombocytopenia may be present secondary to hypersplenism. Red cell inclusion Heinz bodies can be demonstrated by supravital staining with crystal violet either after splenectomy in many cells or, in non-splenectomized patients, in all cells after 48 hr incubation of the blood at 37°C. In the case of Hb Zürich disease drug exposure also produces numerous circulating Heinz bodies. Osmotic fragility is normal or slightly decreased, being reduced by the addition of glucose. Methaemoglobin is present in fresh blood and increases markedly on incubation at 37°C for 18 hr. Heat precipitation of over 10 per cent of the haemoglobin in a haemolysate after 3 hr at 50°C is characteristic of this group of disorders. Details of the technical methods are described by Hutchison (1967).

Comparative features of the different unstable haemoglobinopathies are shown in Table 8.5 from Carroll and Lehmann (1969). Hb Hammersmith disease (Grimes et al., 1964) is a severe form of UHHA and has only been described in children, probably as a new mutation in each case. Its severity may preclude its propagation over many generations. Hb Zürich is probably a mild form of the disease, initially being described by Hitzig, Frick, Betke and Huisman in 1960 in an infant girl and her father following administration of sulphonamides. Severe haemolysis accompanied by numerous circulating Heinz bodies followed drug exposure but at other times the haemolysis was mild (Frick *et al.*, 1962). Other types of UHHA are roughly intermediate between these two extremes including Hb Köln which in general exists as a compensated haemolytic anaemia (Carrell *et al.*, 1966; Hutchison *et al.*, 1964; Jackson *et al.*, 1967; Vaughan-Jones *et al.*, 1967). Infection but not drugs appear to accentuate the haemolysis (Beutler, 1969).

MANAGEMENT

There is no specific therapy but patients should be cautioned against exposure to drugs with known oxidant effects and also, possibly to hyperbaric oxygen (Carrell and Lehmann, 1969). A modest improvement in haemoglobin level, together with correction of thrombocytopenia and neutropenia when present, has been recorded after splenectomy in a number of patients with UHHA due to Hb Köln. In general this operation has been delayed until the patients were in their 'teens.

M-haemoglobinopathies, and other causes of methaemoglobinaemia

Hereditary methaemoglobinaemia can arise as a result of either a structural change in haemoglobin (M-haemoglobinopathy) rendering it abnormally susceptible to oxidation, or to a defect of the methaemoglobin reductase enzyme system. *Acquired* methaemoglobinaemia results from exposure of a normal individual to potentially oxidative agents, such as nitrates or aniline derivatives, which exceed the compensatory capacity of the methaemoglobin reductase system. Neonates are especially susceptible.

Because of similarities in clinical and haematological features, as well as the practical considerations of differential diagnosis, these three types of methaemoglobinaemia are considered together.

HAEMATOLOGICAL ASPECTS

Haemolysis does not occur with hereditary methaemoglobinaemia of either the haemoglobinopathy type or enzyme deficiency type (Gerald and Scott, 1966), but can occur in association with methaemoglobinaemia caused by toxic agents such as the analine derivative TCC (Quie *et al.*, 1962). The asymptomatic laboratory finding of slightly elevated Met Hb in unstable haemoglobin haemolytic anaemias has been mentioned in the previous section. Since both Met Hb and Heinz bodies are the result of oxidative injury the occurrence of these in various haemolytic and non-haemolytic disorders is set out in Table 8.6.

As mentioned earlier some of the M haemoglobins have higher oxygen affinity than normal which may lead to polycythaemia (Ranney *et al.*, 1968).

Under normal conditions the ferrous iron of oxyhaemoglobin is constantly being oxidized to the ferric form, yielding Met Hb in which the iron is no longer available for reversible combination with oxygen necessary for oxygen transport. Accumulation of Met Hb within the red cells is normally prevented by the function of two different Met Hb reductases; one linked to NADP H_2 (Huennekens *et al.*, 1958), the other linked to NADH$_2$ (Scott, 1960). Generation of the reduced forms of the two coenzymes is dependent upon the pentose shunt and glycolytic pathways respectively. Defects of the pentose shunt do not result in methaemoglobinaemia since the alternative NADH$_2$-linked enzyme is the more important source of Met Hb reduction. It is deficiency of this NADH$_2$-linked enzyme that causes hereditary methaemoglobinaemia of the enzymatic type. In this condition methylene blue is capable of stimulating the other, NADPH$_2$-linked, pathway sufficiently to compensate for the block.

Table 8.6 Occurrence of Met Hb, Heinz bodies and haemolysis in haematological disorders

Disorder	Defects of pentose shunt pathway (e.g. G–6–PD)	Unstable haemoglobinopathies (e.g. Hb Köln)	Met Hb opathy	Met Hb reductase defic.	Toxic Met Hb aemia (e.g. analine derivs)
Haemolysis	+	+	—	—	±
Heinz bodies	+	+	—	—	±
% Met Hb (approx).	<1%	up to 10%	10–50%	10–50%	10–70%

Percentage of Met Hb is percentage of circulating Hb in methaemoglobin form in fresh blood. After incubation there is a distinct increase in UHHA.

Ascorbic acid and reduced glutathione may be capable of reducing Met Hb directly without enzymatic participation.

M haemoglobins have amino acid substitutions in the same region of haem attachment as in the unstable haemoglobins. The effect, however, is confined to stabilizing the molecule in the ferrihaem state (Farmer *et al.*, 1964), probably since the additional polar group reacts with the third valency present in Ferric iron. This favours accumulation of Met Hb in the red cells despite an intact reductase system. A number of different M haemoglobins have been described (Gerald and Efron, 1961). These are listed in Table 8.7. In some the abnormality is in the alpha chain, when methaemoglobinaemia may appear at birth; in others it is in the beta chain, when clinical manifestations do not appear until 4–6 months of age.

severe headache. Congestion of the conjunctival and retinal veins may also be present.

In the M haemoglobinopathies cyanosis may be present at birth, but this depends upon whether it is the alpha or beta chain that is affected (*vide supra*). Heterozygotes manifest the disorder (as in UHHA) so inheritance is of the autosomal dominant pattern. There is no clinical response to methylene blue.

In the hereditary reductase deficiency cyanosis is present from birth and the pattern of inheritance is autosomal recessive. There is a strikingly high incidence of mental defect in children with this type of methaemoglobinaemia. Whether this is due to hypoxic brain damage or to an associated genetic defect is not clear (Gerald and Scott, 1966). There is rapid clearing of cyanosis after I.V. methylene blue.

Table 8.7 M Haemoglobinopathies

Haemoglobin	Defective chain	Amino acid substitution		Reference
		Position	Alteration	
^{M}Boston	α	58	His → Tyr	Gerald and Efron (1961)
^{M}Iwate	α	87	His → Tyr	Konigsberg and Legmann (1965)
^{M}Reserve	α	Unknown		Overly *et al.* (1967)
^{M}Saskatoon	β	63	His → Tyr	Gerald and Efron (1961)
^{M}Milwaukee I	β	67	Val → Glu	Ditto
^{M}Milwaukee II	β	Unknown		Ditto
^{M}New York	β	113	Val → Glu	Ranney *et al.* (1967)
^{M}Hyde Park	β	92	His → Tyr	Heller *et al.* (1966)

Data reproduced by permission from A. M. Mauer (1969) Pediatric Hematology. New York: McGraw-Hill.

During the neonatal period there is an exaggerated susceptibility to Met Hb formation even in normal infants. This is both because Hb F is more easily oxidized to the Met Hb form (Martin and Huisman, 1963), and because the $NADH_2$-dependent reductase is reduced to around 60 per cent of the adult level at this age (Ross, 1963). These factors may account for the slightly elevated levels of Met Hb found at birth (mean 1.5 per cent) and especially in premature infants (mean 2.3 per cent) (Kravitz *et al.*, 1956) compared to the adult mean of 0.8 per cent.

CLINICAL FEATURES

Generalized slaty grey cyanosis in the absence of clubbing and cardiorespiratory disease is common to all forms of methaemoglobinaemia (Gerald and Scott, 1966). Cyanosis appears at a level of approx. 15 per cent Met Hb. In severe cases with over 50 per cent of the Hb in the Met Hb form there is dyspnoea on exertion, a tendency to fatigue and

Toxic forms of methaemoglobinaemia are also characteristically seen in the neonatal period because of the biochemical susceptibility described above. Nitrate contamination of well water and even of municipal water supplies has been a well recognized cause of methaemoglobinaemia occurring in the first four months of life (Oski and Naiman, 1972C). These authors also list the following agents as known causes of the condition in the newborn:

Ethyl nitrite,
Analine derivatives (Diaper marking ink, disinfectants, benzocaine),
Acetophenetidin (Analgesic compounds),
Sulphonamides

The occurrence of methaemoglobinaemia at birth should raise the suspicion that the toxic agent has been administered to the mother (e.g. Prilocaine – a local obstetric analgesic).

In older children methaemoglobinaemia may

occur as part of the clinical picture of acute poisoning from a wide variety of oxidizing agents (Chan *et al.*, 1971). Symptoms of acute anoxia may be present in severe cases and will respond to methylene blue or ascorbic acid.

DIAGNOSIS

The major clinical distinction that has to be made is from cyanotic congenital heart disease. Blood in a test tube or even on filter paper is brown and does not become red on exposure to air. Methaemoglobinaemia is confirmed spectroscopically by the presence of a band at 634 mμ which disappears on the addition of cyanide. Quantitative estimation shows Met Hb concentrations of 15–80 per cent in the presence of cyanosis (normal < 1 per cent). The usual method of measurement is that of Evelyn and Mallory (1938), but certain of the abnormal methaemoglobins fail to be detected by this method. If due to an M haemoglobinopathy the absorption peak is nearer 600 mμ and the abnormal Met Hb derivative can be separated from normal Met Hb by electrophoresis on starch gel at pH 7.0 (Gerald, 1958). If it is due to enzyme deficiency the reductase level in red cells will be virtually zero, with intermediate enzyme levels in the (heterozygote) parents.

Intravenous injection of methylene blue (1–2 mg/kg) causes rapid disappearance of the circulating Met Hb within 2 hours in the toxic and enzyme deficient patients, but not in the M haemoglobinopathy patients.

TREATMENT

Correction by methylene blue is permanent in the toxic cases providing the causative agent is removed, but transient in enzyme deficiency. Further treatment with oral methylene blue 3–5 mg/kg/day or oral ascorbic acid 300–400 mg/day may be continued during the neonatal period or in severe cases but is not usually needed beyond the age of a few months. These aspects are discussed by Gerald and Scott (1966) and Oski and Naiman (1972D). Overdosage with methylene blue can cause acute haemolysis in these patients since it is itself an oxidizing agent (Goluboff and Wheaton, 1961).

In the M haemoglobinopathies no specific treatment is needed and the prognosis is good.

Thalassaemia syndromes

These are due to inherited defects of the rate of synthesis of globin chains (Itano, 1957) resulting in unbalanced production of alpha or beta chains. In the common Mediterranean form of thalassaemia beta chain synthesis is impaired (beta thalassaemia) and in a separate disease more common in Orientals and black Americans or Africans alpha chain synthesis is impaired (alpha thalassaemia) (Ingram and Stretton, 1959). There is no evidence of an abnormal form of globin chain synthesis, comparable to that found in the haemoglobinopathies, in any form of thalassaemia (Weatherall, 1969).

BIOCHEMICAL LESIONS IN THALASSAEMIA

The supposition that beta chain synthesis was impaired in Mediterranean or Cooley's anaemia was based on the fact that Hb A (alpha$_2$ beta$_2$) was reduced or absent and that Hb F (alpha$_2$ gamma$_2$) and Hb A$_2$ (alpha$_2$ delta$_2$) were relatively increased in this disorder. This hypothesis has now been confirmed by the direct measurement of the rates of alpha and beta globin chain synthesis in intact blood and marrow cells. This has been possible following the development of chromatographic methods for separation of the individual types of globin chain after short term incubation of reticulocytes or normoblasts with labelled amino acids (Clegg *et al.*, 1965; Heywood *et al.*, 1964). In all forms of beta thalassaemia studied by *in vitro* labelling the rate of alpha chain synthesis has exceeded that of beta chain synthesis (Weatherall, 1968). Furthermore there is a demonstrable accumulation of excess free alpha chains within cells as a result of this unbalanced synthesis. Such free alpha chains are unstable and rapidly precipitate within the cell (Weatherall *et al.*, 1965). They are undoubtedly the source of the large insoluble inclusion bodies present in the majority of marrow normoblasts and first described in this condition by Fessas (1963).

Likewise in alpha thalassaemia it has been confirmed by Clegg and Weatherall (1967) by haemoglobin synthesis studies in reticulocyte preparations that beta chains are produced two to three times faster than alpha chains in the usual form of the disease (Hb H disease). In the most severe, homozygous form of alpha thalassaemia (Hb Bart's hydrops foetalis syndrome) there is a *total absence* of any alpha chain synthesis in the cord blood reticulocytes and normoblasts (Weatherall, *et al.*, 1970). Due to defective alpha chain synthesis there is total replacement of Hb F (alpha$_2$ gamma$_2$) at birth by a tetramer of gamma chains, Hb Bart's (gamma$_4$), in the severe hydrops form of alpha thalassaemia, and partial replacement in milder forms of the disease (Ager and Lehmann, 1958). When there is the normal switch from gamma to beta chain synthesis in the neonatal period (i.e. Hb F→Hb A) Hb Bart's (gamma$_4$) becomes replaced

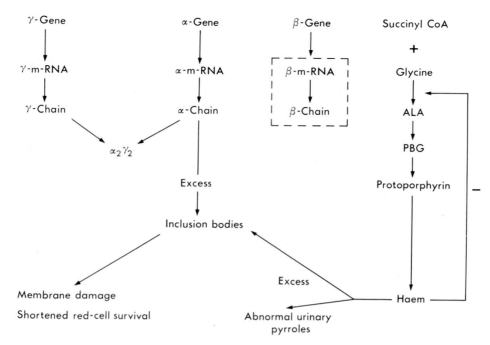

Fig. 8.10 The genetics of the thalassaemias. (Reproduced from Weatherall (1969), *British Medical Bulletin*, **25** 24, by permission).

by Hb H (beta$_4$), a tetramer of beta chains. Because of its instability Hb H is not present in the peripheral blood at the same level as it is being synthesized (Weatherall, 1968). It tends to precipitate in older red cells in the form of inclusion bodies that can be stained supravitally by cresyl blue. (These are removed by pitting as the cells circulate through the spleen so that they are more numerous after splenectomy.)

The fundamental biochemical defect is thought to be a quantitative reduction in the amount of messenger RNA for the affected chain (Clegg et al., 1968). This may imply that thalassaemia is, in fact, a 'controller' gene disease (Weatherall, 1969). The consequences of this are shown schematically in Fig. 8.10. This figure shows also how an excess of haem accumulates which exerts a secondary block of the early stages of haem synthesis by negative feed back inhibition, and how metabolism of this excess haem leads to excretion of dipyrollic pigments in this disease (Kreimer-Birnbaum et al., 1966B).

GENETICS OF DIFFERENT FORMS OF THALASSAEMIA

Beta chain synthesis is controlled by a pair of allelomorphic genes. In beta thalassaemia major both are replaced by β thal genes; in thalassaemia minor only one is replaced. A complication arises from the fact that there are two types of β thal gene which run true within a family, producing different severity of disease. The more severe type (sometimes designated $\beta°$ gene) results in zero synthesis of beta chains in the homozygous state, only Hb F and A$_2$ being synthesized; the other results in only partial suppression of beta chains.

Inheritance of a beta thal gene from one parent and a beta haemoglobinopathy gene (such as β^s) from the other results, for example, in the genetic constitution $a/a/\beta$ thal-β^s. If the β thal gene is of the severe type there is no Hb A, with Hb S accounting for most of the Hb. If it is of the less severe type about 20 per cent of Hb A may be present. The clinical *severity* of the disease in these double heterozygotes is determined, therefore, by the type of thalassaemia gene, and the clinical *manifestations* by the type of inherited haemoglobinopathy (Weatherall, 1969).

Further variants within the group of beta thalassaemia syndromes can occur (a) by virtue of simultaneous suppression of delta chains, delta beta thalassaemia or F thalassaemia (Brancati and Baglioni, 1966), or (b) by simultaneous suppression of gamma chains, gamma beta thalassaemia (Kan et al., 1972B). The former give rise to a condition similar to beta thalassaemia but with only Hb F in the homozygous condition, since no Hb A$_2$ (alpha$_2$ delta$_2$) can be formed. The latter gives rise to a transient severe hypochromic and haemolytic anaemia in the neonatal period, subsequently developing into typical beta thalassaemia (trait). Pure delta thalassaemia in the homozygous state causes only an absence Hb A_2, without anaemia (Ohta et al., 1971). An apparently abnormal type of haemoglobin with electrophoretic mobility similar to Hb S has been found in a small number of individuals with a haematological state similar to beta thalassaemia. The abnormal haemoglobin was named Hb Lepore, after the family name in which it was first found (Gerald and Diamond, 1958). It has been shown to contain normal alpha chains plus non-alpha chains which consist of the N terminal portion of normal delta chains attached to the carboxy-terminal portion of normal beta chains. The gene which is responsible for the synthesis of this hybrid molecule is thought to have arisen by a process of cross-over of the chromosome carrying the closely linked beta and delta loci (Baglioni 1962). Homozygous and heterozygous forms of the disease exist, the former producing a clinical picture identical to severe thalassaemia major. Minor molecular variants have subsequently been reported in a variety of racial groups.

Alpha thalassaemia exists at 3 or 4 levels of clinical severity ranging from hydrops foetalis to an asymptomatic carrier state (Table 8.8). Wasi, Na-Nakorn and Suingdumrong (1964) suggested that alpha thalassaemia genes of two groups of severity exist, designated as alpha thal[1] (severe) and alpha thal[2] (mild), which may occur in homozygous or heterozygous combination to account for the spectrum of haematological severity (Table 8.8). An alternative hypothesis has been proposed by Lehmann and Carrell (1968), viz. that alpha chain synthesis is controlled by two or more pairs of allelomorphic genes, and that the severity depends upon whether 1, 2, 3 or 4 of these alpha genes are replaced by abnormal alpha thal genes. Table 8.8 attempts to relate haematological severity to both these hypotheses since, it must be emphasized, the genetics of alpha thalassaemia are still sub judice. The severity of block in alpha chain synthesis is inversely related to the percentage of Hb Bart's

(gamma$_4$) in the cord blood at birth as described above.

Alpha thalassaemia may be inherited from one parent and an alpha chain haemoglobinopathy from the other. In Hb Q-alpha thalassaemia there was total suppression of normal alpha chains (Dormandy et al., 1961) while in Hb I-alpha thalassaemia some alpha chain synthesis occurred (Atwater et al., 1960). This further suggests that alpha thalassaemia trait effectively occurs at two levels of severity, by analogy with the situation in beta chain heterozygotes described above (Weatherall, 1969).

Combination of alpha thalassaemia with the beta chain haemoglobinopathy Hb E occurs in S.E. Asia producing a clinical picture similar to beta thalassaemia major (Wasi et al., 1967).

A benign condition which interacts genetically with haemoglobinopathies in the same fashion as the thalassaemias is hereditary persistence of foetal haemoblogin (HPFH). A homozygous individual for this condition has only Hb F in his blood without any Hb A or A_2. There is no anaemia but target cells and anisocytosis on the blood film. The condition may arise from a failure of the genetic 'operon' controlling the closely linked beta and delta loci to 'switch-on' close to birth (Conley et al., 1963). Not only is the condition asymptomatic but its inheritance in combination with Hb S may actually reduce sickling. In contradistinction to thalassaemia the Hb F is uniformly distributed among all red cells. African, Greek and Swiss types of HPFH are recognized with approximate Hb F concentrations of 30, 15 and 2 per cent respectively. Also molecular subclasses of their gamma chains may exist (Huisman et al., 1970).

PATHOGENESIS OF THE ANAEMIA

In beta thalassaemia major there is an excess of alpha chains which are rapidly precipitated to form insoluble inclusion bodies in the marrow normoblasts (Fessas, 1963). It is possible that red cell membrane damage results from mechanical trauma

Table 8.8 Hypothetical genotypes in different alpha thalassaemia syndromes

Clinical severity	Percentage of Hb Bart s in cord blood	Wasi et al., (1964)	Lehmann & Carrell (1968)
Hydrops foetalis	100	α thal₁ + α thal₁	4 × α thal
Chronic mild anaemia (Hb H disease)	20–30	α thal₁ + α thal₂	3 × α thal
Asymptomatic trait	5–10	α thal₁ + α (normal)	2 × α thal
Asymptomatic trait	1–2	α thal₂ + α (normal)	1 × α thal

due to the rigidity of the inclusion bodies, but binding of membrane sulphydryl groups may also be important (Weatherall, 1969). The fact that the major precipitation of alpha chains occurs in the marrow is in good agreement with the ineffective erythropoiesis characteristic of this disease and the extreme degree of resulting marrow hyperplasia (Sturgeon and Finch, 1957). Such inclusion bodies as do reach the peripheral blood appear to be removed by the spleen by a process of 'pitting', with the production of 'teardrop' red cells and probable membrane damage accounting for 'leaky' cells with marked increase in potassium flux (Nathan and Gunn, 1966). Good photomicrographs demonstrating this sequence of events are shown in the review by Nathan (1972). The role of alpha chains in the causation of haemolysis is confirmed by the work of Vigi and colleagues (1969) who found a good correlation between red cell survival and excess alpha chain synthesis in different patients with beta thalassaemia.

This intramedullary and peripheral haemolysis is superimposed upon a basic failure of normal haemoglobin production, with decreased cellular content of haemoglobin (hypochromia) and a partial block in haem synthesis (Fig. 8.10).

Very similar considerations apply to Hb H disease in alpha thalassaemia. Hb H (beta$_4$) precipitates as the red cell ages causing premature destruction of the red cells (Rigas and Koler, 1961), presumably through a similar process of 'pitting'. There is increased permeability to cations as in the case of beta thalassaemia (Nathan and Gunn, 1966).

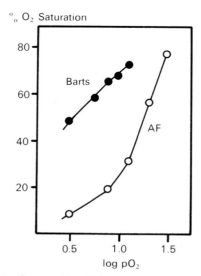

Fig. 8.11 Oxygen dissociation curves of Hb Barts and normal cord blood (AF). (Reproduced from Horton *et al.* (1962), *Blood*, **20**, 302, by permission).

In the case of alpha thalassaemia in the neonatal period there is a further disability due to the unfavourable oxygen dissociation curve of Hb Bart's resulting in impaired release of O_2 to the tissues at low O_2 tension (Fig. 8.11).

HAEMATOLOGICAL FINDINGS AND DIAGNOSIS

Hypochromia and target cell formation are the morphological stigmata of thalassaemia in all its forms except perhaps in the mildest carrier states. The hypochromia distinguishes the thalassaemias from the pure haemoglobinopathies; target cells may be present in a wide variety of disorders including both thalassaemias and haemoglobinopathies (Table 8.9). In thalassaemia major the anaemia is severe (e.g. Hb 4–7 g/100 ml) and there is extreme anisocytosis together with irregularly contracted red cells, 'teardrop' cells, polychromasia or punctate basophilia and circulating normoblasts in addition to the hypochromia and target cells mentioned above. In mild forms of the homozygous disease (thalassaemia intermedia), in the heterozygous thalassaemia minor and in Hb H disease the same morphological changes are present but to a less marked degree. The anaemia may also be mild (e.g. 11 g/100 ml) or absent. Red cell indices show microcytosis, low M.C.H.C. and low M.C.H. Reticulocytes are increased up to 10 per cent. Serum bilirubin may be slightly elevated. A neutrophil leucocytosis is often present and thrombocytopenia if there is hypersplenism. Bone marrow examination shows erythroid hyperplasia which is occasionally megaloblastic due to folate depletion. A proportion of the erythroblasts are PAS-positive.

A key investigation is the osmotic fragility curve, which shows *increased osmotic resistance* due to the thinner, flatter red cells (leptocytes) in thalassaemia. Results should be expressed as the median corpuscular fragility (MCF) for this purpose. In thalassaemia the MCF is below the normal lower limit of 0.4 per cent saline. In severe iron deficiency some of the cells show increased resistance to hypotonic saline but it is unusual for this to be sufficiently marked to affect the median value (Hutchison, 1967).

Distinction from iron deficiency is also readily made by the fasting serum iron, which is usually elevated, and TIBC which is not elevated and shows a good degree of saturation. Stainable iron is also present in both reticulum cells and erythroblasts (sideroblasts) in the marrow. While these findings are typical of thalassaemia major there is no reason why children with thalassaemia minor should be immune from concomitant iron de-

ABNORMALITIES OF HAEMOGLOBIN SYNTHESIS   133

Table 8.9   The more common causes of target cells

Disorder	Approximate incidence of Target cells (per cent of total)
Thalassemia syndromes	
Thalassemia, heterozygous, both α and β	Present
Thalassemia major	30
Thalassemia with hemoglobin variants S, C, or E	30
Thalassemia with other hemoglobin variants	Present
Hemoglobin variants	
Sickle cell trait	Occasional
Sickle cell disease	10
Hemoglobin C trait	Variable, up to 100
Hemoglobin C disease	High, up to 100
SC disease	High, up to 85
Following splenectomy	Occasional
Severe liver disease and jaundice from any cause	Occasional
Iron deficiency	Often present, up to 5
Lead poisoning	Often present, up to 5

Reproduced, by permission, from Van Eys (1970), Pediat. Clin. N. Amer. **17,** 449.

ficiency between 6 months and around 3 years. In such patients the anaemia will largely respond to oral iron, but perhaps to a suboptimal Hb level such as 11 g/100 ml.

Valuable aids to diagnosis are the demonstration of inclusion bodies. Hb H, characteristic of alpha thalassaemia, is seen after supravital staining with one part of 1 per cent brilliant cresyl blue in saline plus two parts of *fresh* anticoagulated blood at 37°C overnight. Large alpha chain inclusion bodies are found in the majority of the normoblasts and in occasional red cells in beta thalassaemia major. Howell-Jolly bodies (nuclear remnants) may also sometimes be seen.

Definitive diagnosis depends upon demonstration of an inappropriate haemoglobin in a red cell lysate. Hb F is measured by the alkali denaturation test of Singer *et al.* (1951), Hb A_2, Hb H, Hb Bart's and Hb Lepore can be identified and measured by starch gel electrophoresis (SGE) in tris-EDTA-borate buffer at pH 8.6 (Huehns and Shooter, 1965). Details of preparation of the haemolysate and the gel, application, staining and interpreting the run are fully described by Hutchison (1967).

In the usual form of beta thalassaemia major Hb F constitutes 60–90 per cent of the total, with a concomitant elevation in Hb A_2 above 3 per cent. In some variants there is no Hb A, in others it is up to 30 per cent. In heterozygous beta thalassaemia Hb A_2 is always increased but Hb F is mildly

elevated in only about half the cases. A Kleihauer stained film from whole blood may, however, disclose the presence of small numbers of Hb F-containing cells in some cases where the percentage of alkali resistant Hb is too low to measure accurately. I have found the Kleihauer film a useful pointer to the diagnosis of thalassaemia minor. This has also been the experience of Raper (1973).

In alpha thalassaemia the cord blood shows Hb Bart's, but after 4–6 months this is replaced by Hb H in similar proportions (i.e. 10–30 per cent) in the patients with chronic mild anaemia (Hb 8–10 g/100 ml) termed Hb H disease. Hb H can be demonstrated by SGE or as inclusion bodies but in either case the blood must be very fresh as it is unstable. It travels ahead of (anodal to) Hb A being described as one of 'fast' haemoglobins.

Mixed thalassaemia haemoglobinopathy syndromes show the additional abnormal Hb, with a reduction in Hb A.

AGE OF PRESENTATION AND EARLY DIAGNOSIS

As in the case of beta chain haemoglobinopathies so beta thalassaemia only becomes clinically manifest after 4–6 months, with most new cases of thalassaemia major being diagnosed by the end of the first year. An exception to this is an infant described by Oski and Naiman (1972E) who developed pallor and anaemia (Hb 8.5 g/100 ml) at 7 weeks, falling to a Hb of 5.2 g/100 ml at 12 weeks when both liver and spleen were clinically enlarged. Five similar cases were found in the literature by these authors.

When one is alerted to the possibility of thalassaemia major by the family history then early diagnosis can frequently be made, if specifically sought. Morphological abnormalities characteristic of the disease may be present to a mild degree at birth and become more prominent with the addition of circulating normoblasts by two to three months. Erlandson and Hilgartner (1959) showed that in five such infants followed from birth the Hb level was abnormally low (less than 10 g/100 ml) between the first and second month in all, and that the rate of fall in percentage of Hb F was markedly slower than in normal infants.

Diagnosis at birth is now technically possible using the newly developed methods of isotopic measurement of alpha and beta chain synthesis in reticulocyte-rich blood, in this case cord blood. This has been achieved both for the heterozygous (Kan and Nathan, 1968) and homozygous (Gaburro et al., 1970) forms of the disease. The same technique made possible the identification of gamma beta thalassaemia (Kan et al., 1972B), a previously hypothetical disorder (Stamatoyannopoulis, 1971).

Antenatal diagnosis may now be attainable by applying this technique to small amounts of foetal blood (i.e. 100 microlitres of blood, 10 per cent foetal and 90 per cent maternal) obtained by placental aspiration (Hollenberg et al., 1971; Kan et al., 1972A). By these means it should be possible to diagnose thalassaemia major as well as sickle cell disease by determining whether or not normal beta chains are being synthesized. Recent progress with these techniques has been described by Hobbins and Mahoney (1974) and Chang et al. (1974).

Two forms of thalassaemia that show distinct clinical and haematological abnormalities in the neonatal period are alpha thalassaemia and gamma beta thalassaemia. Hb Bart's hydrops foetalis syndrome (severe homozygous alpha thalassaemia) typically results in stillbirth at 28 to 38 weeks with occasional infants surviving for an hour or more after birth (Kan et al., 1967). In one case described by Weatherall et al. (1970) antenatal prediction by amniotic fluid spectrophotometry plus the family history led to premature delivery and treatment by exchange transfusion, but the infant did not survive. The clinical picture closely resembles severe rhesus disease except that there is only minimal splenomegaly. Cord blood Hb levels are around 4 g/100 ml. The less severe form of alpha thalassaemia, Hb H disease, sometimes presents as a mild to moderate haemolytic, hypochromic an-

aemia with target cells, but the majority of such infants are clinically and haematologically normal. The case of gamma beta thalassaemia presented with jaundice at 24 hr, a Hb level of 10.4 g/100 ml, bilirubin of 13.7 mg/100 ml, with hypochromia and target cells in the blood film, 400 normoblasts per 100 white cells and a reticulocytosis of 26 per cent. Hb F was reduced to 52 per cent at birth, and this would be one of the more easily determined pointers to impaired gamma chain synthesis. Transient neonatal anaemia would be expected (Stamatoyannopoulos, 1971).

CLINICAL FEATURES OF THALASSAEMIA

Anatomical changes in thalassaemia are caused by the chronic haemolysis and ineffective erythropoiesis leading to gross marrow hyperplasia and to extramedullary erythropoiesis. Destruction of the patient's own cells and of transfused cells results in deposition of iron in such tissues as spleen, liver, kidneys, gonads and myocardium (Fink, 1964).

Clinical diagnosis in thalassaemia major is seldom made before 6 months of age. Most cases present towards the end of the first year with progressive pallor and frequently poor feeding and diarrhoea. Symptoms may also arise from the splenomegaly and protuberant abdomen. On examination the liver may be enlarged as well as the constant splenomegaly (Cooley and Lee, 1925). A characteristic facies is present due to prominence of the malar eminences, frontal 'bossing', depression of the bridge of the nose, a mongoloid slant to the eyes and exposure of the upper central teeth. There is often cardiac enlargement with haemic murmurs. Other features include pericarditis, gallstones and leg ulcers. Growth retardation appears after the age of 4 years (Johnston et al., 1966) and hypogonadism at puberty. Haemosiderosis with a brown pigmentation of the skin and cirrhosis of the liver develops in those children who have required frequent transfusion.

Bone changes are a striking feature of thalassaemia major and were noted in the original description by Cooley and Lee. They are the result of marrow hyperplasia. Radiologically the skull shows a characteristic 'hair-on-end' appearance due to thinning of the outer table and broadening of the diploë similar to sickle cell disease. There is generalized skeletal osteoporosis with thinning of the cortex and trabeculation, prominent in the metacarpals. Pathological fractures of the long bones and vertebral collapse may occur. Skeletal maturation is retarded.

Thalassaemia major is usually fatal in late childhood or early adolescence. This decreased life expectancy is largely due to the long-term hazard of iron overload leading to hepatic and cardiac failure as well as an increased liability to infection (Case 6). Episodes of severe anaemia may be precipitated by infection or folic acid depletion (aplastic or megaloblastic crises).

Double heterozygotes for beta thalassaemia and sickle cell trait show a similarly severe disease with the added complication of sickling crises. Mixed with other beta chain haemoglobinopathies the clinical picture is similar to thalassaemia major but the severity depends upon that of the thalassaemia trait.

Heterozygous thalassaemia minor may be asymptomatic or cause mild anaemia. Facial abnormalities are absent and skeletal changes minimal. Slight splenomegaly is occasionally present. The important point is to distinguish these patients from cases of mild iron deficiency, for which they are often wrongly treated. Some patients with homozygous beta thalassaemia, but from a family with a mild form of the disease, show a similar clinical picture. They are commonly termed 'thalassaemia intermedia'. Recently a family of Swiss-French descent has been described with the haemoglobin analysis picture of heterozygous β thalassaemia but a far more marked anaemia associated with inclusions in the normoblasts consisting of precipitated alpha chains (Stamatoyannopoulos et al., 1974).

Alpha thalassaemia may present as hydrops foetalis with features similar to severe rhesus disease as mentioned above, but without splenomegaly. Haemoglobin H disease may present with mild anaemia in the neonatal period but more typically in later life. Accompanying a mild anaemia there may be slight icterus and moderate splenomegaly. In some of these patients episodes of severe anaemia occur requiring transfusion.

A more complete account of the clinical features of the thalassaemias is given by Mauer (1969) and Weatherall (1965), while a useful review is that of Bird (1972).

MANAGEMENT

The more severe forms of thalassaemia require frequent and regular blood transfusion. Washed, packed red cells are preferable so as to avoid the development of antileucocyte antibodies that can give rise to febrile transfusion reactions. In centres where blood of fully documented blood group phenotype is stored in liquid nitrogen it is possible to select donor blood closely matching the patient's with respect to the common immunogenic antigens (e.g. Kell, Duffy, S, Lewis and Kidd groups) so as to minimize the chance of antibody formation (Mitchell, 1972). This is now the practice in Glasgow. The washing of red cells after storage in nitrogen effectively removes leucocytes as well as senescent red cells which would have a shortened life in vivo. No instance of transmission of serum hepatitis has been recorded following the use of such washed, nitrogen-stored red cells (Tullis et al., 1970).

Criteria for transfusion have recently changed. In the past the recommendation was to determine the haemoglobin level at which symptoms appeared and then to aim to keep it above this level. But Wolman (1964) and more recently Kattamis et al. (1970) have shown that maintenance of the Hb level above 8 g/100 ml results in superior growth performance and improved general health as compared to patients in whom the level is allowed to fall to 6 g/100 ml or lower. This must now be the recommended policy. Bone changes including the facial characteristics can also be prevented by the early institution of an energetic hypertransfusion policy (Piomelli et al., 1969). This is because the alleviation of anaemia removes the stimulus for erythroid hyperplasia which causes the bone changes from marrow expansion. Nathan (1972) shows some striking examples of regression of skeletal changes following the institution of this transfusion régime plus splenectomy (Figs. 8.12 and 13). Although transfusion contributes to iron overload the cardiac toxicity from this iron may be diminished by correction of the anaemia and its resultant hypoxia (Necheles et al., 1969).

Splenectomy can reduce transfusion requirements in those thalassaemia major patients with evidence of hypersplenism, viz. gross splenomegaly, excessive transfusion requirements and thrombocytopenia (Smith et al., 1960; Bouroncle and Doan, 1964). Following splenectomy survival of transfused cells becomes normal but survival of the patient's own cells remains shortened (Shahid and Sahli, 1971). Benefit from splenectomy has also been seen in the more severe types of Hb H disease (Rigas and Koler, 1961). Hazards of splenectomy in thalassaemia, include an increased liability to overwhelming pneumococcal infection (Case 6) (Smith et al., 1964), and a possible increased tendency to parenchymal iron deposition in the liver with greater resultant cirrhosis (Berry et al., 1967). Thus iron overload remains the major long-term problem. Current opinion is that desferrioxamine has not proved very effective at removing excess iron in this disease (Nathan, 1972), especially in the presence of a large spleen, which is a major site of chelatable iron in these patients (Seshadri, Colebatch and Fisher, 1974). Serum ferritin,

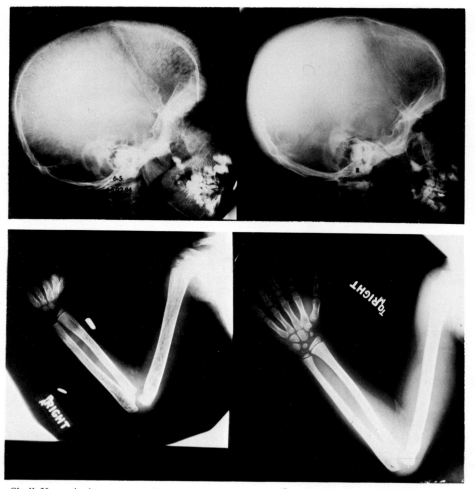

Fig. 8.12 Skull X-ray in homozygous beta-thalassaemia. At the age of 6½ years (*left*), before splenectomy and transfusion therapy, and at the age of 8 years (*right*), after these treatments. Note the decrease of 'hair-on-end' appearance. (Reproduced from *New England Journal of Medicine* (1972), **286**, 588, by permission of the Editors and the author, Professor Nathan).

Fig. 8.13 Arm X-rays in homozygous beta-thalassaemia. This is the same child as described in the legend to Fig. 8.12. Note the growth and re-calcification after splenectomy and transfusion therapy (*right*). (Reproduced from *New England Journal of Medicine* (1972), **286**, 589, by permission of the Editors and the author, Professor Nathan).

which reflects liver iron levels, remains in the range seen in idiopathic haemochromatosis even after 6–7 years on chelation therapy, although a little lower in those on such drugs than in thalassaemic children not given chelating agents (Letsky et al., 1974).*

General management includes the prophylactic administration of folic acid, especially in those patients with poor nutritional status, the avoidance of iron therapy and the energetic treatment of infections to which these patients are unduly prone. There is a case for giving prophylactic penicillin for 2 years after splenectomy since the pneumococcal infections to which such splenectomized patients are particularly susceptible are virtually always penicillin sensitive. Efforts should also be made to improve their general state of nutrition.

The management of thalassaemia has recently been reviewed in a Lancet Editorial (1972), while the different forms of thalassaemia occurring among apparently pure British stock have been reported by Knox-Macaulay et al. (1973).

Case 6. A little girl of Pakistani origin (*No. 95739*) presented at the age of 15 months because the mother had noted an abdominal mass. The parents had not noted pallor or jaundice, and there was no family history of anaemia. On examination she was pale and under-

* See dihydroxybenzoic acid p. 64.

weight with oedema of the feet. The spleen reached below the level of the umbilicus. Haematological investigation showed Hb 4.4 g/100 ml, total nucleated cell count 20,800/mm³ (normoblasts 14 per cent, 2,900/mm³, neutrophils 42 per cent, 8,700/mm³), platelets 40,000/mm³, reticulocytes 10.2 per cent. Direct Coombs test, Heinz body test and Sickling test were negative. Red cell morphology showed marked anisocytosis, polychromasia, some fragmentation and small numbers of target cells. A Kleihauer film showed Hb F in all cells. Starch gel electrophoresis (performed by Dr. H. E. Hutchison at the Western Infirmary) showed Hb F and a trace of Hb A_2, but no Hb A or abnormal Hb. (The parents had Hb levels of 12.8 and 9.7 g/100 ml, with occasional target cells and a small proportion of the RBCs showing Hb F on a Kleihauer film. SGE showed Hb A_2 levels of 5·2 and 5·5 per cent, with Hb F levels of 2·5 per cent and less than 2 per cent respectively in the father and mother, both typical of beta thalassaemia minor.) Serum bilirubin was 4·5 mg/100 ml (all indirect), the Schumm's test strongly positive, serum iron 192 ug/100 ml and TIBC 434 ug/ml.

X-ray examination showed marked generalized osteoporosis with reduction in cortical width particularly at the ends of the long bones, a loose trabecular pattern in the metacarpals and some widening of the diploeic space in the cranial vault. The heart was slightly enlarged (CT ratio 52 per cent).

Transfusion requirements proved excessive with average interval between transfusions of 31 days. Platelets remained around 50,000/mm³. Hypersplenism seemed certain and splenectomy was therefore performed, primarily to reduce transfusion requirements and consequent iron overload. By this time the serum iron was 288 ug/100 ml (over 60 per cent saturated TIBC), after 6 transfusions totalling 1,450 ml and calculated to containing approximately 750 mg of iron.

Within 3 days of splenectomy the platelet count had risen to 171,000/mm³, and was subsequently maintained above 200,000/mm³. She was put on prophylactic penicillin G 250 mg twice daily, and oral folic acid 5 mg per day. Subsequent intervals between transfusions increased to approximately 8 weeks, but height and weight remained below the 3rd per centile. When the iron saturation reached 80 per cent she was started on desferrioxamine 500 mg in 2–3 ml H_2O I.M. twice weekly plus 1 g in 100 ml saline I.V. at the time of each blood transfusion.

Subsequent progress was uneventful until, at the age of 8, $6\frac{1}{2}$ years after splenectomy, she suddenly became seriously ill with vomiting, diarrhoea and loss of consciousness, dying in the ambulance on the way to hospital. Necropsy showed pneumococcal septicaemia and marked haemosiderosis affecting lymph glands, marrow, adrenals, myocardium, kidneys, pituitary, pancreas, salivary glands, thyroid, leptomeninges and liver with associated micronodular cirrhosis.

The desferrioxamine had failed to prevent haemosiderosis and, on this occasion, the prophylactic penicillin had failed to prevent pneumococcal septicaemia. A penicillinase-producing *Staph. aureus* was isolated from the respiratory tract.

REFERENCES

Ager, J. A. M. & Lehmann, H. (1958) Observations on some 'fast' haemoglobins: K.J.N. and Barts. *Brit. med. J.*, **1**, 929.

Allen, D. W., Wyman, J. & Smith, C. A. (1953) The oxygen equilibrium of fetal and adult hemoglobin. *J. Biol. Chem.* **203**, 81.

Allison, A. C. (1954) Protection afforded by sickle-cell trait against subertian malarial infection. *Brit. med. J.*, **1**, 290.

Anderson, R., Cassell, M., Mullinax, G. L. & Chaplin, H. (1963) Effect of normal cells on viscosity of sickle-cell blood. *In vitro* studies and report of six years' experience with a prophylactic program of 'partial exchange transfusion.' *Arch. Intern. Med.*, **111**, 286.

Atwater, J., Schwartz, I. R., Erslev, A. J., Montgomery, T. L. & Tocantins, L. M. (1960) Sickling of erythrocytes in a patient with thalassaemia-haemoglobin-I disease. *New Eng. J. Med.*, **263**, 1215.

Baelen, H., Van, Vandepitte, J. & Eeckels, R. (1969) Observations on sickle-cell anaemia and haemoglobin Bart's in Congolese neonates. *Ann. Soc. belge. Méd. trop.*, **49**, 157.

Baglioni, C. (1962) The fusion of two peptide chains in hemoglobin Lepore and its interpretation as a genetic deletion. *Proc. natn. Acad. Sci.*, **48**, 1880.

Bard, H., Makowski, E. L., Meschia, G. & Battaglia, F. C. (1970) The relative rates of synthesis of hemoglobins A and F in immature red cells of newborn infants. *Pediatrics*, **45**, 766.

Barnes, P. M., Hendrickse, R. G. & Watson-Williams, E. J. (1965) Low-molecular-weight Dextran in treatment of bone-pain crises in sickle-cell disease: A double-blind trial. *Lancet*, **ii**, 1271.

Barnes, M. G., Komarmy, L. & Novack, A. H. (1972) A comprehensive screening program for hemoglobinopathies. *J.A.M.A.*, **219**, 701.

Bauer, C., Ludwig, I. & Ludwig, M. (1968) Different effects of 2, 3–diphosphoglycerate and adenosine triphosphate on oxygen affinity of adult and fetal hemoglobin. *Life Sci.*, **7**, 1339.

Beale, D. & Lehmann, H. (1965) Abnormal hemoglobins and the genetic code. *Nature*, **207**, 259.

Beaven, G. H., Ellis, M. J. & White, J. C. (1960) Studies on human foetal haemoglobin. I. Detection and estimation. *Brit. J. Haemat.*, **6**, 1.

Bellingham, A. J. & Huehns, E. R. (1968) Compensation in haemolytic anaemias caused by abnormal haemoglobins. *Nature*, **218**, 924.

Benesch, R., Benesch, R. E. & Yu, C. I. (1968) Reciprocal binding of oxygen and diphosphoglycerate by human hemoglobin. *Proc. Nat. Acad. Sci.*, **59**, 526.

Berry, C. L., Long, M. B., Marshall, W. C. & Sydney, M. B. (1967) Iron distribution in the liver of patients with thalassaemia major. *Lancet*, **i**, 1031.

Bertles, J. F. & Milner, P. A. (1968) Irreversibly sickled erythrocytes: a consequence of the heterogeneous distribution of hemoglobin types in sickle cell anemia. *J. Clin. Invest.*, **47**, 1731.

Bertles, J. F. & Dobler, J. (1969) Reversible and irreversible sickling: a distinction by electron microscopy, *Blood*, **33**, 884.

Beutler, E. (1969) Drug-induced hemolytic anemia. *Pharmacological Reviews*, **21**, 73.

Binder, R. A. & Jones, S. R. (1970) Prevalance and awareness of sickle cell hemoglobin in a military population: Determination by a rapid screening method. *J.A.M.A.*, **214**, 909.

Bird, G. W. G. (1972) The haemoglobinopathies. *Brit. med. J.*, **1**, 363.

Bird, G. W. G. & Lehmann, H. (1956) Haemoglobin D in India. *Brit. med. J.*, **1**, 514.

B.M.J. (1972) Detecting sickle haemoglobin. *British Medical Journal*, **ii**, 246.

Bouroncle, B. A. & Doan, C. A. (1964) Cooley's anemia: Indications for splenectomy. *Ann. N.Y. Acad. Sci.*, **119**, 709.

Brancati, C. & Baglioni, C. (1966) Homozygous beta-delta thalassaemia (beta-delta microcythaemia). *Nature*, **212**, 262.

Brody, S. & Nilsson, B. (1960) Foetal and adult haemoglobin mass in relation to foetal development. *J. Obst. Gynaec. Brit. Emp.*, **67**, 827.

Bromberg, Y. M., Abrahamov, A. & Salzberger, M. (1956) The effect of maternal anoxemia on the foetal haemoglobin of the newborn. *J. Obst. Gynaec. Brit. Emp.*, **63**, 875.

Bruning, W. & Holtzer, A. (1961) The effect of urea on hydrophobic bonds: the critical micelle concentration of n-Dodecyltrimethylammonium bromide in aqueous solutions of urea. *J. Am. Chem. Soc.*, **83**, 4865.

Canning, D. M. & Huntsman, R. G. (1970) An assessment of sickledex as an alternative to the sickling test. *J. Clin. Path.*, **23**, 736.

Carrell, R. W., Lehmann, H. & Hutchison, H. E. (1966) Haemoglobinopathy Köln (β–98 valine→ methionine): An unstable protein causing inclusion body anaemia. *Nature*, **210**, 915.

Carrell, R. W. & Lehmann, H. (1969) The unstable haemoglobin haemolytic anaemias. *Seminars in Hematology*, **6**, 116.

Cathie, I. A. B. (1952) Apparent idiopathic Heinz body anaemia. *Great Ormond Street Journal*, **2**, 43.

Cawein, M. J., O'Neill, R. P., Danzer, L. A., Lappat, E. J. & Roach, T. (1969) A study of the sickling phenomenon and oxygen dissociation curve in patients with hemoglobins SS, SD, SF and SC. *Blood*, **34**, 682.

Cerami, A. & Manning, J. M. (1971) Potassium cyanate as an inhibitor of the sickling of erythrocytes *in vivo*. *Proc. Natl. Acad. Sci. U.S.A.*, **68**, 1180.

Cerami, A. (1972) Cyanate as an inhibitor of red-cell sickling. *New Eng. J. Med.*, **287**, 807.

Chan, T. K., Mak, L. W. & Ng, R. P. (1971) Methemoglobinemia, Heinz bodies, and acute massive intravascular hemolysis in lysol poisoning. *Blood*, **38**, 738.

Chang, H., Hobbins, J. C., Cividalli, G., Frigoletto, F. D., Mahoney, M. J., Ka , Y. W. & Nathan, D. G. (1974) *In utero* diagnosis of hemoglobinopathies: Hb synthesis in fetal red cells. *New Eng. J. Med.*, **290**, 1067.

Charache, S., Weatherall, D. J. & Clegg, J. B. (1966) Polycythemia associated with a hemoglobinopathy. *J. Clin. Invest.*, **45**, 813.

Charache, S., Conley, C. L., Waugh, D. F., Ugoretz, R. J., Spurrell, R. J. & Gayle E. (1967) Pathogenesis of hemolytic anemia in homozygous hemoglobin C disease. *J. Clin. Invest.*, **46**, 1795.

Charney, E. & Miller, G. (1964) Reticulocytopenia in sickle cell disease. *Am. J. Dis. Child.*, **107**, 450.

Clegg, J. B., Naughton, M. A. & Weatherall, D. J. (1965) An improved method for the characterization of human haemoglobin mutants: identification of $\alpha_2 \beta_2$ 95 GLU haemoglobin N (Baltimore). *Nature*, **207**, 945.

Clegg, J. B. & Weatherall, D. J. (1967) Haemoglobin synthesis in alpha-thalassaemia (Haemoglobin H disease). *Nature*, **215**, 1241.

Clegg, J. B., Weatherall, D. J., Na-Nakorn, S. & Wasi, P. (1968) Haemoglobin synthesis in β-thalassaemia. *Nature*, **220**, 664.

Conley, C. L., Weatherall, D. J., Richardson, S. N., Shepherd, M. K. & Charache, S. (1963) Hereditary persistence of fetal hemoglobin: A study of 79 affected persons in 15 Negro families in Baltimore. *Blood*, **21**, 261.

Conn, H. O. (1954) Sickle-cell trait and splenic infarction associated with high-altitude flying. *New Eng. J. Med.*, **251**, 417.

Cooley, T. B. & Lee, P. (1925) Series of cases of splenomegaly in children with anemia and peculiar bone change. *Trans. Am. Pediat. Soc.*, **37**, 29.

Crosby, W. H. (1959) Normal functions of the spleen relative to the red blood cells. *Blood*, **14**, 399.

Dacie, J. V. (1963) *The haemolytic anaemias. Part 1. The congenital anaemias.* London: Churchill.

Dacie, J. V., Grimes, A. J., Meisler, A., Steingold, L., Hemstead, E. H., Beaven, G. H. & White, J. C. (1964) Hereditary heinz-body anaemia. A report of studies of five patients with mild anaemia. *Brit. J. Haemat.*, **10**, 388.

Delivoria-Papadopoulos, M., Roncevic, N. P. & Oski, F. A. (1971) Postnatal changes in oxygen transport of term, premature, and sick infants: The role of red cell 2, 3–diphosphoglycerate and adult haemoglobin. *Pediat. Res.*, **5**, 235.

Desforges, J. F. (1971) Treatment of sickle crisis. *New Eng. J. Med.*, **284**, 913.

Desforges, J. F. & Wang, M. Y. F. W. (1966) Sickle cell anemia. *Med. Clin. N. Amer.*, **50**, 1519.

Diggs, L. W. (1935) Siderofibrosis of the spleen in sickle cell anemia. *J. Am. Med. Ass.*, **104**, 538.

Diggs, L. W. (1956) The crisis in sickle cell anaemia. Hematologic studies. *Am. J. Clin. Pathol.*, **26**, 1109.

Diggs, L. W. (1965) Sickle cell crises. *Am. J. Clin. Pathol.*, **44**, 1.

Diggs, L. W. (1969) Pulmonary lesions in sickle cell anaemia. In abstracts from the first international sickle cell anaemia conference. *Blood*, **34**, 734.

Diggs, L. W., Kraus, A. P., Morrison, D. B. & Rudnicki, R. P. (1954) Intraerythrocytic crystals in a white patient with hemoglobin C in the absence of other types of hemoglobin. *Blood*, **9**, 1172.

Dormandy, K. M., Lock, S. P. & Lehmann, H. (1961) Haemoglobin Q–alpha thalassaemia. *Brit. med. J.* **1**, 1582.

Erdem, S. & Aksoy, M. (1969) The increase of hemoglobin A_2 to its adult level. *Israel J. Med. Sci.*, **5**, 427.

Erlandson, M. E. & Hilgartner, M. (1959) Hemolytic disease in the neonatal period and early infancy. *J. Pediat.*, **54**, 566.

Evelyn, K. A. & Malloy, H. T. (1938) Microdetermination of oxyhemoglobin, methemoglobin and sulfhemoglobin in a single sample of blood. *J. Biol. Chem.*, **126**, 655.

Eys, J. Van (1970) Recent progress in genetic hemolytic disorders: A practical approach. *Prediat Clinics N. America*, **17**, 449.

Fanelli, A., Antonini, E. & Caputo, A. (1958) I. Physicochemical properties of human globin. *Biochim. Biophys. Acta.*, **30**, 608.

Farmer, M. B., Lehmann, H. & Raine, D. N. (1964) Two unrelated patients with congenital cyanosis due to haemoglobinopathy. *Lancet*, **ii**, 786.

Farrar, J. F. & Blomfield, J. (1963) Alkali-resistant haemoglobin content of blood in congenital heart disease. *Brit. J. Haemat.*, **9**, 278.

Fessas, P. (1963) Inclusion of hemoglobin in erythroblasts and erythrocytes in thalassaemia. *Blood*, **21**, 21.

Fink, H. (1964) Transfusion haemochromatosis in Cooley's anemia. *Annals N.Y. Acad. Sci.*, **119**, 680.

Finch, J. T., Perutz, M. F., Bertles, J. F. & Dobler, J. (1973) Structure of sickled erythrocytes and of sickle-cell hemoglobin fibers. *Proc. Nat. Acad. Sci. U.S.A.*, **70**, 718.

Fraser, I. D. & Raper, A. B. (1962) Observations on the change from foetal to adult erythropoiesis. *Arch. Dis. Childh.*, **37**, 289.

Frick, P. G. Hitzig, W. H. & Betke, K. (1962) Hemoglobin Zürich, a new hemoglobin anomaly associated with acute hemolytic episodes with inclusion bodies after sulphonamide. *Blood*, **20**, 261.

Gaburro, D., Volpato, S. & Vigi, V. (1970) Diagnosis of beta thalassaemia in the newborn by means of haemoglobin synthesis. *Acta Paediat. Scand.*, **59**, 523.

Garby, L., Sjölin, S. & Vuille, J. C. (1962) Studies of erythro-kinetic in infancy II. The relative rate of synthesis of haemoglobin F and haemoglobin A during the first months of life. *Acta Paediatrica*, **51**, 245.

Gerald, P. S. (1958) The electrophoretic and spectroscopic characterization of haemoglobin M. *Blood*, **12**, 936.

Gerald, P. S. & Diamond, L. K. (1958) A new hereditary hemoglobinopathy (the Lepore trait) and its interaction with thalassaemia trait. *Blood*, **13**, 835.

Gerald, P. S. & Efron, M. L. (1961) Chemical studies of several varieties of hemoglobin M. *Proc. Nat. Acad. Sci.*, **47**, 1758.

Gerald, P. S. & Scott, E. M. (1966) The hereditary methemoglobinemias. In *Metabolic Basis of Inherited Disease*. Edited by Stanbury. Wyngaarden & Fredrickson. New York: McGraw-Hill.

Gerbie, A. B., DeCosta, E. J. & Reis, R. A. (1959) Fetal hemoglobin as an index of maturity. *Am. J. Obst. Gynec.*, **78**, 57.

Gillette, P. N., Peterson, C. M., Yang, S. Lu. & Cerami, A. (1974) Sodium cyanate as a potential treatment for sickle-cell disease. *New Eng. J. Med.*, **290**, 654.

Goldring, J. S. R. (1969) The changing pattern of the orthopedic complications of the abnormal hemoglobins. In abstracts from the First International Sickle Cell Anaemia Conference. *Blood*, **34**, 728.

Goldstein, G. W., Hammaker, L. & Schmid, P. (1968) The catabolism of Heinz bodies. *Blood*, **31**, 388.

Goluboff, N. & Wheaton, R. (1961) Methylene blue induced cyanosis and acute hemolytic anemia complicating the treatment of methemoglobinemia. *J. Pediat.*, **58**, 86.

Gray, R. (1969) Clinical features of sickle cell anaemia in Jamaican children. In abstracts from the First International Sickle Cell Anaemia Conference. *Blood*, **34**, 728.

Green, R. L., Huntsman, R. G. & Serjeant, G. R. (1971) The sickle-cell and altitude. *Brit. med. J.*, **iv**, 593.

Greenberg, M. S. & Kass, E. H. (1958) Studies on the production of red blood cells XIII. Observations on the role of pH in the pathogenesis and treatment of painful crisis in sickle-cell disease. *Am. Med. Assoc. Arch. Intern. Med.*, **101**, 355.

Grimes, A. J., Meisler, A. & Dacie, J. V. (1964) Congenital Heinz-body anaemia. Further evidence on the cause of Heinz-body production in red cells. *Brit. J. Haemat.*, **10**, 281.

Haggard, M. E. & Schneider, R. G. (1961) Sickle cell anemia in the first 2 years of life. *J. Pediat.*, **58**, 785.

Harris, J. W. (1959) The role of physical and chemical factors in the sickling phenomenon. *Progr. Hematol.*, **2**, 47.

Heller, P., Yakulis, V. J. & Josephson, A. M. (1962) Immunologic studies of human hemoglobins. *J. Lab. Clin. Med.*, **59**, 401.

Heller, P. (1965) The molecular basis of the pathogenicity of abnormal hemoglobins—some recent developments. *Blood*, **25**, 110.

Heller, P., Coleman, R. D. & Yakulis, V. (1966) Haemoglobin $M_{\text{Hyde Park}}$: A new variant of abnormal methemoglobin. *J. Clin. Invest.*, **45**, 1021.

Heywood, J. D., Karon, M. & Weissman, S. (1964) Amino acid: incorporation into alpha—and beta-chains of hemoglobin by normal and thalassaemic reticulocytes. *Science*, **146**, 530.

Hitzig, W. H., Frick, P. G., Betke, K. & Huisman, T. H. J. (1960) Hämoglobin Zurich: eime meu Hämoglobinanomalie mit sulphonamidin-duzierter Innenkörperanämie. *Helv. Paediat. Acta.*, **15**, 499.

Hobbins, J. C. & Mahoney, M. J. (1974) *In utero* diagnosis of hemoglobinopathies: Technic for obtaining fetal blood. *New Eng. J. Med.*, **290**, 1065.

Hollenberg, M. D., Kaback, M. M. & Kazazian, H. H. (1971) Adult hemoglobin synthesis by reticulocytes from human fetus at midtrimester. *Science*, **174**, 698.

Huehns, E. R. & Shooter, E. M. (1961) Polypeptide chains of haemoglobin A_2. *Nature*, **189**, 918.

Huehns, E. R., Hecht, F., Keil, J. V. & Motulsky, A. G. (1964) Developmental hemoglobin anomalies in a chromosomal triplication: D1-trisomy syndrome. *Proc. Nat. Acad. Sci.*, **51**, 89.

Huehns, E. R. & Shooter, E. M. (1965) Human haemoglobins. *J. Med. Genet.*, **2**, 48.

Huehns, E. R. & Bellingham, A. J. (1969) Annotation: Diseases of function and stability of haemoglobin. *Brit. J. Haemat.*, **17**, 1.

Huennekens, F. M., Caffrey, R. W. & Gabrio, B. W. (1958) Electron transport sequence of methemoglobin reductase. *Ann. N.Y. Acad. Sci.*, **75**, 167.

Hugh-Jones, K., Lehmann, H. & McAlister, J. M. (1964) Some experiences in managing sickle-cell anaemia in children and young adults, using alkalis and magnesium. *Brit. med. J.*, **ii**, 226.

Huisman, T. H. J., Schroeder, W. A., Adams, H. R., Shelton, J. R., Shelton, J. B. & Apell, G. (1970) A possible sub-class of the hereditary persistence of fetal haemoglobin. *Blood*, **36**, 1.

Huntsman, R. G. & Lehmann, H. (1974) Annotation: Treatment of sickle-cell disease. *Brit. J. Haemat.*, **28**, 437.

Hutchison, H. E. (1967) *An Introduction to the Haemoglobinopathies and the Methods Used for Their Recognition.* London: Edward Arnold.

Hutchison, H. E., Pinkerton, P. H., Waters, P., Douglas, A. S., Lehmann, H. & Beale, D. (1964) Hereditary Heinzbody anaemia, thrombocytopenia, and haemoglobinopathy (Hb Köln) in a Glasgow family. *Brit. med. J.*, **ii**, 1099.

Ingram, V. M. (1959) Chemistry of the abnormal human haemoglobins. *Brit. Med. Bull.*, **15**, 27.

Ingram, V. M. (1961) Gene evolution and the haemoglobins. *Nature*, **189**, 704.

Ingram, V. M. & Stretton, A. O. W. (1959) The genetic basis of the thalassaemia diseases. *Nature*, **184**, 1903.

Itano, H. A. (1957) The human hemoglobins. Their properties and genetic control. *Advances in Protein Chem.*, **12**, 215.

Itano, H. A., Bergren, W. R. & Sturgeon, P. (1956) The abnormal human hemoglobins. *Medicine*, **35**, 121.

Jackson, J. M., Way, B. J. & Woodliff, H. J. (1967) A West Australian family with a haemolytic disorder associated with Köln. *Brit. J. Haemat.*, **13**, 474.

Jacob, H. S. (1970) Mechanisms of Heinz body formation and attachment to red cell membrane. *Seminars in Hematology*, **7**, 341.

Jacob, H. S., Brain, M. C., Dacie, J. V., Carrell, R. W. & Lehmann, H. (1968) Abnormal haem binding and globin SH group blockade in unstable haemoglobins. *Nature*, **218**, 1214.

Jensen, W. N. (1969) Fragmentation and the Freakish Poikilocyte. *Amer. J. Med. Sci.*, **257**, 355.

Jensen, W. N. & Lessin, L. (1970) Membrane alterations associated with hemoglobinopathies. *Seminars in Hematology*, **7**, 409.

Johnston, F. E., Hertzog, K. P. & Malina, R. M. (1966) Longitudinal growth in thalassaemia major. *Am. J. Dis. Child.*, **112**, 396.

Kan, Y. W., Allen, A. & Lowenstein, L. (1967) Hydrops fetalis with alpha thalassemia. *New Eng. J. Med.*, **276**, 18.

Kan, Y. W. & Nathan, D. G. (1968) Beta thalassaemia trait: detection at birth. *Science*, **161**, 589.

Kan, Y. W., Dozy, A. M., Alter, B. P., Frigoletto, F. D. & Nathan, D. G. (1972A) Detection of the sickle gene in the ..uman fetus. *New Eng. J. Med.*, **287**, 1.

Kan, Y. W., Forget, B. G. & Nathan, D. G. (1972B) Gamma-beta thalassaemia: A cause of hemolytic disease of the newborn. *New Eng. J. Med.*, **286**, 129.

Kattamis, C., Touliatos, N., Haidas, S. & Matsaniotis, N. (1970) Growth of children with thalassaemia: Effect of different transfusion regimens. *Arch. Dis. Childh.*, **45**, 502.

Keitel, H. G., Thompson, D. & Itano, H. A. (1956) Hyposthenuria in sickle cell anemia: A reversible renal defect. *J. Clin. Invest.*, **35**, 998.

Kirschbaum, T. H. (1962) Fetal hemoglobin content of cord blood determined by column chromatography. *Am. J. Obst. Gynec.*, **84**, 1375.

Kleihauer, E., Braun, H. & Betke, K. (1957) Demonstration von fetalem Hämoglobin in den erythrocyten eines Blutausstrichs. *Klin. Wschr.*, **35**, 637.

Knox-Macauley, H. H. M., Weatherall, D. J., Clegg, J. B. & Pembrey, M. E. (1973) Thalassaemia in the British. *Brit. med. J.*, **3**, 150.

Kraus, A. P., Robinson, H., Cooper, M. R., Felts, J. H., Rhyne, A. L., Porter, F. S., Rosse, W. F. & Grush, O. C. (1974) Clinical trials of therapy for sickle-cell vaso-occlusive crises. *J.A.M.A.*, **228**, 1120.

Kohn, J. (1969) Separation of haemoglobins on cellulose acetate. *J. Clin. Path.*, **22**, 109.

Königsberg, W. & Lehmann, H. (1965) The amino acid substitution in haemoglobin M_{Iwate}. *Biochim. Biophys. Acta*, **107**, 266.

Kravitz, H., Elegant, L. D., Kaiser, E. & Kagan, B. M. (1956) Methemoglobin values in premature and mature infants and children. *Am. J. Dis. Child.*, **91**, 1.

Kreimer-Birnbaum, M., Pinkerton, P. H., Bannerman, R. M. & Hutchison, H. E. (1966A) Dipyrrolic urinary pigments in congenital Heinz-body anemia due to Hb Köln and in thalassaemia. *Brit. med. J.*, **ii**, 395.

Kreimer-Birnbaum, M., Pinkerton, P. H., Bannerman, R. M. & Hutchison, H. E. (1966B) Urinary dipyrroles; their occurrence and significance in thalassemia and other disorders. *Blood*, **28**, 993.

Lancet (1971) Editorial: Treatment and prevention of sickle-cell crisis. *Lancet*, **ii**, 1069.

Lancet (1972) Editorial: Management of thalassaemia. *Lancet*, **ii**, 467.

Lancet (1974) Treatment of sickle-cell crises. *Lancet*, **ii**, 762.

Laszlo, J., Obenour, W. & Saltzman, H. A. (1969) Effects of hyperbaric oxygenation on sickle syndromes. *Sth. Med. J.*, **62**, 453.

Lehmann, H., Story, P. & Thein, H. (1956) Haemoglobin E in Burmese; two cases of haemoglobin E disease. *Brit. med. J.*, **1**, 544.

Lehmann, H., Beale, D. & Boi-Doku, F. S. (1964) Haemoglobin G$_{Accra}$. *Nature*, **203**, 363.

Lehmann, H., Huntsman, R. G. & Ager, J. A. M. (1966) The hemoglobinopathies and thalassemia. In *The Metabolic Basis of Inherited Disease*, ed. Stanbury, J. B., Wyngaarden, J. B. and Fredrickson, D. S. New York: McGraw-Hill.

Lehmann, H. & Carrell, R. W. (1968) Differences between alpha—and beta-chain mutants of human haemoglobin and between alpha- and beta-thalassaemia: possible duplication of the alpha-chain gene. *Brit. med. J.*, **4**, 748.

Lehmann, H. & Carrell, R. W. (1969) Variations in the structure of human haemoglobin—with particular reference to the unstable haemoglobins. *Brit. med. Bull.*, **25**, 14.

Letsky, E. A., Miller, F., Worwood, M. & Flynn, D. M. (1974) Serum ferritin in children with thalassaemia regularly transfused. *J. clin. Path.*, **27**, 652.

Lindenbaum, J. & Klipstein, F. A. (1963) Folic acid deficiency in sickle-cell anemia. *New Eng. J. Med.*, **269**, 875.

Loh, W. P. (1971) Evaluation of a rapid test tube turbidity test for the detection of sickle cell hemoglobin. *Amer. J. Clin. Path.*, **55**, 55.

Lubin, B. H. & Oski, F. A. (1973) Oral urea therapy in children with sickle-cell anemia. *J. Pediat.*, **82**, 311.

Lukens, J. N. (1972) Hemoglobin S, the pneumococcus and the spleen. *Am. J. Dis. Child.*, **123**, 6.

Luzzatto, L., Nwachuku-Jarrett, E. S. & Reddy, S. (1970) Increased sickling of parasitised erythrocytes as mechanism of resistance against malaria in the sickle-cell trait. *Lancet*, **1**, 319.

McCurdy, P. R. 1969) ^{32}DFP and ^{51}Cr for measurement of red cell life span in abnormal hemoglobin syndromes. *Blood*, **33**, 214.

McCurdy, P. R., Binder, R. A., Mahmood, L., Bullock, W. H., Hudson, R. L., Jilly, P. N., Scott, R. B., Garrett, T. A., Schmitz, T. H., & Westerman, M. P. (1974) Treatment of sickle-cell crisis with urea in invert sugar. *J.A.M.A.*, **228**, 1125.

McCurdy, P. R. & Mahmood, L. (1971) Intravenous urea treatment of the painful crisis of sickle-cell disease—a preliminary report. *New Eng. J. Med.*, **285**, 992.

Mann, J. R., Deeble, T. J., Breeze, G. R. & Stuart, J. (1972) Ancrod in sickle-cell crisis. *Lancet*, **i**, 934.

Mann, J. R., Cotter, K. P., Walker, R. A., Bird, G. W. G. & Stuart, J. (1975) Anaemic crisis in sickle cell disease. *J. Clin. Path.*, **28**, 341.

Martin, H. & Huisman, T. H. J. (1963) Formation of ferrihaemoglobin of isolated human haemoglobin types by sodium nitrate. *Nature*, **200**, 898.

Mauer, A. M. (1969) *Pediatric Hematology*. New York: McGraw-Hill.

May, A., Bellingham, A. J., Huehns, E. R. & Beaven, G. H. (1972) Effect of cyanate on sickling. *Lancet*, **i**, 658.

Mitchell, R. (1972) Personal communication.

Mott, M. G., Apley, J. & Raper, A. B. (1969) Congenital (erythroid) hypoplastic anaemia: Modified expression in males. *Arch. Dis. Childh.*, **44**, 757.

Muirhead, H. & Petutz, M. F. (1963) Structure of haemoglobin. A three-dimensional fourier synthesis of reduced human haemoglobin at 5·5 Å resolution. *Nature*, **199**, 633.

Murayama, M. (1962) A sub-molecular mechanism of gel formation in sickle cell haemolysate. *Nature*, **194**, 933.

Murayama, M. (1964) A molecular mechanism of sickled erythrocyte formation. *Nature*, **202**, 258.

Nalbandian, R. M., Henry, R. L., Nichols, B. M., Camp, F. R. & Wolf, P. L. (1970) The Murayama test. Part 1. Evidence for the modified Murayama hypothesis for the molecular mechanism of sickling. *U.S. Army Med. Res. Lab. Report No. 893.*

Nalbandian, R. M., Anderson, J. W., Lusher, J. M., Agustsson, A. & Henry, R. L. (1971) Oral urea and the prophylactic treatment of sickle cell disease—a preliminary report. *Am. J. Med. Sci.*, **261**, 325.

Nalbandian, R. M., Shultz, G., Lusher, J. M., Anderson, J. W. & Henry, R. L. (1971) Sickle cell crisis terminated by intravenous urea in sugar solutions—a preliminary report. *Am. J. Med. Sci.*, **261**, 309.

Nathan, D. H. (1972) Thalassemia. *New Eng. J. Med.*, **286**, 686.

Nathan, D. G. & Gunn, R. B. (1966) Thalassemia: the consequences of unbalanced hemoglobin synthesis. *Amer. J. Med.*, **41**, 815.

Necheles, T. F. & Allen, D. M. (1969) Heinz-body anemias. *New Eng. J. Med.*, **280**, 203.

Necheles, T. F., Beard, M. E. J. & Allen, D. M. (1969) Myocardial hemosiderosis in hypoxic mice. *Ann. N.Y. Acad. Sci.*, **165**, 167.

Neel, J. V. (1951) The inheritance of sickling phenomena, with particular reference to sickle cell disease. *Blood*, **6**, 389.

New England Journal of Medicine (1971) Editorial: Urea therapy in sickle-cell disease. *New Eng. J. Med.*, **285**, 1025.

Ohta, Y., Yamaoka, K., Sumida, I., Fujita, S., Fujimura, T. & Yanase, T. (1971) Homozygous delta-thalassemia first discovered in Japanese family with hereditary persistence of fetal hemoglobin. *Blood*, **37**, 706.

Oppé, T. E. & Fraser, I. D. (1961) Foetal haemoglobin in haemolytic disease of the newborn. *Arch. Dis. Child.*, **36**, 507.

Opio. E. & Barnes, P. M. (1972) Intravenous urea in treatment of bone-pain crises of sickle-cell disease. A double-blind trial. *Lancet*, **ii**, 160.

Orzalesi, M. M. & Hay, W. W. (1971) The regulation of oxygen affinity of fetal blood. 1. *In vivo* experiments and results in normal infants. *Pediatrics*, **48**, 857.

Oski, F. A. and Naiman, J. L. (1972A) *Hematologic Problems in the Newborn*, p. 141. Philadelphia: Saunders.

Oski, F. A. and Naiman, J. L. (1972B) *Hematologic Problems in the Newborn*, p. 153. Philadelphia: Saunders.

Oski, F. A. and Naiman, J. L. (1972C) *Hematologic Problems in the Newborn*, p. 170. Philadelphia: Saunders.

Oski, F. A. and Naiman, J. L. (1972D) *Hematologic Problems in the Newborn*, p. 174. Philadelphia: Saunders.

Oski, F. A. and Naiman, J. L. (1972E) *Hematologic Problems in the Newborn*, p. 166. Philadelphia: Saunders.

Overly, W. L., Rosenberg, A. & Harris, J. W. (1967) Hemoglobin M Reserve: Studies on identification and characterization. *J. Lab. Clin. Med.*, **69**, 62.

Pauling, L., Itano, H. A., Singer, S. J. & Wells, I. C. (1949) Sickle cell anemia, a molecular disease. *Science*, **110**, 543.

Pearson, H. A. & Diamond, L. K. (1971) The critically ill child: Sickle cell disease crises and their management. *Pediat.*, **48**, 629.

Perillie, P. E. & Epstein, F. H. (1963) Sickling phenomenon produced by hypertonic solutions: A possible explanation for the hyposthenuria of sicklemia. *J. Clin. Invest.*, **42**, 570.

Perutz, M. F., Muirhead, H., Cox, J. M. & Goaman, L. C. G. (1968) Three-dimensional fourier synthesis of horse oxyhaemoglobin at 2·8 A resolution: the atomic model. *Nature*, **219**, 902.

Petch, M. C. & Serjeant, G. R. (1970) Clinical features of pulmonary lesions in sickle-cell anaemia. *Brit. med. J.*, **3**, 31.

Pierce, L. E., Rath, C. E. & McCoy, K. (1963) A new hemoglobin variant with sickling properties. *New Eng. J. Med.*, **268**, 862.

Piomelli, S., Danoff, S. J., Becker, M. H., Lipera, M. J. & Travis, S. F. (1969) Prevention of bone malformations and cardiomegaly in Cooley's anemia by early hypertransfusion regimen. *Ann. N.Y. Acad. Sci.*, **165**, 427.

Prindle, K. H. & McCurdy, P. R. (1970) Red cell lifespan in hemoglobin C disorders (with special reference to hemoglobin C trait). *Blood*, **36**, 14.

Quie, P. G., Fisch, R. O. & Raile, R. (1962) Methemoglobinemia and hemolytic anemia in normal newborns and normal prematures. *Lancet*, **82**, 428.

Ranney, H. M. (1970) Clinically important variants of human hemoglobin. *New Eng. J. Med.*, **282**, 144.

Ranney, H. M., Jacob, A. S. & Nagel, R. L. (1967) Haemoglobin New York. *Nature*, **213**, 876.

Ranney, H. M., Nagel, R. L., Heller, P. & Udem, L. (1968) Oxygen equilibrium of hemoglobin M Hyde Park. *Biochim. Biophys. Acta*, **160**, 112.

Raper, A. B. (1973) Differentiation of iron-deficiency anaemia from thalassaemia trait. *Lancet*, **i**, 778.

Reynolds, J. D. H. (1971) Painful sickle cell crisis. Successful treatment with hyperbaric oxygen therapy. *J. Am. Med. Ass.*, **216**, 1977.

Rhodes, R. S., Revo, L., Hara, S., Hartmann, R. C. & Van Eys, J. (1974) Therapy for sickle-cell vaso-occlusive crises. *J.A.M.A.*, **228**, 1129.

Rifkind, R. A. (1965) Heinz-body anemia, ultrastructural study. II. Red cell sequestration and destruction. *Blood*, **26**, 433.

Rigas, D. A. & Koler, R. D. (1961) Decreased erythrocyte survival in hemoglobin H disease as a result of the abnormal properties of hemoglobin H: the benefit of splenectomy. *Blood*, **18**, 1,

Robinson, A. R., Robson, M., Harrison, A. P. & Zuelzer, W. W. (1957) A new technique for differentiation of hemoglobin. *J. Lab. Clin. Med.*, **50**, 745.

Rosemeyer, M. A. & Huehns, E. R. (1967) On the mechanism of the dissociation of haemoglobin. *J. Molec. Biol.*, **25**, 253.

Ross, J. D. (1963) Deficient activity of DPNH-dependent methemoglobin diaphorase in cord blood erythrocytes. *Blood*, **21**, 51.

Rywlin, A. M. & Benson, J. (1961) Massive necrosis of the spleen with the formation of a pseudocyst: Report of a case in a white man with sickle-cell trait. *Amer. J. Clin. Path.*, **36**, 142.

Salvaggio, J. E., Arnold, C. A. & Banov, C. H. (1963) Long-term anticoagulation in sickle-cell disease. A clinical study. *New Eng. J. Med.*, **269**, 182.

Schroeder, W. A., Cua, J. T., Matsuda, G. & Fenninger, W. D. (1962) Hemoglobin F₁, an acetyl-containing hemoglobin. *Biochim. Biophys. Acta*, **63**, 532.

Schroeder, W. A., Huisman, T. H. J., Shelton, J. R., Shelton, J. B., Keihauer, E. F., Dozy, A. M. & Robberson, B. (1968) Evidence for multiple structural genes for the α chain of human fetal hemoglobin. *Proc. Natl. Acad. Sci.*, **60**, 537.

Schwartz, E. & McElfresh, A. E. (1964) Treatment of painful crises in sickle cell disease. A double blind study. *J. Pediat.*, **64**, 132.

Scott, E. M. (1960) The relation of diaphorase of human erythrocytes to inheritance of methaemoglobinaemia. *J. Clin. Invest.*, **39**, 1176.

Serjeant, J. R., Serjeant, B. E. & Milner, P. F. (1969) The irreversibly sickled cell: a determinant of haemolysis in sickle cell anaemia. *Brit. J. Haemat.*, **17**, 527.

Seshadri, R., Colebatch, J. H. & Fisher, R. (1974) Urinary iron excretion in thalassaemia after desferrioxamine administration. *Arch. Dis. Childh.*, **49**, 195.

Shahid, M. J. & Sahli, I. T. (1971) Erythrokinetic studies in thalassaemia. *Brit. J. Haemat.*, **20**, 75.

Shahidi, N. T., Gerald, P. S. & Diamond, L. K. (1962) Alkali-resistant hemoglobin in aplastic anemia of both acquired and congenital types. *New Eng. J. Med.*, **266**, 117.

Shepherd, M. K., Weatherall, D. J. & Conley, C. L. (1962) Semi-quantitative estimation of distribution of fetal hemoglobin in red cell populations. *Bull. John Hopkins Hosp.*, **110**, 293.

Singer, K., Chernoff, A. I. & Singer, L. (1951) Studies on abnormal hemoglobins. I. Their demonstration in sickle cell anemia and other hematological disorders by means of alkali denaturation. *Blood*, **6**, 413.

Smith, C. H., Erlandson, M. E., Stern, G. & Schulman, I. (1960) The role of splenectomy in the management of thalassaemia. *Blood*, **15**, 197.

Smith, C. H., Earlandson, M. E., Stern, G. & Hilgartner, M. W. (1964) Post-splenectomy infection in Cooley's anemia. *Ann. N.Y. Acad. Sci.*, **119**, 748.

Smith, E. W. & Krevans, J. R. (1959) Clinical manifestations of hemoglobin C disorders. *Bull. Hopkins Hosp.*, **104**, 17.

Smits, H. L., Oski, F. A. & Brody, J. I. (1969) The hemolytic crisis of sickle cell disease: The role of glucose–6–phosphate dehydrogenase deficiency. *J. Pediat.*, **74**, 544.

Spaet, T. H., Alway, R. H. & Ward, G. (1953) Homozygous type C hemoglobin. *Pediatrics*, **12**, 483.

Stamatoyannopoulos, G. (1971) Gamma-thalassaemia. *Lancet, ii*, 192.

Stamatoyannopoulos, G., Woodson, R., Papayannopoulou, Th., Heywood, D. & Kurachi, S. (1974) Inclusion-body β-thalassaemia trait. *New Eng. J. Med.*, **290**, 939.

Steadman, J. H., Yates, A. & Huehns, E. R. (1970) Idiopathic heinz body anaemia: Hb-Bristol (β 67 (Ell) Val — Ash). *Brit. J. Haemat.*, **18**, 435.

Stuart, M. J., Stockman, J. A. & Oski, F. A. (1974) Abnormalities of platelet aggregation in the vaso-occlusive crisis of sickle-cell anemia. *J. Pediat.*, **85**, 629.

Sturgeon, P. & Finch, C. A. (1957) Erythrokinetics in Cooley's anemia. *Blood*, **12**, 64.

Tanaka, K. R. & Clifford, G. O. (1958) Homozygous hemoglobin C disease: Report of three cases. *Ann. Intern. Med.*, **49**, 30.

Terry, D. W., Motulsky, A. G. & Rath, C. E. (1954) Homozygous hemoglobin C. A new hereditary hemolytic disease. *New. Eng. J. Med.*, **251**, 365.

Thomas, E. D., Lochte, H. L., Greenough, W. B. & Wales, M. (1960) *In vivo* synthesis of foetal and adult haemoglobin by foetal haematopoietic tissues. *Nature*, **185**, 396.

Thompson, R. B., Rau, P. J., Odom, J. & Bell, W. N. (1965) The sickling phenomenon in a white male without Hb S. *Acta Haematol.*, **34**, 347.

Tullis, J. L., Hinman, J., Sproul, M. T. & Nickerson, R. J. (1970) Incidence of post transfusion hepatitis in previously frozen blood. *J.A.M.A.*, **214**, 719.

Vaughan-Jones, R., Grimes, A. J., Carrell, R. W., & Lehmann, H. (1967) Köln haemoglobinopathy. Further data and a comparison with other hereditary Heinz-body anaemias. *Brit. J. Haemat.*, **13**, 394.

Vigi, V., Volpato, S., Gaburro, D., Conconi, F., Bargellesi, A. & Pontremoli, S. (1969) The correlation between red-cell survival and excess of α-globin synthesis in β-thalassaemia. *Brit. J. Haemat.*, **16**, 25.

Walzer, S., Gerald, P. S., Breau, G., O'Neill, D. & Diamond, L. K. (1966) Hematologic changes in the D_2 trisomy syndrome. *Pediatrics*, **38**, 419.

Wasi, P., Na-Nakorn, S. & Suingdumrong, A. (1964) Haemoglobin H disease in Thailand: a genetical study. *Nature*, **204**, 907.

Wasi, P., Sookanek, M., Pootrakus, S., Na-Nakorn, S. & Suingdumrong, A. (1967) Haemoglobin E and alpha-thalassaemia. *Brit. med. J.*, **4**, 29.

Watson, R. J., Lichtman, H. C. & Shapiro, H. D. (1956) Splenomegaly in sickle cell anaemia. *Am. J. Med.*, **20**, 196.

Watson, R. J., Burko, Megas, H. & Robinson, M. (1963) The hand-foot syndrome in sickle cell disease in young children. *Pediatrics*, **31**, 975.

Weatherall, D. J. (1963) Abnormal haemoglobins in the neonatal period and their relationship to thalassaemia. *Brit. J. Haemat.*, **9**, 265.

Weatherall, D. J. (1965) *The Thalassaemia Syndromes*. Oxford: Blackwell Scientific Publications.

Weatherall, D. J. (1968) Annotation: The biochemical lesion in thalassaemia. *Brit. J. Haemat.*, **15**, 1.

Weatherall, D. J. (1969) The genetics of the thalassaemias. *Brit. Med. Bull.*, **25**, 24.

Weatherall, D. J., Clegg, J. B. & Naughton, M. A. (1965) Globin synthesis in thalassaemia: an *in vitro* study. *Nature*, **208**, 1061.

Weatherall, D. J., Clegg, J. B. & Wong Hock Boon (1970) The haemoglobin constitution of infants with the haemoglobin Bart's hydrops foetalis syndrome. *Brit. J. Haemat.*, **18**, 357.

Wilson, M. G., Schroeder, W. A. & Graves, D. A. (1968) Postnatal change of hemoglobins F and A_2 in infants with Down's syndrome (G trisomy). *Pediatrics*, **42**, 349.

Wolman, I. J. (1964) Transfusion therapy in Cooley's anemia: growth and health as related to long-range hemoglobin levels. A progress report. *Ann. N.Y. Acad. Sci.*, **119**, 736.

W.H.O. (1972) Treatment of haemoglobinopathies and allied disorders. Technical Report No. 509, Geneva: W.H.O.

Wright, C–S. & Gardner, E. (1959) Observations on the genesis of crises in sickle cell anaemia. *Ann. Intern. Med.*, **50**, 1502.

Zilliacus, H. & Ottelin, A–M. (1967) Haemoglobins in the blood of human embryos. *Biol. Neonat.*, **11**, 389.

9. Acquired Haemolytic Anaemias

Microangiopathic haemolytic anaemia (MAHA), *Mechanism of burr cell formation. Pathogenesis of MAHA, Haematological diagnosis* / Red-cell membrane disorders, *Lipid accumulation and stagnation, Lipid peroxidation and haemolysis, Changes in membrane plasticity, Structural defects of red-cell membrane, including dyserythropoietic anaemias* / Autoimmune haemolytic anaemias, *Pathogenesis of the anaemia, Relationship of autoantibodies to underlying disease, Clinical manifestations, Haematological features, Treatment* / Drug-induced and toxic haemolysis, *Immune drug-induced haemolytic anaemia, Haemolytic anaemias due to infection* / Hypersplenism / Haemolytic anaemia secondary to systemic disease

Whereas hereditary haemolytic anaemias are likely to manifest themselves first during childhood the same does not necessarily hold for acquired haemolytic anaemias. Some selectivity has been exercised, therefore, with more emphasis being placed on those forms of acquired haemolytic anaemia that are characteristically seen in children. Those that are confined to the neonatal period are described in the following chapters.

MICROANGIOPATHIC HAEMOLYTIC ANAEMIA (MAHA)

This term was first coined by Symmers (1952) but its true pathogenic significance was first appreciated by Brain, Dacie and Hourihane (1962). It is characterized by the presence 'burr' erythrocytes in the blood film usually, but not invariably,

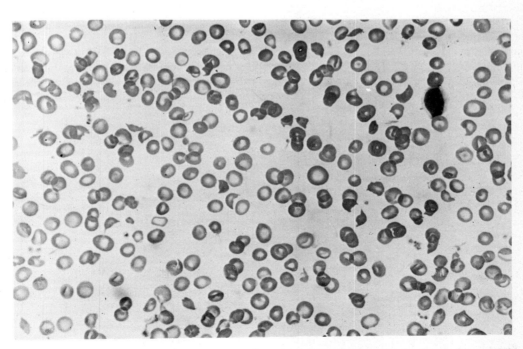

Fig. 9.1 Photomicrograph of burr cells, triangular cells and other small, fragmented red cells from a child with microangiopathic haemolytic anaemia (MAHA) due to the haemolytic uraemic syndrome (× 540).

in association with thrombocytopenia. Burr cells are a type of fragmented or distorted red cell originally described by Schwartz and Motto (1949) and later by Aherne (1957), Allison (1957) and Lock and Dormandy (1961), usually in association with renal disease. Fig. 9.1 shows the appearance of these cells with one or more 'bites' out of the circumference resulting in thorn-like spiny projections. Burr cells have also been called 'helmet cells'. They may be accompanied by small, darkly staining triangular cells and a variable proportion of microspherocytes. Good pictures of all these variations are given by Brain *et al.* (1962) They are not an artefact due to the making of the film (as is crenation) since burr cells can be recognized when the erythrocytes are suspended in their plasma or other fluid medium.

Mechanism of burr cell formation; pathogenesis of MAHA

Not only do burr cells and MAHA occur in association with diseases where there is demonstrable vasculitis with deposition of fibrin within arterioles and capillaries (Brain *et al.*, 1962) but there is also good *in vivo* and *in vitro* evidence that the red cell fragmentation and the resulting haemolysis are due to the mechanical trauma of rapidly moving red cells impinging upon intravascular fibrin strands. Experimental infusion of thrombin or *E. coli* endotoxin in rabbits produced acute intravascular haemolysis and burr cell formation proportionate to the extent of fibrin thrombi formed in renal glomeruli and other microvasculature (Brain *et al.*, 1967). Defibrination produced by coagulant Malayan pit-viper venom

in rabbits caused similar haemolysis and red cell changes associated with the formation of loose, porous fibrin thrombi and microclots with which red cells interacted (Rubenberg *et al.*, 1968). Anticoagulation prevented the fibrin deposition and the haemolysis. Finally the *in vitro* perfusion of red cells through artificial 'clots' of glass fibre and nylon, mimicking the *in vivo* situation, also caused the formation of typical burr cells (Bull *et al.*, 1968). It is easy to extend this concept of mechanical haemolysis to the other clinical disorders listed in Table 9.1 which are associated with either vascular abnormality, intravascular fibrin deposition or the presence of a foreign surface (e.g. Teflon graft) in a part of the circulation where it is exposed to a high pressure stream of blood (Sayed *et al.*, 1961; Eyster *et al.*, 1968).

Haematological diagnosis

This depends solely upon the morphological recognition of significant numbers of burr cells (Fig. 9.1) on a well-made blood film in association with evidence of haemolysis and usually with thrombocytopenia. The severity of both the anaemia and thrombocytopenia as well as the degree of compensatory erythroid response varies greatly. This is because MAHA can be secondary to so many different diseases and the rate of haemolysis ranges from hyperacute (e.g. in septicaemia) to chronic (e.g. in cardiac prostheses). In common with other forms of intravascular haemolysis plasma haemoglobin levels may be elevated, haptoglobins absent, haemosiderinuria present and urinary iron excretion increased in the more chronic forms (Sears *et al.*, 1966).

Table 9.1   Causes of MAHA in childhood

Haemolytic uraemic syndrome	Gasser *et al.*, 1955
Thrombotic thrombocytopenic purpura	McWhinney *et al.*, 1962
Renal vein thrombosis	Murphy and Willoughby, 1976
Renal transplant rejection	Hutton *et al.*, 1970
Radiation nephritis	Beck (1958)
Chronic renal failure	Aherne, 1957
Severe hepatocellular disease	Grahn *et al.*, 1968
Malignant hypertension	Capelli *et al.*, 1966
Giant haemangioma	Propp *et al.*, 1966
Coarctation of aorta	Ravenel *et al.*, 1969
Severe valvular heart disease	Dameshek & Roth, 1964
SBE of aortic valve	Starobin & Castleman, 1970
Intracardiac prostheses	Sears & Crosby, 1965
Severe burns	Topley & Jackson, 1957
Disseminated herpes infection	Miller *et al.*, 1970
Meningococcal septicaemia	Dacie, 1967A
Cerebral falciparum malaria	Borochovitz *et al.*, 1970
Disseminated intravascular coagulation of any cause, including septicaemia	Deykin (1970) Hathaway (1960)

An increase in burr cells is also seen after splenectomy (Smith & Khakoo, 1970)

Serum fibrin degradation products (FDPs) are elevated in MAHA due to renal disease or malignant hypertension, when small blood vessels are involved, but not in the haemolysis due to prosthetic heart valves (Slater *et al.*, 1973).

I^{131}-fibrinogen catabolism can be shown to be increased in some patients with MAHA even although their plasma fibrinogen levels are normal (Baker *et al.*, 1968). The thrombocytopenia is due to consumption of platelets in the microthrombi and is an example of excessive platelet destruction rather than a failure of production. The marrow therefore shows normal numbers of megakaryocytes together with erythroid hyperplasia. Acute forms of MAHA are sometimes accompanied by demonstrable consumption of circulating coagulation factors (consumptive coagulopathy) apparently reversible by heparin. This has been shown in the case of acute hepatic necrosis (Rake *et al.*, 1970) and severe examples of the haemolytic uraemic syndrome (Willoughby *et al.*, 1972). In other patients with this syndrome, as well as in renal transplants, MAHA with selective thrombocytopenia without coagulation or FDP changes has been found (Harker and Slichter, 1972; Pillay *et al.*, 1973). The relevance of this to the treatment of these disorders is discussed under the treatment of consumptive coagulopathy (Chap. 19). In many instances the MAHA is of only secondary importance to the underlying disease.

A practical point regarding diagnosis is that the presence of burr cells must be confirmed on further fresh films made from a finger stab. The possibility of artefactual red cell fragmentation or crenation due to such factors as slow drying of the film,

be the key to diagnosis (e.g. haemolytic uraemic syndrome). Sequential haemoglobin measurements and platelet counts during the day will also indicate whether the process is fulminating as in the case of gram-ve septicaemia.

Related forms of mechanical or traumatic haemolysis but not accompanied by burr cells in the blood and usually occurring in young adults include March or exertional haemoglobinuria (Davidson, 1969) and a similar form of haemolysis due to karate exercises (Streeton, 1967) attributed to traumatic intravascular fragmentation of red cells, particularly the older cells, by the unaccustomed exposure of tissues to pounding by hard surfaces.

RED CELL MEMBRANE DISORDERS

A number of membrane changes, either acquired or secondary to hereditary diseases, can result in abnormal red cell morphology, loss of red cell plasticity and in some instances haemolysis. These changes include (a) lipid accumulation and stagnation, (b) lipid peroxidation, (c) impaired ATP function and (d) ultrastructural deformation of the membrane.

Lipid accumulation and stagnation

Renewal systems involving lipid interchange between the plasma lipoproteins and the red cell membrane normally preserve the membrane lipid constitution (Cooper, 1970). The membrane phospholipids, especially phosphatidylethanolamine, are subject to continuous peroxidative

Table 9.2 Variations in red cell lipids in disease

	Normal	Target cells in liver disease	Spur cells in liver disease	Acanthocytosis in abeta-lipoproteinaemia
Cholesterol $\mu g/10^8$ cells	12.24	18.10	20.90	12.68
Phospholipid $\mu g/10^8$ cells	29.58	36.98	32.15	27.10
Cholesterol: lecithin molar ratio	2.59	2.17	3.64	4.46

Data abbreviated from Cooper (1970).

Reproduced, by permission of the author and publishers from Seminars in Hematology **7**, *296–322 (1970).*

detergent or fat on the slide, degeneration changes (or heating) of an anticoagulated blood sample or cell damage due to forceful extrusion of blood through a fine needle must be excluded. This is important since the presence of true burr cells can

destruction particularly in the absence of vitamin E (Cooper and Shattil, 1971). Under certain pathological conditions there is an increase in membrane lipid (especially cholesterol) or alternatively an increase in cholesterol: lecithin ratio (Table 9.2).

This results in actual membrane acquisition with an increase in the amount of membrane per cell. Resulting morphological changes include spur cells and acanthocytes with surface spicules or target cells; in each case there is a relative increase in surface area of the cell in question or 'wrinkling' of the membrane.

ACANTHOCYTOSIS

This disorder is mentioned again (cf. Chapter 6) since acanthocytes are morphologically identical to spur cells of hyperlipaemic liver disease and similar to the red cells in infantile pycnocytosis and vitamin E deficient haemolytic anaemia. Similar factors may also be operative in the formation of these distorted cells (viz. lipid stagnation and peroxidation – *vide infra*). Acanthocytes differ, however, from burr cells found in MAHA. There is potential confusion here since both *burr* cells and *spur* cells (like acanthocytes) can occur in severe liver disease. For instance Grahn *et al.* (1968) made the distinction that the 'acanthoid' cells reverted to normal if suspended in normal serum but that the burr cells did not. Both types of cell were present in a patient with hepatic cirrhosis.

McBride and Jacob (1970) suggested a common pathogenesis for the formation of acanthocytes whether due to hereditary abetalipoproteinaemia, acquired hypobetalipoproteinaemia or severe hepatic failure. They found a 15–20 per cent increase in membrane cholesterol in all these conditions and pointed out that the normal bidirectional flow of cholesterol between red cell and plasma is blocked in the patients with abetalipoproteinaemia. They concluded that lipid stagnation and less importantly accumulation, caused the membrane changes responsible for acanthocyte or spur cell formation and increased cell rigidity which in turn shortened the life span of the cells in the circulation. The case of acquired hypobetalipoproteinaemia was an infant who suffered severe brain damage at birth, could not suck and as a result had severe deprivation of dietary lipids until the age of 10 weeks. It was postulated that this had removed the normal stimulus for lipoprotein synthesis. This was accompanied by the progressive appearance of acanthocytes and haemolysis.

SPUR CELL HAEMOLYTIC ANAEMIA

This has been well documented in severe hepatocellular disease in adults (Smith *et al.*, 1964; Silber *et al.*, 1966). Membrane cholesterol and cholesterol: phospholipid ratio have been grossly increased in these patients (Cooper, 1970) and it seems likely that this accounts for the more marked haemolysis compared to that seen in hereditary acanthocytosis, although the pathogenesis may be similar as suggested by McBride and Jacob (1970). Other endogenous or exogenous hyperlipaemias do not appear to cause haemolysis (Bagdade and Ways, 1970).

Recently Cooper *et al.* (1974) have produced evidence that the spur cell phenomenon is a 2-stage process: First the RBC acquires extra cholesterol from serum lipoproteins; secondly the cell surface is conditioned by the spleen. Splenectomy decreased haemolysis in one patient.

TARGET CELLS IN LIVER DISEASE

The occurrence of target cells is particularly associated with jaundice, especially of the obstructive type (Cooper and Jandl, 1966). Accumulation of both cholesterol and lecithin increases their surface area with an accompanying increased resistance to lysis in hypotonic saline. Bile salts are present in the plasma in obstructive jaundice and alter the partition of free cholesterol between plasma lipoproteins and red cell membranes (Cooper and Jandl, 1968). They also inhibit a serum enzyme lecithin: cholesterol acyltransferase (LCAT) which normally contributes to loss of cholesterol from the red cell by converting free cholesterol to a fatty acid ester of cholesterol which is then lost to the plasma (Turner *et al.*, 1953). It is of some interest therefore that the rare hereditary deficiency of LCAT activity in plasma is associated with target cells with an increased cholesterol content and moderate anaemia with a haemolytic component (Gjone *et al.*, 1968).

Target cells in liver disease are not usually associated with a haemolytic anaemia. An exception is in Zieve's syndrome when there is additional gross elevation of the serum triglycerides, a large, tender fatty liver and splenomegaly. The association of haemolytic anaemia with the above features has been described in young adult alcoholics (Zieve, 1958).

Recent reviews of haemolysis and changes in red cell membrane lipids are those by Shohet (1972) and (1974), the latter entitled 'Acanthocytogenesis – or how the red cell won its spurs'!

Lipid peroxidation and haemolysis

It is probable that peroxidation by free radicals, a process similar to spontaneous rancidification of fat, plays a major role in the normal ageing process of red cells or even the ageing process in general (Dormandy, 1971). If a free radical, which may itself be generated by H_2O_2, reaches a lipid double bond in the presence of O_2 unstable lipoperoxides are formed. The process then becomes autocatalytic being accelerated by ferrous or cuprous ions or ascorbic acid but inhibited by vitamin E (alpha-tocopherol) which is a free radical scavenger (Shohet, 1972). There is some evidence that red cell membrane lipid peroxidation plays a part in many types of haemolytic anaemia (Stocks *et al.*, 1971; Melhorn *et al.*, 1971) including paroxysmal nocturnal haemoglobinuria (PNH), in which haemolysis is aggravated by parenteral iron therapy (Mengel *et al.*, 1967), and acanthocytosis, in which there may be a secondary deficiency of vitamin E because of the accompanying malabsorption (Dodge *et al.*, 1967). Of greatest paediatric interest, however, is its probable relation to vitamin E deficiency and haemolysis in premature infants.

It has been known for some time that there was a relationship between low serum tocopherol levels and increased red cell sensitivity to haemolysis by H_2O_2 in premature infants (Mackenzie, 1954). This was confirmed by Nitowsky *et al.* (1956). The first observation of a spontaneous clinical haemolytic anaemia that could be attributed to vitamin E deficiency was made by Oski and Barness (1967). They found evidence of haemolysis between the age of 6 to 10 weeks in premature babies associated with low serum tocopherol levels and increased *in vitro* haemolysis with H_2O_2. The anaemia in these infants was characterized morphologically by the presence of a small number of spherocytes, variable numbers of irregularly contracted, spiculated red cells, red cell fragments, anisocytosis and polychromasia. The abnormal forms appeared at approximately one month of age and were generally maximal at 6 to 10 weeks. A shortened ^{51}Cr survival of the infants' red cells was confirmed. A rapid rise in haemoglobin occurred following treatment with 200–800 mg (270 to 1,090 i.u.) of d-alpha tocopherol orally over 1 to 4 days. Prophylaxis with 9 mg per day in similar infants largely prevented the anaemia. Additional features of oedema and thrombocytosis in some cases were described by Ritchie *et al.* (1968).

The cause of vitamin E deficiency in these infants can be related to an impaired intestinal absorption of the vitamin which is directly related to the degree of prematurity. Progressive improvement in absorption occurs in severely premature babies mature to a chronological age equivalent to full term (Melhorn and Gross, 1971A). Since vitamin E deficiency alone in later childhood, due to cytic fibrosis or malabsorption disorders, does not cause anaemia (Binder *et al.*, 1965) a second factor must be necessary to account for the haemolysis occurring between 6 and 10 weeks in these infants. One such additional factor has been

shown to be oral iron therapy (10–20 mg/day) (Melhorn and Gross 1971B) which is indeed almost invariably given to such babies to prevent the 'late' anaemia of prematurity. A combination of oral iron plus parenteral vitamin E may eventually prove to be the optimum therapy for severely premature babies. Gross and Melhorn (1974) have recently shown that water-soluble alpha tocopherol, polyethylene glycol-1,000-succinate (TPGS), 25 i.u./day, is much better absorbed by these infants than the normal fat-soluble vitamin E in the same dosage.

RELATIONSHIP TO INFANTILE PYCNOCYTOSIS

It was pointed out by Oski and Barness (1967) and more recently by Oski and Naiman (1972) that the red cells in vitamin E deficiency are morphologically indistinguishable from those in infantile pycnocytosis. Infantile pycnocytosis appears to be an exaggeration of the normal occurrence of pycnocytes in newborn babies, more particularly in premature babies (Tuffy *et al.*, 1959). It is accompanied by haemolysis which has been shown to affect transfused cells to the same extent as the patients cells (Keimowitz and Desforges, 1965). It is possible that vitamin E deficiency may also contribute to the haemolysis in this disorder since serum vitamin E levels are particularly low in premature infants (Wright *et al.*, 1951) as well as the morphological similarities mentioned above. Infantile pycnocytosis can mimic rhesus disease in its clinical presentation. It is further discussed in chapter 12, as is vitamin E deficiency.

Changes in membrane plasticity

It has recently been stressed that diminished red cell plasticity may account for the shortening of cell survival in many types of haemolytic anaemia including hereditary spherocytosis and elliptocytosis, glycolytic enzyme defects such as PK deficiency as well as that associated with spur cells in liver disease and acanthocytosis discussed above (La Celle, 1970; Cooper and Shattil, 1971).

Hypophosphataemia, due to a transientary metabolic imbalance, has been reported as causing an acute haemolytic anaemia due to demonstrable red cell rigidity. Numerous microspherocytes were present and diminished red cell survival, both returning to normal after parenteral phosphate supplementation (Jacob and Amsden, 1971). The phosphate deficiency resulted in low ATP levels in the red cell (below 15 per cent). There is evidence that an actomyosin-like microfilamentous protein is present in the red cell membrane and may be responsible for maintenance of its normal shape

150 PAEDIATRIC HAEMATOLOGY

and plasticity (Ohnishi, 1962; Weed et al., 1969). Impaired ATP production could result in loss of this plasticity. This could be a final common factor in defects of the glycolytic enzyme system, as well as hypophosphataemia and possibly magnesium depletion, which can cause red cell rigidity and haemolysis in rats (Oken et al., 1971). A genetic mutation in the actomyosin-like protein is the probable cause of hereditary spherocytosis in man (Jacob et al., 1971).

Structural defects of red cell membrane including dyserythropoietic anaemias

Paroxysmal nocturnal haemoglobinuria (PNH) is a rare haemolytic anaemia probably related to an acquired red cell membrane defect (Weinstein and McNutt, 1970). There is electron microscopic evidence of pitting and irregularity of the membrane and the suggestion has been made that this is the result of a defect of protein synthesis (Lewis et al., 1965). Other workers have failed to confirm this abnormality of the membrane (Weinstein and Williams, 1967). However it is indisputable that the membrane in PNH is functionally altered (Ham and Dingle, 1939), susceptibility to lysis by complement being increased about 30-fold (Rosse and Dacie, 1966). There has been the suggestion, mentioned above, that these cells are unduly sensitive to peroxidation. Dacie (1967B) has suggested that the disease arises as a result of a somatic mutation giving rise to a defective clone of erythroblasts.

Accompanying these changes there is intermittent or chronic intravascular haemolysis with haemoglobinuria. Typically this is noted in the morning perhaps due to an exaggeration of haemolysis due to a tendency to acidosis or other metabolic changes during sleep. Intermittent haemoglobinuria gives rise to haemosiderin deposits in the urine and on occasions to a hypochromic anaemia due to iron loss. The possibility of more widespread membrane or metabolic abnormality in haemic cells is suggested by the inconstant associated features of neutropenia and thrombocytopenia. There is also an unexplained relation with aplastic anaemia whereby pancytopenia can precede or coexist with PNH as has been discussed in Chap. 4. PNH presenting initially as aplastic anaemia has been reported in a girl of $7\frac{1}{2}$ years (Ross and Rosenbaum, 1964).

The disease may present not only as haemolytic anaemia or intermittent haemoglobinuria, but also with episodes of thrombosis, with hemiplegia (Pierce and Aldrich, 1943) or slurred speech and facial weakness (McDougal et al., 1959). In addition it may present either as thrombocytopenic purpura or as iron deficiency anaemia (Dacie, 1967C). Clinically the spleen may be slightly enlarged and mild jaundice may be present. Haemolysis is accentuated by infections and blood transfusions unless the cells are washed free of plasma, since this contains complement.

PNH is predominantly a disease of adults in their 3rd to 5th decade and the disease has been reported in children on only a small number of occasions (Pierce and Aldrich, 1943; Marks, 1949; Hinz et al., 1956; McDougal et al., 1959; Resegotti and Givone, 1962; Ross and Rosenbaum, 1964; Miller et al., 1967).

Laboratory diagnosis depends upon the abnormal susceptibility of PNH red cells to lysis by dilute acid (Ham, 1937) or by thrombin (Crosby, 1950). A recent test, the sugar water test (Hartman and Jenkins, 1966), depends upon the aggregation of IgG molecules that occurs at low ionic concentrations. In their aggregated state the IgG activates complement to which PNH cells are extremely sensitive (Mollison, 1970).

A family has been described by Danon et al. (1962), in which electron microscopy disclosed a similar type of structural abnormality to that in PNH. It appeared that this rendered the cells susceptible to haemolysis by drugs and possibly virus infections, but there was normal red cell survival at other times. A non-familial haemolytic anaemia with decreased lecithin content of the red cell membrane associated with dwarfism and mental retardation has been reported from Japan (Arakawa et al., 1966).

Abnormality of the red cell membrane is also probably present in the group of disorders termed congenital dyserythropoietic anaemias since increased sensitivity to lysis by complement-binding abtibodies has been demonstrated (Lewis et al., 1970).

AUTOIMMUNE HAEMOLYTIC ANAEMIAS

In this group of haemolytic anaemias shortened red cell survival is caused by the action of immunoglobulins (Ig) with or without the participation of complement (C), upon the red cell membrane. The red cell autoantibodies may be of the 'warm' type (usually IgG), 'cold' type (usually IgM) or the 'cold-warm', Donath-Landsteiner type (Table 9.3). Complement participation is usually confined to the IgM type of antibody, only rarely is it associated with IgG, although this is the case with the

Donath-Landsteiner antibody in paroxysmal cold haemoglobinuria (PCH) (Cooper and Shatill, 1971). This is because a *single* IgM molecule attached to two antigenic sites on the red cell membrane, can activate complement but in the case of IgG *two* molecules on *adjacent* antigen sites are needed (Humphrey and Dourmashkin, 1965; Borsos and Rapp, 1965). It has been calculated that as many as 1,000 IgG molecules would have to react with a single cell for there to be an even chance of two adjacent sites to be involved with resultant complement activation. Furthermore, of the sub-classes of IgG (gamma-G_{1-4}) only gamma G_1 and gamma G_3 readily activate complement (Müller-Eberhard *et al.*, 1967)

Pathogenesis of the anaemia

IgG antibodies, the usual 'warm' incomplete 7S type of autoantibody, cause haemolysis and spherocytosis of red cells *in vivo* but not *in vitro*. This is because interaction of macrophages of the reticuloendothelial system, particularly in the spleen, with the antibody-coated cell is a prerequisite to haemolysis. Monocytes partially ingest IgG-coated red cells and it is only after contact with these phagocytic cells that the remainder of the red cell becomes spherocytic due to loss of membrane (Jandle and Tomlinson, 1958; Archer, 1965; Lo Buglio *et al.*, 1967). Both the phagocytosis and also the sphering of the residual red cell fragment, which will impede its transit through the circulation, contribute to the shortened red cell survival (Cooper and Shatill, 1971). The rate at which the cells are destroyed depends upon the amount of antibody on the cell surface (Mollison *et al.*, 1965).

In the case of complement-activating IgM antibodies, mostly 'cold', complete, 19 S autoantibodies, structural damage to the red cell membrane is produced. This takes the form of 'holes' visible by electron microscopy (Dourmashkin and Rosse, 1966). These lesions first appear as C5 (the fifth component of complement) becomes

fixed to the cell. Details of the 9 different components of complement and their sequential interactions finally leading to lysis of the cell have recently been reviewed by Mollison (1970) and Rosse and Lauf, (1970). Antibodies of the IgM class also agglutinate red cells by overcoming the Zeta potential electrostatic forces that normally cause mutual cell repulsion. This agglutination typically occurs at low temperatures (cold agglutinins) whereas complement fixation is greatest at body temperature and haemolysis may be quite mild (Cooper and Shatill, 1971). It is when the thermal amplitude of the antibody is such that agglutination occurs at 31°C or higher that *clinical haemolysis* occurs, as opposed to haemagglutination. The cold haemagglutinin syndrome typically causes the Raynaud phenomena plus intermittent mild haemolysis and haemoglobinuria related to exposure to the cold.

In the case of Donath-Landsteiner antibodies the antibody reacts with red cells and fixes complement in the cold (below 15°C). It is only after subsequent warming to 37°C that complement-induced lysis occurs (Dacie, 1962A). Clinically this results in intravascular haemolysis and haemoglobinuria after exposure to the cold (paroxysmal cold haemoglobinuria PCH).

Relationship of autoantibodies to underlying disease

The majority of autoimmune haemolytic anaemias are 'idiopathic', especially in childhood, but a minority are associated with and apparently secondary to reticuloses, infections and, in the case of warm autoantibodies, with disseminated lupus erythematosus (DLE). The reticuloses concerned are predominantly lymphoma and reticulosarcoma (Rosenthal *et al.*, 1955; Sacrez *et al.*, 1963) since chronic lymphatic leukaemia hardly ever occurs in children. The incidence of AHA is approximately 5 per cent in the lymphomas (Miller, 1967). AHA in association with ovarian tumours has been

Table 9.3   Numbers of patients with different categories of AHA

Type of antibody	Idiopathic	Reticulosis	Infections	DLE
Warm (20 were under 15 years)	89	16	12	6
Cold (none were under 15 years)	19	6	11	
Donath-Landsteiner (4 were under 15 years)			7	

Data from Dacie (1962B), representing all cases of AHA (children plus adults) seen between 1947 and 1961 at the P.G.M. Hammersmith.

attributed to lymphoid tissue in these mixed tumours (de Bruyere *et al.*, 1971). One case has been reported in a child of 5 years (Allibone and Collins, 1951). Infections that can cause AHA are mycoplasma (primary atypical pneumonia), viral, including measles, glandular fever and infectious hepatitis, and bacterial, including subacute bacterial endocarditis and pneumonia (Dacie, 1962B). Paroxysmal cold haemoglobinuria due to the Donath-Landsteiner antibody has been reported after measles (O'Neill and Marshall, 1967) and after measles immunization (Bunch *et al.*, 1972). The relative proportions of patients with autoimmune haemolytic anaemia falling into these various categories are shown in Table 9.3.

It is apparent that few cases of cold AHA are found in childhood other than paroxysmal cold haemoglobinuria due to the Donath-Landsteiner cold-warm antibody.

Clinical manifestations

Warm antibodies are associated with haemolysis of variable severity but typically resulting in pallor, jaundice, dark stools and urine, and definite splenomegaly (Dameshek and Schwartz, 1950). Gangrene of the skin and fingers has occasionally been reported (Kölbl, 1955).

The cold haemagglutinin syndrome due to cold antibodies is characteristically associated with Raynaud-like phenomena including painful swelling of the ears and digits in cold weather. The anaemia is mild and intermittent, again related to cold exposure. Jaundice and splenomegaly are less frequent but cold-induced haemoglobinuria can occur (Dacie, 1962C).

Haematological features

In warm AHA prominent spherocytosis is present together with the associated features of a haemolytic anaemia, viz. polychromasia and pseudomacrocytosis. In cold AHA all these features are less marked. Both may show autoagglutination in blood samples and on smears. Either type may occasionally have neutropenia or thrombocytopenia. Increased osmotic fragility and autohaemolysis is roughly proportional to the degree of spherocytosis. Red cell survival is reduced with sequestration predominantly in the spleen in most cases, but largely in the liver when the haemolysis is hyperacute.

A key investigation is the direct Coombs test (or antihuman globulin test) on the patient's red cells. Between 300 and 500 molecules of gamma G

per red cell are needed for a positive reaction to be obtained with most anti-gamma G sera. More sensitive methods such as antiglobulin consumption techniques (Gilliland *et al.*, 1970) are capable of detecting down to around 50 gamma G molecules per cell. Gilliland, Baxter and Evans (1971) have reported six patients with acquired AHA in whom the direct Coombs test was persistently negative but whose red cells had between 70 and 434 molecules of gamma G per cell as measured by their antiglobulin consumption technique. In the light of this report a negative direct Coombs test can no longer be taken to exclude warm AHA. Another way in which the test can be made more sensitive is by using the 'build-up' or 'lattice' technique with Coombs reagents from a series of animal species (Coombs *et al.*, 1951). A patient has been described whose cells were positive by this test but negative by the normal test (Miescher and Holländer, 1956). When the direct Coombs test is positive the cell-bound antibody in warm AHA can be characterized as gamma G by the fact that the reaction of Coombs reagent (anti-human gamma globulin) with the patient's red cells is inhibited by premixing with small amounts of pure gamma G globulin (the gamma globulin inhibition test). In cold types of AHA there is a considerable non-gamma component to the globulin coating of the red cells (e.g. the beta globulins of complement) and their reaction with Coombs reagent is less completely blocked by pure gamma G (Dacie, 1951). A similar distinction can be made by using Coombs reagents that have been prepared against different globulin fractions (e.g. anti-gamma G or anti-beta IgG) (Dacie, 1960).

7S IgG autoantibody is present in serum as well as on the red cells in many patients with warm AHA and in all with cold AHA. Trypsinized normal red cells were agglutinated at $37°C$ in 65 per cent of the series of patients with warm AHA seen by Dacie (1962D), and in 47 per cent autoantibodies could be detected in the serum by the indirect Coombs reaction at $37°C$. The autoantibodies both in the serum or recovered in an eluate from the circulating red cells often show specificity within the rhesus system, reacting with an antigen such as ē present on the patient's cells. There may be a non-specific component in addition. These points are relevant to the selection of blood for transfusion in such patients. By cross-matching against an eluate from the patient's cells it may be possible to select blood which, although not wholly compatible, lacks the antigen to which the patient has a specific autoantibody (e.g. R_2R_2 cells for a patient with anti-ē). Such blood may survive in the circulation better than the patient's own cells.

In the cold type of AHA (cold haemagglutinin syndrome) the serum characteristically contains 19S IgM complete antibodies capable of agglutinating normal red cells in saline at $4°C$ to a titre of 1 in 1,000 or much more. For this test to be valid it is essential that the blood should be collected into a warm container and kept at $37°C$ until the serum is separated from the red cells, to prevent auto-absorption. Cold reacting non-specific antibody is commonly present in normal individuals (up to a titre of $1/64$). It is the high titre, or concentration, and also the broader range of 'thermal amplitude' that renders cold agglutinins pathological. Those that are active to as high a temperature as $29-31°C$ are capable of causing haemolysis *in vivo* (Ferriman *et al.*, 1951). This is probably because the skin temperature can fall as low as these temperatures. Many high titre cold agglutinins show haemolytic activity at acid pH and in the presence of complement (Dacie, 1950). PNH cells are particularly susceptible to such lysis. Complement appears to be essential for the firm binding of some cold agglutinins and such cells can then give a positive reaction with Coombs serum of the non-gamma type (*vide supra*). In some intances high titre cold agglutinins are identical with cryoglobulins. Blood group specificity of cold agglutinins is related to the I antigen (Weiner *et al.*, 1956), the great majority of adults have I-positive red cells that react strongly with these cold agglutinins, but a minority have I-negative or i cells which react much less strongly (Jenkins *et al.*, 1960). The I antigen only develops during the first year of life, all infants cells behaving as if they were I-negative (Marsh, 1961). In some cases of cold AHA secondary to malignant reticulosis or infectious mononucleosis it has been found that the specificity of the cold agglutinin is anti-i, rather than the anti-I seen in idiopathic cases (Marsh and Jenkins, 1960).

The Donath-Landsteiner cold-warm antibody is unique in that it reacts with red cells and binds complement in the cold but only lyses the red cells upon warming to $37°C$. No lysis, for instance, occurs with the reverse sequence. The antibody sensitizes red cells to non-gamma Coombs reagent mainly by virtue of the attached complement (Dacie *et al.*, 1957). The blood group specificity is anti-P, which is a very high frequency antigen. The direct Coombs test becomes transitorily positive in patients with paroxysmal cold haemoglobinuria who have recently been exposed to cold. It is of the non-gamma pattern, i.e. not inhibited by traces of pure gamma G, and preferentially demonstrated by Coombs reagent prepared against whole serum or complement (Dacie, 1962E).

For a more detailed discussion of the serology of autoimmune haemolytic disorders reference should be made to The Haemolytic Anaemias, Part 2, The Autoimmune Anaemias, by Dacie (1962). Some more recent observations are described by the same author (Dacie, 1969; 1970). Drug-induced autoantibodies or drug-haptene disease are described below under haemolytic anaemias due to toxic agents and drugs.

Treatment

In paediatric practice it is mainly the treatment of idiopathic AHA of the warm type with which we are concerned. Post infective PCH is usually self-limiting as is the rare cold haemagglutinin syndrome after primary atypical pneumonia or infectious mononucleosis. Protection from chilling plus initial transfusion if the anaemia is severe may be all that is needed. If complement-dependent, washed red cells should be used for transfusion. In other secondary forms of AHA therapy must also be directed to the underlying disease.

Steroids are the first line of treatment in idiopathic Coombs positive AHA of the warm type. A suitable initial dose is prednisolone 60 $mg/m^2/day$ in divided doses, with progressive reduction to the smallest dose which will maintain an adequate haemoglobin level and minimal reticulocytosis. When and if the direct Coombs test becomes negative the steroids are stopped. Unfortunately not all patients respond and fewer are cured by steroids (Case 7). Damashek and Komninos (1956) treated 43 patients with idiopathic or secondary warm AHA with high doses of ACTH, cortisone or prednisone. Twenty eight had a full clinical and haematological response, 12 had a partial response and 3 failed to respond. More than half of those who had responded well relapsed when this treatment was stopped.

Splenectomy is reserved for patients showing an inadequate response to steroids. Dausset and Colombani (1959), who obtained a rather low rate of response from steroids alone, found that over half their patients benefited from splenectomy although it did not result in cure. It is also of value in AHA secondary to malignant reticuloses (Rosenthal *et al.*, 1955) and DLE (Sarles and Levin, 1959).

Immunosuppressive drugs, particularly 6-mercaptopurine and azathioprine (Imuran) are also reserved for patients refractory to steroids. Hitzig and Massimo (1966) reported good responses in three young children aged 4 months, 6 months and 2 years in whom large doses of steroids had produced only partial and temporary improvement. Azathioprine, 2 to 5 mg/kg/day, produced a complete cure in one, and allowed a marked decrease in steroid dose in two. The closely related drug 6-mercaptopurine proved curative in Case 7.

Case 7. A little girl aged 2 (*No. 168595*) presented with a 2-month history of pallor and mild jaundice. Her spleen was 3 inches below the costal margin. The haemoglobin was 4 g/100 ml, the blood film showed polychromasia, spherocytes and normoblasts. The direct Coombs test was positive, ESR 77, L. E. cell test negative and reticulocytes ranged between 35 and 52 per cent. Serological investigations at the Regional Blood Transfusion Centre (Dr. John Wallace) showed that the auto-antibody was of the warm type and that the eluate from the RBCs did not show blood group specificity.

Treatment was commenced with oral prednisolone (30 mg/day) which resulted in a rapid rise in Hb. to 12 g /100 ml and a fall in reticulocytes to normal. Over the next $2\frac{1}{2}$ years numerous attempts were made to reduce the steroid dose because of increasingly severe Cushingoid effects, but on each occasion this was followed in about a month's time by a precipitous fall in haemoglobin sometimes to as low as 3–4 g/100 ml, accompanied by jaundice and requiring emergency transfusion. Two brief trials of azothioprine 25 mg/day were without benefit. By this time there were prominent cutaneous striae and X-ray of the bones showed severe generalized osteoporosis.

A trial was therefore given of 6-mercaptopurine initially at a dose of 25 mg/day, later increased to 50 mg/ day. This was followed by maintenance of haemoglobin with a fall in reticulocyte count in spite of gradual reduction and final stopping of prednisolone 2 months after 6–MP had been instituted. A month later the direct Coombs test became negative. The 6-MP was then reduced and finally stopped 3 months after the Coombs test became negative. By this time her Cushingoid features had regressed. She has remained off all drugs for 18 months now without recurrence of anaemia.

One episode of increased haemolysis in the early course of this patient appeared to be precipitated by a pertussis vaccination, and the same has been seen on two occasions in another child with AHA.

I am indebted to Dr. W. R. McAinsh for referral of this interesting patient.

The growth curve, which is retarded during prednisone therapy, may catch up while on azathioprine (Hitzig and Massimo, 1966). Other workers, however, have found a low rate of response with this drug (Corley *et al.*, 1966). The apparent hazard of malignancy in patients on this and other immunosuppressive drugs (*B.M.J.*, 1972) should caution their uncritical use in young children unless steroid therapy fails, as in Case 7.

Thymectomy has been performed in three infants with severe AHA and was shortly followed by remission (Dacie, 1970). In a further infant thymectomy at 14 weeks of age produced no immediate response so splenectomy was performed 2 weeks later, and 10 days later she went into remission (Oski and Abelson, 1965). At present thymectomy or thymic irradiation are experimental.

In urgent situations at diagnosis or during the course of the disease blood that is incompatible by indirect Coombs cross-match against the patient's serum may have to be given since no compatible cells can be found and delay could be fatal. Such blood will not usually be any more incompatible than the patient's own cells. If more time is available cross-matching can also be performed against an eluate from the patient's cells and the least incompatible blood selected, especially if the eluate shows rhesus specificity as described earlier. Packed cells or, better, washed cells should be given if the haemolysis is suspected of being complement-dependent.

DRUG-INDUCED AND TOXIC HAEMOLYSIS

Drug-induced haemolysis in patients with red cell enzyme defects (Chap. 7) and unstable haemoglobinopathies (Chap. 8) have already been described. Even normal red cells are susceptible to the same drugs if present in higher concentrations as well as to other toxic agents, such as lead, listed in Table 9.4. The higher concentrations may follow overdosage or renal failure (Hayes and Felts, 1964).

Of perhaps greatest paediatric importance is chronic lead poisoning which may present in the surgical wards as colicky abdominal pain or, as lead encephalopathy, may mimic acute medical or neurosurgical disorders. The characteristic haematological features are a mild hypochromic anaemia with evidence of slight haemolysis and punctate basophilia (also known as 'basophilic stippling') on a well-stained blood film (Watson *et al.*, 1958; Waldron, 1966). In spite of the hypochromic anaemia the marrow shows stainable iron in sideroblasts (Kaplan *et al.*, 1954) since there is an associated block in porphyrin synthesis.

Diagnosis may be suspected if there is a history of pica, and confirmed by a serum lead level.

Immune drug-induced haemolytic anaemia

This represents a further group of drug-induced haemolytic anaemias not so far considered, yet with many features in common with AHA discussed above.

ACQUIRED HAEMOLYTIC ANAEMIAS 155

Table 9.4 The more important drugs, past and present, which have caused (or have been thought to cause) acute haemolytic anaemia

Inorganic chemicals
Arsine, lead, chlorate, copper sulphate
Organic chemicals
Acetylphenylhydrazine and phenylhydrazine, naphthalene
Aniline, benzene, carbon tetrachloride, dialuric acid, disulphides, hydroxylamine, insecticides, nitrobenzene, para-dichlorbenzene, phenols, trinitrotoluene, zinc ethylene bisthiocarbamate
Compounds of vegetable origins
Male fern and mushrooms, onion juice, penny royal, quinine
Animal venoms
Certain spider bites and bee stings
Drugs
Antimalarials
Plasmochin(e) (plasmoquin(e), pamaquin(e)), primaquine, chloroquine
Sulphonamides
Sulphanilamide, sulphapyridine, sulphadiazine, sulphadimidine, dimethylbenzoylsulphanilamide (Irgafan), sulphamethoxypyridazine, salicylazosulphapyridine (Salazopyrin), etc.
Antibiotics
Penicillin, Amphotericin B, chloramphenicol, Novobiocin, oxytetracycline, streptomycin

Anthelminthics
Phenothiazine, β-napthol, stibophen (Fouadin)
Antileprotics
Glucosulphone sodium (Promin), diaminophenylsulphone Dapsone), sulfoxone
Antipyretics
Penacetin (acetophenetidin)
Acetanilide, Cryogènine (phenylsemicarbazide)
Aspirin
Antituberculosis drugs
Para-aminosalicylic acid, sodium salt (PAS), isonicotinic acid hydrazide (INAH)
Vitamin K and synthetic analogues
Synkavit
Miscellaneous drugs
Antihistamines, barbiturates, benzedrine, BZ 55, chlorpromazine, mesontoin, methylene blue, neoarsphenamine, nalidixic acid, neodymium (Thrombodym), nitrofurantoin (Furadantin), nitrofurazone, para-phenylenediamine quinidine, resorcin, thiazides

Reproduced, by permission of Professor J. V. Dacie (1967) The Haemolytic Anaemias, Part 4, p. 1031.

Table 9.5 Drugs reported as provoking immune haemolysis

Penicillin
Cephalosporins
Tetracycline
Rifampicin

Sulphonamides
Para-Aminosalicylic acid
Isonicotinic acid hydrazide
Stibophen
Quinine

Quinidine
Antistin
Phenacetin
Chlorpromazine
Pyramidone
Dipyrone
Melphalan
Insecticides
Sulphonylurea derivatives
Insulin

Data from Worlledge (1973) Seminars in Hematology, 10, 327–344 by permission of the author and the publishers.

There are two distinct groups of immune drug-induced haemolytic anaemia, referred to by Worlledge (1969) as 'immune' and 'autoimmune' respectively.

IMMUNE OR DRUG-HAPTENE TYPE

Table 9.5 shows the drugs reported as causing this type of haemolysis. The number of cases are very few with the exception of penicillin. The more recent additions are two patients with haemolysis associated with cephalothin (Gralnick *et al.*, 1971) and one with tetracycline (Wenz *et al.*, 1974). It is possible that a similar mechanism was operative in a child with insulin-resistant diabetes and a Coombs positive haemolytic anaemia attributed to immune insulin-anti-insulin complexes in his serum (Tomsovic *et al.*, 1971).

The pattern and mechanism of haemolysis appears to be similar for all the drugs with the possible exceptions of penicillin and cephalosporins. Haemolytic anaemia develops after normal dosage but only after recurrent administration. The clinical picture is usually that of acute intravascular haemolysis with haemoglobinaemia and haemoglobinuria, sometimes with acute renal failure. Spherocytosis and increased osmotic fragility are transitorily present. The direct Coombs test is usually only weakly positive and can be shown to be due to complement components on the red cell surface rather than IgG. Recovery with reticulocytosis typically follows a few days after the haemolytic insult. The antibodies present in these patients react with red cells *only in the presence of the drug in question.*

In the case of penicillin (Petz and Fudenberg, 1966) haemolysis only follows large doses, usually 20 mega units per day. Haemolysis appears to be due to sequestration in the spleen rather than intravascular haemolysis. Spherocytosis has been reported less frequently and the direct Coombs test is strongly positive due to IgG which probably represents antibody specific to penicillin and which has become strongly bound to the red cell membrane (Levine and Redmond, 1967). The possible serological mechanisms are fully discussed by Worlledge (1969, 1973).

AUTOIMMUNE DRUG-INDUCED TYPE

Only a few drugs are known to cause this type of haemolysis: Methyldopa, of which there are very numerous reports (Carstairs *et al.*, 1966; LoBuglio and Jandl, 1967), mefenamic acid (Ponstan), an anti-rheumatic drug of which there is only one report (Scott *et al.*, 1968), hydantoins, methysergide and chlorpromazine (Worlledge, 1973).

A positive direct Coombs test is found in approximately 15 per cent of patients on methyldopa but overt haemolysis has been found in less than 0.8 per cent (Worlledge, 1969). Patients have usually been on the drug for 3 to 6 months before the direct Coombs test has become positive. The haematological and serological findings are the same as those of an idiopathic warm AHA. Spherocytosis is present, the red cells are coated with IgG and free IgG autoantibodies are present in the serum which react with enzyme-treated red cells, often showing specificity within the rhesus system (Bakemeier and Leddy, 1968). The antibody induced by methyldopa treatment therefore reacts with both the patients' and normal red cells *in the absence of the drug*. The same situation applies to mefenamic acid. Various hypotheses concerning the genesis of these autoimmune states are discussed by Worlledge (1969, 1973). They have obvious relevance to the origin of idiopathic AHA.

The clinical picture and the haemolysis usually rapidly improve on stopping the drug (Ewing *et al.*, 1968) but if necessary steroids may be given with a rapid response in 4 to 5 days (Hamilton, 1968). Although the antihypertensive drug methyldopa is seldom used in paediatrics we have encountered one patient with the haemolytic uraemic syndrome who developed a positive Coombs test due to this drug (Willoughby *et al.*, 1972).

Haemolytic anaemias due to infection

During the neonatal period haemolysis can be caused by a variety of infections including toxoplasmosis, cytomegalovirus, congenital syphilis and congenital rubella (Chap. 12). Of these chronic toxoplasmosis can also cause haemolysis in later life (Kalderon *et al.*, 1964). Also the intra-erythrocytic infections, Oroya fever and malaria, can cause haemolysis at any age. In the case of malignant tertian malaria (*Plasmodium Falciparum*) acute intravascular haemolysis may occur leading to massive haemoglobinuria and the clinical picture of Blackwater fever. This has to be distinguished from haemolysis induced by the administration of an 8-aminoquinoline drug such as pamaquine (used for the treatment of benign tertian malaria) in a patient who is fortuitously G-6-PD deficient. It is a good practice to exclude G-6-PD deficiency in Black or Mediterranean patients before starting antimalarial therapy. Reviews of the haematological manifestations of Oroya fever and malaria are those of Reynafarje and Ramos (1961) and Zuckerman (1964) respectively. The latter author emphasized the role of hypersplenism as a cause of anaemia in chronic malaria. This may also be a factor in the anaemia of infections such as tuberculosis, histoplasmosis (Mauer, 1969) and other infections (Jandl *et al.*, 1961).

Of particular relevance to paediatrics are Lederer's anaemia and haemolysis due to septicaemia. Lederer in 1925 and 1930 described the association of an acute, self-limiting haemolytic anaemia associated with infection and constitutional symptoms of lethargy, abdominal pain and vomiting. There is no certainty that this syndrome represented a single entity but the term is useful in practice if other recognizable types of haemolytic anaemia can be excluded. A single transfusion is often all that is required to tide the patient over the initial phase of anaemia, and haemolysis may prove self-limiting. The triggering event often appears to be a gram negative infection of the urinary tract (Horowitz *et al.*, 1960). Splenomegaly and a haemolytic blood picture with spherocytosis may be present.

Predisposing causes of septicaemia in paediatric patients include leukaemia, aplastic anaemia and infected Spitz-Holter valves. A microangiopathic blood picture and rapidly falling haemoglobin level may be found in all these conditions, especially when the organism is a gram negative bacillus. Meningococcal septicaemia (Nussbaum and Dameshek, 1957), subacute bacterial endocarditis (Jandl *et al.*, 1961) and a range of gram positive coccal infections (Gasser, 1951) have been reported as causing haemolysis and this is in accord with my own experience.

HYPERSPLENISM

Whether splenic enlargement is caused by infection or is secondary to such diseases as thalassaemia, portal hypertension, reticulosis or storage disease a shortened red cell survival with excessive sequestration can be demonstrated in many patients with clinical splenomegaly (Crosby, 1962). Typically hypersplenism is accompanied by moderate neutropenia and thrombocytopenia (in the range of 50,000 to 75,000/mm³) with active erythropoiesis, myelopoiesis and thrombopoiesis in the marrow. The final proof of hypersplenism is that splenectomy is followed by a return to normal of the peripheral blood values.

The normal function of the spleen is to remove senescent blood cells and it appears that a greatly increased splenic mass, with enlargement of the pulp spaces and hyperplasia of the phagocytic cells (Dacie, 1967D) quite simply exaggerates this function. This concept is supported by the haemolytic anaemia that follows injection of methyl cellulose, with resultant splenic hyperplasia, in experiment animals (Rowley *et al.*, 1962).

A decision as to whether splenectomy should be performed requires consideration of (a) the degree of clinical handicap imposed by the anaemia, neutropenia and thrombocytopenia, and (b) the nature and prognosis of the underlying disease. In general if the consequences of hypersplenism are dominating the clinical manifestations of an otherwise relatively benign disorder then splenectomy should be considered.

HAEMOLYTIC ANAEMIA SECONDARY TO SYSTEMIC DISEASES

There remain a small number of disorders which cause haemolysis without a demonstrable autoimmune element nor MAHA nor hypersplenism. These include the haemolytic anaemia due to hereditary systemic disorders such as Wilson's disease (McIntyre *et al.*, 1967), erythropoietic porphyria (Schmid, 1966; Kramer *et al.*, 1965), familial haemophagocytic reticulosis (Farquhar *et al.*, 1958) and osteopetrosis (Sjölin, 1959).

Buchanan (1975) has pointed out that any children of over 6 or 7 years of age who develop acute haemolytic anaemia of obscure origin should be investigated for Wilson's disease, including slit-lamp examination of the cornea for Kayser-Fleischer rings. Red cell changes and standard diagnostic tests for haemolytic anaemia are unrewarding. It is thought that episodes of hepatic copper release cause direct toxicity to the red cells, possibly by membrane damage, resulting in periodic haemolysis.

REFERENCES

Aherne, W. A. (1957) The 'burr' red cell and azotaemia. *J. Clin. Path.*, **10**, 252.

Allibone, E. C. & Collins, D. H. (1951) Symptomatic haemolytic anaemia associated with ovarian teratoma in a child. *J. Clin. Path.*, **4**, 412.

Allison, A. C. (1957) Acute haemolytic anaemia with distortion and fragmentation of erythrocytes in children. *Brit. Haemat.*, **3**, 1.

Arakawa, T., Katsushima, N. & Fujiwara, T. (1966) A hemolytic anemia with abnormality of erythrocyte lipids and dwarfism—probably a new syndrome. *Tohoku J. Exptl. Med.*, **88**, 35.

158 PAEDIATRIC HAEMATOLOGY

Archer, G. T. (1965) Phagocytosis by human monocytes of red cells coated with Rh antibodies. *Vox Sang.*, **10**, 590.

Bagdade, J. D. & Ways, P. O. (1970) Erythrocyte membrane lipid composition in exogenous and endogenous hyper-triglyceridemia. *J. Lab. Clin. Med.*, **75**, 53.

Bakemeier, R. F. & Leddy, J. P. (1968) Erthrocyte autoantibody associated with alpha-methyldopa: heterogeneity of structure and specificity. *Blood*, **32**, 1.

Baker, L. R. I., Rubenberg, M. L., Dacie, J. V. & Brain, M. C. (1968) Fibrinogen catabolism in microangiopathic haemolytic anaemia. *Brit. J. Haemat.*, **14**, 617.

Beck, J. S. (1958) Acute radiation nephritis in childhood. *Brit. med. J.*, **ii**, 489.

Binder, H. J., Herting, D. C., Hurst, V., Finch, S. C. & Spiro, H. M. (1965) Tocopherol deficiency in man. *New Eng. J. Med.*, **273**, 1289.

Borochovitz, D., Crosley, A. L. & Metz, J. (1970) Disseminated intravascular coagulation with fatal haemorrhage in cerebral malaria. *Brit. med. J.*, **ii**, 710.

Borsos, T. & Rapp, H. J. (1965) Complement fixation on cell surfaces by 19 S and 7 S antibodies. *Science*, **150**, 505.

Brain, M. C., Dacie, J. V. & Hourihane, D.O'B. (1962) Microangiopathic haemolytic anaemia: the possible role of vascular lesions in pathogenesis. *Brit. J. Haemat.*, **8**, 358.

Brain, M. C., Esterly, J. R. & Beck, E. A. (1967) Intravascular haemolysis with experimentally produced vascular thrombi. *Brit. J. Haemat.*, **13**, 868.

British Medical Journal (1972) Editorial: Immunosuppression and malignancy. *Brit. med. J.*, **3**, 713.

Buchanan, G. R. (1975) Acute hemolytic anemia as a presenting manifestation of Wilson disease. *J. Pediat.*, **86**, 245.

Bull, B. S., Rubenberg, M. L., Dacie, J. V. & Brain, M. C. (1968) Microangiopathic haemolytic anaemia: Mechanisms of red-cell fragmentation: *in vitro* studies. *Brit. J. Haemat.*, **14**, 643.

Bunch, C., Schwartz, F. C. M. & Bird, G. W. G. (1972) Paroxysmal cold haemoglobinuria following measles immunization. *Arch. Dis. Childh.*, **47**, 299.

Capelli, J. P., Wesson, L. G. & Erslev, A. V. (1966) Malignant hypertension and red cell fragmentation syndrome. Report of a case. *Ann. Intern. Med.*, **64**, 128.

Carstairs, K., Worlledge, S., Dollery, C. T. & Breckenridge, A. (1966) Methyldopa and haemolytic anaemia. *Lancet*, **i**, 201.

Coombs, R. R. A., Gleeson-White, M. H. & Hall, J. G. (1951) Factors influencing the agglutinability of red cells. II. The agglutination of bovine red cells previously classified as 'inagglutinable' by the building up of an anti-globulin: globulin lattice' on the sensitized cells. *Brit. J. Exp. Path.*, **32**, 195.

Cooper, R. A. (1970) Lipids of human red cell membrane: Normal composition and variability in disease. *Seminars in Hematology*, **7**, 296.

Cooper, R. A. & Jandl, J. H. (1966) Mechanism of 'target cell' formation in jaundice. *Clin. Res.*, **14**, 314.

Cooper, R. A. & Jandl, J. H. (1968) Bile salts and cholesterol in the pathogenesis of target cells in obstructive jaundice. *J. Clin. Invest.*, **47**, 809.

Cooper, R. A. & Shattil, S. J. (1971) Mechanism of hemolysis—The minimal red-cell defect. *New Eng. J. Med.*, **285**, 1514.

Cooper, R. A., Kimball, D. B. & Durocher, J. R. (1974) Role of the spleen in membrane conditioning and hemolysis of spur cells in liver disease. *New Eng. J. Med.*, **290**, 1279.

Corley, C. C., Lesner, H. E. & Larsen, W. E. (1966) Azathioprine therapy of Autoimmune disease. *Am. J. Med.*, **41**, 404.

Crosby, W. H. (1950) Paroxysmal nocturnal hemoglobinuria. A specific test for the disease based on the ability of thrombin to activate the hemolytic factor. *Blood*, **5**, 843.

Crosby, W. H. (1962) Hypersplenism. *Ann. Rev. Med.*, **13**, 127.

Dacie, J. V. (1950) The presence of cold haemolysins in sera containing cold haemagglutinins. *J. Path. Bact.*, **62**, 241.

Dacie, J. V. (1951) Differences in the behaviour of sensitized red cells to agglutination by antiglobulin sera. *Lancet*, **ii**, 954.

Dacie, J. V. (1960) Acquired haemolytic anaemia. In *Lectures on Haematology*, p. 1. Edited by F. H. J. Hayhoe. Cambridge: University Press.

Dacie, J. V. (1962) *The Haemolytic Anaemias*. London: Churchill.

Dacie, J. V. (1962A) *The Autoimmune Anaemias*. Part 2, p. 568. London: Churchill.

Dacie, J. V. (1962B) *The Autoimmune Anaemias*. Part 2, p. 343. London: Churchill.

Dacie, J. V. (1962C) *The Autoimmune Anaemias*. Part 2, p. 371. London: Churchill.

Dacie, J. V. (1962D) *The Autoimmune Anaemias*. Part 2, p. 434. London: Churchill.

Dacie, J. V. (1962E) *The Autoimmune Anaemias*. Part 2, p. 560. London: Churchill.

Dacie, J. V. (1967A) *The Haemolytic Anaemia*. Part 3, p. 909, London: Churchill.

Dacie, J. V. (1967B) *The haemolytic anaemias. Congenital and Acquired*. Part 4, p. 1220. London: Churchill.

Dacie, J. V. (1967C) *The haemolytic anaemias. Congenital and Acquired*. Part 4, p. 1142. London: Churchill.

Dacie, J. V. (1967D) The haemolytic anaemias. Secondary or symptomatic haemolytic anaemias. Part 3, p. 929. London: Churchill.

Dacie, J. V. (1969) Editorial: The haemolytic anaemias—A brief review of recent advances. *Seminars in Hematology*, **6**, 109.

Dacie, J. V. (1970) Autoimmune haemolytic anaemias. *Brit. med. J.*, **ii**, 381.

Dacie, J. V., Crookston, J. H. & Christenson, W. N. (1957) 'Incomplete' cold antibodies: role of complement in sensitization to antiglobulin serum by potentially haemolytic antibodies. *Brit. J. Haemat.*, **3**, 77.

Dameshek, W. & Schwartz, S. O. (1940) Acute hemolytic anemia (acquired hemolytic icterus, acute type). *Medicine*, **19**, 231.

Dameshek, W. & Komninos, Z. D. (1956) The present status of treatment of autoimmune hemolytic anemia with ACTH and cortisone. *Blood*, **11**, 648.

Dameshek, W. & Roth, S. I. (1964) Hemolytic anemia and valvular heart disease. *New Eng. J. Med.*, **271**, 898.

Danon, D., DeVries, A., Djaldetti, M. & Kirschmann, C. (1962) Episodes of acute haemolytic anaemia in a patient with familial ultrastructural abnormality of the red-cell membrane. *Brit. J. Haemat.*, **8**, 274.

Dausset, J. & Colombani, J. (1959) The serology and prognosis of 128 cases of autoimmune hemolytic anemia. *Blood*, **14**, 1280.

Davidson, R. J. L. (1969) March or exertional haemoglobinuria. *Seminars in Hematology*, **6**, 150.

DeBruyère M., Sokal, G., Devoitille, J. M., Fauchet-Dutrieux, M. Ch. & Spa, V. de (1971) Autoimmune haemolytic anaemia and ovarian tumour. *Brit. J. Haemat.*, **20**, 83.

Deykin, D. (1970) The clinical challenge of disseminated intravascular coagulation. *New Eng. J. Med.*, **283**, 636.

Dodge, J. T., Cohen, G., Kayden, H. J. & Phillips, G. B. (1967) Peroxidative hemolysis of red blood cells from patients with abetalipoproteinemia (acanthocytosis). *J. Clin. Invest.*, **46**, 357.

Dormandy, T. L. (1971) Annotation: The autoxidation of red cells. *Brit. J. Haemat.*, **20**, 457.

Dourmashkin, R. R. & Rosse, W. F. (1966) Morphologic changes in the membrane of red blood cells undergoing hemolysis. *Am. J. Med.*, **41**, 699.

Ewing, D. J., Hughes, C. J. & Wardle, D. F. (1968) Methyldopa induced autoimmune haemolytic anaemia—a report of two further cases. *Guy Hosp. Rep.*, **117**, 111.

Eyster, E., Mayer, K. & McKenzie, S. (1968) Traumatic hemolysis with iron deficiency anemia in patients with aortic valve lesions. *Ann. Intern. Med.*, **68**, 995.

Farquhar, J. W., MacGregor, A. R. & Richmond, J. (1958) Familial haemophagocytic reticulosis. *Brit. med. J.*, ii, 1561.

Ferriman, D. G., Dacie, J. V., Keele, K. D. & Fullerton, J. M. (1951) The association of Raynaud's phenomena, chronic haemolytic anaemia, and the formation of cold antibodies. *Quart. J. Med.*, **20**, 275.

Gasser, C. (1951) *Die hämolytischen Syndrome im Kindersalter*, p. 55. Stuttgart: G. Thieme.

Gasser, C., Gautier, E., Steck, A., Siebenmann, R. E. & Oechslin, R. (1955) Hämolytischururämische Syndrome: bilaterale Nierenrindennekorsen bei akuten erworbenen hämolytischen Anämien. *Schweiz. Med. Wschr.*, **85**, 905.

Gilliland, B. C., Turner, E. R. & Evans, R. S. (1970) Quantitation of red cell antibodies in acquired hemolytic disease by complement fixing antibody consumption test. *Clin. Res.*, **18**, 155.

Gilliland, B. C., Baxter, E. & Evans, R. S. (1971) Red-cell antibodies in Coombs negative hemolytic anemia. *New Eng. J. Med.*, **285**, 252.

Gjone, E., Torsvik, H. & Norum, K. R. (1968) Familial plasma cholesterol ester deficiency: a study of the erythrocytes. *Scand. J. Clin. Lab. Invest.*, **21**, 327.

Grahn, E. P., Dietz, A. A., Stefani, S. S. & Donnelly, W. J. (1968) Burr cells, hemolytic anemia and cirrhosis. *Amer. J. Med.*, **45**, 78.

Gralnick, H. R., McGinniss, M., Elton, W. & McCurdy, P. (1971) Hemolytic anemia associated with cephalothin. *J.A.M.A.*, **217**, 1193.

Gross, S. & Melhorn, D. K. (1974) Vitamin E-dependent anemia in the premature infant. *J. Pediat.*, **85**, 753.

Ham, T. H. (1937) Chronic hemolytic anemia with paroxysmal nocturnal hemoglobinuria. Study of the mechanism of hemolysis in relation to acid-base equilibrium. *New Eng. J. Med.*, **217**, 915.

Ham, T. H. & Dingle, J. H. (1939) Studies on destruction of red cells. II. Chronic hemolytic anemia with paroxysmal nocturnal hemoglobinuria: Certain immunological aspects of the hemolytic mechanism with special reference to serum complement. *J. Clin. Invest.*, **18**, 657.

Hamilton, M. (1968) Some aspects of the long-term treatment of severe hypertension with methyldopa. *Postgrad. Med. J.*, **44**, 66.

Harker, L. A. & Slichter, S. J. (1972) Platelet and fibrinogen consumption in man. *New Eng. J. Med.*, **287**, 999.

Hartmann, R. C. & Jenkins, D. E. (1966) The Sugar-water test for paroxysmal nocturnal hemoglobinuria. *New Eng. J. Med.*, **275**, 155.

Hathaway, W. E. (1970) Care of the critically ill child: The problem of disseminated intravascular coagulation. *Pediatrics*, **46**, 767.

Hayes, D. M. & Felts, J. H. (1964) Sulphonamide methaemoglobinemia and hemolytic anemia during renal failure. *Am. J. Med. Sci.*, **247**, 552.

Hinz, C. F., Weisman, R. & Hurley, T. H. (1956) Paroxysmal nocturnal hemoglobinuria. Relationship of *in vitro* and *in vivo* hemolysis to clinical severity. *J. Lab. Clin. Med.*, **48**, 495.

Hitzig, W. H. & Massimo, L. (1966) Treatment of autoimmune hemolytic anemia in children with azathioprine (Imuran). *Blood*, **28**, 840.

Horowitz, H. I., Javid, J. & Spaet, T. H. (1960) Lederer's anemia accompanying urinary tract infection. Report of a case, with a note on the diagnostic use of haptoglobin determination. *Am. J. Dis. Child.*, **99**, 757.

Humphrey, J. H. & Dourmashkin, R. R. (1965) Electron microscope studies of immune cell lysis. In *Ciba Foundation Symposium on Complement*. London: Churchill.

Hutton, M. M., Prentice, C. R. M., Allison, M. E. M., Duguid, W. P., Kennedy, A. C., Struthers, N. W. & McNicol, G. P. (1970) Renal homotransplant rejection associated with microangiopathic haemolytic anaemia. *Brit. med. J.*, **3**, 87.

Jacob, H. S. & Amsden, T. (1971) Acute hemolytic anemia with rigid red cells in hypophosphatemia. *New Eng. J. Med.*, **285**, 1446.

Jacob, H., Amsden, T. & White, J. (1971) Experimental production of hereditary spherocytosis (HS): role of defective membrane microfilaments in the disorder. *J. Clin. Invest.*, **50**, 48a.

Jandl, J. H., Jacob, H. S. & Daland, G. A. (1961) Hypersplenism due to infection. A study of five cases manifesting haemolytic anaemia. *New Eng. J. Med.*, **264**, 1063.

Jandl, J. H. & Tomlinson, A. S. (1958) The destruction of red cells by antibodies in man. II. Pyrogenic, leukocytic and dermal responses to immune hemolysis. *J. Clin. Invest.*, **37**, 1202.

Jenkins, W. J., Marsh, W. L., Noades, J., Tippett, P., Sanger, R. & Race, R. R. (1960) The I antigen and antibody. *Vox. Sang.*, **5**, 97.

Kalderon, A. E., Kikkawa, Y. & Bernstein, J. (1964) Chronic toxoplasmosis associated with severe hemolytic anemia. Case report with electron microscopic studies. *Arch. Intern. Med.*, **114**, 95.

Kaplan, E., Zuelzer, W. W. & Mouriquand, C. (1954) A study of stainable non-hemoglobin iron in marrow normoblasts. *Blood*, **9**, 203.

Keimowitz, R. & Desforges, J. F. (1965) Infantile pycnocytosis. *New Eng. J. Med.*, **273**, 1152.

Kölbl, H. (1955) Klinik und Therapie der akuten erworbenen hämolytischen Anämien im Kindersalter. *Ost. Z. Kinderheilk*, **11**, 27.

Kramer, S., Viljoen., E., Meyer, A. M. & Metz, J. (1965) The anaemia of erythropoietic porphyria with the first description of the disease in an elderly patient. *Brit. J. Haemat.*, **11**, 666.

LaCelle, P. L. (1970) Alteration of membrane deformability in hemolytic anemias. *Seminars in Hematology*, **7**, 358.

Levine, B. B. & Redmond, A. P. (1967) Immune mechanisms of penicillin-induced Coombs positivity in man. *Clin. Invest.*, **46**, 1085.

Lewis, S. M., Danon, D. & Marikovsky, Y. (1965) Electron-microscope studies of the red cell in paroxysmal nocturnal haemoglobinuria. *Brit. J. Haemat.*, **11**, 689.

Lewis, S. M., Grammaticos, P. & Dacie, J. V. (1970) Lysis by Anti-I in dyserythropoietic anaemias: Role of increased uptake of antibody. *Brit. J. Haemat.*, **18**, 465.

LoBuglio, A. F., Cotran, R. S. & Jandl, J. H. (1967) Red cells coated with immunoglobulin G: binding and sphering by mononuclear cells in man. *Science*, **158**, 1582.

LoBuglio, A. F. & Jandl, J. H. (1967) The nature of the alpha-methyldopa red-cell antibody. *New Eng. J. Med.*, **276**, 658.

Lock, S. P. & Dormandy, K. M. (1961) Red-cell fragmentation syndrome. A condition of multiple aetiology. *Lancet*, **1**, 1020.

McBride, J. A. & Jacob, H. S. (1970) Abnormal kinetics of red cell membrane cholesterol in acanthocytes: Studies in genetic and experimental abetalipoproteinaemia and in spur cell anaemia. *Brit. J. Haemat.*, **18**, 383.

McDougal, R. A., Shively, J. A. & Palmer, C. (1959) Paroxysmal nocturnal hemoglobinuria in a negro child. *J. Dis. Child.*, **97**, 92.

McIntyre, N., Clink, H. M., Levi, A. J., Cummings, J. N. & Sherlock, S. (1967) Hemolytic anemia in Wilson's disease. *New Eng. J. Med.*, **276**, 439.

Mackenzie, J. B. (1954) Relation between serum tocopherol and hemolysis in hydrogen peroxide of erythrocytes in premature infants. *Pediatrics*, **13**, 346.

MacWhinney, J. B., Packer, J. T., Miller, G. & Greendyke, R. M. (1962) Thrombotic thrombocytopenic purpura in childhood. *Blood*, **19**, 181.

Marks, J. (1949) The Marchiafava Micheli syndrome (paroxysmal nocturnal haemoglobinuria). *Quart. J. Med.*, **18**, 105.

Marsh, W. L. & Jenkins, W. J. (1960) Anti-i: a new cold antibody. *Nature*, **188**, 753.

Marsh, W. L. (1961) Anti-i: a cold antibody defining the Ii relationship in human red cells. *Brit. J. Haemat.*, **7**, 200.

Mauer, A. M. (1969) *Pediatric Hematology*, p. 187. New York: McGraw Hill.

Melhorn, D. K. & Gross, S. (1971A) Vitamin E-dependent anemia in the premature infant. II. Relationships between gestational age and absorption of vitamin E. *J. Pediat.*, **79**, 581.

Melhorn, D. K. & Gross, S. (1971B) Vitamin E-dependent anemia in the premature infant. I. Effects of large dose of medicinal iron. *J. Pediat.*, **79**, 569.

Melhorn, D. K., Gross, S., Lake, G. A. & Leu, J. A. (1971) The hydrogen peroxide fragility test and serum tocopherol level in anemias of various etiologies. *Blood*, **37**, 438.

Mengel, C. E., Kann, H. E. & Meriwether, W. D. (1967) Studies of paroxysmal nocturnal hemoglobinuria erythrocytes: increased lysis and lipid peroxide formation by hydrogen peroxide. *J. Clin. Invest.*, **46**, 1715.

Miescher, P. & Höllander, L. (1956) Positiver modifizierter antiglobulintest (Antiglobulin-Globulin-Kette) bei einem Fall von subakuter Splenomegalie. *Vox Sang*, **1**, 265.

Miller, D. G. (1967) The association of immune disease and malignant lymphoma. *Ann. Intern. Med.*, **66**, 507.

Miller, D. R., Baehner, R. L. & Diamond, L. K. (1967) Paroxysmal nocturnal hemoglobinuria in childhood and adolescence. Clinical and erythrocyte metabolic studies in two cases. *Pediatrics*, **39**, 675.

Miller, D. R., Hanshaw, J. B., O'Leary, D. S. & Hnilicka, J. V. (1970) Fatal disseminated *Herpes simplex* virus infection and haemorrhage in the neonate. *J. Pediat.*, **76**, 409.

Mollison, P. L. (1970) Annotation: The role of complement in antibody-mediated red-cell destruction. *Brit. J. Haemat.*, **18**, 249.

Mollison, P. L., Crome, P., Hughes-Jones, N. C. & Rochna, E. (1965) Rate of removal from the circulation of red cells sensitized with different amounts of antibody. *Brit. J. Haemat.*, **11**, 461.

Müller-Eberhard, H. J., Hadding, U. & Calcott, M. A. (1967) Current problems in complement research. In *Immunopathology, Fifth International Symposium*, p. 179. Basel: Schwabe.

Murphy, A. V. & Willoughby, M. L. N. (1976), to be published.

Nitowsky, H. M., Cornblath, M. & Gordon, H. H. (1956) Studies of tocopherol deficiency in infants and children. II. Plasma tocopherol and erythrocyte hemolysis in hydrogen peroxide. *Am. J. Dis. Child.*, **92**, 164.

Nussbaum, M. & Dameshek, W. (1957) Transient hemolytic and thrombocytopenic episode (? acute transient thrombohemolytic thrombocytopenic purpura), with probable meningococcemia. Report of a case. *New Eng. J. Med.*, **256**, 448.

Ohnishi, T. (1962) Extraction of actin- and myosin-like proteins from erythrocyte membranes. *J. Biochem.*, **52**, 307.

Oken, M. M., Lichtman, M. A., Miller, D. R. & Leblond, P. (1971) Spherocytic hemolytic disease during magnesium deprivation in the rat. *Blood*, **38**, 468.

O'Neill, B. J. & Marshall, W. C. (1967) Paroxysmal cold haemoglobinuria and measles. *Arch. Dis. Childh.*, **42**, 183.

Oski, F. A. & Abelson, N. M. (1965) Autoimmune hemolytic anemia in an infant. *J. Pediat.*, **67**, 752.

Oski, F. A. & Barness, L. A. (1967) A previously unrecognized cause of hemolytic anemia in the premature infant. *J. Pediat.*, **70**, 211.

Oski, F. A. & Naiman, J. L. (1973) *Hematologic Problems in the Newborn.* 2nd Edn., Philadelphia: p. 126. Saunders.

Petz, L. D. & Fudenberg, H. H. (1966) Coombs-positive hemolytic anemia caused by penicillin administration. *New Eng. J. Med.*, **274**, 171.

Pierce, P. P. & Aldrich, C. A. (1943) Chronic hemolytic anemia with paroxysmal nocturnal hemoglobinuria (Marchiafava-Micheli syndrome). Report of a case with marked thrombocytopenia in a five-year-old child. *J. Pediat.*, **22**, 30.

Pillay, V. K. G., Kurtzman, N. A., Manaligod, J. R. & Jonasson, O (1973) Selective thrombocytopenia due to localised microangiopathy of renal allografts. *Lancet*, **ii**, 988.

Piomelli, S., Danoff, S. J., Becker, M. H. *et al.* (1969) Prevention of bone malformations and cardiomegaly in Cooley's anemia by early hypertransfusion regimen. *Ann. N.Y. Acad. Sci.*, **165**, 427.

Propp, R. P. & Scharfman, W. B. (1966) Hemangioma-thrombocytopenia syndrome associated with microangiopathic hemolytic anemia. *Blood*, **28**, 623.

Rake, M. O., Flute, P. T., Pannell, G. & Williams, R. (1970) Intravascular coagulation in acute hepatic necrosis. *Lancet*, **1**, 533.

Ravenel, S. D., Johnson, J. D. & Sigler, A. T. (1969) Intravascular hemolysis associated with coarctation of the aorta. *J. Paediatrics*, **75**, 67.

Resegotti, L. & Givone, S. (1962) Paroxysmal nocturnal haemoglobinuria. Report of a case in a two-year-old boy. *Acta Haematol.*, **27**, 120.

Reynafarje, C. & Ramos, J. (1961) The hemolytic anemia of human Bartonellosis. *Blood*, **17**, 562.

Ritchie, J. H., Fish, M. B., McMasters, V. & Grossman, M. (1968) Edema and hemolytic anemia in premature infants. A vitamin E deficiency syndrome. *New Eng. J. Med.*, **279**, 1185.

Rosenthal, M. C., Pisciotta, A. V., Komnios, Z. D., Goldenberg, H. & Dameshek, W. (1955) The autoimmune hemolytic anemia of malignant lymphocytic disease. *Blood*, **10**, 197.

Ross, J. D. & Rosenbaum, E. (1964) Paroxysmal nocturnal hemoglobinuria presenting as aplastic anemia in a child. Case report with evidence of deficient leucocyte acetylcholinesterase activity. *Am. J. Med.*, **37**, 130.

Rosse, W. F. & Dacie, J. V. (1966) Immune lysis of normal human and paroxysmal nocturnal hemoglobinuria (PNH) red cells. I. The sensitivity of PNH red cells to lysis by complement and specific antibody. *J. Clin. Invest.*, **45**, 736.

Rosse, W. F. & Lauf, P. K. (1970) Effects of immune reactions on the red cell membrane. *Seminars in Hematol.*, **7**, 323.

Rowley, D. A., Fitch, F. W. & Bye, I. J. (1962) Anaemia produced in the rat by methylcellulose. I. Repeated intraperitoneal injections of methylcellulose. *Arch. Path.*, **74**, 331.

Rubenberg, M. L., Regoeczi, E., Bull, B. S., Dacie, J. V. & Brain, M. C. (1968) Microangiopathic haemolytic anaemia the experimental production of haemolysis and red-cell fragmentation by defibrination *in vivo*. *Brit. J. Haemat.*, **14**, 627.

Sacrez, R., Fruhling, L., Levy, J–M., Beauvais, P. & Dourovin, N. (1963) Lymphatose à évolution sarcomateuse avec syndrome hémolytique et hypergammaglobulinemie chez un garçon de 14 ans. *Arch. Franc. Pediat.*, **20**, 531.

Sarles, H. E. & Levin, W. C. (1959) The role of splenectomy in the management of acquired autoimmune hemolytic anemia complicating systemic lupus erythematosus. *Am. J. Med.*, **26**, 547.

Sayed, H. M., Dacie, Handley, D. A., Lewis, S. M. & Cleland, W. P. (1961) Haemolytic anaemia of mechanical origin after open heart surgery. *Thorax*, **16**, 356.

Schmid, R. (1966) The porphyrias. In *The Metabolic Basis of Inherited Disease*, 2nd edn, p. 813. Edited by Stanbury, J. B., Wyngaarden, J. B. and Fredrickson, D. S. New York: McGraw-Hill.

Schwartz, S. O. & Motto, S. A. (1949) The diagnostic significance of 'burr' red blood cells. *Amer. J. Med. Sci.*, **218**, 563.

Scott, G. L., Myles, A. B. & Bacon, P. A. (1968) Autoimmune haemolytic anaemia and mefenamic acid therapy. *Brit. med. J.*, **3**, 534.

Sears, D. A. & Crosby, W. H. (1965) Intravascular hemolysis due to intracardiac prosthetic devices: diurnal variations related to activity. *Am. J. Med.*, **39**, 341.

Sears, D. A., Anderson, P. R., Foy, A. L., Williams, H. L. & Crosby, W. H. (1966) Urinary iron excretion and renal metabolism of hemoglobin in hemolytic diseases. *Blood*, **28**, 708.

Shohet, S. B. (1972) Hemolysis and changes in erythrocyte membrane lipids. *New Eng. J. Med.*, **286**, 577 & 638.

Shohet, S. B. (1974) Acanthocytogenesis—or how the red cell won its spurs. *New Eng. J. Med.*, **290**, 1316.

Silber, R., Amorosi, E., Lhowe, J. & Kayden, H. J. (1966) Spur-shaped erythrocytes in Laennec's cirrhosis. *New Eng. J. Med.*, **275**, 639.

Sjölin, S. (1959) Studies on osteopetrosis. II. Investigations concerning the nature of the anaemia. *Acta Paediat.*, **48**, 529.

Slater, S. D., Prentice, C. R. M., Bain, W. H. & Biggs, J. D. (1973) Fibrinogen-fibrin degradation product levels in different types of intravascular haemolysis. *Brit. med. J.*, **iii**, 471.

Smith, C. H. & Khakoo, Y. (1970) Burr cell: Classification and effect of splenectomy. *J. Pediatrics*, **76**, 99.

Smith, J. A., Lonergan, E. T. & Sterling, K. (1964) Spur-cell anemia: hemolytic anemia with red cells resembling acanthocytes in alcoholic cirrhosis. *New Eng. J. Med.*, **271**, 396.

Starobin, O. E. & Castleman, B. (1970) Aortic-valve disease with hemolysis and thrombocytopenia. *New Eng. J. Med.*, **283**, 1042.

Stocks, J., Kemp, M. & Dormandy, T. L. (1971) Increased susceptibility of red-blood-cell lipids to autoxidation in haemolytic states. *Lancet*, **1**, 268.

Streeton, J. A. (1967) Traumatic haemoglobinuria caused by karate exercises. *Lancet*, **2**, 191.

Symmers, W. St. C. (1952) Thrombotic microangiopathic haemolytic anaemia (thrombotic microangiopathy). *Brit. med. J.*, **ii**, 897.

Tomsovic, E. J., Page Faulk, W. & Fudenberg, H. H. (1971) Anaphylaxis and red-cell survival studies in a child with insulin-resistant diabetes mellitus. *Acta Paediat. Scand.*, **60**, 647.

Topley, E. & Jackson, D. MacG. (1957) The clinical control of red cell loss in burns. *J. Clin. Path.*, **10**, 1.

Tuffy, P., Brown, A. K. & Zuelzer, W. W. (1959) Infantile pycnocytosis: common erythrocyte abnormality of the first trimester. *Am. J. Dis. Child.*, **98**, 227.

Turner, K. B., McCormack, G. H. & Richards, A. (1953) The cholesterol- esterifying enzyme of human serum. I. In liver disease. *J. Clin. Invest.*, **32**, 801.

Waldron, H. A. (1966) The anaemia of lead poisoning: a review. *Brit. J. Industr. Med.*, **23**, 83.

Watson, R. J., Decker, E. & Lichtman, H. C. (1958) Hematologic studies of children with lead poisoning. *Pediatrics*, **21**, 40.

Weed, R. I., LaCelle, P. L. & Merrill, E. W. (1969) Metabolic dependence of red cell deformability. *J. Clin. Invest.*, **48**, 795.

Weiner, A. S., Unger, L. J., Cohen, L. & Feldman, J. (1956) Type-specific cold auto-antibodies as a cause of acquired hemolytic anemia and hemolytic transfusion reactions: a biologic test with bovine red cells. *Ann. Intern. Med.*, **44**, 221.

Weinstein, R. S. & Williams, R. A. (1967) Freeze-cleaning of red cell membranes in paroxysmal nocturnal hemoglobinuria. *Blood*, **30**, 785.

Weinstein, R. S. & McNutt, N. S. (1970) Ultrastructure of red cell membranes. *Seminars in Hematol.*, **7**, 259.

Wenz, B., Klein, R. L. & Lalezari, P. (1974) Tetracycline-induced immune hemolytic anemia. *Transfusion*, **14**, 265.

Willoughby, M. L. N., Murphy, A. V., McMorris, S. & Jewell, F. G. (1972) Coagulation studies in haemolytic uraemic syndrome. *Arch. Dis. Childh.*, **47**, 766.

Worlledge, S. M. (1969) Immune drug-induced haemolytic anaemias. *Seminars in Hematol.*, **6**, 181.

Worlledge, S. M. (1973) Immune drug-induced hemolytic anemias. *Seminars in Hematol.*, **10**, 327–344.

Wright, S. W., Filer, L. J. & Mason, K. E. (1951) Vitamin E blood levels in premature and full term infants. *Pediatrics*, **7**, 386.

Zieve, L. (1958) Jaundice, hyperlipemia hemolytic anemia: A heretofore unrecognized syndrome associated with alcoholic fatty liver and cirrhosis. *Ann. Intern. Med.*, **48**, 471.

Zuckerman, A. (1964) Autoimmunization and other types of indirect damage to host cells as factors in certain protozoan diseases. *Exp. Parasit.*, **15**, 138.

10. Anaemias in the Neonatal Period 1. Rhesus Disease (Rhesus Isoimmunization)

Synonyms / Pathogenesis and prevention / Antenatal detection and prediction of severity of Rh disease / Clinical findings / Laboratory findings / Management and treatment, *Intrauterine transfusion.*

Severe anaemia in the neonatal period is usually due to haemolysis, occasionally due to haemorrhage, and only very rarely due to failure of red cell production. Haemolytic anaemia at this age is typified by Rhesus disease in which there is a rapid onset of jaundice within the first 24 hours, with pallor and hepatosplenomegaly. This disorder will be described first, followed by a number of other neonatal causes of haemolysis which can to some extent mimic Rhesus disease and can be included under the general term of 'Haemolytic anaemia of the newborn' (Table 12.1).

Haemorrhage in the perinatal period simulates at least some of the findings of Rhesus disease, including anaemia, erythroblastosis and reticulocytosis, and can even produce jaundice if the haemorrhage is into tissues with resulting bruising or haematoma formation (Davis and Schiff, 1966). The causes and types of blood loss are described in later chapters.

SYNONYMS

Hydrops foetalis (universal oedema of the foetus) hrs been recognized for centuries; *icterus gravis neonatorum* recognized since the late nineteenth century; *erythroblastosis foetalis* was a term introduced around 1910 to describe the excess of erythroblasts seen microscopically in blood and tissues; *congenital anaemia of the newborn* was only recognized in the 1930's as a result of haematological study of newborn infants (Diamond, Blackfan and Baty, 1932). It was these authors who first proposed that there was a common pathological basis for these four entities. Haemolytic disease of the newborn (HDNB) is a term that is often used synonymously with Rhesus disease, but also includes other forms of haemolysis in the newborn (e.g. ABO haemolytic disease). Likewise it should be pointed out that a degree of erythroblastosis is seen both in haemolysis and foetal blood loss such as massive foeto-maternal haemorrhage.

PATHOGENESIS AND PREVENTION

For a full account of this aspect good recent reviews are available (Clarke, 1968; Clarke, 1969; Finn, 1970). It has been realized since 1940, when the Rhesus blood group system was defined, that Rhesus isoimmunization occurs when an Rh —ve mother carries an Rh +ve foetus. Since the Rh antigens are bound to the red cell membrane it was presumed that maternal immunization necessitated the crossing of foetal red cells into the mother's circulation. Precise information regarding the timing and magnitude of such foetomaternal haemorrhage, or transplacental haemorrhage (TPH), was lacking until the development of the Kleihauer staining technique (Kleihauer *et al.,* 1957) whereby small numbers of foetal cells could be detected in the maternal circulation (Chap. 8). It was Zipursky and colleagues (1959) who first used this technique to detect foetal red cells in the maternal circulation after delivery. Woodrow and Donohoe (1968) later showed that the *number* of foetal red cells in the mother's circulation just after delivery correlated well with the incidence of development of anti-D over the subsequent 6 months (Fig. 10.1). The 'foetal cell score' of 5 used by these workers roughly corresponded to a TPH of 0.25 ml. In general it can therefore be said that a TPH of 0.25 ml or more results in immunization in approximately 20 per cent of Rh negative mothers if they have an ABO compatible Rhesus +ve baby. A TPH of this magnitude is found in approximately one fifth of all deliveries (Clarke, 1967), but in a higher proportion after obstetric procedures such as manual removal of the placenta

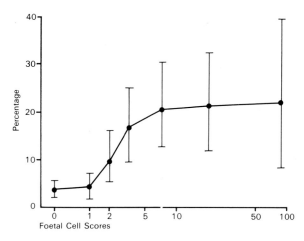

Fig. 10.1 Relationship between Kleihauer film findings and development of Rh antibodies. The incidence of anti-D development during the 6 months following delivery of an ABO-compatible Rh-positive baby. The 90 per cent confidence limits on the percentages are given. (A foetal-cell score of 10 corresponds to approx. 0·4 ml of foetal blood). (Reproduced from *British Medical Journal* (1968), **4**, 139, by permission of Dr Woodrow).

(Queenan and Nakamoto, 1964), external cephalic version (Pollack, 1968) or placental injury during delivery or amniocentesis (Zipursky et al., 1963). Caesarian section, breech delivery, toxaemia of pregnancy and a short interval between immunising and subsequent pregnancy are further determinants of Rh sensitization (Knox, 1968). The pathology of placental lesions related to TPH have been discussed by Wentworth (1964). Foetal red cells spilt into the maternal peritoneal cavity after ruptured ectopic pregnancy or caesarian section are slowly absorbed and constitute a further means of immunization (Lancet, 1972).

The protective effect of maternal ABO incompatibility to the foetal red cells (e.g. mother group O and foetus group A) was suspected by the observation of Levine in 1943 that there was a deficiency of ABO incompatible matings in families where Rhesus disease occurred. More particularly the sensitizing foetus was shown usually to be ABO compatible with the mother (Clarke et al., 1958). The implication that protection was due to destruction of foetal cells by the maternal anti-A or anti-B lead to the concept that a similar type of protection might be achieved by the administration of concentrated anti-D at the time of greatest hazard of TPH, viz. at delivery. Protection has been extended to second and subsequent pregnancies as well as to abortions (when the Rh group of the foetus is indeterminable). A gamma globulin fraction containing IgG anti-D (anti-D immunoglobulin) is given IM within 60 hr of delivery. Unlike whole plasma this is free from the risk of serum hepatitis transmission.

Recent research has been directed to determining the minimum effective dose for the average sized TPH (MRC, 1974) and the additional dose that is needed in mothers with an unusually large TPH. It is to detect this group of patients that the Kleihauer test should be routinely performed. Methods have been described to allow more accurate calculation of the volume of TPH (Jones, 1969; Mollison, 1972). Whereas the standard dose of 100 μg of anti-D immunoglobulin is adequate protection for a TPH of up to 4 ml of foetal red cells, which includes the great majority of deliveries, an additional 25–50 μg should be given for every additional ml TPH (Mollison, 1972). Failures in protection after massive TPH are described by Woodrow et al (1968), Hughes-Jones and Mollison (1968) and Dudok de Wit and Borst-Eilers (1968).

A small number of apparent failures in protection after normal TPH may be due to the mother already being 'primed' by a recent TPH earlier in pregnancy even although anti-D cannot be detected in her serum by available techniques. This is especially likely to be the case in multiparae (Clarke, 1969). The high degree of protection from anti-D immunoglobulin given shortly after delivery argues in favour of this being the usual time of maternal isoimmunization. Chown's group, however, has advocated the administration of anti-D at 28–34 weeks' gestation, *before* delivery (Bowman, 1970). This small dose has no adverse effect on the baby (Zipursky and Israels, 1967).

ANTENATAL DETECTION AND PREDICTION OF SEVERITY OF Rh DISEASE

It is my practice to screen all antenatal patients at their first clinic visit for both Rhesus and non-Rhesus antibodies (e.g. Duffy, Kidd, Kell, S, etc.) whatever their blood group. This policy immediately brings to light Rh +ve patients with, for instance, anti-c̄ who would not otherwise be suspected. The great majority of Rhesus-affected pregnancies can likewise be detected at their first clinic visit providing a sensitive antibody screening test is used, e.g. papainized R_1R_2 or R_2R_2 red cells. If the patient is Rh negative and no antibodies are found early in pregnancy they are tested for again at 28 weeks, 36 weeks and at delivery (this last test being relevant to whether or not she is given prophylactic anti-D after delivery).

Once an immune antibody is detected in the mother's serum her history is considered, the husband's blood is obtained for grouping and genotyping and a provisional decision is made regarding the need for amniocentesis and its timing. The specificity of the antibody is also important since it is only anti-D and occasionally anti-c̄ that can cause foetal death *in utero*; other antibodies such as anti-E, and Kell, Duffy etc., produce a less severe disease, sometimes causing haemolysis and jaundice in the neonatal period but not intra-uterine foetal death. Often the non-Rhesus antibodies have arisen from previous blood transfusion rather than pregnancies. When this is the case the father may well lack the offending antigen and if this fact is determined at an early stage it can confidently be stated that the foetus is free from haemolytic hazard, e.g. if the mother has acquired anti-Kell from a previous transfusion and her husband is Kell-negative, k/k, their offspring must also be Kell-negative, k/k, and will be un-

shortly after delivery due to extreme anaemia at birth (e.g. Hb of 4 g/100 ml). The latter babies can be described as cases of 'living hydrops'. In either instance it is thought that the severity of anaemia leads to cardiac failure. Kernicterus is a later sequelae consequent upon an excessive rise in concentration of unbound bilirubin during the first few days of life. This complication is normally prevented by exchange transfusion.

To some extent the probable severity of Rhesus disease can be judged from the history and the maternal antibody titre (Allen *et al.*, 1950, 1954). In large series reported by these authors the incidence of stillbirth has been 9 per cent in first affected pregnancies, 40 per cent in subsequent pregnancies and 56 per cent where there is a history of previous stillbirth. There was no general tendency to increasing severity after the second baby. There is a statistical relationship between maternal antibody titre and foetal outcome, as shown in Table 10.1.

Bowman and Pollock (1965) found that their prediction of severe Rh disease when based upon

Table 10.1 Outcome in 469 cases of Rh disease related to highest prepartum anti-D titre by albumin technique

Titre:	Up to 1/8 per cent	1/16–1/32 per cent	1/64–1/128 per cent	1/256–1/512 per cent	1/1,000+ per cent
Stillbirth	4	14	25	42	48
Hydrops foetalis	0	2	6	9	11
Death without hydrops	4	6	4	3	0
Kernicterus	10	3	6	1	11
Survival	81	76	59	45	30
No in group	68	131	141	77	27

Data reprinted, by permission, from Allen et al., *(1954) New England Journal of Medicine, 251, 435.*

affected by maternal anti-K. Antibodies of the Lewis system (anti-Le^a anti-Le^b) seldom affect the foetus since their Lewis antigens are not well developed until after birth.

The problem with the management of Rhesus disease is that some babies are only mildly affected and are best delivered at term; others are more severely affected and may perish in the last few weeks of gestation, yet would have survived if delivered prematurely; while other still more severely affected babies would die *in utero* before reaching a stage of maturity at which survival after delivery is possible. A proportion of babies in the last category may be salvaged by intra-uterine transfusion (Lilly, 1965).

In the severely affected baby death may take place *in utero*, when a hydropic stillbirth results, or

history and antibody titre alone was correct in 62 per cent of cases. The errors were chiefly in first affected pregnancies and in cases where there was a history of severe Rh disease but a heterozygous husband (i.e. heterozygous for 'D' antigen as in R_1r, CDe/cde). When the information from examination of the amniotic fluid was added to that of the history and antibody titre the accuracy of their prediction increased from 62 to 96.8 per cent. This latter figure is in agreement with our own experience at the Queen Mother's Hospital, Glasgow. Examples could be quoted where patients with a history of previous Rh stillbirths have been referred for intrauterine transfusion, yet the combination of this history plus high antibody titres, a heterozygous husband and a low amniocentesis reading (*vide infra*) has led to the correct prediction that the baby was Rh—ve, avoiding the hazards of intra-uterine transfusion or premature delivery and allowing the birth of an unaffected mature baby at term.

The severity of haemolysis in the foetus appears to be reflected by the level of bilirubin and biliburin-like pigment in the liquor amnii. The potential value of perabdominal amniocentesis in the management of Rh disease was first suggested by Bevis (1953 and 1956), who described the spectrophotometric characteristics of bilirubin and blood pigments in amniotic fluid and their relation to foetal outcome. This approach was extended by Walker (1957) and Lilly (1961, 1963) who related the height of the bilirubin 'bulge' above the 'constructed' base line corresponding to pigment-free amniotic fluid (Fig. 10.2). to the severity of Rh

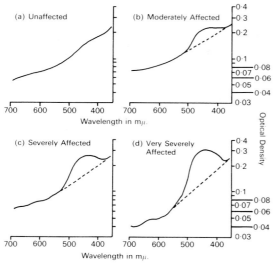

Fig. 10.2 Spectrophotometric curves of amniotic fluid in different severities of Rh disease. (Reproduced from *British Medical Journal* (1964), **3**, 147, by permission of Dr J. G. Robertson and the Editor).

disease in a large series of infants. Lilly's chart (Fig. 10.3) takes into account the fact that, for a given severity of Rh disease, the optical density bulge decreases as gestation advances. This is probably due to increase in volume of amniotic fluid and decreasing concentrations of bilirubin-binding protein. The validity of this method of prediction has been repeatedly confirmed (Alvey, 1964; Walker *et al.*, 1964; Robertson, 1964; Freda, 1965; Bowman and Pollock, 1965 and Little *et al.*, 1966). The trend of results in serial readings have

greater significance than individual readings (Lilly, 1963; Pomerance *et al.*, 1968). It is my policy to repeat amniocentesis at approximately 3-week intervals while the results fall into Lilly's Zone I, at 2-week intervals if in Mid Zone II, but at 7–10 day intervals if close to the junction of Zones II and III. The procedure is not done after 35 weeks' gestation. An upward or horizontal trend entering Zone III on Lilly's prediction graph indicates the need for immediate action; either premature delivery or intrauterine transfusion. A steady trend within Zone II confirms the need for induction at 36 weeks. A downward trend into Zone I confirms that it is safe to leave delivery to term.

Modifications of the original Lilly's method of measuring the amniotic pigment have included the ratio of transmittance at 490 μ to that at 520 mμ (Knox *et al.*, 1965), adaptations of chemical methods of bilirubin estimation to the low concentrations of around 0.2 mg/100 ml found in amniotic fluid (Stewart and Taylor, 1964) and the ratio of bilirubin to protein in the liquor (Morris *et al.*, 1967). The spectrophotometric method is, however, generally preferred (Walker 1970). It is probably better for one obstetric unit to become

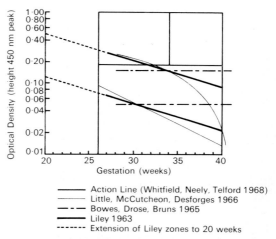

Fig. 10.3 Different methods of interpreting liquor bilirubin. (Reproduced from *British Medical Journal* (1970), **2**, 220, by permission of Dr W. Walker and the Editor).

totally familiar with a single system of interpretation and to follow the trend over 2–4 spaced tests between about 28 and 34 weeks, rather than to try to unravel the significance of multiple analyses (e.g. bilirubin concentration, bilirubin/protein ratio, transmittance ratio at 490 and 520 mμ or the various systems for interpreting spectrophotometry tracings shown in Fig. 10.3 on a single sample of amniotic fluid). At a single point in time these

ANAEMIAS IN THE NEONATAL PERIOD. 1. RHESUS DISEASE (RHESUS ISOIMMUNIZATION) 167

different measurements can give different predictions of severity. Our experience over 10 years at the Queen Mother's Hospital with the original Lilly's method is remarkably satisfactory.

The main sources of erroneous interpretation are incorrect assessment of gestation and contamination of the liquor with blood, usually caused by placental trauma. The latter can be reduced by placental localization prior to amniocentesis. Haemoglobin pigment distorts the spectrophotometric tracing since the Soret band of Hb O_2 at 415 mμ is close to the bilirubin peak at 450 mμ. If the blood is foetal a further error is introduced since the accompanying foetal plasma contains sufficient bilirubin to seriously invalidate liquor assessment (Pridmore *et al.*, 1972). Other sources of error are discussed by Lilly (1963), including the problem of twin amniotic sacs necessitating separate aspiration from each sac. Also gross changes in the volume of the amniotic fluid, such as the development of hydramnios, may falsify pigment concentrations (Queenan *et al.*, 1968). Technical handling of the fluid must also be standardized for consistence of results. The fluid must be transported to the laboratory in a brown bottle to protect the pigment from photo-oxidation, kept at 4° C until analysis, centrifuged and filtered through a small standardized Seitz filtre and analysed preferably within 12 hours of collection. It is a good practice to make a Kleihauer film of any portion of the centrifuged deposit that appears to contain red cells. In this way foetal bleeding into the liquor will be detected. Such bleeding not only tends to invalidate interpretation of the bilirubin level, but if the contamination by foetal blood is gross it may indicate that the foetus is at some hazard due to continuing haemorrhage. A possible bonus is that it may be possible to Rhesus group the foetal cells, perform a direct Coombs test and even make some assessment of the degree of erythroblastosis from a stained film of the deposit.

Hazards of amniocentesis are essentially to the foetus rather than to the mother. Maternal infection is extremely rare. Puncture of the placenta has been mentioned as a cause of foetal haemorrhage into the liquor amnii, which may be fatal on occasions. Foetal haemorrhage may also be retro-placental (Walker, 1970). Foetal bleeding into the maternal circulation (TPH) was found in 4 out of 13 women after amniocentesis by Zipursky *et al.* (1963) but a more recent investigation by Cassady *et al.* (1967) showed a TPH exceeding 0.1 ml in only 2 instances out of 54 amniocenteses (4 per cent). They concluded that the hazard of increasing

maternal immunization was no greater than that of pregnancy. However, Rh +ve foetal cells will be rapidly removed from the circulation in immunized mothers and their presence may therefore be underestimated. Rises in maternal antibody titre have been observed following amniocentesis (Queenan and Adams, 1964), as well as pyrexia and rigors shortly after the procedure, also probably due to small TPH. Because amniocentesis is not entirely without hazard to the existing and subsequent foetuses it is reserved for pregnancies where the history and maternal antibody level are such that there is a real hazard of stillbirth or neonatal death due to Rh disease. Criteria for performing amniocentesis proposed by Lilly (1965), and Bowman and Pollock (1965) can be summarized as follows:

1. A history of previous Rh disease severe enough to require exchange transfusion or to cause stillbirth,

or

2. A maternal titre of anti-D, anti-c̄ or anti-Kell greater than 1:8 by indirect Coombs or albumen titration.

In practice the great majority of patients with the above history have antibody titres in excess of 1:8. This level is taken because it is extremely unlikely that there will be intrauterine death or neonatal death (living hydrops) due to Rh disease unless the titre is higher than this at 35 weeks' gestation – the latest time for amniocentesis. Each laboratory should, however, determine the lowest titre which in their hands is found to be associated with Rhesus foetal loss and be prepared to modify their criteria for amniocentesis in the light of their accumulating experience. Bowman also advises amniocentesis in any immunized mother with a history of previous stillbirth, cause unknown. When the maternal antibody is measured as μg/ml by autoanalyser technique rather than titre the level at which amniocentesis becomes indicated is 1.5 μg/ml or more before 35 weeks' gestation in first affected pregnancies or 1.0 μg/ml. when there has been a previously affected baby (Fraser, Tovey, Lockyer and Sobey, 1972). There were no instances of severe Rh disease below these levels in 600 pregnancies. Timing of the first amniocentesis is suggested between 28 and 31 weeks' gestation by Lilly, but earlier if there is a bad history. There is no advantage in performing an amniocentesis at a much earlier stage of gestation than it is technically possible to give an intrauterine transfusion. In most hands this is approximately 25 weeks.

In ABO haemolytic disease there is no necessity for accurate antenatal prediction since foetal loss never occurs from this cause alone. In particular, amniocentesis is *never* indicated. It is, however, useful for the presence of alpha or beta haemolysins (the immune, IgG, 7S forms of anti-A and anti-B) to be recorded when found in the maternal serum. In this way the neonatal unit can be forewarned that the baby is a candidate for this form of neonatal jaundice enabling determination of its ABO group at birth and observation over the first few days of life. Although seldom needed there are schemes for the accurate antenatal prediction of ABO haemolytic disease using pig A^D cells (Tovey et al., 1962) or standardized tests for alpha and beta haemolysins plus an indirect Coombs reaction on the patient's serum tested against A and B cells after partial neutralization by A and B blood group substance (Ames and Lloyd, 1964).

CLINICAL FINDINGS

The most severely affected infants with Rhesus disease suffer from generalized oedema, ascites and pleural effusions resulting in either stillbirth or a living but hydropic infant with negligible chance of survival. The oedema is thought to be due to cardiac failure secondary to the severe anaemia (3–4 g Hb/100 ml) that is invariably present in such infants. Radiological evidence of Rhesus IUD includes a 'Buddha position' of the foetus, due to its distended abdomen, oedema of the subcutaneous tissue visible over the scalp and a grossly enlarged placenta, seen in all cases of severe Rhesus disease. Maternal signs that develop in a proportion of patients with Rhesus IUD include hydramnios, PET, oedema of the legs and obstetric defibrination after long-retained I.U.D.

Rhesus affected babies of more moderate severity show hepatosplenomegaly, variable pallor and occasionally cutaneous petechiae at birth with rapidly developing jaundice within the first 24 hours. This is often apparent at 4 to 5 hours, and increases in severity over the first 3 to 4 days if untreated. The onset of jaundice within the first 24 hours distinguishes Rh disease from 'physiological' jaundice and most other causes of neonatal jaundice such as ABO haemolytic disease. Cardiac enlargement and cardiac failure may be present or develop in the more anaemic babies. Recent puncture wounds may be present in those born after intrauterine transfusions and the abdomen may still be distended with blood if delivery inadvertently takes place within a few days of this procedure.

Kernicterus constitutes the main hazard for those Rhesus babies delivered in a non-hydropic state and potentially capable of survival. The classical signs of kernicterus are opisthotonus, a high-pitched cry, an absent Moro reflex appearing in the first week followed by generalized convulsions in the most severe cases. Surviving infants with kernicterus inevitably have permanent brain damage (Jones et al., 1954). This is manifest in later life by choreoathetosis, asymmetrical spasticity and high frequency hearing loss. More recently it has also been appreciated that there may be long-term impairment of I.Q. and cognitive functions after severe neonatal hyperbilirubinaemia even when the clinical features of kernicterus were not detected at the time (Odell et al., 1970).

Kernicterus should seldom be encountered nowadays since its pathogenesis is better understood and exchange transfusion is widely available. The brain damage is due to bilirubin encephalopathy as a consequence of unconjugated and unbound bilirubin penetrating the blood-brain barrier. Intracellularly bilirubin inhibits respiration and 'uncouples' oxidative phosphorylation (Ernster et al., 1957). For many years it has been known that the basal ganglia and other areas of the brain were stained with bilirubin in this condition (Claireaux, 1950). The development of kernicterus is closely related to the peak serum level of unconjugated ('indirect') bilirubin insofar as this complication is seldom seen unless the level exceeds 20 mg/100 ml (Vaughan et al., 1950; Hsia et al., 1952). Levels as high as this are never reached until after birth since foetal bilirubin is rapidly cleared into the maternal circulation via the placenta (Lester et al., 1963).

The work of Odell and coworkers (1969, 1970) has emphasized that it is free bilirubin, unbound to albumin, which is toxic to cells and mitochondria and which is associated with brain damage in the neonatal period. When finer degrees of cognitive function are assessed at the age of 5 years it is found that this is related to the degree of albumin saturation by bilirubinin in the neonatal period rather than to the peak bilirubin level. In this context it is relevant that anionic drugs, such as sulphonamides, salicylates and heparin, certain naturally occurring organic anions, such as haematin, as well as acidosis and hypoalbuminaemia can increase the hazard of kernicterus (Odell et al., 1969). These workers also showed that the *duration* of hyperbilirubinaemia is more important than the peak level.

Kernicterus is not confined to Rh disease but can occur with any form of neonatal jaundice if the level of unconjugated bilirubin rises above 20 mg/100 ml.

The 'inspissated' bile syndrome refers to the secondary appearance of obstructive jaundice superimposed upon the initial phase of haemolytic jaundice. It is not now thought that the term accurately describes its pathogenesis. The obstructive phase may be caused by intense intrahepatic erythropoiesis. Clinical features include a greenish discoloration of the skin, pale stools and persistence of firm hepatosplenomegaly for up to 15 weeks (Hsia et al., 1952; Harris et al., 1954).

Late anaemia may develop at between 2 and 8 weeks not only in severely affected infants but also in those who did not require exchange transfusion in their early course. This fact necessitates careful monitoring of the haemoglobin level over the first 2 months of life.

Occasionally older children are encountered with portal hypertension and a history of exchange transfusion in infancy. This is a consequence of thrombosis of the portal vein due to trauma or infection (Oski et al., 1963).

LABORATORY FINDINGS

Clotted and anticoagulated samples of cord blood should be collected in all Rh immunized pregnancies and tested without delay to determine if the baby is affected and, if so, how severely. Affected babies are Rh positive and direct Coombs positive. On rare occasions the maternal anti-D in her serum is too weak to react by indirect Coombs technique, being detected only by enzyme-treated D positive cells. In these circumstances the baby's red cells may be found to be Rh positive but direct Coombs test negative. It is a fortunate coincidence that the amount of antibody needed to sensitize red cells to the Coombs reagent (anti-human globulin) corresponds closely to the amount needed to render the cells susceptible to reticuloendothelial phagocytosis and consequent shortened survival. Infants with negative direct Coombs tests do not therefore usually show other clinical or haematological evidence of haemolysis.

Free maternal anti-D can also be detected in the baby's serum, in a similar titre to that in the mother's serum. Its rate of decline in the baby's serum after birth is exponential (Fig. 10.4), persisting up to 7–8 weeks.

The anticoagulated specimen of cord blood is used to determine the haemoglobin concentration, perform a reticulocyte count and make a blood film for assessment of the degree of erythroblastosis. Findings indicative of haemolysis in the newborn are a reticulocytosis in excess of 10 per cent, 10 or more normoblasts per 100 white cells in the film and a haemoglobin level less than 15 g/100 ml. The cord serum bilirubin is usually greater than 3.0 mg/100 ml in the presence of significant haemolysis. It is upon these initial findings that the severity of the Rh disease is assessed and the need for early exchange transfusion determined. It is essential that the results of the above tests (Rh group, DCT, Hb and bilirubin) should be correlated and should be internally consistent, e.g. a negative direct Coombs test in an Rh positive baby when the mother has anti-D should not be accepted without confirmation. On occasions foetal RBC's heavily coated with maternal anti-D may show a 'blocked' reaction with anti-D grouping serum, and may initially be grouped as Rh negative. Babies born after intrauterine transfusions may have predominantly Rh—ve adult RBCs in their circulation which are direct Coombs negative. Nevertheless the serum bilirubin is usually above 3 mg/100 ml and rises rapidly during the first hours after birth.

Severely affected babies may have haemoglobin levels as low as 4 g/100 ml with intense erythroblastosis in the blood film (Fig 10.6) and a bilirubin level of 7 mg/100 ml or more. Moderately severely affected infants may have haemoglobin levels up to 15 g/100 ml but bilirubin levels usually above 3.0 mg/100 ml and a degree of erythroblastosis proportionate to the anaemia. Mildly affected infants, perhaps requiring no specific treatment, may have a haemoglobin level above 15 g/100 ml and a bilirubin below 3 mg/100 ml. The bilirubin is entirely 'indirect' unconjugated in type except in those severely affected infants liable to the inspissated bile syndrome (Dunn, 1963). The blood film in Rh disease does not usually show spherocytes, as are found in ABO haemolytic disease and certain other types of haemolysis. In severe cases megaloblastic features may be found, but these are usually

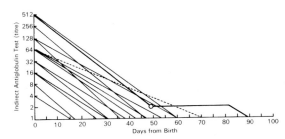

Fig. 10.4 Disappearance of Rh-antibody from infants' serum. ———, Rh-positive (15 cases) T½ = 7 days (range 6–9 days); - - - -, Rh-negative infant, T½ = 12 days. (Reproduced from the British Journal of Haematology (1965), in a paper by Hurdle and Davies, by permission of the Editor and Dr Davis).

170 PAEDIATRIC HAEMATOLOGY

unrelated to folate deficiency. Also in severe cases thrombocytopenia may be found, correlating with the presence of petechiae. In some cases the thrombocytopenia is caused by intravascular coagulation in these severely affected infants (Chessells and Wigglesworth, 1971).

MANAGEMENT AND TREATMENT

If antenatal prediction of the severity of Rhesus disease has been successful many babies will be delivered with haemoglobin levels of around 10 g/100 ml and bilirubin levels of 5–8 mg/100 ml, this being at term in the 'Zone I' babies and at 35–36 weeks in the Zone II babies. Among the Zone I babies some will have milder disease with minimal anaemia and some will be Rh—ve and unaffected. Severely affected 'living hydrops' babies with haemoglobin levels around 5 g/100 ml should seldom be encountered and then only in the Zone III cases where intrauterine transfusion has failed or been followed by unintended premature labour.

There is a particular hazard of hyaline membrane disease or (idiopathic) respiratory distress syndrome (RDS) in infants delivered prematurely because of Rh disease (Phibbs *et al.*, 1972). Yet premature delivery is needed in the infants with Zone II amniocentesis results. A valuable guide in determining the optimum time of delivery so as to avoid the separate hazards of Rh disease on the one hand and RDS on the other is measurement of the lecithin: sphingomyelin ratio in amniotic fluid (Gluck *et al.*, 1971). Dipalmitoyl lecithin is the main pulmonary surfactant and is deficient in RDS. This deficiency is reflected in the amniotic fluid. A lecithin: sphingomyelin ratio below 1.5 is usually associated with the development of RDS after delivery but a ratio of over 2.0 indicates a negligible hazard of RDS (Whitfield *et al.*, 1972).

After delivery the single most contributory therapeutic procedure is exchange transfusion (ET) and the first decision facing the paediatrician is whether to perform an early ET or whether to defer this until after a period of observation (Naiman, 1972). In either case the prime objective is to prevent the serum bilirubin rising above 20 mg/100 ml, at which level there arises the danger of kernicterus. Early ET reduces this hazard primarily by replacing the infant's antibody-coated Rh +ve cells, destined for haemolysis, by compatible Rh -ve transfused cells which will have an essentially normal survival in the circulation. Later on subsequent ET achieves the added effect

of washing out the plasma bilirubin, which at such time is usually elevated to between 15 and 20 mg/100 ml. Maternal antibody is also removed during ET, of probable minor benefit. In practice the red cell mass is exchanged to the extent of 80–90 per cent (Fig. 10.5) but the bilirubin concentration is reduced only by about 50 per cent during ET (Odell *et al.*, 1962). This is probably because more bilirubin is extracted from extravascular pools during the process of ET. A further possible benefit from ET lies in the fact that a small amount of unconjugated bilirubin can be absorbed on to the surface of the normal, transfused cells but not by the original antibody-coated cells (Oski and Naiman, 1963). A rise in the infant's haemoglobin level is not consistently found after ET since the blood used for the procedure may well have a Hb concentration of 12 g/100 ml. It is therefore only in the relatively anaemic babies that any immediate improvement in Hb level is found; in those with a Hb of say 14 g/100 ml at birth it may fall during ET. Nevertheless the baby is always left with an adequate Hb level after ET. In the severely anaemic hydropic infant with cardiac failure it has generally been felt that immediate clinical benefit can be achieved by creating an initial 20–40 ml deficit during ET, thereby reducing plasma volume and central venous pressure. Recent work by Brans *et al.* (1974) has, however, shown that the blood volume in Coombs positive premature infants is normal, and that in term infants hypovolaemic. They suggest that maintenance of a volume deficit after ET should be avoided.

Indications for immediate ET vary somewhat from one department to another but are largely based upon the cord blood haemoglobin and bilirubin levels. History and maternal antibody titre are less precise indices of severity. McKay (1964) considers a cord blood haemoglobin below 12 g/100 ml or a cord blood bilirubin above 5 mg/100 ml indications for immediate ET. Dunn (1966) regarded a cord Hb below 13.5 g/100 ml plus a cord bilirubin above 3.5 mg/100 ml indicative. At the Queen Mother's Hospital, Glasgow, a haemoglobin below 14 g/100 ml or bilirubin above 4 mg/100 ml are taken as indications for ET within a few hours of birth. Clinical evidence of severe disease such as gross hepatosplenomegaly, golden liquor and especially oedema or ascites is an indication for ET as early as possible. It is our practice to have fresh Rh negative blood already cross-matched against the mother's serum and available at birth for those infants in whom severe disease is expected, so as to obviate any delay in

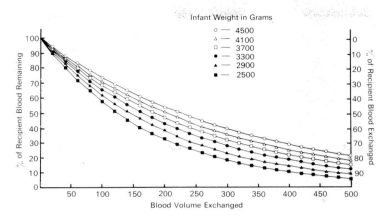

Fig. 10.5 Predicted percentage of blood exchanged in E.T. based on infant weight. An infant blood volume of 75 ml/kg has been assumed. Percentage is based on the equation $\%\,R = \left(\frac{v-s}{v}\right)^N$. (Reproduced from *Journal of Pediatrics* (1974), **84**, 1, by permission of Dr D. H. Buchholz and the publisher).

ET. In less severely affected infants a few hours' delay is not deleterious.

The indications for later ET, or for repeat ET are a rising level of unconjugated bilirubin which, when plotted on a graph, projects a level of 20 mg/100 ml within 72–96 hours for a full-term infant or 18 mg/100 ml for a premature infant (Naiman, 1972). Because of immaturity of the glucuronyl transferase system and possibly also of impaired hepatic excretion the premature infant is at greater risk of bilirubin intoxication than the full-term infant.

Estimation of the degree of saturation of serum with bilirubin may give further help in assessing the hazard of bilirubin levels above 15 mg/100 ml (Odell *et al.*, 1970). This is especially so after an ET in which albumin has also been administered (Waters and Porter, 1964) since the increased binding capacity of this may allow one to permit the bilirubin to rise to 23–24 mg/100 ml in full-term infants and 20–22 mg/100 ml in premature infants (Bowman, 1967). Techniques for measuring the bilirubin binding capacity include the HABA (HABA is a derivative of benzoic acid) binding method (Porter and Waters, 1966) and the salicylate displacement method of Odell and co-workers (1969).

Exchange transfusion is performed with whole blood under 5 days old that is compatible by cross-match against the mother's (or baby's) serum and has been warmed to 37° C before use. A total volume of 160–180 ml/kg body weight is used in aliquots of 20 ml via a two-way syringe. The group of the transfused blood is Rh negative and ABO-compatible with the baby if it is possible to satisfy this without incompatibility with the mother's serum (against which it is cross-matched to exclude incompatibility from a second maternal antibody outside the Rhesus system). For instance, an A baby with an A mother is given A Rh −ve blood but an A baby with an O mother has to have O Rh −ve blood. The disadvantage of the latter choice is that O blood will contain anti-A which can react with the baby's A cells, slightly increasing the rate of haemolysis of these cells.

Details of the technique of ET are well described by Allen and Diamond (1957), Mauer (1969), Bowman and Friesen (1970) and Oski and Naiman (1972A). Superior release of oxygen to the tissues with fresh whole blood has been shown by Delivoria-Papadopoulos *et al.* (1971), and superior removal of bilirubin if 1 g albumin per kg body weight is given 1–2 hr before ET (Odell *et al.*, 1962B). 50 ml of salt poor (25 per cent) albumin may be used to replace 50 ml of supernatant plasma in the blood used for ET (Waters and Porter, 1964) in severely affected babies in whom a second ET is expected. Oski and Naiman (1972B), however, point out that the addition of albumin could aggravate congestive cardiac failure in the hydropic infant. These authors also give detailed additional measures that should be undertaken in such hydropic infants.

Hazards of ET include acidosis, hyperkalaemia, hypocalcaemia, hypoglycaemia, hypothermia, bacteraemia and portal vein thrombosis. Other hazards are listed by Odell *et al.* (1962A). The overall mortality should be less than 1 per cent but has been reported as 5–10 per cent (Wilson, 1969).

Acidosis is the consequence of the acid-citrate-dextrose (ACD) anticoagulant used in the donor blood, and is a special danger in the small premature infant with RDS or sepsis. This can largely be prevented by either sodium bicarbonate, 1 mEq injected after each 100 ml of blood (Barrie, 1965), or THAM added to the blood immediately before use (Pierson et al., 1968). Alternatively citrate-phosphate-dextrose (CPD) can be used as the original anticoagulant. Hyperkalaemia is avoided by using blood not more than 4 days old, since loss of red cell potassium into the plasma becomes significant in older blood. Hypocalcaemia, due to calcium binding by the citrate of ACD, can be prevented by giving 1 ml of 10 per cent calcium gluconate I.V. after every 100–150 ml of blood exchanged (Naiman, 1972). Hypoglycaemia may exist both before and a few hours after ET (Barrett and Oliver, 1968). Two hours after ET a screening test (Dextrostix) should be performed. Treatment is with hypertonic glucose. Other hazards are avoided by warming the blood to 37°C, ensuring an ambient temperature of 28° to 30°C, and employing good aseptic technique.

Late anaemia may occur up to the age of 8 weeks whether or not ET has been given (Fig. 10.6). The occurrence of this anaemia is poorly correlated with the initial severity of the haemolytic disease, but more closely correlated with the post ET haemoglobin level, being commoner when this is below 14 g/100 ml (Hurdle and Davis, 1965). These authors suggest that the most likely mechanism is that the marrows of all infants pass through a stage of erythroid hypoplasia and that

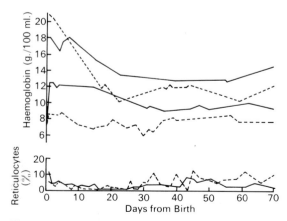

Fig. 10.6 Development of late anemia in Rh disease. The limits of haemoglobin and the max. reticulocyte counts in 19 infants with haemolytic disease of the newborn in the first 70 days. ———, 7 Cases showing min. haemoglobin > 9 g/100 ml; - - - -, 12 cases showing min. haemoglobin < 9 g/100 ml. (Reproduced from the *British Journal of Haematology* (1965), from a paper by Hurdle and Davis, by permission of the Editor and Dr Davis).

the natural decay of transfused red cells renders them liable to later anaemia, especially when the post ET haemoglobin level is relatively low. Treatment is simple transfusion if the haemoglobin level falls below around 7 g/100 ml especially if the anaemia is accompanied by lethargy, poor feeding and persisting reticulocytopenia.

Phototherapy and barbiturate therapy are of value in reducing the bilirubin level in infants with mild jaundice due to prematurity or ABO haemolytic disease, in which context they are discussed in more detail in chapter 11. They play a much smaller part in the management of hyperbilirubinaemia due to Rh disease but may constitute an adjunct to ET in the more mildly affected babies, perhaps reducing the need for second or late ETs. McMullin et al. (1970) have claimed a beneficial effect of large doses of phenobarbitone in Rh disease but this is not universally accepted (Oski and Naiman, 1972C).

Intrauterine transfusion

Those babies whose Rh disease is of such severity that they would perish *in utero* before they have reached a stage of gestation at which premature delivery is feasible may be salvaged by intrauterine transfusion (Lilly, 1963; 1965). Since the survival rate with this procedure hardly ever exceeds 50 per cent (Table 10.2) and since at least some of the foetal loss is caused by direct trauma to the foetus or placenta (Walker and Ellis, 1970), great care must be taken in selecting only those babies who would not survive otherwise. This selection is made primarily from the results of serial amniocenteses, but all other relevant facts including history, husband's genotype and maternal antibody titre may contribute to the accuracy of prediction, as described above. The gestational age at which it becomes safer to induce delivery rather than give an intrauterine transfusion is that at which the chance of loss from prematurity is less than that of intrauterine transfusion. This is likely to be somewhere between 32 and 34 weeks but will vary with the experience of the units concerned, tending towards a later gestation as greater expertise is gained in the technique of intrauterine transfusion. In practice an unexpected source of error may be that due to a wrong estimate of the period of gestation unless this possibility is constantly borne in mind. The recent advances in prediction of foetal lung maturity from the lecithin: sphingomyclin ratio should also play a part in deciding between early induction and intrauterine transfusion.

ANAEMIAS IN THE NEONATAL PERIOD. 1. RHESUS DISEASE (RHESUS ISOIMMUNIZATION)

Table 10.2 Results of intrauterine transfusion in various series

Centre	No. of cases	Average no. of IUTs per patient	Stillbirths (per cent of cases treated)	Survivors (per cent of cases treated)	Neonatal deaths (per cent livebirths)
U.S.A. co-operative study	591	1·8	51	34	30
Lewisham	172	1·6	55	40	42
Auckland	171	2·0	49	37	28
Newcastle upon Tyne	104	2·0	50	38	26
Winnipeg	100	2·2	45	48	13
Connecticut	58	2·1	48	35	33
Hammersmith	22	2·2	27	45	38

Data reproduced by permission of Dr. W. Walker and the Editor of the British Medical Journal, B.M.A. House, Tavistock Square, London, W.C.1., from Brit. med. J. ii, 223 (1970).

An even more contentious question is whether certain babies can be judged to be too severely affected, i.e. already hydropic, for attempted salvage by intrauterine transfusion to be attempted (Naiman, 1972).

The technique of intrauterine transfusion has been described in many publications (Lilly, 1965; Little *et al.*, 1966; Queenan *et al.*, 1966; Fairweather *et al.*, 1967; Queenan, 1967; Walker and Ellis, 1970), and will not be given in detail here. It depends upon the fact that red cells injected into the foetal peritoneal cavity are slowly absorbed into the circulation via the lymphatics (Mellish and Wolman, 1958). Absorption appears to be delayed in the presence of foetal ascites in hydropic infants. Fresh O Rh negative blood, compatible with the mother's serum, is used partially packed to a concentration of 20 g/100 ml. It is preferably washed so as to remove immunocompetent lymphocytes, although the incidence of graft versus host reaction is extraordinarily low, very few instances being known (Cohen *et al.*, 1965; Naiman *et al.*, 1969). The origin of the lymphocytes causing the graft versus host disease can sometimes be shown to be an ET in infants having previous IUT (Parkman *et al.*, 1974). Maximum absorption of the red cells occurs in around 10 days, so transfusions are initially given at 14 day intervals, and are then repeated at 2–3 week intervals until 10–14 days before delivery at 36–38 weeks' gestation. The volume of blood injected is related to the foetal age, i.e. 20 ml at 20–22 weeks to 75 ml at 33 weeks, these volumes being smaller than those originally used (Naiman, 1972).

At birth it is important to make sure that an intrauterine transfusion has not been given within the previous few days as immediate peritoneal aspiration would then be needed to avoid difficulties in respiration secondary to abdominal distention. Cord blood results are atypical after successful intrauterine transfusion insofar as the great majority of circulating red cells should be transfused, O Rh negative, direct Coombs negative and adult in type. A Kleihauer film should always be made to document the degree of efficiency of the intrauterine transfusions. Neither reticulocytosis nor erythroblastosis are present if the haemoglobin level is near to normal. The cord blood bilirubin level, however, is usually elevated and the serum bilirubin may rise rapidly after birth. In spite of deceptively normal initial haematological findings these infants require very careful monitoring over their first hours and days, frequently requiring several ETs to combat rising bilirubin levels. There is great variability in this respect from case to case. Later development was normal in 21 out of 24 such infants studied by Phibbs *et al.* (1971), but there is a high incidence of late inguinal hernias.

Intrauterine exchange transfusion by various techniques (Adamsons *et al.*, 1965; Asensio *et al.*, 1968; Seelen *et al.*, 1966) must be regarded as at the experimental stage and have no established place in the management of Rh disease.

The place of intensive plasmapheresis, using a cell-separator, instead of intrauterine transfusion in highly selected cases of severe Rh disease is currently being investigated (Graham Pole *et al.*, 1974A; 1974B).

REFERENCES

Adamsons, K., Freda, V. J., James, L. S. & Towell, M. E. (1965) Prenatal treatment of erythroblastosis fetalis following hysterotomy. *Pediatrics*, **35**, 848.

Ahuja, G. L., Willoughby, M. L. N., Kerr, M. M. & Hutchison, J. H. (1969) Massive subaponeurotic haemorrhage in infants born by vacuum extraction. *Brit. med. J.*, **iii**, 743.

Akerman, B. D. (1969) Infantile pyknocytosis in Mexican-American infants. *Amer. J. Dis. Child.*, **117**, 417.

Allen, F. H., Diamond, L. K. & Vaughan, V. C. (1950) Erythroblastosis Fetalis. II. Prognosis in relation to history, maternal titre and length of fetal gestation. *Pediatrics*, **6**, 441.

Allen, F. H., Diamond, L. K. & Jones, A. R. (1954) Erythroblastosis Fetalis. IX. The problems of stillbirth. *New Eng. J. Med.*, **251**, 453.

Allen, F. H. & Diamond, L. K. (1947) *Erythroblastosis Fetalis.* Boston: Little, Brown & Co.

Allison, A. C. (1957) Acute haemolytic anaemia with distortion and fragmentation of erythrocytes in children. *Brit. J. Haemat.*, **3**, 1.

Alvey, J. P. (1964) Obstetrical management of Rh incompatibility based on liquor amnii studies. *Amer. J. Obstet. Gynec.*, **90**, 769.

American Academy of Pediatrics (1961) Vitamin K compounds and the water-soluble analogues. Use in therapy and prophylaxis in pediatrics. *Pediat.*, **28**, 501.

Ames, A. C. & Lloyd, R. S. (1964) A scheme for the ante-natal prediction of ABO haemolytic disease of the newborn. *Vox Sang*, **9**, 712.

Anders, D., Kinderman, G. & Pfeifer, U. (1973) Neuroblastoma metastases in placenta simulating erythroblastosis. Report of two cases. *J. Pediat.*, **82**, 50.

Andrews, B. F. & Thompson, J. W. (1962) Materno-fetal transfusion. A common phenomenon. *Pediatrics*, **29**, 500.

Asensio, S. H., Figueroa-Longo, J. G. & Pelegrina, I. A. (1968) Intrauterine exchange transfusion. A new technic. *Obstet. Gynec.*, **32**, 350.

Austin, R. F. & Desforges, J. F. (1969) Hereditary elliptocytosis: An unusual presentation of haemolysis in the newborn associated with transient morphological abnormalities. *Pediatrics*, **44**, 196.

Bajpai, P. C., Tripathi, T. K. & Agarwala, S. C. (1972) A study of erythrocyte life span in galactosemia using CR[51]. *J. Pediat.*, **80**, 835.

Barrett, C. T. & Oliver, T. K. (1968) Hypoglycemia and hyperinsulinism with erythroblastosis fetalis. *New Eng. J. Med.*, **278**, 1260.

Barrie, H. (1965) Acid-base control during exchange transfusion. *Lancet*, **ii**, 712.

Beckett, R. S. & Flynn, F. J. (1953) Toxoplasmosis: report of two new cases, with a classification and a demonstration of the organism in the human placenta. *New Eng. J. Med.*, **249**, 345.

Bernard, J., Seligmann, M., Chassigneux, J. & Dresch, C. (1962) Anémie de Blackfan-Diamond. *Nouv. Rev. Franc. Hémat.*, **2**, 721.

Bevis, D. C. A. (1953) Composition of liquor amnii in haemolytic disease of the newborn. *J. Obstet. Gynaec. Brit. Emp.*, **60**, 244.

Bevis, D. C. A. (1956) Blood pigments in haemolytic disease of the newborn. *J. Obstet. Gynaec. Brit. Emp.*, **63**, 68.

Bowman, J. M. (1967) *Modern Management of the Rh Problem*, p. 230. Edited by Queenan, J. T. Haebner Medical Division. New York: Harper and Row.

Bowman, J. M. (1970) Annotation: Prevention of haemolytic disease of the neborn. *Brit. J. Haemat.*, **19**, 653.

Bowman, J. M. & Pollock, J. M. (1965) Amniotic fluid spectrophotometry and early delivery in the management of erythroblastosis fetalis. *Pediatrics*, **35**, 815.

Bowman, J. D. & Friesen, R. F. (1970) Haemolytic disease of the newborn. In *Current Pediatric Therapy*, Vol. 4, p. 405. Edited by S. S. Gellis and B. M. Kagan. Philadelphia: Saunders.

Brans, Y. W., Milstead, R. R., Bailey, P. E. & Cassady, G. (1974) Blood-volume estimates in Coombs-test-positive infants. *New Eng. J. Med.*, **290**, 1450.

Bulova, S. I. (1972) Hydrops fetalis and congenital syphilis. *Pediat.*, **49**, 285.

Burman, D. (1958) Congenital spherocytosis in infancy. *Arch. Dis. Childh.*, **33**, 335.

Cassady, G. Cailleteau, J., Lockard, D. & Milstead, R. (1967) The hazard of fetal-maternal transfusion after transabdominal amniocentesis. *Amer. J. Obstet. Gynec.*, **99**, 284.

Cathie, I. A. B. (1952) Apparent idiopathic Heinz body anaemia. *Gt. Ormond St. J.*, **3**, 43.

Chessells, J. M. & Wigglesworth, J. S. (1971) Haemostatic failure in babies with rhesus isoimmunization. *Arch. Dis. Childh.*, **46**, 38.

Claireaux, A. (1950) Haemolytic disease of the newborn. Part I: A clinico-pathological study of 157 cases. *Arch. Dis. Childh.*, **25**, 61.

Clarke, C. A. (1967) Prevention of Rh-Haemolytic disease. *Brit. med. J.*, **4**, 7.

Clarke, C. A. (1968) Prevention of Rhesus iso-immunisation. *Lancet*, **1**, 1.

Clarke, C. A. (1969) Prevention of Rhesus iso-immunisation. *Seminars in Hematology*, **6**, 201.

Clarke, C. A., Finn, R., McConnell, R. B. & Sheppard, P. M. (1958) The protection afforded by ABO incompatibility against erythroblastosis due to Rhesus anti-D. *Int. Arch. Allerg.*, **13**, 380.

Clayton, E. M., Pryor, J. A., Wierdsma, J. G. & Whitacre, F. E. (1964) Fetal and maternal components in third-trimester obstetric hemorrhage. *Obstet. Gynec.*, **24**, 56.

Cohen, F., Zuelzer, W. W., Gustafson, D. C. & Evans, M. M. (1964) Mechanisms of Isoimmunisation. I. The transplacental passage of fetal erythrocytes in homospecific pregnancies. *Blood*, **23**, 621.

Cohen, F., Zuelzer, W. W., Kadowski, J., Thompson, R. & Kennedy, D. (1965) Temporary persistence of replicating donor cells after intrauterine transfusions. *J. Pediat.*, **67**, 937.

Davis, J. A. & Schiff, D. (1966) Bruising as a cause of neonatal jaundice. *Lancet*, **1**, 636.

Delivoria-Papadopoulos, M., Morrow, G. & Oski, F. A. (1971) Exchange transfusion with fresh and 'old' blood: The role of storage on 2, 3-diphosphoglycerate, hemoglobin-oxygen affinity, and oxygen release. *J. Pediat.*, **79**, 898.

Desmond, M. (1968) Clinical pathological conference. *J. Pediat.*, **73**, 283.

Diamond, L. K., Blackfan, K. D. & Baty, J. M. (1932) Erythroblastosis fetalis and its association with universal edema of fetus, icterus gravis neonatorum, and anaemia of the newborn. *J. Pediat.*, **1**, 269.

Diamond, L. K., Allen, D. M. & Magill, F. B. (1961) Congenital (erythroid) hypoplastic anemia. *Am. J. Dis. Child.*, **102**, 149.

Doxiadis, S. A., Fessas, P., Valaes, T. & Mastrokalos, N. (1961) Glucose–6–phosphate dehydrogenase deficiency; a new aetiological factor of severe neonatal jaundice. *Lancet*, **i**, 297.

Doxiadis, S. A. & Valaes, T. (1964) The clinical picture of glucose–6–phosphate dehydrogenase deficiency in early infancy. *Arch. Dis. Childh.*, **39**, 545.

Driscoll, S. G. (1966) Hydrops foetalis. *New Eng. J. Med.*, **275**, 1432.

Dudok de Wit, C. & Borst-Eilers, E. (1968) Failure of anti-D immunoglobulin injection to protect against Rhesus immunization after massive foeto-maternal haemorrhage. Report of 4 cases. *Brit. med. J.*, **i**, 152.

Dunn, P. M. (1963) Obstructive jaundice and haemolytic disease of the newborn. *Arch. Dis. Childh.*, **38**, 54.

Dunn, P. M. (1966) The unnecessary exchange transfusion: A study of Rh hemolytic disease of the newborn. *J. Pediat.*, **69**, 829.

Eichenwald, H. F. (1957) Congenital toxoplasmosis. A study of 150 cases. *A.M.A. J. Dis. Child.*, **94**, 411.

Embil, J. A., Ozere, R. L. & Haldane, E. V. (1970) Congenital cytomegalovirus infection in two siblings from consecutive pregnancies. *J. Pediat.*, **77**, 417.

Ernster, L., Herlin, L. & Zetterström, R. (1957) Experimental studies on the pathogenesis of kernicterus. *Pediatrics*, **20**, 647.

Eshaghpour, E., Oski, F. A. & Naiman, J. L. (1966) Iron deficiency anemia in a newborn infant. *J. Pediat.*, **68**, 806.

Eshaghpour, E., Oski, F. A. & Williams, M. (1967) The relationship of erythrocyte glucose–6–phosphate dehydrogenase deficiency to hyperbilirubinemia in Negro premature infants. *J. Pediat.*, **70**, 595.

Fairweather, D. V. I., Tacchi, D., Coxon, A., Hughes, M. I., Murray, S. & Walker, W. (1967) Intrauterine transfusion in Rh-isoimmunization. *Brit. med. J.*, **ii**, 189.

Finn, R. (1970) Rh haemolytic disease.—Recent advances in Rh isoimmunization prevention. *Brit. med. J.*, **1**, 219.

Fraser, I. D., Tovey, G. H., Lockyer, W. J. & Sobey, D. F. (1972) Antibody protein levels in the maternal serum in rhesus iso-immunization. *J. Obstet. Gynec. Brit. Cmwlth.*, **79**, 1074.

Freda, V. J. (1965) The Rh problem in obstetrics and a new concept of its management using amniocentesis and spectrophotometric scanning of amniotic fluid. *Amer. J. Obstet. Gynec.*, **92**, 341.

Garica, A. G. P. (1968) Congenital toxoplasmosis in two successive sibs. *Arch. Dis. Childh.*, **43**, 705.

Gasser, C. (1953) Die hämolytischen Frühgeburtenämie mit spontaner Innenkörperbildung; ein neue Syndrom, beobachtet an 14 Fälle. *Helv. paediat. Acta*, **8**, 491.

Gasser, C. (1957) Aplasia of erythropoiesis. *Pediat. Clin. N. Amer.*, **4**, 445.

Gasser, C. (1959) Heinz body anemia and related phenomena. *J. Pediat.*, **54**, 673.

Gasser, C. & Willi, H. (1952) Spontane Innenkörpebildung bei Milzagenesie. *Helvet. paediat. Acta*, **7**, 369.

Gluck, L., Kulovich, M. V., Borer, R. C., Brenner, P. H., Anderson, C. G. & Spellacy, W. N. (1971) Diagnosis of the respiratory distress syndrome by amniocentesis. *Am. J. Obstet. Gynec.*, **109**, 440.

Goodall, H. B., Grahan, F. S., Miller, M. C. & Cameron, C. (1958) Transplacental bleeding from the foetus. *J. Clin. Path.*, **11**, 251.

Graham Pole, J. R., Barr, W. & Willoughby, M. L. N. (1974A) Continuous-flow exchange plasma-pheresis in severe rhesus isoimmunisation. *Lancet*, **i**, 1051.

Graham Pole, J. R., Donald, I., Barr, W. & Willoughby, M. L. N. (1974B) Plasmapheresis in rhesus isoimmunisation. *Lancet*, **ii**, 1459.

Grimes, A. J., Meisler, A. & Dacie, J. V. (1964) Congenital Heinz-body anaemia: further evidence of the cause of Heinz-body production in red cells. *Brit. J. Haemat.*, **10**, 281.

Gross, R. T., Bracci, R., Rudolph, N. Schroeder, E. & Kochen, J. A. (1967) Hydrogen peroxide toxity and detoxification in the erythrocytes of newborn infants. *Blood*, **29**, 481.

Gross, G. P. & Hathaway, W. E. (1972) Fetal erythrocyte deformability. *Pediat. Res.*, **6**, 593.

Harris, R. C., Anderson, D. H. & Day, R. L. (1954) Obstructive jaundice in infants with normal biliary tree. *Pediatrics*, **13**, 293.

Harvey, B., Remington, J. S. & Sulzer, A. J. (1969) IgM malaria antibodies in a case of congenital malaria in the United States. *Lancet* **1**, 333.

Hathaway, W. E., Mull, M. M. & Pechet, G. S. (1969) Disseminated intravascular coagulation in the newborn. *Pediatrics*, **43**, 233.

Helz, M. K. & Menten, M. L. (1944) Elliptocytosis, a report of two cases. *J. Lab. Clin. Med.*, **29**, 185.

Hsia, D. Y–Y., Allen, F. H., Gellis, S. S. & Diamond, L. K. (1952) Erythroblastosis fetalis. *VIII*. Studies of serum bilirubin in relation to kernicterus. *New Eng. J. Med.*, **247**, 668.

Hsia, D. Y–Y., Patterson, P., Allen, F. H., Diamond, L. K. & Gellis, S. S. (1952) Prolonged obstructive jaundice in infancy. I. General survey of 156 cases. *Pediatrics*, **10**, 243.

Hsia, D. Y. & Walker, F. A. (1961) Variability in clinical manifestation of galactosemia. *J. Pediat.*, **59**, 872.

Hughes-Jones, N. C. & Mollison, P. L. (1968) Failure of a relatively small dose of passively administered anti-Rh to suppress primary immunization by a relatively large dose of Rh-positive red cells. *Brit. med. J.*, **1**, 150.

Hurdle, A. D. F. & Davis, J. A. (1965) The 'late' anemia of haemolytic disease of the newborn. *Brit. J. Haemat.*, **11**, 247.

Jones, P. (1969) Assessment of size of small volume foeto-maternal bleeds. A new method of quantification of the Kleihauer technique. *Brit. med. J.*, **ii**, 85.

176 PAEDIATRIC HAEMATOLOGY

Jones, M. H., Sands, R., Hyman, C. B., Sturgeon, P. & Koch, F. P. (1954) Longitudinal study of the incidence of central nervous system damage following erythroblastosis fetalis. *Pediatrics*, **14**, 346.

Kabat, D. (1974) An elution procedure for visualization of adult hemoglobin in human blood smears. *Blood*, **43**, 239.

Kan, Y. W., Allen, A. & Lowenstein, L. (1967) Hydrops fetalis with alpha thalassemia. *New Eng. J. Med.*, **276**, 18.

Kan, Y. W., Forget, B. G. & Nathan, D. G. (1972) Gamma-beta thalassemia: A cause of hemolytic disease of the newborn. *New Eng. J. Med.*, **286**, 129.

Keimowitz, R. & Desforges, J. F. (1965) Infantile pycnocytosis. *New Eng. J. Med.*, **273**, 1152.

Kerr, M. M. (1959) Anaemia and polycythaemia in uni-ovular twins. *Brit. med. J.*, **i**, 902.

Kirkman, H. N. & Riley, H. D. (1959A) Posthemorrhagic anemia and shock in the newborn. A review. *Pediatrics*, **24**, 97.

Kirkman, H. N. & Riley, H. D. (1959B) Posthemorrhagic anemia and shock in the newborn due to hemorrhage during delivery. Report of 8 cases. *Pediatrics*, **24**, 92.

Kleihauer, E., Braun, H. & Betke, K. (1957) Demonstration von fetalen Hämoglobin in Erythrozyten eines Blutaus-striches. *Klin. Wschr.*, **35**, 637.

Knox, E. (1968) Obstetric determinants of Rh sensitisation. *Lancet*, **i**, 433.

Knox, E. G., Fairweather, D. V. I. & Walker, W. (1965) Spectrophotometric measurements on liquor amnii in relation to the severity of haemolytic disease of the newborn. *Clin. Sci.*, **28**, 147.

Lancet (1972) Editorial: Fetal/Maternal incompatibility. *Lancet*, **ii**, 958.

Lausecker, C., Heidt, P., Fischer, D., Hartleyb, H. & Löhr, G. E. (1965) Anémie hémolytique constitutionelle avec déficite en phosphogluconate dehydrogenase. *Arch. Fr. Pediat.*, **22**, 789.

Lee-Potter, J. P., Deacon-Smith, R. A., Simpkiss, M. J., Kamuzora, H. & Lehmann, H. (1975) A new cause of haemolytic anaemia in the newborn. *J. Clin. Path.*, **28**, 317.

Lester, R., Behrman, R. E. & Lucey, J. F. (1963) Transfer of bilirubin—C14 across monkey placenta. *Pediatrics*, **32**, 416.

Levine, P. (1943) Serological factors as possible causes in spontaneous abortion. *J. Hered.*, **34**, 71.

Lilly, A. W. (1961) Liquor amnii analysis in management of pregnancy complicated by rhesus sensitization. *Amer. J. Obstet. Gynec.*, **82**, 1359.

Lilly, A. W. (1963) Errors in the assessment of hemolytic disease from amniotic fluid. *Am. J. Obstet. Gynec.*, **86**, 485.

Lilly, A. W. (1963) Intrauterine transfusion of the foetus in haemolytic disease. *Brit. med. J.*, **ii**, 1107.

Lilly, A. W. (1965) The use of amniocentesis and fetal transfusion in erythroblastosis fetalis. *Pediatrics*, **35**, 836.

Little, B., McCutcheon, E. & Desforges, J. F. (1966) Amniocentesis and intrauterine transfusion in Rh-sensitized pregnancy. *New Eng. J. Med.*, **274**, 332.

Loos, L. (1892) Die Anämie bei hereditärer Syphiles. *Wien klin. Wchnschr.*, **5**, 291.

Lopez, R. & Cooperman, J. M. (1971) Glucose–6–phosphate dehydrogenase deficiency and hyperbilirubinemia in the newborn. *Amer. J. Dis. Child.*, **122**, 66.

Lunay, G. G., Edwards, R. F. & Thomas, D. B. (1970) Chronic transplacental haemorrhage causing acute fetal distress. *Brit. med. J.*, **ii**, 218.

McGovern, J. J., Driscall, R., Dutiot, C. H., Grove-Rasmussen, M. & Bedell, R. F. (1958) Iron deficiency anemia resulting from fetomaternal transfusion. *New Eng. J. Med.*, **258**, 1149.

McKay, R. J. (1964) Current status of exchange transfusion in newborn infants. *J. Pediat.*, **33**, 763.

McMullin, G. P., Hayes, M. F. & Arorar, S. C. (1970) Phenobarbitone in Rhesus haemolytic disease. A controlled trial. *Lancet*, **ii**, 949.

Mauer, A. M. (1969) *Pediatric Hematology*. New York: McGraw Hill.

Medearis, D. N. (1957) Cytomegalic inclusion disease. An analysis of the clinical features based on the literature and six additional cases. *Pediatrics*, **19**, 467.

Medical Research Council (1974) Controlled trial of various anti-D dosages in suppression of Rh sensitization following pregnancy. *Brit. med. J.*, **ii**, 75.

Mellish, P. & Wolman, I. J. (1958) Intraperitoneal blood transfusions. *Am. J. Med. Sci.*, **235**, 717.

Miles, R. M., Maurer, H. M. & Valdes, O. S. (1971) Iron-deficiency anemia at birth: Two examples secondary to chronic fetal-maternal hemorrhage. *Clinical Pediatrics*, **10**, 223.

Miller, D. R., Hanshaw, J. B., O'Leary, D. S. & Hnilicka, J. V. (1970) Fatal disseminated herpes simplex virus infection and hemorrhage in the neonate. *J. Pediatrics*, **76**, 409.

Moe, P. J. & Skjaeveland, A. (1969) Therapeutic studies in osteopetrosis—Report of 4 cases. *Acta Paediat. Scand.*, **58**, 593.

Mollison, P. L. (1972) Quantitation of transplacental haemorrhage. *Brit. med. J.*, **ii**, 31.

Morris, E. D., Murray, J. & Ruthven, C. R. J. (1967) Liquor bilirubin levels in normal pregnancy: A basis for accurate prediction of haemolytic disease. *Brit. med. J.*, **ii**, 352.

Naiman, J. L. & Kosoy, M. H. (1964) Red cell glucose–6–phosphate dehydrogenase deficiency—A newly recognized cause of neonatal jaundice and kernicterus in Canada. *Canad. M.A.J.*, **91**, 1243.

Naiman, J. L. (1972) Current management of hemolytic disease of the newborn infants. *J. Pediat.*, **80**, 1049.

Naiman, J. L., Punnett, H. H., Lischer, H. W., Destinè, M. I. & Arey, J. V. (1969) Possible graft-versus host reaction after intrauterine transfusion for Rh erythroblastosis fetalis. *New Eng. J. Med.*, **281**, 697.

Necheles, T. F., Boles, T. A. & Allen, D. M. (1968) Erythrocyte glutathione peroxidase deficiency and haemolytic disease of the newborn infant. *J. Pediat.*, **72**, 319.

Necheles, T. F. & Allen, D. M. (1969) Heinz-body anemias. *New Eng. J. Med.*, **280**, 203.

Neligan, G. A. & Russell, J. K. (1955) Anaemia of the newborn following anterior placenta praevia. *Brit. med. J.*, **i**, 164.

Odell, G. B., Bryan, W. B. & Richmond, M. D. (1962A) Exchange transfusion. *Ped. Clin. N. Amer.*, **9**, 605.

Odell, G. B., Cohen, S. N. & Gordes, E. H. (1962B) Administration of albumin in the management of hyperbilirubinemia by exchange transfusions. *Pediat.*, **30**, 613.

Odell, G. B. (1967) Physiologic hyperbilirubinemia in the neonatal period. *New Eng. J. Med.*, **277**, 193.

Odell, G. B., Cohen, S. N. & Kelly, P. C. (1969) Studies in kernicterus. II. The determination of the saturation of serum albumin with bilirubin. *J. Pediat.*, **74**, 214.

Odell, G. B., Storey, G. N. B. & Rosenberg, L. A. (1970) Studies in kernicterus. III. The saturation of serum proteins with bilirubin during neonatal life and its relationship to brain damage at five years. *J. Pediat.*, **76**, 12.

Oski, F. A. & Diamond, L. K. (1963) Erythrocyte pyruvate kinase deficiency: Report of three cases. *New Eng. J. Med.*, **269**, 763.

Oski, F. A., Allen, D. M. & Diamond, L. K. (1963) Portal hypertension—a complication of umbilical vein catheterization. *Pediatrics*, **31**, 297.

Oski, F. A. & Naiman, J. L. (1963) Red cell binding of bilirubin. *J. Pediat.*, **63**, 1034.

Oski, F. A., Nathan, D. G., Sidel, V. W. & Diamond, L. K. (1964) Extreme haemolysis and red cell distortion in erythrocyte pyruvate kinase deficiency. I. Morphology, erythrokinetics and family enzyme studies. *New Eng. J. Med.*, **270**, 1023.

Oski, F. A. & Barness, L. A. (1967) Vitamin E deficiency: A previously unrecognized cause of hemolytic anemia in the premature infant. *J. Pediat.*, **70**, 211.

Oski, F. A. & Naiman, J. L. (1972A) Hematologic problems in the newborn 2nd edn., p. 73. Vol. IV. *Major Problems in Clinical Pediatrics*. Philadelphia: Saunders.

Oski, F. A. & Naiman, J. L. (1972B) Hematologic problems in the newborn, 2nd edn., p. 78, Vol. IV. In *Major Problems in Clinical Pediatrics*. Philadelphia: Saunders.

Oski, F. A. & Naiman, J. L. (1972D) Hematologic problems in the newborn, 2nd edn., p. 125, Vol. IV. In *Major Problems in Clinical Pediatrics*. Philadelphia: Saunders.

Oski, F. A. & Naiman, J. L. (1972E) Hematologic problems in the newborn, 2nd edn., p. 127, Vol. IV. In *Major Problems in Clinical Pediatrics*. Philadelphia: Saunders.

Oski, F. A. & Naiman, J. L. (1972F) Hematologic problems in the newborn, 2nd edn., p. 154, Vol. IV. In *Major Problems in Clinical Pediatrics*. Philadelphia: Saunders.

Oski, F. A. & Naiman, J. L. (197C) Hematologic problems in the newborn, 2nd edn., p. 117, Vol. IV. In *Major Problems in Clinical Pediatrics*. Philadelphia: Saunders.

Paglia, D. E., Holland, P., Baughan, M. A. & Valentine, W. N. (1969) Occurrence of defective hexomonophosphate isomerization in human erythrocytes and leukocytes. *New Eng. J. Med.*, **280**, 66.

Paloheimo, J., Essen, R. von, Klemola, E., Kääriänen, L. & Siltanen, P. (1968) Subclinical cytomegalovirus infections and cytomegalovirus mononucleosis after open heart surgery. *Am. J. Cardiol.*, **22**, 624.

Parkman, R., Mosier, D., Umansky, I., Cochran, W., Carpenter, C. B. & Rosen, F. S. (1974) Graft–versus–host disease after transfusions for hemolysis in newborn. *New Eng. J. Med.*, **290**, 359.

Pasternak, A., Furuhjelm, V., van Knoring, J., Skrefvars, B. & Kuhlbäck, B. (1966) Acute renal failure after haemolysis, probably due to foeto-maternal transfusion. *Acta Med. Scand.*, **180**, 13.

Pearson, H. A. & Diamond, L. K. (1959) Fetomaternal transfusion. *A.M.A. J. Dis. Child.*, **97**, 267.

Pearson, H. A. (1967) Life span of the fetal red blood cell. *J. Pediat.*, **70**, 166.

Petersen, H. S. (1972) Pycnocytotic haemolytic anaemia of the newborn. *Acta Pediat. Scand.*, **61**, 362.

Phibbs, R. H., Harvin, D., Jones, G., Talbot, C., Cohen, C., Crowther, D. & Tooley, W. H. (1971) Development of children who had received intrauterine transfusions. *Pediatrics*, **47**, 689.

Phibbs, R. H., Johnson, P., Kitterman, J. A., Gregory, G. A. & Tooley, W. H. (1972) Cardiorespiratory status of erythroblastic infants. I. Relationship of gestational age, severity of hemolytic disease, and birth asphyxia to idiopathic respiratory distress syndrome and survival. *Pediat.*, **49**, 5.

Pierson, W. E., Barrett, C. T. & Oliver, T. K. (1968) The effect of buffered and non-buffered ACD blood on electrocyte and acid-base homeostatis during exchange transfusion. *Pediatrics*, **41**, 802.

Pochedly, C. & Ente, G. (1969) Fetal bleeding: A dual menace. *Postgrad. Med.*, **45**, 157.

Pollack, A. (1968) Transplacental haemorrhage after external cephalic version.

Pomerance, W., Moltz, A., Biezenski, J. J. & Wolf, L. (1968) Spectrophotometric analysis of amniotic fluid in Rh-negative women. *Obstet. Gynec.*, **31**, 390.

Porter, E. G. & Waters, W. J. (1966) A rapid micromethod for measuring the reserve albumin binding capacity in serum from newborn infants with hyperbilirubinemia. *J. Lab. Clin. Med.*, **67**, 660.

Preston, F. E., Malia, R. G., Sworn, M. J. & Blackburn, E. K. (1973) Intravascular coagulation and *E. coli* septicaemia. *J. clin. Path.*, **26**, 120.

Pridmore, B. R., Robertson, E. G. & Walker, W. (1972) Liquor bilirubin levels and false prediction of severity in rhesus haemolytic disease. *Brit. med. J.*, **iii**, 136.

Queenan, J. T. (1967) *Modern Management of the Rh Problem*, p. 152. Hoeber Medical Division. New York: Harper and Row.

Queenan, J. T. & Nakamoto, M. (1964) Postpartum immunization: the hypothetical hazard of manual removal of the placenta. *Obstet. Gynec.*, **23**, 392.

Queenan, J. T. & Adams, D. W. (1964) Amniocentesis: a possible immunizing hazard. *Obstet. Gynec.*, **24**, 530.

Queenan, J. T., Anderson, G. G. & Mead, P. B. (1966) Intrauterine transfusion by the multiple-needle technique. *J.A.M.A.*, **196**, 664.

Queenan, J. T., Lanzkowsky, P. & Golobow, J. (1968) Significance of amniotic fluid volume in the interpretation of amniotic fluid-spectrophotometric analysis in antenatal management of erythroblastosis foetalis. Abstract. Soc. Pediat. Research, Atlantic City, May, 1968, p. 128.

Ratten, G. J. (1969) Spontaneous haematoma of the umbilical cord. *Austral. New Zeal. J. Obstet. Gynec.*, **9**, 125.

Rausen, A. R. Seki, M. & Strauss, L. (1965) Twin transfussion syndrome. A review of 19 cases studied at one institution. *J. Pediat.*, **66**, 613.

Rausen, A. R., Richter, P., Tallal, L. & Cooper, L. Z. (1967) Hematologic effects of intrauterine rubella. *J.A.M.A.*, **199**, 75.

Raye, J. R., Gutberlet, R. L. & Stahlman, M. (1970) Symptomatic posthemorrhagic anemia in the newborn. *Ped. Clin. N.A.*, **17**, 401.

Reider, R. F., Zinkham, W. H. & Holtzman, N. A. (1965) Hemoglobin Zürich. Clinical, chemical and kinetic studies. *Amer. J. Med.*, **39**, 4.

Robertson, J. G. (1964) Examination of amniotic fluid in Rhesus isoimmunization. *Brit. med. J.*, **ii**, 147.

Robinson, G. C. (1957) Hereditary spherocytosis in infancy. *J. Pediat.*, **50**, 446.

Roddy, R. (1954) Two cases of hereditary spherocytosis manifest in the newborn period. *J. Pediat.*, **44**, 213.

Ross, J. D. (1963) Deficient activity of DPNH-dependent methemoglobin diaphorase in cord blood erythrocytes. *Blood*, **21**, 51.

Sacks, M. O. (1959) Occurrence of anemia and polycythemia in phenotypically dissimilar single ovum human twins. *Pediat.*, **24**, 604.

Saigal, S., O'Neill, A., Surainder, Y., Chua, Le-B. & Usher, R. (1972) Placental transfusion and hyperbilirubinemia in the premature. *Pediatrics*, **49**, 406.

Schafer, W. B. (1951) Acute hemolytic anemia related to naphthalene. Report of a case in a newborn infant. *Pediatrics*, **7**, 172.

Schmid, R., Brecher, G. & Clemens, T. (1959) Familial hemolytic anemia with erythrocyte inclusion bodies and a defect in pigment metabolism. *Blood*, **14**, 991.

Schröter, W. (1965) Kongenital nichtsphärocytare hämolytische Anämie bei 2, –3 diphospho-glyceramutase-mangel der Erythrocyten im fruhen Säuglingsalter. *Klin. Wschr.*, **43**, 1147.

Schulman, I. (1959) The anemia of prematurity. *J. Pediat.*, **54**, 663.

Scott, J. L., Haut, A., Carwright, G. E. & Wintrobe, M. M. (1960) Congenital hemolytic anemia associated with red cell inclusion bodies, abnormal pigment metabolism and an electrophoretic hemoglobin abnormality. *Blood*, **16**, 1239.

Seelen, J., Van Kessel, H., Eskes, T., Van Leusden, H., Been, J., Evers, J., Van Gent., I., Peeters, L., Van Der Velden, W. & Zonderland, F. (1966) A new method of exchange transfusion *in utero*. Cannulation of vessels on the fetal side of the human placenta. *Am. J. Obstet. Gynec.*, **95**, 872.

Stamey, C. C. & Diamond, L. K. (1957) Congenital hemolytic anemia in the newborn. Relation to kernicterus. *Am. J. Dis. Child.*, **94**, 616.

Stern, H. & Tucker, S. M. (1973) Prospective study of cytomegalovirus infection in pregnancy. *Brit. med. J.*, **2**, 268.

Stewart, A. G. & Taylor, W. C. (1964) Amniotic fluid analysis as an acid to the antepartum diagnosis of haemolytic disease. *J. Obstet. Gynec. Brit. Cwlth.*, **71**, 604.

Stocks, J., Kemp, M. & Dormandy, T. L. (1971) Increased susceptibility of red-blood-cell lipids to autoxidation in haemolytic states. *Lancet*, **i**, 266.

Sullivan, J. F., Peckham, N. H. & Jennings, E. R. (1967) Rh isoimmunization. Its incidence, timing and relationship to fetal-maternal hemorrhage. *Am. J. Obstet. Gynec.*, **98**, 877.

Sweet, L., Reid, W. D. & Roberton, N. R. C. (1973) Hydrops with placental chorioangioma. *J. Pediat.*, **82**, 91.

Thumasathit, B., Nondasuta, A., Jilpisornkosol, S., Lousuebsakul, B., Unchalipongse, P. & Mangkornkanok, M. (1968) Hydrops fetalis associated with Bart's hemoglobin in Northern Thailand. *J. Pediat.*, **73**, 132.

Todd, D., Lai, M. C. S., Braga, C. A. & Soo, H. N. (1969) Alpha-thalassaemia in Chinese: cord blood studies. *Brit. J. Haemat.*, **16**, 551.

Tovey, G. H., Lockyer, J. W., Blades, A. N. & Flavell, H. C. G. (1962) Antenatal prediction of ABO haemolytic disease. *Brit. J. Haemat.*, **8**, 251.

Tovey, L. A. D. & Haggas, W. K. (1971) Prediction of the severity of Rhesus haemolytic disease by means of antibody titrations performed on the autoanalyser. *Brit. J. Haemat.*, **20**, 25.

Trucco, J. T. & Brown, A. K. (1967) Neonatal manifestations of hereditary spherocytosis. *Am. J. Dis. Child.*, **113**, 263.

Tuffy, P., Brown, A. K. & Zuelzer, W. W. (1959) Infantile pyknocytosis. A common erythrocyte abnormality of the first trimester. *Am. J. Dis. Child.*, **98**, 227.

Valaes, T., Karaklis, A., Stravrakakis, D., Bavela-Stravrakakis, K., Perakis, A. & Doxiadis, S. A. (1969) Incidence and mechanism of neonatal jaundice related to glucose-6–phosphate dehydrogenase deficiency. *Pediat. Res.*, **3**, 448.

Valentine, W. N., Oski, F. A., Paglia, D. E., Baughan, M. A., Schneider, A. S. & Naiman, J. L. (1967) Hereditary hemolytic anemia with hexokinase deficiency. Role of hexokinase in erythrocyte ageing. *New Eng. J. Med.*, **276**, 1.

Vaughan, V. C., Allen, F. H. & Diamond, L. K. (1950) Erythroblastosis fetalis. IV. Further observations on kernicterus. *Pediatrics*, **6**, 706.

Walker, A. H. C. (1957) Liquor amnii studies in the prediction of haemolytic disease of the newborn (101 cases). *Brit. med. J.*, **ii**, 376.

Walker, W. (1970) Rh haemolytic disease. Role of liquor examination. *Brit. med. J.*, **ii**, 220.

Walker, W., Fairweather, D. V. I. & Jones, P. (1964) Examination of liquor amnii as a method of predicting severity of haemolytic disease of the newborn. *Brit. med. J.*, **ii**, 141.

Walker, W. & Ellis, M. I. (1970) Intrauterine transfusion. *Brit. med. J.*, **ii**, 223.

Wang, M. Y. F., McCutcheon, E. & Desforges, J. F. (1967) Fetomaternal hemorrhage from diagnostic transabdominal amniocentesis. *Amer. J. Obstet. Gynec.*, **97**, 1123.

Waters, W. J. & Porter, E. G. (1964) Indications for exchange transfusion based upon the role of albumin in the treatment of hemolytic disease of the newborn. *Pediatrics*, **33**, 749.

Weil, M. H., Shubin, N. & Biddle, M. (1964) Shock caused by gram-negative microorganisms. *Annals Intern. Med.*, **60**, 384.

Weisert, O. & Marstrander, J. (1960) Severe anemia in a newborn caused by protracted foeto-maternal 'transfusion'. *Acta Paediat.*, **49**, 426.

Wentworth, P. (1964) A placental lesion to account for foetal haemorrhage into the maternal circulation. *J. Obstet. Gynaec. Brit. Cwlth.*, **71**, 379.

Whitaker, J. A., Sartain, P. & Shaheedy, M. (1965) Hematological aspects of congenital syphilis. *J. Pediat.*, **66**, 629.

White, J. M. & Jones, R. W. (1969) Management of pregnancy in a woman with Hb H disease. *Brit. med. J.*, **iv**, 474.

Whitfield, C. R., Chan, W. H., Sproule, W. B. & Stewart, A. D. (1972) Amniotic fluid lecithin: sphingomyelin ratio and fetal lung developement. *Brit. med. J.*, **ii**, 85.

Willi, H. & Hartmeier, F. (1950) Spontane Innenkörperbildung beim Neugeborenen. *Schweiz. med. Wschr.*, **80**, 1091.

Wilson, J. T. (1969) Phenobarbital in the perinatal period. *Pediatrics*, **43**, 324.

Wong, T. T. T. & Chan, M. C. K. (1972) Transfusion reaction following ABO–incompatible maternal transfusion. *J. Pediat.*, **80**, 479.

Woodrow, J. C., Bowley, C. C., Gilliver, B. E. & Strong, S. J. (1968) Prevention of Rh immunization due to large volumes of Rh-positive blood. *Brit. med. J.*, **i**, 148.

Woodrow, J. C. & Donohoe, W. T. A. (1968) Rh immunisation by pregnancy: Results of a survey and their relevance to prophylactic therapy. *Brit. med. J.*, **ii**, 139.

Zannos-Mariolea, L., Kattamis, C. & Paidouces, M. (1962) Infantile pyknocytosis and glucose–6–phosphate dehydrogenase deficiency. *Brit. J. Haemat.*, **8**, 258.

Zinkham, W. H. (1963) Peripheral blood and bilirubin values in normal full-term primaquine sensitive Negro infants. *Pediatrics*, **31**, 983.

Zipursky, A., Hull, A., White, F. D. & Israels, L. G. (1959) Foetal erythrocytes in the maternal circulation. *Lancet*, **1**, 451.

Zipursky, A., Pollock, J., Chown, B. & Israels, L. G. (1963) Transplacental foetal haemorrhage after placental injury during delivery or amniocentesis. *Lancet*, **2**, 493.

Zipursky, A. & Israels, L. G. (1967) The pathogenesis and prevention of Rh immunization. *Canad. Med. Assoc. J.*, **97**, 1245.

Zuelzer, W. W. & Apt, L. (1949) Acute hemolytic anemia due to naphthalene poisoning: A clinical and experimental study. *J. Amer. Med. Ass.*, **141**, 185.

Zuelzer, W. W. & Mudgett, R. T. (1950) Kernicterus. Etiological study based on an analysis of 55 cases. *Pediatrics*, **6**, 452.

II. Anaemias in the Neonatal Period. 2. ABO Haemolytic Disease of the Newborn (ABO HDNB)

Pathogenesis / Clinical features / Laboratory findings / Management, *Photototherapy and phenobarbitone therapy* / Other blood group incompatibilities

---

Halbrecht, in 1944, first recognized that a hitherto unexplained form of neonatal jaundice (icterus praecox) was usually associated with ABO incompatibility between the infant and its mother. Like Rh disease (icterus gravis) ABO HDNB can cause jaundice in the first 24 hours after birth but the severity of jaundice, anaemia and hepatosplenomegaly are in general much less. Reports of stillbirth, such as that of Miller and Petrie (1963), are quite exceptional. The rarity of severe foetal anaemia in this disease makes antenatal assessment unnecessary, unlike the situation in Rh disease. Neonatal investigations are primarily concerned with confirming the diagnosis of ABO HDNB in infants showing early jaundice, since alternative causes such as infection would otherwise have to be pursued. Management is primarily concerned with the prevention of kernicterus and the treatment of late anaemia.

PATHOGENESIS

Approximately 20 per cent of pregnancies are ABO incompatible, the foetus possessing an A or B antigen which its mother lacks. In all such instances the naturally occurring anti-A or anti-B will be present in the mother's serum, yet in only about 10 per cent of such ABO incompatible pregnancies do the maternal antibodies affect the foetus. Furthermore it is almost exclusively among group O mothers that ABO haemolytic disease is found (Rosenfield, 1955).

Whereas the normal ABO isoagglutinins are predominantly of the macroglobulin 19S (or IgM) type which do not cross the placenta, 'immune' anti-A or anti-B which are 7S (or IgG) in type are found in about 10 per cent of unselected adults, but in all of those mothers with a history of ABO haemolytic disease (Kochwa et al., 1961). These smaller antibodies appear to be in equilibrium on both sides of the placenta, as are Rhesus antibodies (Table 11.1). The isoagglutinins (anti-A or anti-B) found in group O individuals are more likely to contain an 'immune' fraction than are those of group A or B individuals (Abelson and Rawson, 1961; Polley et al., 1963), accounting for the rarity of ABO haemolytic disease in group B or A mothers. Immune anti-A or anti-B may be found in individuals of either sex, being independent of transplacental passage of foetal cells or

---

Table 11.1   Properties of two types of ABO isoantibodies compared

	Naturally occurring	Immune
Cross placenta	—	+
Lyse A or B cells *in vitro*	+	+ +
Sensitize A or B cells to Coombs reagent	—	+
Agglutination *in vitro* enhanced by serum	—	+
Lysis of A^p (PIG) cells	—	+
Agglutination of A or B cells in saline	+	—
Agglutination inhibited by soluble A/B substance	+	—
Immunoglobulin type	IgM	IgG
Sedimentation units	19 S (with minor 11 S and 12 S components)	7 S
Elution from DEAE column (by phosphate buffer at pH 8·1)	0·12–0·3 M	0·01–0·02 M
Inhibition of reactivity by 2-mercaptoethanol	+	—

Data largely from Polley et al., 1963 and Fong et al., 1966.

CLINICAL FEATURES

As indicated above the usual presentation is jaundice occurring in the first 24 hours of life, but it may appear later than this in mild forms of the disease. ABO HDNB is not confined to second and subsequent pregnancies (cf. Rh disease), approximately half the affected babies being first-born. Neither is there any consistent tendency for subsequent babies to be more severely affected, sometimes they are less so (Oski and Naiman, 1972). Premature infants seem less prone to ABO HDNB perhaps due to the weaker A and B red cell antigens present before birth (Mauer, 1969). Neither hepatosplenomegaly nor haemorrhagic manifestations were recorded in the original series of Halbrecht and only 3 out of 12 infants had mild anaemia. Marked anaemia and hepatosplenomegaly, however, may occasionally occur in more severe forms of the disease (Boineau and Hallock, 1971).

Kernicterus has been well-documented in early reports such as that of Grumbach and Gasser (1948). It is probable that the hazard appears when serum bilirubin levels reach 20 mg per 100 ml as in Rh disease.

Late anaemia, appearing at 2 to 6 weeks, is seldom severe (Crawford et al., 1953) but exceptions occur among infants in whom ET was narrowly avoided. ET would have provided a population of group O cells resistant to premature haemolysis. Widespread use of phototherapy may increase this problem (Lanzkowsky et al., 1971).

LABORATORY FINDINGS

Many of these infants develop elevated indirect serum bilirubin levels without anaemia. There is usually, however, evidence of compensated haemolysis with more than 10 normoblasts per 100 white cells and more than 7 per cent reticulocytes. These figures represent the upper limit of normal in term infants at birth (Javert, 1939; Zinkham, 1963).

Spherocytes are present in 80 per cent of infants with ABO HDNB by contrast with Rh disease in which they are absent. Morphologically these are indistinguishable from the cells in hereditary spherocytosis (HS). Both will give increased osmotic fragility and autohaemolysis, but added glucose corrects the autohaemolysis in HS and not in ABO HDNB (Kostinas et al., 1967). In practice, examination of the parents' blood for spherocytosis and a compensated haemolytic anaemia, together with a consideration of their blood groups, will readily achieve this distinction in the majority of cases. Distinction may also have to be made from the acquired spherocytes that occur in haemolytic anaemias due to virus infections such as congenital rubella, when they are accompanied by red cell fragmentation and burr cells (Raussen et al., 1967). Thrombocytopenia does not usually occur in ABO HDNB although well recognized in severe Rh disease and in the group of congenital infections that cause haemolysis in the newborn, viz. cytomegalovirus, rubella, syphilis and toxoplasmosis.

Blood grouping shows that the mother is almost invariably group O and the baby is group A or B. A_2 babies can occasionally be affected (Grundbacher, 1965). The ability of the mother's serum to cause visible haemolysis of adult A or B cells at 37°C (in the presence of fresh complement) is strongly suggestive of 'immune' isoagglutinins (alpha- or beta-haemolysins) but is unfortunately not entirely specific, also occurring with some 19S, non-immune forms of antibody (Polley et al., 1963). Even a 'battery' of tests on the mother's serum, such as those shown in Table 11.1, fail to correlate completely with the presence of ABO HDNB (Fong et al., 1966). The chief value of tests for immune anti-A or B in the mother's serum is that ABO HDNB is excluded if the tests are entirely negative.

A more specific finding is the demonstration of free anti-A in the serum of a group A baby, or anti-B in a group B baby. This is proof that the antibody has crossed from the mother's to the baby's circulation and is therefore 'immune'. In order to ensure maximum sensitivity in this test adult A_1 or B cells should be used since their antigens are more strongly developed than foetal cells. Almost all ABO affected infants show incompatible antibody in their serum in the first 48 hours of life either by the Löw papain or indirect Coombs technique (Gunson, 1957). After 48 hours the test may be negative. Alternatively, antibody can be eluted from the infant's red cells and similarly identified (Yunis and Bridges, 1964; Haberman et al., 1960).

The direct Coombs test is not dependably positive in ABO HDNB. Although the sensitivity is increased with certain selected Coombs sera and modifications of technique the prime source of variability in the direct Coombs reaction is the greater distance between A/B antigenic sites on the foetal red cell compared to adult cells (Voak and Williams, 1971). Foetal A_1 cells correspond to adult A_2 cells in this respect, paralleling their weaker agglutination. The eluted antibodies, however, will react strongly with adult A_1 cells explaining their detection in this way by the indirect Coombs reaction even although the direct Coombs test on the baby's cells is negative.

When the mother is found to have an alpha or beta haemolysin at antenatal blood grouping, or if she has a past history of ABO HDNB it is useful to determine the baby's ABO group and direct Coombs test on cord blood at birth. A technical point to remember is that the ABO antigens are often distinctly weaker at birth than in later life and can lead to the baby being falsely grouped as O; neither can one depend upon the serum 'back-check' in the newborn, viz. the presence of anti-B in group A babies, etc.

MANAGEMENT

Unlike Rh disease there is never any need to consider premature delivery in ABO HDNB. After delivery, however, the keystone of management is the same as in Rh disease, viz. serial bilirubin determinations so as to prevent the serum bilirubin level exceeding 20 mg/100 ml by the use of ET. The peak level is often not reached until the 3rd or 4th day. The indications for ET and the technique are as for Rh disease but group O blood of the same Rh group as the baby are used. The so-called 'dangerous group O donor' with a high titre of alpha haemolysins in their blood clearly should not be used, since these could accentuate the haemolysis of the baby's cells. There has not been found to be any advantage in using group O cells suspended in AB plasma (Goldfarb *et al.*, 1964). In severe cases where multiple ETs are anticipated it has been suggested that there is advantage in adding albumen to the donor blood (see under Rh disease).

Appropriate follow-up is necessary to detect late anaemia for which a straight blood transfusion may occasionally be needed.

Phototherapy and phenobarbitone therapy

These two forms of therapy were introduced to lessen the need for ET by lowering the level of indirect bilirubin in the jaundice of prematurity and in 'physiological jaundice' of term babies. The success in these categories of neonatal jaundice has led to an exploration of the value of these forms of therapy in milder cases of ABO and Rh HDNB.

Since both phenobarbitone and phototherapy

are relatively slow to produce any lowering of the bilirubin they are only appropriately considered when the rate of rise of bilirubin is similarly slow, and will never replace ET when the rise is rapid.

PHENOBARBITONE

This drug can cause enzyme induction of glucuronyl transferase and related enzymes concerned with bilirubin excretion (Wilson, 1969). Glucuronyl transferase activity is often low in newborns, particularly if premature, and catalyses the rate-limiting step in convertion of the potentially neurotoxic, lipid-soluble bilirubin to the harmless, water-soluble glucuronide. Phenobarbitone administration to either the mother, for two weeks before delivery, or to the infant for 3–4 days after birth result in lowering of the serum bilirubin level. Early trials such as that of Trolle (1968) suggested that administration of the drug to the mother was more effective than to the infant. In one recent trial, however, the reverse was found (Yeung *et al.*, 1971). Treating the infant is also more practical since the milder forms of neonatal jaundice are not usually anticipated, especially that due to prematurity.

The value of phenobarbitone therapy in reducing the number of ETs in jaundice associated with prematurity has been established (Vest *et al.*, 1970).

High doses of phenobarbitone given to the infant have also apparently reduced the need for ET in Chinese infants with ABO HDNB or G-6-PD deficiency (Yeung and Field, 1969) as well as in mild Rh disease (McMullin *et al.*, 1970). A recent trial and review of the literature (Carswell *et al.*, 1972) suggests that even the modest reduction of serum bilirubin level attained may be of value, particularly in the pre-term infant in whom kernicterus can develop with a bilirubin level of only 9 mg/100 ml.

Final assessment of the place that phenobarbitone therapy will occupy as an adjunct in the treatment of neonatal jaundice must take account of the lowered levels of prothrombin complex found in infants whose mothers have taken barbiturates (Mountain *et al.*, 1970) and that in one trial phototherapy has proved more efficacious (Valdes *et al.*, 1971).

PHOTOTHERAPY

Light from the blue-violet and yellow-green portions of the spectrum (300–600 mμ) causes progressive photo-oxidation of lipid-soluble bilirubin, first to biliverdin and then to a series of water-soluble, colourless derivatives which do not give the diazo reaction of bilirubin, and which are rapidly excreted in the bile and urine. Animal experiments suggest that these colourless derivatives are non-toxic. A symposium on the effect of light upon bilirubin metabolism and its clinical application forms the basis of a fundamental review on the subject by Behrman and Hsia (1969). Clinical indications and technical details of phototherapy are fully described in this review.

As with phenobarbitone the clearest evidence of clinical benefit has been in the jaundice of prematurity (Lucey et al., 1968). A recent randomized trial in low birth weight Black infants showed that the serum bilirubin exceeded 10 mg per 100 ml in none of the group given phototherapy compared to 26 per cent in those given phenobarbitone (5 mg/kg/day) and 67 per cent in those having neither treatment (Valdes et al., 1971). In the case of ABO HDNB Sisson et al. (1971) found that phototherapy (visible blue light 410–490 mμ) caused a marked decline of serum bilirubin at a time when such levels were rising in control infants with this disease. Five out of 16 of the control group required ET, but none out of the 19 given phototherapy. Kaplan et al. (1971) similarly found a benefit in ABO HDNB but warned that in severely affected infants the institution of phototherapy must not exclude consideration of ET. Failure of phototherapy to control the rise in serum bilirubin has also been reported in ABO and Rh disease (Sisson et al., 1971; Patel et al., 1970). It is important that the phototherapy is monitored by serial serum bilirubin levels since clinical jaundice may be masked in the presence of hyperbilirubinaemia during this treatment. The skin is decolorized before serum levels are affected (Lucey, 1972). Continuous phototherapy is more effective than intermittent (Maurer et al., 1973).

Caution has been expressed regarding phototherapy on the following scores: (a) possible red cell damage increasing haemolysis (Odell et al., 1972), (b) an increased incidence of severe late anaemia when there is an underlying haemolytic state (Lanzkowsky et al., 1971), (c) the development of kernicterus in spite of apparent control of the bilirubin level in small, sick premature infants (Keenan et al., 1972), (d) a late effect of growth retardation including reduced head circumference and (e) eye damage. These problems have recently been reviewed (Lucey, 1972; B.M.J. 1972). The place of phototherapy in the management of haemolytic disease of the newborn has not therefore been finally delineated but it appears to be capable of reducing the need for ET in the milder forms of haemolysis. It may also prove of greater applicability and efficacy than phenobarbitone therapy.

OTHER BLOOD GROUP INCOMPATIBILITIES

Although a foetus will often differ from its mother in the possession of red cell antigens such as c̄, ē, E, Duffy (Fy [a and b]), Kell (K) Kidd (Jk [a and b]), M or S it is seldom that the mother develops immune antibodies to these 'minor' blood groups. The antigens are far less immunogenic than 'D' and the immunizing event in the mother is more often a previous blood transfusion (involving 400–500 ml of blood) rather than a foeto-maternal haemorrhage (involving only 0·2 ml or so). If a subsequent foetus should by chance possess the corresponding antigen it will be liable to haemolysis although, in general, this is less severe than that in Rh disease, due to anti-D. Postnatal hyperbilirubinaemia and late anaemia (7·5 g/100 ml at 49 days) can occur even although ET was not required, for instance with anti-S (Feldman et al., 1973).

The problem will come to light if a suitable antibody screening test both for Rh and non-Rh antibodies is routinely included in the blood grouping procedure for all antenatal patients. The presence of these antibodies will remain unknown if antibody tests are restricted to Rh negative mothers. Since anti-c̄, for instance, can produce quite severe haemolytic disease of the newborn it is desirable that the presence of these maternal antibodies is known.

Alternatively the antibodies may come to light during investigation of neonatal jaundice. In many instances the direct Coombs test on the baby's cells will be positive yet the mother may be Rh positive and the baby ABO compatible with its mother. Testing the mother's serum against papainized O R_1R_2 cells (CDe/cDE) will detect antibodies to any of the Rhesus antigens (c̄, ē, C,D,E) while testing it by indirect Coombs reaction against a group of O cells selected to contain S, Duffy, Kell, Lewis and Kidd antigens will detect most other immune antibodies. Those antibodies that have produced recognizable haemolytic disease of the newborn are shown in Table 11.2. Anti-Lewis antibodies are, in fact, very unlikely to produce disease or a positive direct Coombs test since the antigens, Le^a and Le$_b$, are not normally developed until some time after birth. Many instances of anti-Kell can likewise be disregarded since 9 out of 10 fathers will be Kell negative, in which case the baby will be

ANAEMIAS IN THE NEONATAL PERIOD. 2. ABO HAEMOLYTIC DISEASE OF THE NEWBORN

Table 11.2 Erythroblastosis foetalis due to maternal antibodies outside the RH and ABO systems

System	Severity of HDNB	Reference
Kell	Usually mild but occasionally severe or fatal	Coombs et al. (1946)
Duffy	Mild to severe	Baker et al. (1956)
Kidd	Mild	Zodin and Anderson (1965)
S	Can cause kernicterus	Levine et al. (1952)
M	Mild to severe, with stillbirths. Spherocytosis can occur	Stone and Marsh (1959)
Lewis	Mild: direct Coombs −ve. Spherocytes present	Schwenzer and Spielmann (1957)

Mild Rh disease may be caused by anti-E and relatively severe disease by anti-$\bar{c}$, both within the Rh system although the antibodies occur in Rh positive mothers, usually R_1R_1.

unaffected. As mentioned above, the antibody will usually have been induced by previous blood transfusion. It is clear that on discovering any immune antibody in a mother's serum the next investigative step is to determine whether the husband possesses the corresponding antigen in single (heterozygous) or double (homozygous) dose. If he possesses the antigen then maternal antibody titres are performed throughout pregnancy as in Rh disease. If the titre of anti-$\bar{c}$ or anti-Kell rises above 1 in 8 by indirect Coombs or if there is a history of a previously affected baby then amniocentesis is performed at around 30 weeks and the subsequent management is as described under Rh disease (Lilly, 1965; Naiman, 1972).

Occasionally a mother may develop immune antibodies to a rare or unique or 'private' antigen present in her husband and children. In these circumstances the baby may show a positive direct Coombs test but testing the mother's serum against even a large panel of cells may fail to detect the antibody. The key investigation is to test her serum against the husband's cells or those of her other children, when the antibody should be detected (Finney et al., 1973).

REFERENCES

Abelson, N. M. & Rawson, A. J. (1961) Studies of blood group antibodies. *V. Transfusion*, **1**, 116.

Baker, J. B., Grewar, D., Lewis, M., Ayukawa, H. & Chown, B. (1956) Haemolytic disease of the newborn due to anti-Duffy (Fyª). *Arch. Dis. Childh.*, **31**, 298.

Behrman, R. E. & Hsia, D. Y. Y. (1969) Summary of a symposium on phototherapy for hyperbilirubinaemia. *J. Pediat.*, **75**, 718.

Boineau, F. G. & Hallock, J. A. (1971) Two examples of severe fetal disease due to ABO incompatibility. *Clin. Pediat.*, **10**, 180.

British Medical Journal (1972) Leading Article: Phototherapy in neonatal jaundice. *Brit. med. J.*, **ii**, 62.

Carswell, F., Kerr, M. M. & Dunsmore, I. R. (1972) Sequential trial of effect of phenobarbitone on serum bilirubin of preterm infants. *Arch. Dis. Childh.*, **47**, 621.

Coombs, R. R. A., Mourant, A. E. & Race, R. R. (1946) *In vivo* isosensitisation of red cells in babies with haemolytic disease. *Lancet*, **1**, 264.

Crawford, H., Cutbush, M. & Mollison, P. L. (1953) Hemolytic disease of the newborn due to anti-A. *Blood*, **8**, 620.

Feldman, R., Luhby, A. L. & Gromisch, D. S. (1973) Anti-S erythroblastosis fetalis. *J. Pediat.*, **82**, 88.

Finney, R. D., Blue, A. M. & Willoughby, M. L. N. (1973) Haemolytic disease of the newborn caused by the rare rhesus antibody anti-Cˣ. *Vox Sang.*, **25**, 39.

Fong, S. W., Nuckton, A. & Fudenberg, H. H. (1966) Characterization of maternal isoagglutinins in ABO hemolytic disease of the newborn. *Blood*, **27**, 17.

Goldfarb, D. L., Ginsberg, V., Kaufman, M., Robinson, M. G. & Watson, R. J. (1964) Hemolytic disease of the newborn due to ABO incompatibility: A study of the use of group O erythrocytes in AB plasma. *Pediatrics*, **34**, 664.

Gunson, H. H. (1957) An evaluation of the immunohematological tests used in the diagnosis of AB hemolytic disease. *Am. J. Dis. Child.*, **94**, 123.

Grumbach, A. & Gasser, C. (1948) ABO-Inkompatibilitäten und morbus haemolyticus neonatorum. *Helv. Paediat. Acta.*, **3**, 447.

Grundbacher, F. J. (1965) ABO hemolytic disease of the newborn: A family study with emphasis on the strength of the A antigen. *Pediat.*, **35**, 916.

Haberman, S., Krafft, J., Luecke, P. E. & Peach, R. O. (1960) ABO isoimmunization: the use of the specific Coombs and heat elution tests in the detection of haemolytic disease. *J. Pediat.*, **56**, 471.

Halbrecht, I. (1944) Role of hemagglutinins anti-A and anti-B in pathogenesis of jaundice of the newborn (icterus neonatorum precox). *Am. J. Dis. Child.*, **68**, 248.

Javert, C. T. (1939) The occurrence and significance of the nucleated erythrocytes in the fetal vessels of the placenta. *Am. J. Obst. Gynec.*, **37**, 184.

Kaplan, E., Herz, F., Scheye, E. & Robinson, D. (1971) Phototherapy in ABO hemolytic disease of the newborn infant. *J. Pediat.*, **79**, 911.

Keenan, W. J., Perlstein, P. H., Light, I. J. & Sutherland, J. M. (1972) Kernicterus in small sick premature infants receiving phototherapy. *Pediatrics*, **49**, 652.

Kochwa, S., Rosenfield, R. E., Tallal, L. & Wasserman, L. R. (1961) Isoagglutinins associated with ABO erythroblastosis. *J. Clin. Invest.*, **40**, 874.

Kostinas, J. E., Cantow, E. F. & Wetzel, R. A. (1967) Autohaemolysis of cord blood in congenital spherocytosis and ABO incompatibility. *J. Pediat.*, **70**, 273.

Lanzkowsky, P., Salemi, M. & Gootman, N. (1971) Phototherapy – A note of caution. *Pediatrics*, **48**, 969.

Levine, P., Ferraro, L. R. & Koch, E. (1952) Hemolytic disease of the newborn due to anti-S. A case report with a review of 12 anti-S sera cited in the literature. *Blood*, **7**, 1030.

Lilly, A. W. (1965) The use of amniocentesis and fetal transfusion in erythroblastosis fetalis. *Pediatrics*, **35**, 836.

Lucey, J. F. (1972) Neonatal jaundice and phototherapy. *Pediat. Clin. N. Am.*, **19**, 827.

Lucey, J. F., Ferreiro, M. & Hewitt, J. (1968) Prevention of hyperbilirubinemia of prematurity by phototherapy. *Pediat.*, **41**, 1047.

McMullin, G. P., Hayes, M. F. & Arora, S. C. (1970) Phenobarbitone in rhesus haemolytic disease. A controlled trial. *Lancet*, **ii**, 949.

Mauer, A. M. (1969) *Pediatric Hematology*, p. 62. New York: McGraw-Hill.

Maurer, H. M., Shumway, C. N., Draper, D. A. & Hossaini, A. A. (1973) Controlled trial comparing agar, intermittent phototherapy and continuous phototherapy for reducing neonatal hyperbilirubinemia. *J. Pediat.*, **82**, 73.

Miller, D. F. & Petrie, S. J. (1963) Fatal erythroblastosis fetalis secondary to ABO incompatibility. *Obst. Gynec.*, **22**, 773.

Mountain, K. R., Hirsh, J. & Gallus, A. S. (1970) Neonatal coagulation defect due to anticonvulsant drug treatment in pregnancy. *Lancet*, **1**, 265.

Naiman, J. L. (1972) Current management of hemolytic disease of the newborn infant. *J. Pediat.*, **89**, 1049.

Odell, G. B., Brown, R. S. & Kopelman, A. E. (1972) The photodynamic action of bilirubin on erythrocytes. *J. Pediat.*, **81**, 473.

Oski, F. A. & Naiman, J. L. (1972) *Hematologic Problems in the Newborn*, p. 228. Philadelphia: Saunders.

Patel, D. A., Pildes, R. S. & Behrman, R. E. (1970) Failure of phototherapy to reduce serum bilirubin in newborn infants. *J. Pediat.*, **77**, 1048.

Polley, M. J., Adinolfi, M. & Mollison, P. L. (1963) Serological characteristics of anti-A related to type of antibody protein (7 Sγ or 19 Sγ). *Vox Sang.*, **8**, 385.

Rausen, A. R., Richter, P., Tallal, L. & Cooper, L. Z. (1967) Hematologic effects of intrauterine rubella. *J.A.M.A.*, **199**, 75.

Rosenfield, R. E. (1955) A–B hemolytic disease of the newborn. Analysis of 1480 cord blood specimens, with special reference to the direct antiglobulin test and to the group O mother. *Blood*, **10**, 17.

Schwenzer, A. W. & Spielmann, W. (1957) Über einen Fall von morbus haemolyticus neonatorum, wahrscheinlich bedingt durch Antikorper des Lewis-Blutgruppensystems. *Vox Sang.*, **2**, 428.

Sisson, T. R. C., Kendall, N., Glanser, S. C., Knutson, S. & Bunyaviroch, E. (1971) Phototherapy of jaundice in newborn infants. I. ABO blood group incompatibility. *J. Pediat.*, **79**, 904.

Stone, B. & Marsh, W. L. (1959) Haemolytic disease of the newborn caused by anti-M. *Brit. J. Haematol.*, **5**, 344.

Trolle, D. (1968) Decrease of total serum-bilirubin concentration in newborn infants after phenobarbitone treatment. *Lancet*, **ii**, 705.

Valdes, O. S., Maurer, H. M., Shumway, C. N., Draper, D. A. & Hossaini, A. A. (1971) Controlled clinical trial of phenobarbital and/or light in reducing neonatal hyperbilirubinemia in a predominantly negro population. *J. Pediat.*, **79**, 1015.

Vest, M., Signer, E., Weisser, K. & Olafsson, A. (1970) A double blind study of the effect of phenobarbitone on neonatal hyperbilirubinaemia and frequency of exchange transfusion. *Acta Paediat. Scand.*, **59**, 681.

Voak, D. & Williams, M. A. (1971) An explanation of the failure of the direct antiglobulin test to detect erythrocyte sensitization in ABO haemolytic disease of the newborn and observations on pinocytosis of 1gG anti-A antibodies by infant (cord) red cells. *Brit. J. Haemat.*, **20**, 9.

Wilson, J. T. (1969) Phenobarbital in the perinatal period. *Pediatrics*, **43**, 324.

Yeung, C. Y. & Field, C. E. (1969) Phenobarbitone therapy in neonatal hyperbilirubinaemia. *Lancet*, **ii**, 135.

Yeung, C. Y., Tam, L. S., Chan, A. & Lee, K. H. (1971) Phenobarbitone prophylaxis for neonatal hyperbilirubinemia. *Pediat.*, **48**, 372.

Yunis, E. & Bridges, R. (1964) The serologic diagnosis of ABO hemolytic disease of the newborn. *Am. J. Clin. Path.*, **41**, 1.

Zinkham, W. H. (1963) Peripheral blood and bilirubin values in normal full-term primaquine sensitive Negro infants. *Pediatrics*, **31**, 983.

Zodin, V. & Anderson, R. E. (1965) Hemolytic disease of the newborn due to anti-Kidd (Jk^b): Case report and review of the literature. *Pediatrics*, **36**, 420.

12. Non-immune Anaemias in the Neonatal Period

Infantile pycnocytosis / Neonatal haemolysis due to infection, *Syphilis, Toxoplasmosis and cytomegalovirus, Rubella, Coxsackie B, Herpes Simplex, Malaria, Bacterial infections* / Heinz-body anaemias in the newborn / Neonatal manifestations of hereditary haemolytic anaemias, *Hereditary spherocytosis (HS), Hereditary elliptocytosis (HE), Hereditary red-cell enzyme defects, Thalassaemias and haemoglobinopathies* / Neonatal anaemia due to blood loss, *Chronic foetal blood loss* / Aplastic anaemia in the neonatal period.

The neonate is unduly susceptible to haemolytic insult. Not only is the red cell survival normally shorted to 2/3rd of that in adults (Pearson, 1967) but its red cell metabolism affords less protection against oxidative injury to haemoglobin and cell membrane (Ross, 1963; Gross *et al.*, 1967). Red cell membrane lipids show greatly increased susceptibility to autoxidation (Stocks *et al.*, 1971)

and excrete bilirubin (Odell, 1967). These factors may explain why certain types of haemolytic anaemia, e.g. infantile pycnocytosis and vitamin E deficiency, are confined to the early weeks of life; why the newborn baby is especially susceptible to haemolytic anaemia from infections (e.g. cytomegalovirus, toxoplasmosis), acidosis or drug exposure; and why many of the hereditary hae-

Table 12.1 Causes of haemolysis in the newborn

Isoimmune
  Rh disease, ABO HDNB, minor blood groups (K, M, S, Fy, Jk, Le, 'family')
Congenital infections
  Cytomegalovirus, toxoplasmosis, rubella, syphilis, malaria
Diseases accompanied by MAHA $\pm$ DIC
  Disseminated herpes simplex and Coxsackie B infections, Gm $-$ve septicaemia, renal vein thrombosis, maternal obstetric accidents, certain cases of RDS
Infantile pycnocytosis
Vitamin E deficiency in premature infants
Toxic exposure (drug, chemicals) $\pm$G-6-PD deficiency $\pm$prematurity
  Synthetic vitamin analogues, maternal thiazide diuretics, antimalarials, sulphonamides, nitrofurantoins, naphthalene (moth balls), analine dye marking ink
Hereditary enzyme defects $\pm$drug exposure
  G-6-PD (Caucasian and Oriental) and other enzymes concerned with GSS-G reduction or synthesis
  Pyruvate kinase, and other enzymes of glycolytic pathway, including galactosaemia
Hereditary haemolytic anaemias with characteristic morphology
  Hereditary spherocytosis
  Hereditary elliptocytosis
  Hereditary stomatocytosis
Hereditary abnormalities of haemoglobin synthesis
  Alpha thalassaemia
  Gamma-beta thalassaemia
  Unstable haemoglobins (congenital Heinz body anaemias)

and *in vitro* haemolysis by H_2O_2 is increased. Foetal red cells are also more 'rigid' than adult cells, leading to greater haemolysis and splenic sequestration, this tendency being increased by acidosis and hypoxia (Gross and Hathaway, 1972). Furthermore, the consequence of haemolysis is more conspicuous in the neonate by virtue of reduced ability of the immature liver to conjugate

molytic anaemias, e.g. hereditary spherocytosis, G-6-PD deficiency, cause more severe jaundice in the neonatal period than in later childhood.

Table 12.1 lists the main causes of haemolysis in the neonatal period. Fig. 12.1 shows the normal range of haemoglobin, red cell count and reticulocyte count during the first 12 weeks of life.

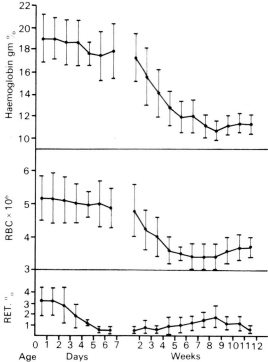

Fig. 12.1 Haemoglobin concentration, red-cell count and reticulocyte count in the first 12 post-natal weeks. Vertical bars indicate standard deviations. (Reproduced from *Acta Paediatric Scandinavia* (1971), **60**, 317, by permission of Prof. Matoth).

INFANTILE PYCNOCYTOSIS

Tuffy, Brown and Zuelzer (1959) described 11 full-term infants with a syndrome which they named infantile pycnocytosis. Seven presented with jaundice in the first or second day of life, mostly accompanied by hepatosplenomegaly and acute haemolytic anaemia. In two of these the bilirubin rose to over 20 mg per 100 ml and exchange transfusion was performed. The four infants who did not show significant neonatal jaundice presented with anaemia (Hb 4·6 to 6·6 g/100 ml) at the age of 3–4 weeks. The syndrome mimicked Rh disease or ABO HDNB but serological incompatibility between the mother's serum and the baby's red cells was excluded.

A constant morphological finding was the presence of small, distorted red cells with several to many spiny projections. Because the authors were impressed by the dense staining of these cells, resembling spherocytes, they named them 'pycnocytes', although recognizing their general similarity to 'burr cells' as described by previous authors, usually in association with renal disease. Photomicrographs showing such 'pycnocytes' are to be found in the papers of Tuffy et al. (1959), Zannos-Mariolea et al. (1962), Akerman (1969), Mauer (1969), Petersen (1972) and the book of Oski and Naiman (1972E). Most of these illustrations show cells which are smaller and darker than normal with multiple radial spikes around their periphery. Pycnocytes differ somewhat from the type of 'burr cell' seen in renal failure or MAHA but are morphologically identical to the cells seen in vitamin E deficiency (Oski and Barness, 1967), and very similar to those in acanthocytosis due to abetalipoproteinaemia.

The percentage of pycnocytes ranged from approximately 6 to 50 per cent in the series of infants reported by Tuffy et al. (1959) and 10 to 34 per cent in the series of Ackerman (1969). The frequency of distorted red cells roughly correlated with the severity of haemolysis. Up to 1·9 per cent of pycnocytes were found in normal full term infants, however, and up to 5·6 per cent in premature infants during their first 2–3 months of life (Tuffy et al., 1959). The syndrome of infantile pycnocytosis appears, therefore, to be an accentuation of a normal process. It appears to be extracorpuscular in origin, perhaps vascular, since transfused cells acquire the same abnormal morphology (Ackerman, 1969) and have a similarly reduced survival in the circulation (Keimowitz and Desforges, 1965). The process is self-limiting since pycnocytes have disappeared and haemolysis ceased by the age of 6 months (Petersen, 1972).

Infantile pycnocytosis may not be a single entity since similar changes have been described in Greek newborn infants with G-6-PD deficiency (Zannos-Mariolea et al., 1962) while more typical 'burr cells' may occur in neonatal haemolysis due to drugs or toxic agents (Allison, 1957) and in disseminated infections such as herpes simplex (Miller et al., 1970) and Gram negative septicaemia, when they usually reflect intra-vascular coagulation (Preston et al., 1973). There is also some possible overlap with the red cell changes attributed to vitamin E deficiency (Fig. 12.2) which appears to cause a morphologically similar type of haemolytic anaemia at 6–10 weeks of age in premature infants (Oski and Barness, 1967). It is tempting to attribute the high 'pycnocyte' count in premature infants recorded by Tuffy et al. (1959) to vitamin E deficiency in the light of current knowledge.

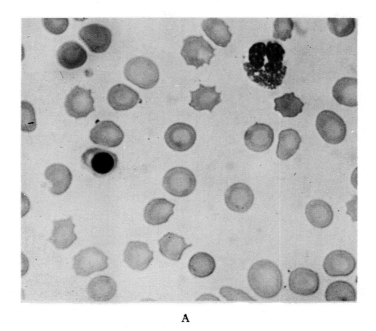

A

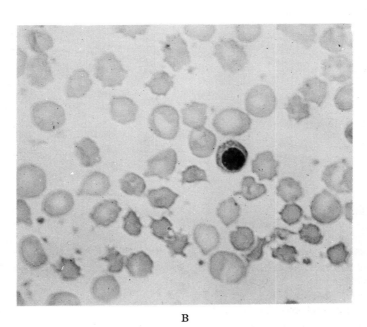

B

Fig. 12.2 Pycnocytes in 3 paediatric situations. x 2,700 in all. A, As normal finding in prematurity (28-week gestation newborn); B, Associated with vitamin E deficiency haemolytic anaemia developing at 5 weeks in a low birthweight (1 kg) twin. (Hb 6·4 g/100 ml,) serum vit E 0·6 mg/100 ml; C, In Infantile Pycnocytosis in a term. Newborn infant developing jaundice, anaemia and hepatosplenomegaly at 16 hrs. (Case history 8).

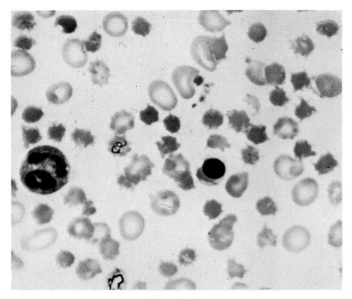

Fig. 12.2C

NEONATAL HAEMOLYSIS DUE TO INFECTION

Driscoll (1966) listed the congenital infections syphilis, toxoplasmosis and cytomegalovirus as possible causes of hydrops foetalis, the most severe form of neonatal anaemia. Zuelzer and Mudgett (1950) in a retrospective analysis of causes of kernicterus found that severe bacterial infections and diarrhoeal diseases predisposed to hyper-bilirubinaemia in premature infants. Hathaway et al. (1969) included congenital rubella and cytomegalovirus with neonatally acquired herpes simplex as viral causes of disseminated intravascular coagulation in the newborn. This may cause a microangiopathic type of haemolytic anaemia.

Syphilis

Congenital syphilis was recognized as a cause of neonatal anaemia by Loos as long ago as 1892. After being a rare disease for many years it is now returning with sufficient frequency to be once again included in differential diagnosis. Whitaker (1965) found hepatosplenomegaly and haemolytic anaemia during the first 2–3 weeks of life in 8 out of 9 infants with congenital syphilis. Thrombocytopenia was present in 4. Elevation of both indirect and direct bilirubin occurred in 6 reflecting both haemolysis and syphilitic hepatitis. Exchange transfusion was needed in 3 infants. The classical clinical features of snuffles, rhagades, mucocutaneous lesions and pseudoparalysis were seldom present in this series. Bulova (1972) has reported a recent case of hydrops foetalis due to this infection with anaemia, thrombocytopenia, hyperbilirubinaemia and 200 normoblasts per 100 WBC on the blood film.

Toxoplasmosis and cytomegalovirus

Neonatal haemolytic anaemia and thrombocytopenia may also be caused by congenital toxoplasmosis or cytomegalovirus infections. The clinical pictures are similar to Rh disease with hepatosplenomegaly, jaundice (sometimes in the first day of life), purpura, intracranial calcification, choroidoretinitis and microcephaly. Not all features are necessarily present. A good review of toxoplasmosis is that of Beckett and Flynn (1953). They point out that there are a number of different clinical syndromes including not only the congenital infection, which mimics Rh disease, but also infections in later life which can cause encephalitis or can present as glandular fever with a negative Paul Bunnell. A good review of cytomegalovirus infection in the newborn is that of Medearis (1957). Of 42 infants with a syndrome resembling severe Rh disease or neonatal sepsis 30 developed jaundice, 26 had either hepatomegaly or splenomegaly or both and 31 had a haemorrhagic state. Some infants escape this neonatal syndrome but show evidence of brain damage subsequently. The overall incidence of subsequent mental retardation is 10–20 per cent (Stern and Tucker,

1973). In later life cytomegalovirus can also cause a glandular fever-like illness with negative Paul Bunnell especially after multiple blood transfusion at times of open heart surgery (Paloheimo *et al.*, 1968). The similarity in clinical and haematological manifestations of the above two infections, one protozoal, the other viral, is striking. Rare instances have been recorded where consecutive pregnancies have resulted in infected infants both in the case of toxoplasmosis (Garica, 1968) and in the case of cytomegalovirus (Embil *et al.*, 1970).

Haematological findings in both include a variable degree of anaemia, erythroblastosis and red cell distortion, with a particular liability to severe thrombocytopenia ($< 20,000/mm^3$) in the case of cytomegalovirus. Moderate numbers of blast cells (Beckett and Flynn, 1953) and also eosinophilia (Eichenwald, 1957) have been observed in the case of toxoplasmosis. Both direct and indirect bilirubin levels may be elevated since hepatitis may be present as well as haemolysis.

Diagnosis is made by the demonstration of cytomegalic 'owl's eye' inclusion bodies in the nucleus and cytoplasm of renal tubular cells from the urine or mononuclear cells from the CSF, by isolation of the virus from the urine or by serological investigations on the mother and the infant. Elevated antibody titres to either agent in the infant's serum may simply reflect passively acquired antibody from the mother. It is necessary to demonstrate a rising titre in the infant during the month after birth in order to be certain that it is evidence of infection in the infant. An elevated neonatal IgM level is found in these and other congenital infections.

Rubella, Coxsackie B, herpes simplex, malaria

Other congenitally acquired virus infections, including rubella and Coxsackie B, may produce the combination of anaemia, jaundice, thrombocytopenia and haemorrhage. The jaundice is at least partly due to hepatic damage which may also cause a deficiency of the prothrombin complex thereby contributing to the haemorrhagic tendency. In the case of congenital rubella syndrome a true haemolytic anaemia with red cell fragmentation and spherocytes has been reported (Rausen *et al.*, 1967). It may persist, with the thrombocytopenia, for several months. Intravascular coagulation has been suggested as the cause of thrombocytopenia and haemorrhage in Coxsackie septicaemia (Desmond, 1968).

Disseminated herpes simplex infection in the newborn is thought to be acquired during birth from contact with a vulval herpetic lesion in the mother. The infant may develop anaemia, jaundice, haemorrhage and hepatosplenomegaly during the first two weeks of life. A recent report by Miller *et al.* (1970) shows prominent red cell fragmentation together with 5 circulating normoblasts per 100 WBC in a 10-day-old infant. From a review of the literature these authors found that 40 per cent of such infants have a haemorrhagic diathesis, and that the thrombocytopenia and coagulation abnormalities suggest both DIC and liver failure. The red cell fragmentation and haemolysis could be secondary to the DIC.

Intrauterine infection with quartan malaria has been recorded by Harvey *et al.* (1969), perhaps transmitted via a small maternal to foetal haemorrhage. As in other intrauterine infections the foetus had been stimulated to form IgM antibodies. There was no jaundice in the neonatal period but hepatosplenomegaly was present at 9 weeks, followed by intermittent fever and a fall of haemoglobin to 7·6 g/100 ml with reticulocytosis at 12 weeks.

Bacterial infections

Gram negative infections with bacteraemia or septicaemia are particularly liable to cause DIC (Weil *et al.*, 1964) and associated MAHA (Preston *et al.*, 1973). Such an infection may be acquired in the first days of life and can give rise to purpura and pallor due to a rapidly falling platelet count and haemoglobin level, the blood film showing red cell fragmentation.

HEINZ BODY ANAEMIAS IN THE NEWBORN

These have many causes. Red cells of the newborn, especially of the premature newborn, are unduly susceptible to oxidative insult and Heinz body formation (Fig. 12.2). In a survey by Willi and Hartmeier (1950) 18 per cent of 1,250 newborn infants showed Heinz bodies in more than 20 per cent of their red cells. Eighty four per cent of those with Heinz bodies were premature. This Heinz body formation is not necessarily accompanied by haemolysis and the phenomenon disappears within the first weeks of life (Gasser, 1959). The presence of circulating Heinz bodies may partly be due to hypofunction of the spleen in the premature infant (Fig. 12.3).

Agenesis of the spleen can occur as part of the syndrome of situs inversus and congenital defects of the heart and great vessels. Gasser and Willi

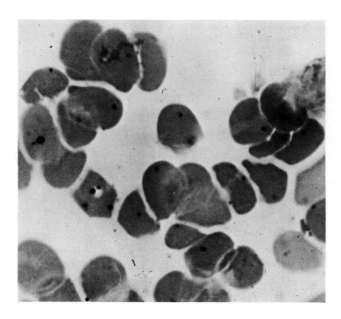

Fig. 12.3 Heinz bodies in a 3-day-old infant with congenital absence of the spleen and partial situs inversus (Gasser's Syndrome). x 5,000. Supravital stain with Methyl Violet.

(1952) pointed out the association of this triad with spontaneous and persistent Heinz body formation in full term infants. Heinz bodies were present in greatest numbers (11–20 per cent) during the first 2 months of life and then persisted in smaller numbers (5 per cent). They were accompanied by an erythroblastosis and Howell Jolly bodies but without evidence of haemolysis or anaemia. There is a poor prognosis because of the cardiovascular anomalies (Gasser, 1959).

Heinz body haemolytic anaemia of the premature infant following administration of synthetic water soluble vitamin K preparations (Synkavite, Hykinone, Menadione) has had great significance in the practice of neonatal paediatrics. In 1953 Gasser described 14 premature infants developing severe jaundice, usually beginning after the first 24 hours, followed by progressive anaemia during the 2nd to 3rd week. Heinz bodies were present in 20–40 per cent of the red cells at the end of the 1st week and during the 2nd week, preceding the anaemia. Prominent red cell fragmentation plus some spherocytes were also present. The only factor common to these infants was the preceding administration of the synthetic, water soluble vitamin K derivative 'Synkavite' in doses of 5–10 mg daily, usually for the first 5 days of life. Other points of note were the absence of splenomegaly, the absence of Heinz bodies at birth, reticulocytopenia at the height of Heinz body formation, the possible development of kernicterus and the good response to blood transfusion. Allison (1957) described a further infant with this syndrome and suggested that the low vitamin E levels in premature infants might be a contributory factor in its genesis.

It was concluded that the dose of vitamin K should not exceed 1 mg daily in premature infants and that the less toxic vitamin K_1 (Konakion) should be substituted for synthetic derivatives. Even the safer K_1 has caused jaundice and a Heinz body haemolytic anaemia when given in the dose of 8 mg to a premature infant (Gasser, 1959). The current recommendation of the American Academy of Pediatrics (1961) is a dose of 1 mg of vitamin K_1 intramuscularly for the prevention of haemorrhagic disease of the newborn in both full term and premature infants. Other drugs and chemicals to which the newborn may be exposed, and which may similarly cause Heinz body haemolytic anaemia, include sulphonamides, chloramphenicol, aniline dyes used for marking nappies and naphthalene used as moth balls.

Unstable haemoglobinopathies (e.g. Hb Köln, Hb Zürich) result in hereditary and life-long forms of 'congenital Heinz body haemolytic anaemia' which may also first present in the neonatal period. As described in Chapter 8 the increased susceptibility to oxidative injury results from structural abnormality of the globin chain in the region of the haem plate. It is possible that the case of 'apparent idiopathic Heinz body anaemia' described in 1952 by Cathie as well as Case 1 of Allison (1957) were the first recorded examples of this type (Grimes *et al.*, 1964). Certainly cases described by Schmid *et al.* (1959) and Scott *et al.* (1960) were early reports of Heinz body haemolytic anaemias due to unstable haemoglobinopathies. Both reports mention abnormal pigment excretion of the meso-bilifuscin type characteristic of these disorders. The father was jaundiced from birth and son jaundiced and anaemic at 20 months in the report of Schmid *et al.* (1959). The case of Scott *et al.* (1960) had pallor at 4 months with splenomegaly and anaemia requiring transfusion at 2- years. Necheles and Allen (1969) in a recent review of Heinz body anaemias point out that circulating Heinz bodies are not found in the unstable haemo-globinopathies unless either the spleen has been removed or the patient has been exposed to an oxidizing drug or chemical. In the case of Hb Zürich the administration of a sulphonamide can cause an acute Heinz body haemolytic anaemia in a previously well-compensated asymptomatic haemolytic state (Reider *et al.*, 1965). The simul-taneous formation of methaemoglobin following drug exposure in these unstable haemoglobin-opathies can give rise to a 'grey' cyanosis clinically. The blood picture is essentially that of a chronic non-spherocytic haemolytic anaemia. During acute drug-induced haemolysis red cell fragmentation may also appear. Special investigations show haemoglobin instability to heat with increased methaemoglobin formation and Heinz body formation on incubation of blood. An unstable foetal haemoglobin (F Poole) has recently been described as a new cause of haemolytic anaemia limited to the newborn period (Lee-Potter *et al.*, 1975).

Alpha thalassaemia should perhaps be included with haemoglobinopathies that predispose to Heinz body formation (Necheles and Allen, 1969). In the form with intermediate severity, Hb 'H' disease, a moderate haemolytic anaemia may be present at birth. There is a reticulocytosis, hypo-chromia and target cells (Fig. 12.1). Because of the relative impairment of alpha chain synthesis there is an accumulation of unstable gamma chain tetramers (Hb 'Barts') at birth (5–25 per cent) followed by similarly unstable beta chain tetramers (Hb H) when significant beta chain synthesis develops over the first few months of life. These unstable tetramers form intracellular precipitates which may be demonstrated microscopically

(Fig. 12.1) by incubation with brilliant cresyl blue and which can form Heinz bodies in the presence of oxidizing agents (Necheles and Allen, 1969). It is probably advisable for patients with Hb H disease to be protected from drugs known to predispose to Heinz body formation.

Hereditary red cell enzyme deficiencies of the hexose monophosphate shunt will also predispose to Heinz body haemolytic anaemia not only in the neonatal period but also in later life (Necheles and Allen, 1969). The commonest deficiency of this type if G-6-PD. In the Mediterranean and Oriental forms there is a severe deficiency of the enzyme, predisposing to apparently spontaneous haemolytic anaemia and jaundice in the newborn, as well as to a marked susceptibility to drug-induced hae-molysis. In Greece, approximately one third of exchange transfusions for neonatal jaundice are because of G-6-PD deficiency (Doxiadis *et al.*, 1961). In the form of G-6-PD deficiency which occurs in Africans and black Americans the enzyme deficiency is less severe, the sensitivity to drugs is less and there is no increased incidence of neonatal jaundice in *full term* infants (Zinkham, 1963). In Black *premature* infants, however, some increased predisposition to neonatal jaundice and exchange transfusions has been found (Eshaghpour *et al.*, 1967).

Clinically the jaundice due to G-6-PD deficiency does not usually appear within the first 24-hours of life (Doxiadis and Valaes, 1964) unlike Rh or ABO HDNB. Also hepatosplenomegaly is un-common in G-6-PD deficiency. The hazard of kernicterus exists, however (Naiman and Kosoy, 1964). As mentioned above there may or may not be a precipitating factor such as drug exposure (e.g. to Synkavite), hypoxia or acidosis (Lopez and Cooperman, 1971). Exposure to naphthalene from moth balls, aniline or nitrobenzene derivatives from nappy marking ink, sulphonamides or resorcin skin lotions can result in jaundice appearing as late as the second week of life.

Investigations may show a slightly low Hb and elevated bilirubin at birth (Valaes *et al.*, 1969), with the Hb later falling to as low as 7 g/100 ml. The red cells may show fragmentation with spherocytes and circulating normoblasts, while Heinz bodies are demonstrable by supravital staining with brilliant cresyl blue or methyl crystal violet. (Fig. 12.2).

Exchange transfusion may be needed. An important aspect of management is avoidance of exposure of either mother or infant to drugs or toxic agents known to induce haemolysis. In the Black infant with G-6-PD deficiency there is less

194   PAEDIATRIC HAEMATOLOGY

sensitivity to drugs and it is safe to administer vitamin K analogues in a dose of 1 mg or vitamin K_1 (Konakion) in even larger doses (Zinkham, 1963). In the more sensitive Caucasian infant the safe dose of vitamin K has not been precisely determined but 1 mg I.M. of the least toxic form (K_1) is recommended in the present state of knowledge (Oski and Naiman, 1972C).

Toxic Heinz body haemolytic anaemia may also be caused in normal, full term infants without red cell enzyme deficiencies if the dose of drug or chemical is large enough (Gasser, 1959). Schafer (1951) reported a case of naphthalene-induced haemolytic anaemia in a full term newborn infant while Zuelzer and Apt (1949) reported four apparently normal older (Black) children (2 to $2\frac{1}{2}$ years) who developed severe Heinz body anaemia after ingestion of naphthalene. A difficulty with these early reports is that it is not possible to exclude G-6-PD deficiency for certain since its existence was unknown at the time. Many of the agents which can cause Heinz body haemolytic anaemias also cause methaemoglobinaemia, (although others such as nitrates may cause methaemoglobinaemia without Heinz body haemolytic anaemia). The most important early clinical sign may therefore be a grey cyanosis rather than jaundice (Gasser, 1959). Whenever methaemoglobinaemia is diagnosed it is profitable to look for a Heinz body haemolytic anaemia.

NEONATAL MANIFESTATIONS OF HEREDITARY HAEMOLYTIC ANAEMIAS

Hereditary spherocytosis (HS)

Burman (1958) collected from the literature 35 cases where the diagnosis of HS had been made in the first year of life. Neonatal jaundice was present in 23 but could have been accounted for by prematurity in 3. Stamey and Diamond (1957) reported four infants with HS who developed jaundice at 14 to 36 hours, all requiring exchange transfusion for hyperbilirubinaemia. Trucco and Brown (1967) described a further 7 infants with HS presenting with jaundice at 5 to 105 hours together with mild anaemia (10·6 to 15·1 g/100 ml). Exchange transfusion was needed in four out of the seven. Kernicterus has been recorded at four days in another infant with HS, while the identical twin was saved by an exchange transfusion (Roddy, 1954).

The high incidence of neonatal jaundice (over 50 per cent) in the series collected by Burman is probably an overestimate since all the cases referred to had been diagnosed in the first year of life and may therefore have been more severe than average. Nevertheless, an incidence of neonatal jaundice close to 50 per cent was also found in a retrospective survey of patients with HS by Stamey and Diamond (1957).

The clinical and haematological features of neonatal jaundice of this cause are very similar to ABO HDNB, with only a minority of infants showing hepatosplenomegaly. Spherocytosis and increased osmotic fragility are present in both conditions. The key to diagnosis is the known presence of HS in another member of the family. In Burman's series at least 60 per cent had a positive family history. When a parent or sibling is known to have HS the newborn infant should be observed in the neonatal period with the same care as if it was a Rhesus baby (Stamey and Diamond, 1957).

Even in the absence of neonatal jaundice HS may cause severe anaemia in the months following birth, with a haemoglobin level as low as 6 g/100 ml by four weeks (Robinson, 1957). Recurrent episodes of severe anaemia may also occur throughout the first year of life, necessitating early splenectomy. This operation is normally deferred until after the age of 4 years because of the possible hazard of later overwhelming infection. The dangers of repeated episodes of severe anaemia whether due to uncompensated haemolysis or to aplastic crises probably exceeds the hazards of splenectomy, making this operation justifiable in these unusually severe cases (Stamey and Diamond, 1957).

Case 7 (No. 10056). A mother had no past history of anaemia or jaundice but a routine full blood examination performed three days after Caesarian section showed her to have a Hb of 9·8 g/100 ml with numerous spherocytes on the blood film. Reticulocytes were 23 per cent, suggesting that she had a well-compensated form of HS. Immediate arrangements were made for the baby to be transferred to the neonatal unit for observation. This suggestion had, however, been overtaken by events since jaundice had been noted at 48 hr and the baby was already in transit to the neonatal unit. On arrival the unconjugated bilirubin was 20·3 mg/100 ml, Hb 17·8 g/100 ml, retics. 10 per cent, and the film showed numerous spherocytes with 2 normoblasts per 100 WBC. The baby was deeply jaundiced with the liver just palpable below the costal margin and the spleen tip palpable. The mother's blood group was AB +ve and the baby's B −ve. The direct Coombs test was negative on the baby's RBCs and these were compatible with the mother's serum by saline, enzyme and Coombs X-match. An exchange transfusion was given on the 4th day but blood collected prior to this showed an increased osmotic fragility curve similar to that given by the mother's blood. Subsequent progress was uneventful. An older sibling was later found to have HS with a compensated haemolytic anaemia but had not shown neonatal jaundice.

Hereditary elliptocytosis (HE)

Austin and Desforges (1969) described 3 infants with HE presenting as neonatal jaundice and moderate anaemia (Hb 11 to 13·5 g/100 ml). All three required exchange transfusion. In the immediate neonatal period the red cell morphology was more like infantile pycnocytosis than elliptocytosis. These distorted cells were, however, transient and gave way to the appearance of typical elliptocytes from the age of 4 weeks onwards. In other infants the typical blood picture of elliptocytosis may not become fully developed until the age of 4–6 months (Helz and Menten, 1944). Haemolytic anaemia may be present in the first few months of life but disappears after the age of one year (Oski and Naiman, 1972D). In later life haemolysis is unusual in HE.

Hereditary red cell enzyme defects

G-6-PD deficiency has already been described as a possible cause of neonatal haemolytic anaemia under the heading of Heinz body anaemias. Other enzyme deficiencies may also first manifest themselves as haemolysis and jaundice in the neonatal period.

Among the other enzymes involved in maintenance of adequate levels of reduced glutathione (GSH) 6-phosphogluconate dehydrogenase deficiency has been associated with neonatal jaundice and anaemia requiring exchange transfusion (Lauseker et al., 1965) and glutathione peroxidase deficiency was associated with haemolysis and hyperbilirubinaemia in 3 out of 4 newborn infants, one requiring exchange transfusion (Necheles et al., 1968).

Enzyme defects of the glycolytic pathway such as pyruvate kinase (PK) deficiency may also cause haemolysis and jaundice in the newborn. Oski and Diamond (1963) described neonatal hyperbilirubinaemia, haemolysis and splenomegaly in 10 infants with PK deficiency, with four requiring exchange transfusion. Kernicterus has also been recorded (Oski et al., 1964). The blood film at birth may show spherocytes and grossly contracted spiculated red cells similar to pycnocytes, as well as the features of haemolysis, i.e. increased normoblasts, polychromasia and macrocytosis. Severe anaemia can develop in the first months of life. Hexokinase deficiency (Valentine et al., 1967),

phosphohexose isomerose deficiency (Paglia et al., 1969) and 2,3-diphosphoglyceromutase deficiency (Schröter, 1965) have been associated with neonatal haemolytic anaemia and jaundice sometimes requiring exchange transfusion.

Galactosaemia, due to a systemic deficiency of the enzyme galactose-1-phosphate uridyl transferase, may cause neonatal jaundice either because of liver damage from galactose accumulation or because of haemolytic anaemia (Hsia and Walker, 1961). Bajpai et al. (1972) investigated an infant with galactosaemia presenting with jaundice on the third day, hepatosplenomegaly and a haemoglobin level between 5 and 8·5 g/100 ml. The serum bilirubin reached 10 mg/100 ml at 15 days. Osmotic fragility was normal. Red cell survival studies showed a shortened half-life in the infant (14 days) but not if the infant's cells were injected into the father unless he was fed a galactose load, when an increased rate of haemolysis of the transfused cells temporarily occurred.

Thalassaemias and haemoglobinopathies

Neonatal anaemia can occur with alpha but not beta thalassaemia since the major fraction of circulating haemoglobin at birth, Hb F, contains alpha but not beta chains.

The most severe form of homozygous alpha thalassaemia regularly results in hydrops foetalis due to severe anaemia. Most such infants die *in utero* but a few live for an hour or less after birth (Kan et al., 1967; Thumasthit et al., 1968). Clinically there is generalized oedema, ascites and hepatomegaly, but minimal splenomegaly. Haematologically there is a severe anaemia, with haemoglobin levels as low as 3 g/100 ml, with marked reticulocytosis, numerous circulating normoblasts and marked hypochromia of the red cells with target cell formation. Hb Barts, a tetramer formed from the excess of gamma chains, precipitates intracellularly during incubation with brilliant cresyl blue forming similar inclusion bodies to those seen in Hb H disease. Hb Barts can also be identified electrophoretically as a fast moving band at alkaline pH. Normal Hb A and Hb F are absent. Pseudosickling may be seen after incubation of the blood.

The less severe form of alpha thalassaemia, Hb H disease in later life, may show milder anaemia and haemolysis in the neonatal period. The red cells are hypochromic with small numbers of target cells and Hb Barts is present in up to 25 per cent compared to 100 per cent in the severe form (Todd et al., 1969). Alpha thalassaemia is predominantly seen among Oriental races where the incidence is similar to that of beta thalassaemia in Mediterranean races.

A further form of thalassaemia, gamma-beta thalassaemia, has also recently been described as a cause of haemolytic anaemia in the newborn (Kan *et al.*, 1972). The family had beta thalassaemia but the baby also had impaired synthesis of gamma chains. She presented with jaundice at 24 hours, a haemoglobin of 10·4 g/100 ml, reticulocytes of 26 per cent and 400 normoblasts per 100 WBC. The red cells showed hypochromia and target cells. Neither Hb Barts nor Hb H was present. The disease is transient, becoming indistinguishable from beta thalassaemia as beta chains replaces gamma chains after the age of a few months. Antenatal prediction by the use of amniocentesis is discussed by White and Jones (1969).

A number of alpha and gamma chain haemoglobinopathies have been discovered in survey analyses of cord bloods but these are not associated with clinical or haematological disease. In general the beta chain haemoglobinopathies do not produce manifestations until after the neonatal period but occasional mild anaemia and jaundice has been recorded in newborns homozygous for Hb S (Oski and Naiman, 1972F).

NEONATAL ANAEMIA DUE TO BLOOD LOSS

The commonest cause of non-haemolytic anaemia in the newborn is blood loss, accounting for perhaps 5–10 per cent of all neonatal anaemias (Raye *et al.*, 1970). Acute foetal blood loss usually occurs during labour and delivery (Kirkman and Riley, 1959A); chronic foetal blood loss occurs over a protracted period before delivery (Pearson and Diamond, 1959).

The report by Kirkman and Riley (1959B) of 8 cases of acute intrapartum haemorrhage due to such causes as incision or disruption of the placenta, and tearing of aberrant vessels from velamentous insertion of cord or a succenturiate lobe focused attention upon the multiplicity of predisposing factors (Table 12.2). The infants in this series had haemoglobin levels of 5·5 to 13·5 g/100 ml at 30 min to 20 hours after birth.

Rupture of the cord has usually been associated with precipitous delivery and is seldom seen in present day obstetrics. Haematoma of the cord may still be seen, however (Ratten, 1969). Anomalous vessels may particularly occur when there is a velamentous insertion of the cord remote from the placenta. The vessels lie between chorion and amnion unprotected by Wharton's jelly. This abnormality occurs in 1 per cent of all pregnancies and in 10 per cent of multiple births (Raye *et al.*, 1970). Similar vessels occur when the placenta is multilobed or has a satellite succenturiate lobe. The greatest hazard exists when the aberrant vessels course across the internal cervical os, then being termed vasa praevia and resulting in a mortality of at least 50 per cent (Pochedly and Ente, 1969).

Incision of the placenta, particularly of the lower segment for placenta praevia, has resulted in foetal haemorrhage in 7 out of 20 such deliveries with one infant dying of shock (Neligan and Russell, 1955). Accidental damage to the placenta during attempted diagnostic amniocentesis can result in placental haemorrhages of up to 50 ml (Wang *et al.*, 1967). Significant foeto-maternal haemorrhage may also occur after external cephalic version (Pollack, 1968). Abruptio placenta, placenta praevia and partial separation of a normally implanted placenta can all result in intrapartum foetal haemorrhage (Clayton *et al.*, 1964). In the case of abruptio and placenta praevia foetal anoxia and perhaps coagulation disturbance also play a major part in foetal shock and loss. Foeto-maternal haemorrhage of the order of 0·2 ml is extremely common, being the genesis of Rh isoimmunization. At the other end of the spectrum foeto-maternal haemorrhage of 40 ml or more may occur in only approx. 1 per cent of pregnancies (Cohen *et al.*, 1964). Since the foetal blood volume is only 200–300 ml these larger haemorrhages may cause acute anaemia and shock if they occur shortly before delivery.

The clinical features and management of the infant have been described in reviews by Kirkman and Riley (1959A) and Raye *et al.* (1970). Although the causes of acute intrapartum foetal blood loss are diverse (Table 12.2) the foetal result and management are similar. The newborn infant is pale with no hepatosplenomegaly or oedema. The more severe cases show tachycardia, weakness and distress out of proportion to any cyanosis. Initially the haemoglobin level may be normal since several hours are necessary for haemodilution to occur. Immediate treatment is to give approximately 20 ml/kg of any available I.V. fluid, so as to restore the blood volume followed by a further 10–20 ml/kg of whole blood when there has been time to assess the clinical situation.

Diagnosis may be facilitated by using the Kleihauer technique for the detection of foetal red cells in either vaginal blood loss or circulating maternal blood. Clayton *et al.* (1964) quantitated the amount of foetal blood loss in third trimester bleeding and related this to foetal outcome. When the bleeding was cervical in origin and the foetus was unaffected no foetal cells were found. In those conditions, including 4 instances of stillbirth, where foetal blood loss could be implicated foetal red cells could be detected in the vaginal blood in

can be invalidated when the baby's red cells carry antigens (e.g. A, B or D) to which the mother has potent antibodies since these will rapidly clear the incompatible foetal cells from the maternal circulation. When this is the case the mother may manifest chills and fever (Goodall *et al.*, 1958) or even acute renal failure (Pasternak *et al.*, 1966) as a result of the incompatible transfusion.

Table 12.2   Causes of haemorrhage in the newborn

Obstetric accidents, malformations of the placenta and cord
    Rupture of a normal umbilical cord
        Precipitous delivery
        Entanglement
    Haematoma of the cord or placenta
    Rupture of an abnormal umbilical cord
        Varices
        Aneurysm
    Rupture of anomalous vessels
        Aberrant vessel
        Velamentous insertion
        Communicating vessels in multilobed placenta
    Incision of placenta during Caesarean section
    Placenta previa
    Abruptio placentae
Occult haemorrhage prior to birth
    Foetomaternal
        Traumatic amniocentesis
        Spontaneous
        Following external cephalic version
    Twin to twin
Internal haemorrhage
    Intracranial
    Giant cephalohaematoma, caput succedaneum
    Retroperitoneal
    Ruptured liver
    Ruptured spleen

Reproduced, by permission of the authors and publishers, from F. A. Oski and J. L. Naiman (1972), Hematologic Problems in the Newborn. Philadelphia : Saunders.

proportions of between 1:100 and 1:5 adult cells. When several ml of such blood are available for analysis a rapid Singer's test for alkali resistant (foetal) haemoglobin will also give evidence of ante- or intrapartum foetal haemorrhage. In cases of unexplained foetal shock or neonatal anaemia massive foetomaternal haemorrhage may be confirmed by a Kleihauer film performed on the mother's circulating blood (venepuncture or finger prick). Other methods of detecting a minor population of foetal red cells are applicable, including immunofluorescent, or serological techniques when the blood group of the foetus differs from that of the mother, and also a Singer test to estimate the percentage of Hb F in the mother's circulation (Cohen *et al.*, 1964; Pearson and Diamond, 1959). None of these are as simple or as sensitive as the Kleihauer technique. All methods

Chronic foetal blood loss

Twin transfusion syndrome represents a unique situation whereby one twin may suffer from anaemia and the other polycythaemia (Kerr, 1959). Both donor and recipient infants may suffer. For this to occur the twins must be monozygous (identical) and monochorial. Approximately 70 per cent of monozygous twins share monochorial placentas, and of 130 monochorial twins twin-transfusion was found in 19 (15 per cent) (Rausen *et al.*, 1965). Two thirds of these were lost in the perinatal period. A haemoglobin difference between the twins of 5 g/100 ml or more was taken to indicate twin transfusion in Rausen's study. In a comparable series of dizygous twins the haemoglobin difference never exceeded 3·3 g/100 ml. From histological and perfusion studies it appears that it is only when a placental artery anastomoses with a placental vein of the other twin that this syndrome occurs. Therapy may require not only transfusion of the anaemic twin but a partial exchange using plasma in the polycythaemic twin so as to reduce its red cell mass. The polycythaemic twin may suffer from cardio-respiratory difficulties, hyperbilirubinaemia and kernicterus (Sacks, 1959).

Polycythaemia can also occur as a result of materno-foetal transfusion in approx. 1 per cent of single pregnancies (Andrews and Thompson, 1962). By the Kleihauer technique individual adult RBCs can readily be identified on blood films of foetal blood. Very few RBCs contain exclusively Hb A in normal newborn blood, but these would be grossly increased. When the maternal cells are incompatible with a foetus who has already developed appropriate isoagglutinins it may suffer from an ABO-incompatible transfusion reaction (Wong and Chan, 1972). A neonatal venous haematocrit greater than 65 per cent or haemoglobin greater than 22·0 g/100 ml is considered evidence of polycythaemia (Oski and Naiman, 1972B). Placental transfusion due to delayed clamping of the cord by increasing red cell volume also greatly enhances the severity of neonatal hyperbilirubinaemia (Saigal et al., 1972).

Chronic foeto-maternal haemorrhage produces a different clinical and haematological picture from acute foetal or foeto-maternal haemorrhage (Pearson and Diamond, 1959). Pallor, tachycardia and even hepatic and cardiac enlargement may occur but the anaemia is well-compensated and the infant does not show shock (Raye et al., 1970). The blood shows a hypochromic anaemia with reticulocytosis and an increase in circulating normoblasts. This is by contrast with the shock and the normochromic anaemia seen with acute foetal blood loss. The hypochromic anaemia of chronic foeto-maternal haemorrhage constitutes the unique cause of true iron deficiency anaemia present in the neonatal period (McGovern et al., 1958; Eshaghpour et al., 1966; Miles et al., 1971). The haemoglobin levels have been as low as 4·5 and 5·2 g/100 ml in these reports with reticulocytes up to 31 per cent and numerous circulating normoblasts. Iron is absent from the marrow and the serum iron is low. Weisert and Marstrander (1960) reported a hydropic infant due to this condition, and pointed out the clinical similarity with severe Rhesus disease. Diagnosis is confirmed by the presence of large numbers of foetal red cells in the mother's blood, as shown by the Kleihauer technique, or even by the chemical demonstration of Hb F, in concentra-

tions as high as 6·9 per cent in the mother's circulation, using the Singer's technique. Treatment is by transfusion of packed cells if the anaemia is marked, together with iron supplementation to replete the iron stores (Eshaghpour et al., 1966). If the anaemia is sufficiently severe to cause cardiac failure then exchange transfusion is indicated (Weisert and Marstrander, 1960).

It is possible that some of the variation in the cord blood haemoglobin levels of apparently normal or premature infants may be due to foeto-maternal haemorrhages of intermediate severity before or during delivery. Schulman (1959) has pointed out that of all the factors involved in contributing to the exhaustion of iron stores and resulting late anaemia in premature infants the initial circulating haemoglobin mass appears to be the most important single variable. It has been suggested that a search for foetal cells in maternal circulation should be made whenever an infant is born anaemic without obvious blood loss (Lunay et al., 1970).

Rare causes of foetal anaemia and erythroblastosis are tumours involving the placenta. Anders et al. (1973) have described two newborn infants with congenital neuroblastoma metastasizing to the liver and placenta with a clinical picture suggesting hydrops foetalis due to severe Rh disease. In one the haemoglobin was 10·4 g/100 ml with 68 normoblasts per 100 WBC. Sweet et al. (1973) have described an infant with hydrops, anaemia (Hb 11·6 g/100 ml) and hypoalbuminaemia (1·2 g/100 ml) due to placental chorioangioma.

Foetal trauma or haemorrhagic states can result in internal or external blood loss in the neonatal period. Massive subaponeurotic haematomas arising after ventouse extraction in the presence of low vitamin K dependent coagulation factors constitute one such cause of potentially fatal haemorrhage which can be prevented by appropriate therapy (Ahuja et al., 1969). Gastrointestinal blood loss in the newborn has to be distinguished from ingested maternal blood during delivery. If the blood passed per rectum is still red in colour it is sometimes possible to distinguish between adult and foetal red cells again by the use of the Kleihauer technique.

APLASTIC ANAEMIA IN THE NEONATAL PERIOD

By contrast with the anaemia of blood loss or haemolysis there is an absence of reticulocytosis and erythroblastosis when failure of red cell production is the cause of the anaemia. The only anaemia of this type occurring in the neonatal period is pure red cell aplasia (congenital hypoplastic anaemia, erythrogenesis imperfecta, Blackfan-Diamond syndrome). In this disease there is an isolated depression or absence of erythropoiesis, with normal myelopoiesis and megakaryocyte function. Typically the diagnosis is not made until the age of 6 weeks or more when severe anaemia is apparent and normoblasts are virtually absent from the marrow. Chance observations have indicated the presence of pallor at birth in approximately one quarter of infants later diagnosed as having this disease (Diamond *et al.*, 1961; Bernard *et al.*, 1962). One infant in Diamond's series had a haemoglobin of 9·4 g/100 ml at the age of one day with 0·3 per cent reticulocytes. The condition is described more fully in Chapter 4. Oski and Naiman (1972A) point out that this disease should be suspected in any anaemic newborn with a reticulocyte count less than 2·0 per cent in the absence of an obvious cause such as overwhelming infection, which can cause temporary marrow depression (Gasser, 1957).

Rare instances of marble bone disease (osteopetrosis, Albers-Schonberg disease) have also shown anaemia at as early an age as 6 weeks when this has been specially sought (Moe and Skjaeveland, 1969).

Other aplastic states such as Fanconi's anaemia do not present in the neonatal period although one form of constitutional aplastic anaemia (Diamond Type II) may cause thrombocytopenia in the neonatal period, with pancytopenia developing a year or more later.

Case 8 (No. 135). A newborn full term male infant developed deep jaundice, with 17 mg/100 ml of indirect bilirubin, at the age of 16 hours. Neonatal jaundice had not occurred in three earlier female siblings. The spleen was firm and enlarged 2 fingers below the costal margin and the liver 3 fingers. Both mother and baby were group O Rh positive with the baby's cells direct Coombs negative and no serological incompatibility demonstrable between the mother's serum and the baby's red cells (by indirect Coombs and enzyme cross-match). The Hb was 19·4 g/100 ml, reticulocytes 8·4 per cent, normoblasts 22 per 100 white cells (WBC count 25,000/mm^3). Blood films consistently showed pycnocytes and spherocytes (Fig. 12.1). Because of the rising bilirubin level an exchange transfusion was performed. The mother's Hb level and red cell morphology was normal, as was her osmotic fragility.

A second ET was narrowly avoided, with a bilirubin level of 17 mg on the 3rd day of life. By the 4th day the jaundice was fading. By the 10th day the spleen was smaller (one finger breadth) but the Hb had fallen to 10·1 g/100 ml. Serological investigations for toxoplasmosis, and CMV were negative. Tests for G-6-PD deficiency and galactosaemia were negative.

By the age of two weeks the Hb level had fallen to 7·8 g/100 ml, the film still showing pycnocytes, spherocytes and nucleated red cells. Serum cholesterol and betalipoprotein levels were normal, excluding acanthocytosis. A top-up tranfusion of 90 ml was given. Subsequent progress was uneventful but splenomegaly persisted until 6 months of age. At that time the Hb level was 12·2 g/100 ml, with only small numbers of pycnocytes and no spherocytes. Reticulocytes were 2·9 per cent, osmotic fragility and autoahemolysis were normal.

Tests for unstable haemoglobin were negative.

Subsequent development over a period of 10 years has been normal.

REFERENCES

Ahuja, G. L., Willoughby, M. L. N., Kerr, M. M. & Hutchinson, J. H. (1969) Massive subaponeurotic haemorrhage in Infants born by Vacuum Extraction. *Brit. Med. J.*, **iii**, 743.

Akerman, B. D. (1969) Infantile pyknocytosis in Mexican-American infants. *Amer. J. Dis. Child.*, **117**, 417.

Allison, A. C. (1957) Acute haemolytic anaemia with distortion and fragmentation of erythrocytes in children. *Brit. J. Haemat.*, **3**, 1.

American Academy of Pediatrics (1961) Vitamin K compounds and the water-soluble analogues. Use in therapy and prophylaxis in pediatrics. *Pediat.*, **28**, 501.

Anders, D., Kinderman, G. & Pfeifer, U. (1973) Neuroblastoma metastases in placenta simulating erythroblastosis. Report of two cases. *J. Pediat.*, **82**, 50.

Austin, R. F. & Desforges, J. F. (1969) Hereditary elliptocytosis: An unusual presentation of haemolysis in the newborn associated with transient morphological abnormalities. *Pediatrics*, **44**, 196.

Bajpai, P. C., Tripathi, T. K. & Agarwala, S. C. (1972) A study of erythrocyte life span in galactosemia using Cr^{51}. *J. Pediat.*, **80**, 835.

Beckett, R. S. & Flynn, F. J. (1953) Toxoplasmosis: report of two new cases, with a classification and a demonstration of the organism in the human placenta. *New Eng. J. Med.*, **249**, 345.

Bernard, J., Seligmann, M., Chassigneux, J. & Dresch, C. (1962) Anémie de Blackfan-Diamond. *Nouv. Rev. Franc. Hémat.*, **2**, 721.

Bulova, S. I. (1972) Hydrops fetalis and congenital syphilis. *Pediat.*, **49**, 285.

Burman, D. (1958) Congenital spherocytosis in infancy. *Arch. Dis. Childh.*, **33**, 335.

Cathie, I. A. B. (1952) Apparent idiopathic Heinz body anaemia. *Gt. Ormond St. J.*, **3**, 43.

Clayton, E. M., Pryor, J. A., Wierdsma, J. G. & Whitacre, F. E. (1964) Fetal and maternal components in thirdtrimester obstetric hemorrhage. *Obstet. Gynec.*, **24**, 56.

Cohen, F., Zuelzer, W. W., Gustafson, D. C. & Evans, M. M. (1964) Mechanisms of Isoimmunisation. I. The transplacental passage of fetal erythrocytes in homospecific pregnancies. *Blood*, **23**, 621.

Desmond, M. (1968) Clinical Pathological Conference. *J. Pediat.*, **73**, 283.

Diamond, L. K., Allen, D. M. & Magill, F. B. (1961) Congenital (erythroid) hypoplastic anemia. *Am. J. Dis. Child.*, **102**, 149.

Doxiadis, S. A., Fessas, P., Valaes, T. & Mastrokalos, N. (1961) Glucose-6-phosphate dehydrogenase deficiency; a new aetiological factor of severe neonatal jaundice. *Lancet*, **i**, 297.

Doxiadis, S. A. & Valaes, T. (1964) The clinical picture of glucose-6-phosphate dehydrogenase deficiency in early infancy. *Arch. Dis. Childh.*, **39**, 545.

Driscoll, S. G. (1966) Hydrops foetalis. *New Eng. J. Med.*, **275**, 1432.

Eichenwald, H. F. (1957) Congenital toxoplasmosis. A study of 150 cases. *A.M.A. J. Dis. Child.*, **94**, 411.

Embil, J. A., Ozere, R. L. & Haldane, E. V. (1970) Congenital cytomegalovirus infection in two siblings from consecutive pregnancies. *J. Pediat.*, **77**, 417.

Eshaghpour, E., Oski, F. A. & Naiman, J. L. (1966) Iron deficiency anemia in a newborn infant. *J. Pediat.*, **68**, 806.

Eshaghpour, E., Oski, F. A. & Williams, M. (1967) The relationship of erythrocyte glucose-6-phosphate dehydrogenase deficiency to hyperbilirubinemia in Negro premature infants. *J. Pediat.*, **70**, 595.

Garica, A. G. P. (1968) Congenital toxoplasmosis in two successive sibs. *Arch. Dis. Childh.*, **43**, 705.

Gasser, C. (1953) Die hämolytischer Frühgeburtenämie mit spontaner Innenkörperbildung; ein neue Syndrom, beobachtet an 14 Fälle. *Helv. paediat. Acta.*, **8**, 491.

Gasser, C. (1957) Aplasia of erythropoiesis. *Pediat. Clin. N. Amer.*, **4**, 445.

Gasser, C. (1959) Heinz body anemia and related phenomena. *J. Pediat.*, **54**, 673.

Gasser, C. & Willi, H. (1952) Spontane innenkörpebildung bei milzagenesie. *Helvet. paediat. acta.*, **7**, 369.

Goodall, H. B., Grahan, F. S., Miller, M. C. & Cameron, C. (1958) Transplacental bleeding from the foetus. *J. Clin. Path.*, **11**, 251.

Grimes, A. J., Meisler, A. & Dacie, J. V. (1964) Congenital Heinz-body anaemia: further evidence of the cause of Heinz-body production in red cells. *Brit. J. Haemat.*, **10**, 281.

Gross, R. T., Bracci, R., Rudolph, N., Schroeder, E. & Kochen, J. A. (1967) Hydrogen peroxide toxicity and detoxification in the erythrocytes of newborn infants. *Blood*, **29**, 481.

Gross, G. P. & Hathaway, W. E. (1972) Fetal erythrocyte deformability. *Pediat. Res.*, **6**, 593.

Harvey, B., Remington, J. S. & Sulzer, A. J. (1969) IgM malaria antibodies in a case of congenital malaria in the United States. *Lancet*, **1**, 333.

Hathaway, W. E., Mull, M. M. & Pechet, G. S. (1969) Disseminated intravascular coagulation in the newborn. *Pediatrics*, **43**, 233.

Helz, M. K. & Menten, M. L. (1944) Elliptocytosis, a report of two cases. *J. Lab. Clin. Med.*, **29**, 185.

Hsia, D. Y. & Walker, F. A. (1961) Variability in clinical manifestation of galactosemia. *J. Pediat.*, **59**, 872.

Kabat, D. (1974) An elution procedure for visualization of adult hemoglobin in human blood smears. *Blood*, **43**, 239.

Kan, Y. W., Allen, A. & Lowenstein, L. (1967) Hydrops fetalis with alpha thalassemia. *New Eng. J. Med.*, **276**, 18.

Kan, Y. W., Forget, B. G. & Nathan, D. G. (1972) Gamma-Beta thalassemia: a cause of hemolytic disease of the newborn. *New Eng. J. Med.*, **286**, 129.

Keimowitz, R. & Desforges, J. F. (1965) Infantile pycnocytosis. *New Eng. J. Med.*, **273**, 1152.

Kerr, M. M. (1959) Anaemia and polycythaemia in uni-ovular twins. *Brit. med. J.*, **i**, 902.

Kirkman, H. N. & Riley, H. D. (1959[A]) Posthemorrhagic anemia and shock in the newborn. A review. *Pediatrics*, **24**, 97.

Kirkman, H. N. & Riley, H. D. (1959[B]) Posthemorrhagic anemia and shock in the newborn due to hemorrhage during delivery. Report of 8 cases. *Pediatrics*, **24**, 92.

Lausecker, C., Heidt, P., Fischer, D., Hartleyb, H. & Löhr, G. E. (1965) Anémie hémolytique constitutionelle avec déficite en phosphogluconate dehydrogenase. *Arch. Fr. Pediat.*, **22**, 789.

Loos, L. (1892) Die Anämie bei hereditärer Syphiles. *Wien klin. Wchnschr.*, **5**, 291.

Lopez, R. & Cooperman, J. M. (1971) Glucose-6-phosphate dehydrogenase deficiency and hyperbilirubinemia in the newborn. *Amer. J. Dis. Child.*, **122**, 66.

Lunay, G. G., Edwards, R. F. & Thomas, D. B. (1970) Chronic transplacental haemorrhage causing acute fetal distress. *Brit. med. J.*, **ii**, 218.

McGovern, J. J., Driscall, R., Dutiot, C. H., Grove-Rasmussen, M. & Bedell, R. F. (1958) Iron deficiency anemia resulting from fetomaternal transfusion. *New Eng. J. Med.*, **258**, 1149.

Mauer, A. M. (1969) *Pediatric Haematology*, Philadelphia: McGraw-Hill.

Medearis, D. N. (1957) Cytomegalic inclusion disease. An analysis of the clinical features based on the literature and six additional cases. *Pediatrics*, **19**, 467.

Miles, R. M., Maurer, H. M. & Valdes, O. S. (1971) Iron-deficiency anemia at birth: Two examples secondary to chronic fetal-maternal hemorrhage. *Clinical Pediatrics*, **10**, 223.

Miller, D. R., Hanshaw, J. B., O'Leary, D. S. & Hnilicka, J. V. (1970) Fatal disseminated herpes simplex virus infection and hemorrhage in the neonate. *J. Pediatrics*, **76**, 409.

Moe, P. J. & Skjaeveland, A. (1969) Therapeutic studies in osteopetrosis—Report of 4 cases. *Acta Paediat. Scand.*, **58**, 593.

Naiman, J. L. & Kosoy, M. H. (1964) Red cell glucose-6-phosphate dehydrogenase deficiency—A newly recognized cause of neonatal jaundice and kernicterus in Canada. *Canad. M. A. J.*, **91**, 1243.

Necheles, T. F., Boles, T. A. & Allen, D. M. (1964) Erythrocyte glutathione peroxidase deficiency and haemolytic disease of the newborn infant. *J. Pediat.*, **72**, 319.

Necheles, T. F. & Allen, D. M. (1969) Heinz-body anemias. *New Eng. J. Med.,* **280,** 203.

Neligan, G. A. & Russell, J. K. (1955) Anaemia of the newborn following anterior placenta praevia. *Brit. med. J.,* **i,** 164.

Odell, G. B. (1967) 'Physiologic' hyperbilirubinemia in the neonatal period. *New Eng. J. Med.,* **277,** 103.

Oski, F. A. & Diamond, L. K. (1963) Erythrocyte pyruvate kinase deficiency: report of three cases. *New Eng. J. Med.,* **269,** 763.

Oski, F. A., Nathan, D. G., Sidel, V. W. & Diamond, L. K. (1964) Extreme haemolysis and red cell distortion in erythrocyte pyruvate kinase deficiency. I. Morphology, erythrokinetics and family enzyme studies. *New Eng. J. Med.,* **270,** 1023.

Oski, F. A. & Barness, L. A. (1967) Vitamin E deficiency: A previously unrecognized cause of hemolytic anemia in the premature infant. *J. Pediat.,* **70,** 211.

Oski, F. A. & Naiman, J. L. (1972[A]) Hematologic problems in the newborn, vol. iv, 2nd edn. In the series *Major Problems in Clinical Pediatrics.* Philadelphia: Saunders, p. 73.

Oski, F. A. & Naiman, J. L. (1972[B]), p. 78.

Oski, F. A. & Naiman, J. L. (1972[C]), p. 117.

Oski, F. A. & Naiman, J. L. (1972[D]), p. 125.

Oski, F. A. & Naiman, J. L. (1972[E]), p. 127.

Oski, F. A. & Naiman, J. L. (1972[F]), p. 154.

Paglia, D. E., Holland, P., Baughan, M. A. & Valentine, W. N. (1969) Occurrence of defective hexomonophosphate isomerization in human erythrocytes and leukocytes. *New Eng. J. Med.,* **280,** 66.

Paloheimo, J., Essen, R. von, Klemola, E., Kääriänen, L. & Siltanen, P. (1968) Subclinical cytomegalovirus infections and cytomegalovirus mononucleosis after open heart surgery. *Am. J. Cardiol.,* **22,** 624.

Pasternak, A., Furuhjelm, V., Knoring, J. van, Skerfvars, B. & Kuhlbäck, B. (1966) Acute renal failure after haemolysis, probably due to foeto-maternal transfusion. *Acta Med. Scand.,* **180,** 13.

Pearson, H. A. & Diamond, L. K. (1959) Fetomaternal transfusion. *A.M.A. J. Dis. Child.,* **97,** 267.

Pearson, H. A. (1967) Life span of the fetal red blood cell. *J. Pediat.,* **70,** 166.

Petersen, H. S. (1972) Pycnocytotic haemolytic anaemia of the newborn. *Acta Pediat. Scand.,* **61,** 362.

Pochedly, C. & Ente, G. (1969) Fetal bleeding: A dual menace. *Postgrad. Med.,* **45,** 157.

Pollack, A. (1968) Transplacental haemorrhage after external cephalic version. *Lancet,* **1,** 612.

Preston, F. E., Malia, R. G., Sworn, M. J. & Blackburn, E. K. (1973) Intravascular coagulation and *E. Coli* septicaemia. *J. clin. Path.,* **26,** 120.

Ratten, G. J. (1969) Spontaneous haematoma of the umbilical cord. *Austral. New Zeal. J. Obstet. Gynec.,* **9,** 125.

Rausen, A. R., Seki, M. & Strauss, L. (1965) Twin transfusion syndrome. A review of 19 cases studied at one institution. *J. Pediat.,* **66,** 613.

Rausen, A. R., Richter, P., Tallal, L. & Cooper, L. Z. (1967) Hematologic effects of intrauterine rubella. *J.A.M.A.,* **199,** 75.

Raye, J. R., Gutberlet, R. L. & Stahlman, M. (1970) Symptomatic posthemorrhagic anemia in the newborn. *Ped. Clin. N.A.,* **17,** 401.

Reider, R. F., Zinkham, W. H. & Holtzman, N. A. (1965) Hemoglobin Zürich. Clinical, chemical and kinetic studies. *Amer. J. Med.,* **39,** 4.

Robinson, G. C. (1957) Hereditary spherocytosis in infancy. *J. Pediat.,* **50,** 446.

Roddy, R. (1954) Two cases of hereditary spherocytosis manifest in the newborn period. *J. Pediat.,* **44,** 213.

Ross, J. D. (1963) Deficient activity of DPNH-dependent methemoglobin diaphorase in cord blood erythrocytes. *Blood,* **21,** 51.

Sacks, M. O. (1959) Occurrence of anemia and polycythemia in phenotypically dissimilar single ovum human twins. *Pediat.,* **24,** 604.

Saigal, S., O'Neill, A., Surainder, Y., Chua, Le-B. & Usher, R. (1972) Placental transfusion and hyperbilirubinemia in the premature. *Pediatrics,* **49,** 406.

Schafer, W. B. (1951) Acute hemolytic anemia related to naphthalene. Report of a case in a newborn infant. *Pediatrics,* **7,** 172.

Schröter, W. (1965) Kongenital nichtsphärocytare hämolytische anämie bei 2,-3 diphosphoglyceramutase-mangel der erythrocyten im frühen säuglingsalter. *Klin. Wschr.,* **43,** 1147.

Schmid, R., Brecher, G. & Clemens, T. (1959) Familial hemolytic anemia with erythrocyte inclusion bodies and a defect in pigment metabolism. *Blood,* **14,** 991.

Schulman, I. (1959) The anemia of prematurity. *J. Pediat.,* **54,** 663.

Scott, J. L., Haut, A., Cartwright, G. E. & Wintrobe, M. M. (1960) Congenital hemolytic anemia associated with red cell inclusion bodies, abnormal pigment metabolism and an electrophoretic hemoglobin abnormality. *Blood,* **16,** 1239.

Stamey, C. C. & Diamond, L. K. (1957) Congenital hemolytic anemia in the newborn. Relation to kernicterus. *Am. J. Dis. Child.,* **94,** 616.

Stern, H. & Tucker, S. M. (1973) Prospective study of cytomegalovirus infection in pregnancy. *Brit. med. J.,* **2,** 268,

Stocks, J., Kemp, M. & Dormandy, T. L. (1971) Increased susceptibility of red-blood-cell lipids to autoxidation in haemolytic states. *Lancet,* **i,** 266.

Sweet, L., Reid, W. D. & Robertson, N. R. C. (1973) Hydrops with placental chorioangioma. *J. Pediat.,* **82,** 91.

Thumasathit, B., Nondasuta, A., Jilpisornkosol, S., Lousuebsakul, B., Unchalipongse, P. & Mangkornkanok, M. (1968) Hydrops fetalis associated with Bart's hemoglobin in Northern Thailand. *J. Pediat.,* **73,** 132.

Todd, D., Lai, M. C. S., Braga, C. A. & Soo, H. N. (1969) Alpha-thalassaemia in Chinese: cord blood studies. *Brit. J. Haemat.*, **16**, 551.

Trucco, J. T. & Brown, A. K. (1967) Neonatal manifestations of hereditary spherocytosis. *Am. J. Dis. Child.*, **113**, 263.

Tuffy, P., Brown, A. K. & Zuelzer, W. W. (1959) Infantile pyknocytosis. A common erythrocyte abnormality of the first trimester. *Am. J. Dis. Child.*, **98**, 227.

Valaes, T., Karaklis, A., Stravrakakis, D., Bavela-Stravrakakis, K., Perakis, A. & Doxiadis, S. A. (1969) Incidence and mechanism of neonatal jaundice related to glucose-6-phosphate dehydrogenase deficiency. *Pediat. Res.*, **3**, 448.

Valentine, W. N., Oski, F. A., Paglia, D. E., Baughan, M. A., Schneider, A. S. & Naiman, J. L. (1967) Hereditary hemolytic anemia with hexokinase deficiency. Role of hexokinase in erythrocyte ageing. *New Eng. J. Med.*, **276**, 1.

Wang, M. Y. F., McCutcheon, E. & Desforges, J. F. (1967) Fetomaternal hemorrhage from diagnostic transabdominal amniocentesis. *Amer. J. Obstet. Gynec.*, **97**, 1123.

Weil, M. H., Shubin, N. & Biddle, M. (1964) Shock caused by gram-negative microorganisms. *Annals Intern. Med.*, **60**, 384.

Weisert, O. & Marstrander, J. (1960) Severe anaemia in a newborn caused by protracted foeto-maternal 'transfusion'. *Acta Paediat.*, **49**, 426.

Whitaker, J. A., Sartain, P. & Shaheedy, M. (1965) Hematological aspects of congenital syphilis. *J. Pediat.*, **66**, 629.

White, J. M. & Jones, R. W. (1969) Management of pregnancy in a woman with Hb H disease. *Brit. med. J.*, **iv**, 474.

Willi, H. & Hartmeier, F. (1960) Spontane innénkörperbilding beim neugeborenen. *Schweiz. med. Wschr.*, **80**, 1091.

Wong, T. T. T. & Chan, M. C. K. (1972) Transfusion reaction following ABO-incompatible maternal transfusion. *J. Pediat.*, **80**, 479.

Zannos-Mariolea, L., Kattamis, C. & Paidouces, M. (1962) Infantile pyknocytosis and glucose-6-phosphate dehydrogenase deficiency. *Brit. J. Haemat.* **8**, 258.

Zinkham, W. H. (1963) Peripheral blood and bilirubin values in normal full-term primaquine sensitive Negro infants. *Pediatrics*, **31**, 983.

Zuelzer, W. W. & Apt, L. (1949) Acute hemolytic anemia due to naphthalene poisoning—A clinical and experimental study. *J. Amer. Med. Ass.*, **141**, 185.

Zuelzer, W. W. & Mudgett, R. T. (1950) Kernicterus. Etiological study based on an analysis of 55 cases. *Pediatrics*, **6**, 452.

13. Secondary Anaemias

Anaemias of prematurity / Anaemias due to chronic infections / Rheumatoid arthritis and collagen diseases / Renal failure / Liver disease / Endocrine disorders / Malignant disease and bone marrow encroachment, *Marble-bone disease* / Sideroblastic anaemias.

A number of clinical situations apparently unrelated to the haemopoietic system predispose to anaemia. There is not usually any real diagnostic problem provided that the underlying condition is recognized; and the anaemia is seldom sufficiently severe to provide the major clinical problem in management. The importance of these anaemias stems from their relative frequency in paediatric practice, the fact that many are refractory to haematinic therapy and the insight into haemopoietic function that has resulted from their study.

ANAEMIAS OF PREMATURITY

At least four different factors have been incriminated as contributing to anaemia during the first year of life in premature or low birth weight infants. Some of these have already been discussed, viz. the 'late' anaemia of prematurity from the age of 4 months onwards due to iron deficiency, the liability to folate deficiency from 6 weeks onwards and the haemolytic anaemia attributed to vitamin E deficiency from about 6 to 10 weeks (Table 13.1).

At birth the premature infant has a slightly lower haemoglobin level than the term baby (16.4 ± 2.2 g/100 ml compared to 17.1 ± 1.7 g/100 ml) as well as higher reticulocyte counts (8.8 ± 2.3 per cent cf. 3.2 ± 1.4 per cent) and more circulating normoblasts (21/100 WBC cf. 7.3/100 WBC) (Matoth *et al.*, 1971; Gill and Schwartz, 1972). Small for dates babies, however, have higher than usual haemoglobin levels (Humbert *et al.*, 1969) yet the expected degree of reticulocytosis for their gestation (Lockridge *et al.*, 1971).

Whereas the late anaemia can be prevented by prophylactic iron administration (Gorten and Cross, 1964) and theoretically the megaloblastic and haemolytic anaemias could be prevented by folate (Hoffbrand, 1970) and vitamin E supplements (Oski and Barness, 1967) the early anaemia cannot be prevented or corrected by haematinics. Indeed Schulman (1959), in an excellent review of the subject, pointed out that the early anaemia occurs at a time when the iron stores in the marrow are actually increasing. The precise sequence appears to be as follows: During the first 7–8 weeks of life there is an arrest of erythropoiesis as is normal at this age (Seip, 1955). When pulmonary respiration is established at birth the new level of oxygen saturation of the relatively polycythaemic blood removes the previously existing stimulus for erythropoietin secretion (Halvorsen, 1963). An additional factor may be an impaired erythropoietic response by the marrow in premature infants

Table 13.1   Anaemias of prematurity

Type	Mechanism	Time of max. incidence
Early	Erythropoietic arrest + expanding blood volume	4–8 weeks
Intermediate	Erythropoiesis under stress from expanding blood volume	8–16 weeks
Late	Exhaustion of iron stores by expanding red cell mass	16 weeks onwards
Megaloblastic	Folate deficiency in face of precarious balance + infection	6–8 weeks
Haemolytic	Vitamin E deficiency at time of red cell susceptibility to oxidation	6–10 weeks

(Buchanan and Schwartz, 1974). Over these first weeks the haemoglobin level falls rapidly (Fig. 13.1), partly because of the shortened life span of foetal red cells, especially premature foetal cells (Gill and Schwartz, 1972), and partly because of the disproportionately rapid rate of weight and

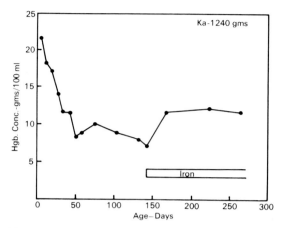

Fig. 13.1 Typical course of haemoglobin concentration in a premature infant. (Reproduced from Schulman (1959), *Journal of Pediatrics*[2] **54**, 663, by permission of the author and the publishers).

blood volume increase in the premature baby compared to the term baby, e.g. as shown by the shorter time taken to double its birth weight. The anaemia therefore results from the combination of these factors of shortened red cell survival plus unduly rapid expansion of blood volume at a time of relative cessation of erythropoiesis (Seip, 1955). Iron is present in the marrow and reticuloendothelial system throughout this early anaemia of prematurity and is in fact *increasing* due to the shrinking circulating red cell mass (Schulman, 1959).

The early phase is terminated by the return of erythropoiesis as a consequence of erythropoietin secretion in response to the development of anaemia (Mann et al., 1965). This is shown by the appearance of reticulocytes in the peripheral blood, absent earlier. Schulman has named this the 'intermediate' phase. The fall in haemoglobin is largely halted by the return of erythropoiesis but the continuing factors of haemolysis and increasing blood volume may delay an actual rise in haemoglobin concentration occurring (Fig. 13.1). The iron stores, however, are now being consumed and these are inevitably smaller than normal in proportion to the birth weight. By 16–20 weeks the iron stores become exhausted (Seip and Halvorsen, 1956) and at that point hypochromic red cells are formed for the first time, indicative of an actual iron deficiency anaemia which will result in a further fall in haemoglobin, the 'late' anaemia of prematurity, unless iron therapy is instituted (Fig. 13.1). From this description of the mechanisms involved it is clear that it is only this late anaemia which can be corrected or prevented by the administration of iron. Prophylactic iron is now universal practice in premature babies, e.g. 2.5 ml Sytron b.d. equivalent to 25 mg elemental iron per day, started within a few weeks of birth.

Term infants also have a falling haemoglobin level during their first 8–10 weeks of life, this being named the 'physiological anaemia of the newborn'. It is caused by similar mechanisms as those causing the 'early' anaemia of prematurity (O'Brien and Pearson, 1971) but the shortened red cell survival and the rate of blood volume expansion are less marked, resulting in a less severe anaemia. In the smaller premature infant the haemoglobin level may fall to as low as 8 g/100 ml, reaching this level at around 5 weeks, whereas in term infants the haemoglobin seldom falls below 10 g/100 ml and its lowest level is reached at 8–10 weeks (Gill and Schwartz, 1972).

Transfusion is seldom required for the anaemias of prematurity and never for the physiological anaemia of the newborn, since they are essentially self-limiting. Iron supplementation is essential, however, for low birth weight babies and folic acid and vitamin E supplementation have also recently been recommended (Dallman, 1974). Copper deficiency has also been recognized in premature babies on an iron fortified diet (Seely et al., 1972). A premature infant of birth weight 1.14 kg who trebled its weight in 7 weeks while on a copper poor cow's milk formula and had an episode of bacterial infection became severely anaemic and neutropenic. The haemoglobin was 4.3 g/100 ml, neutrophils 120/mm^3, and the marrow megaloblastic and vacuolation of erythroblasts while on iron and folic acid. The serum copper was 14 μg/ml. A remarkable response in Hb and neutrophils followed administration of 10 drops of 1 per cent $CuSO_4$ per day (Al-Rashid and Spangler, 1971).

ANAEMIAS DUE TO CHRONIC INFECTIONS

Haemolytic anaemias due to acute infections have been discussed in Chapter 9, neonatal anaemias due to infection in Chapter 12 and aplastic anaemias following viral infection in Chapter 4.

Chronic infection of duration greater than a month also commonly causes a relatively mild anaemia with a haemoglobin level usually between 9 and 11 g/100 ml. In the pre-antibiotic era infection accounted for approximately half the cases of anaemia in paediatric practice (Baty, 1947). Although the incidence is now considerably lower chronic infections do still occur and they are then a potent cause of anaemia.

The morphological features of the anaemia are non-specific, the blood film often showing only anisocytosis and rouleaux formation (indicative of an elevated ESR). In a recent review of this type of anaemia Cartwright and Lee (1971) describe this as most frequently normochromic and normocytic, less frequently hypochromic and normocytic, and occasionally, particularly in patients

(b) impaired marrow response to anaemia; and (c) impaired flow of iron from reticulendothelial cells to the marrow erythroblasts (Cartwright and Lee, 1971). The shortened red cell survival appears to be due to an extracorpuscular factor, and over-activity of the RES has been suggested. Bush et al. (1956) emphasized that there was only a moderate shortening of red cell survival for which a normal, healthy marrow with its six to eight-fold reserve for erythropoiesis could easily compensate. Inadequate function of the marrow was therefore suggested as the main factor determining the development of overt anaemia. The rate of erythropoiesis is found to be increased only two-fold in such anaemias. Recent work suggests that this failure of appropriate marrow response is due to impaired erythropoietin release in response to

Table 13.2 Values for iron, copper and porphyrins in normal subjects and in patients with the anaemia of chronic disorders

Determination	Normal subjects	Chronic disease
Plasma iron (μg/100 ml)	100 (70–150)	30 (10–70)
Total iron-binding capacity (μg/100 ml)	350 (300–400)	290 (100–300)
Transferrin saturation (%)	30 (25–50)	15 (10–25)
Sideroblasts (%)	40 (30–50)	10 (5–20)
Reticuloendothelial iron	2+ (1 to 2+)	3+ (2 to 6+)
Plasma copper (μg/100 ml)	114 (81–147)	191 (118–267)
Free erythrocyte protoporphyrin (μg/100 ml)	36 (14–79)	180 (36–634)

Data reproduced, by permission of Dr. G. E. Cartwright and the Editor, from Brit. J. Haemat. (1971) 21, 147.

with very long-standing disease, it is both hypochromic and microcytic. The hypochromia precedes the microcytosis (the opposite to iron deficiency) and is less marked than seen in pure iron deficiency. Other studies (Cartwright and Wintrobe, 1952; Bush et al., 1956) and reviews (Mitus, 1966; Cartwright, 1966) have characterized the anaemia of infection as having a low serum iron, a low TIBC, decreased marrow sideroblasts and normal or increased marrow reticuloendothelial iron (Table 13.2). The percentage of iron saturation is often low and if less than 16 per cent is associated with the production of hypochromic red cells. The low serum copper and increased erythrocyte protoporphyrin also simulate iron deficiency. A new test which promises to be of distinguishing value is the serum ferritin estimation since this is high in hypochromic secondary anaemia and low in iron deficiency (Chapter 1).

Kinetic and other studies have shown that at least three factors are involved in the pathogenesis of the anaemia: (a) shortened red cell survival;

anaemia in the presence of chronic inflammation (Ward et al., 1971). In experimental animals the anaemia of chronic inflammation will respond to erythropoietin, and in man such anaemias will respond to cobalt, a known stimulus of erythropoietin secretion. (Cobalt is not, however, recommended therapeutically because of its toxicity.)

The third factor of reticuloendothelial iron block was suggested by the combination of diminished iron in erythroblasts plus increased iron in marrow reticulum cells already mentioned. Kinetic radio iron studies in the closely related anaemia of rheumatoid arthritis have shown that a much lower proportion of the iron from red cell turnover is reutilized for erythropoiesis, only 40 per cent compared to 55–70 per cent in normals (Freireich et al., 1957). Presumably this is the cause of the hypochromia seen in a proportion of anaemias due to chronic disease. The cause of the RE iron block is unknown (Murdoch and Smith, 1972). A further factor which may contribute to iron deficiency changes in these patients is the depression of iron absorption during pyrexia that has recently been demonstrated (Beresford et al., 1971).

Therapy must be directed to controlling the underlying disease. Small blood transfusions have been recommended in preference to iron therapy, which is ineffective for anaemias of both acute (Mengel et al., 1967) and chronic infections (Adams and Mayet, 1966). The rise in plasma iron is minimal after administration of oral iron, while injected iron is rapidly removed from the blood (Murdoch and Smith, 1972).

RHEUMATOID ARTHRITIS AND COLLAGEN DISEASES

A very similar type of anaemia is seen in other inflammatory states including rheumatoid arthritis and collagen diseases. Haemoglobin levels below 10 g/100 ml have been found in approximately 40 per cent of children with rheumatoid arthritis (Kelley, 1960; Brewer, 1970). A similarly high incidence of anaemia in the Hb range of 9–10 g/100 ml is seen in acute rheumatic fever (Taylor, 1972) and systemic lupus erythematosus in childhood (Cook et al., 1960). The latter disease, however, includes instances of secondary auto-immune haemolytic anaemia (Chapter 9) and anaemia due to renal failure.

The anaemia is often normochromic and normocytic but sometimes moderately hypochromic and microcytic. As in the anaemia of chronic infection the serum iron is relatively low but the TIBC low rather than high. There is a correlation between Hb concentration and ESR. The red cell life span is moderately shortened but the main factor in determining anaemia is defective compensatory marrow response rather than haemolysis per se (Weinstein, 1959; Roberts et al., 1963). This appears to be due to impaired erythropoietin secretion in the presence of anaemia in this disease (Ward et al., 1969). The similarity in haematological findings and pathogenesis, including reticuloendothelial iron block, has led to the anaemias of rheumatoid arthritis and chronic infection being grouped together in recent years under the title 'anaemia of chronic disorders' (Cartwright, 1966; Cartwright and Lee, 1971).

Additional factors that may contribute to anaemia in children with acute rheumatoid arthritis are occult intestinal blood loss, due to steroid or salicylate therapy, and folate depletion. Omer and Mowat (1968) found a serum folate below 2·0 ng/ml in 46 per cent, a red cell folate below 130 ng/ml in 37 per cent and early megaloblastic changes in the marrow in 22 per cent of adults with rheumatoid arthritis. They attributed the findings to a combination of increased folate needs due to cellular proliferation, an exaggeration of the folate deficiency by iron deficiency and the reduced release of folate from effete erythrocytes (Mowat, 1971; Mowat, 1972).

While the disease is still active there is seldom a haematological response to oral iron although sometimes a partial response to parenteral iron. The latter effect probably reflects the ability of these larger quantities of circulating iron to overcome the avidity of the reticuloendothelial system for iron (Mowat, 1972). A trial of iron therapy during the active phase of the disease becomes more justified if the child is in the age group ($\frac{1}{2}$–3 years) when pre-existing iron deficiency is common, or if the serum iron is very low, with less than 16 per cent saturation. Control of the activity of the disease, for instance with corticosteroids or ACTH, results in a rapid rise in serum iron (Fig. 13.2) and an increase in transport of iron to the marrow (Mowat et al., 1969).

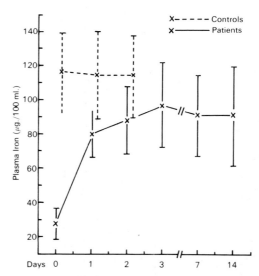

Fig. 13.2 The effect of 20 i.u. of ACTH/day on plasma iron values in rheumatoid arthritis. (Reproduced from *Annals of the Rheumatic Diseases* (1969), **28**, 303, by permission of Dr Mowat and the Editor).

Felty's syndrome of rheumatoid arthritis, splenomegaly and leucopenia is rare in children. Although splenomegaly occurs in 20 per cent of patients there is usually a prominent neutrophil leucocytosis. The splenomegaly may, however, contribute to the anaemia by haemodilution from the expanded plasma volume rather than by hypersplenism and haemolysis (Mowat, 1972).

RENAL FAILURE

The anaemia of chronic renal failure has many features in common with that of chronic infection and chronic inflammatory states described above. It is usually normochromic and normocytic and is primarily due to a failure of the marrow to respond adequately to the associated mild haemolysis (Brown, 1966; Desforges, 1970; Magid and Hilden, 1967). Impaired renal secretion or activation of erythropoietin is thought to be the major cause of the hypoproliferative marrow (Brown 1965). It is also possible that the uraemic environment impairs marrow erythropoiesis. In certain circumstances other factors may, however, operate to increase the severity of the anaemia. These include the presence of an associated microangiopathic haemolytic anaemia secondary to vascular changes and shown by the additional presence of numerous Burr cells on the blood film (Aherne, 1957; Brain et al., 1962), the presence of pyelonephritis which may be suspected from excessive rouleaux formation on the blood film (de Gruchy, 1970), or the presence of iron deficiency, caused by blood loss from the haemorrhagic state of uraemia and perhaps from diminished iron absorption.

There are difficulties in assessing the total body iron stores from the marrow erythroblast iron in these patients but it is probably true that reduced marrow iron indicates that the haemoglobin level will show some improvement after iron therapy (Mallick and Geary, 1972). Recently it has been suggested that histidine acts as a rate limiting metabolite in uraemia and haematological responses have been obtained after its administration in a dose of 300 mg/day for an 8-year-old child (Giordano et al., 1973).

In acute renal failure such as acute glomerulonephritis there is often a mild anaemia but the mechanism here is probably one of increase in plasma volume causing haemodilution (Verel et al., 1959). In another characteristically paediatric cause of acute renal failure, the haemolytic uraemic syndrome, the anaemia is due to acute haemolysis of the microangiopathic type. Although there is renal failure the reticulocytosis and the circulating normoblasts seen in these patients are evidence of normal marrow stimulation and capability (Adamson et al., 1968). Erythropoietin secretion in response to anaemia appears to be normal in acute renal failure (Miller and Denny, 1968) although defective in chronic renal failure.

Haemodialysis during the course of chronic renal failure may affect erythropoiesis in several ways. Kurtides et al. (1964) demonstrated an improvement in marrow function following haemodialysis. After a period of one or two years of regular dialysis the rate of red cell production can double (Esbach et al., 1967). Loss of blood and mechanical haemolysis associated with the procedure may, however, lead to iron depletion which can be prevented by giving iron dextran (Imferon) 200 to 250 mg per month, intravenously, during the dialysis therapy (Mallick and Geary, 1972). Megaloblastic changes and folic acid deficiency have also been reported after regular dialysis (Hampers et al., 1967) and may likewise be prevented by an oral maintenance dose. A controlled trial of androgen therapy (100 mg nandrolone decanoate IM per week in adults) has shown an increase in red cell mass and haematocrit, with a fall in transfusion requirements in patients on maintenance haemodialysis (Hendler et al., 1974). Blood transfusions are best avoided as much as possible in these patients because of the hazards of introducing the hepatitis B (serum hepatitis) virus or cytomegalovirus. Should future transplantation be contemplated the leucocyte and platelet components of a normal blood transfusion will almost certainly induce immunization to HLA antigens foreign to the patient. These infective and immunogenic complications may be considerably reduced by the use of red cells for transfusion which have been kept stored in liquid nitrogen and extensively washed prior to transfusion (Tullis et al., 1970). Nevertheless there remains the long-term liability to iron overload if

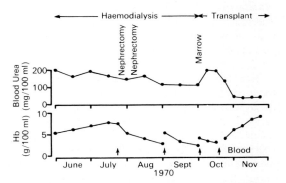

Fig. 13.3 Erythropoietic response after renal transplantation in a patient who had polycystic kidneys. After these were removed the haemoglobin fell steadily and the bone marrow showed no evidence of red-cell production. Repeated transfusion was necessary. After urgent and successful renal transplantation, the haemoglobin rose to normal levels which were maintained 18 months later. Sternal marrow aspiration (Marrow) showed delayed maturation of the erythroid series. (Reproduced from Clinics in Haematology (1972), 1, 569, by permission of Dr C. G. Geary and the publishers).

repeated transfusions are given and it proves possible to manage the majority of these patients without transfusion with the haemoglobin level lying between 6 and 12 g/100 ml. Following successful renal transplantation there is a rise in haemoglobin level in parallel with the return to normal of renal function (Fig. 13.3). These aspects are discussed in recent reviews by Mallick and Geary (1972) and by Taylor (1972).

LIVER DISEASE

Anaemia may arise by a number of different mechanisms in liver disease. Cirrhosis may be associated with a form of red cell fragmentation 'spur cell anaemia' (Smith *et al.*, 1964) and shortened red cell survival (Sjolin, 1964), especially if there is elevation of the serum lipids (Zieve, 1966). In the presence of secondary obstructive splenomegaly there is an additional element of hypersplenism with splenic sequestration of red cells as well as possible intermittent blood loss from oesophageal varices, resulting in iron deficiency (Kimber *et al.*, 1965). Hypoproteinaemia can accentuate the anaemia by increasing the plasma volume (Sjolin, 1964). In certain specific hepatic disorders other mechanisms of anaemia are operative: In Wilson's disease there is an intrinsic chronic haemolytic anaemia due to accumulation of copper in the red cells (McIntyre *et al.*, 1967; Deiss *et al.*, 1970); in acute viral hepatitis aplastic anaemia may develop (Schwartz *et al.*, 1966); if nutritional deficiency is present a megaloblastic anaemia due to folic acid deficiency may occur (Klipstein and Lindenbaum, 1965). This is also true in kwashiorkior (Spector and Metz, 1966).

The anaemia is sometimes slightly macrocytic in chronic liver disease but the marrow is then macronormoblastic, due to compensatory increased erythropoiesis, rather than megaloblastic (Nunnally and Levine, 1961). Target cells are present if there is an obstructive element to the liver failure, but they do not seem to be directly related to the development of anaemia. Folate deficiency is rare except in the context mentioned above. The serum B_{12} level is pathologically high in the presence of severe liver disease due to leaking out of the vitamin from the liver cells.

Treatment of the anaemia is unsatisfactory if the underlying liver disease cannot be improved. Acute gastrointestinal haemorrhage necessitates blood and perhaps platelet transfusion. A portocaval or lienorenal shunt can relieve the blood loss from oesophageal varices and a simultaneous splenectomy will alleviate the element of hypersplenism. In the minority of patients with associated folic acid deficiency this should be corrected.

ENDOCRINE DISORDERS

Anaemia is frequently present in hypothyroidism whether congenital (cretinism) or acquired. It is usually normochromic and normocytic but is sometimes hypochromic due to associated iron deficiency, and occasionally macrocytic due to B_{12} deficiency. In an adult series the incidence of anaemia was 32 per cent, with half of these showing iron deficiency and a quarter B_{12} deficiency (Tudhope and Wilson, 1960). There is no evidence of haemolysis (McClelland *et al.*, 1958), although the level of G-6-PD is low in children with hypothyroidism (Root *et al.*, 1967) and irregularly contracted red cells, similar to pycnocytes, are seen on the blood film in 60–70 per cent of cases (Wardrop and Hutchison, 1969).

The bone marrow is usually fatty and hypocellular, and erythropoiesis is usually normoblastic (Axelrod and Berman, 1951). It has been suggested that the marrow hypoplasia is due to erythropoietin deficiency (Nakao *et al.*, 1965).

The coincidence of hypothyroidism and iron deficiency may be fortuitous due to the high incidence of the latter, or may be related to impaired iron absorption (Taylor, 1972). A practical point is that there is a suboptimal response to iron therapy in these patients until thyroid replacement therapy is added (Bomford, 1938).

The finding of a macrocytic anaemia and megaloblastic marrow in children with hypothyroidism should raise the possibility of an autoimmune disease with antibodies against parietal cells as well as against the thyroid, leading to B_{12} deficiency (Taylor, 1972). The association of pernicious anaemia and hypothyroidism in adults is discussed by Tudhope (1972). In the uncomplicated anaemia of hypothyroidism a slow haemopoietic response occurs to thyroxine alone (Fig. 13.4).

Hypopituitarism produces a mild anaemia with similar haematological features to that of hypothyroidism. In Addison's disease some degree of anaemia is also present but may be masked by coexisting haemoconcentration (Taylor, 1972). In general these anaemias will respond only to appropriate endocrine replacement therapy. Again the association of Addison's disease and a megaloblastic anaemia raises the possibility of an in-

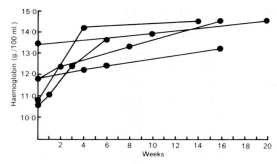

Fig. 13.4 Response to thyroxine in five cases of anemia of hypothyroidism. (Reproduced from Tudhope and Wilson (1960), Anaemia in Hypothyroidism. Incidence, pathogenesis and response to treatment, *Quarterly Journal of Medicine*, **29**, 513, by permission of the authors and the publishers, Oxford University Press).

herited autoimmune disease directed against multiple tissues including parietal cells (Hung et al., 1963).

MALIGNANT DISEASE AND BONE MARROW ENCROACHMENT

Many factors may contribute to the development of anaemia in malignant disease (Table 13.3) and these have recently been reviewed by Crowther and Batemen (1972). Maron and Shahidi (1970) have described a refractory hypochromic seen in children with lymphoma or Hodgkin's disease. This has many of the biochemical and morphological stigmata of iron deficiency but does not respond to iron. The defect appears to be a failure to transfer iron from the malignant reticuloendothelial system to the plasma and appears to have much in common with the 'anaemia of chronic disorders' delineated by Cartwright and coworkers. It is a rather striking fact that, by contrast, children with acute leukaemia hardly ever show iron deficiency during the active stage of their disease or at presentation.

The unique anaemia associated with malignant disease is that due to involvement of the bone marrow by the malignant process. The commonest non-haemic malignancy in paediatric practice that metastasizes to the marrow is neuroblastoma. Less frequent tumours are retinoblastoma and rhabdomyosarcoma. Nephroblastoma (Wilm's tumour) by contrast seldom involves the marrow. Among reticuloendothelial tumours Letterer-Siwe disease demonstrably infiltrates the marrow in approximately 10 per cent of patients (Mauer, 1969), lymphosarcoma in 30 per cent (Jones et al., 1972) at some stage of the disease and Hodgkin's disease in 5 per cent (Rosenberg, 1971). Marrow infiltration is suspected when a 'leucoerythroblastic anaemia' (Vaughan, 1936) is found. This term signifies the presence of myelocytes and normoblasts with anaemia, reticulocytosis and, at a late stage, thrombocytopenia and neutropenia (i.e. pancytopenia). The probable explanation of the leucoerythroblastic blood picture is that extramedullary erythropoiesis occurs when the marrow is infiltrated and that this allows escape of early myeloid and erythroid cells into the circulation (Gross and Marymont, 1963). Although anaemia is usually present this is not necessarily so at an early stage (Crowther and Bateman, 1972) and the term 'leucoerythroblastic blood picture' is then more appropriate. The reticulocytosis, and accompanying polychromasia, is to be noted since confusion with a haemolytic state may be made if this association is not appreciated. Bone marrow examination frequently demonstrates infiltration with tumour cells in the presence of the above mentioned peripheral blood findings (Clifford, 1966). Normal peripheral blood findings, however, do not exclude marrow secondaries. Contreras et al. (1972) have reported that bone marrow aspiration showed the presence of metastatic carcinoma in only one half of those with tumour cells detectable by biopsy with histological assessment.

Table 13.3 Causes of anaemia in malignant disease

1. Haemorrhage
2. Deficiency states
3. Dyserythropoietic anaemias
    (a) Anaemia similar to that seen in chronic inflammation
    (b) Sideroblastic anaemia
    (c) Erythroid hypoplasia
4. Haemodilution
5. Haemolysis
6. Leucoerythroblastic anaemia and marrow infiltration
7. Cytotoxic drug therapy

Data reproduced, by permission of Professor D. Crowther and the publishers, from Clinics in Haematology (1972) **1**, *448.*

Similarly Rosenberg (1971) found in the case of Hodgkin's disease that among 36 cases with demonstrable marrow involvement aspiration yielded 1 positive result, Westerman-Jensen needle biopsy yielded 12 positive results and in the remaining 23 patients only the open biopsy gave positive evidence of involvement. Wedge-biopsy of the iliac crest is the recommended procedure for detection of marrow involvement in the staging of Hodgkin's disease, performed at the same time as laparotomy.

As in other secondary anaemia there is little chance of correcting the anaemia, other than temporarily by transfusion, unless the underlying process can be controlled. In the case of malignant disease with marrow involvement the only possibility of improvement will lie with chemotherapy and, at least initially, this may accentuate the tendency to anaemia. This is particularly so in advanced neuroblastoma of patients on multidrug chemotherapy.

Marble bone disease

Also known as Albers-Schönberg disease or osteopetrosis this is a hereditary disorder that may present as a severe form (autosomal recessive) or a mild form (autosomal dominant) (Cocchi, 1952). The severe form presents in the first months of life with pallor, hepatosplenomegaly, generalized lymphadenopathy and a leucoerythroblastic blood picture with variable pancytopenia. These children tend to have an angular facies (Fig. 13.5). Great difficulty is found in obtaining marrow by aspiration, which can be an important clue to diagnosis (see Case 9). Radiological changes are characteristic and diagnostic consisting of generalized osteosclerosis with clubbing of the metaphyses (Fig. 13.5) (Kneal and Sante, 1951). The milder form of the disease shows the same features but not usually until late childhood or adolescence. One of the most distressing aspects of this disease is the progressive narrowing of the cranial foramina resulting ultimately in blindness due to optic atrophy and other cranial nerve lesions.

The haematological findings of circulating normoblasts and early myelocytes plus progressive pancytopenia including thrombocytopenia indicate encroachment on the haemopoietic marrow by the overgrowth of bone and compensatory extramedullary haemopoiesis, accounting for the hepatosplenomegaly and lymphadenopathy. If marrow can be obtained it is hypoplastic. An additional component of haemolysis has more recent been demonstrated in 4 cases by Sjolin (1959) and in 2 by Gamsu et al. (1961). The defect is extracorpuscular, affecting transfused normal cells to the same extent as the patient's cells. It is attributed to splenic sequestration of red cells and perhaps to general overactivity of the reticuloendothelial system. Splenectomy resulted in improvement in haemolysis in at least 2 out of Sjolin's 4 patients and in a further patient reported by Besselman (1966). Thrombocytopenia was consistently corrected by splenectomy in these reports. Prednisolone 7·5 to 10·0 mg on alternate days has also been reported as causing improvement in both the haematological status and the deranged mineral metabolism (Moe and Skjaeveland, 1969).

Case 9. A baby girl (No. 166061) developed twitching and was found to be hypocalcaemic in the neonatal period. At the age of 3 months she was found to be pale and to have hepatosplenomegaly. Investigation showed Hb 8·2 g/100 ml, WBC 23,000/mm³, platelets 50,000/mm³, with normoblasts, myelocytes and myeloblasts present on the film.

She was transferred for further investigation. The liver was 2 fingers and spleen 3 fingers below the costal margin, with no lymphadenopathy. Bone marrow aspiration was attempted from both Rt. and Lt. posterior iliac crests but was unusually difficult and yielded only a small amount of material with similar cellular content to the peripheral blood. The degree of bony resistance encountered during these attempts led to the suggestion of marble bone disease. A further feature suggesting this diagnosis was the angular facies (Fig. 13.5). The diagnosis was confirmed by a skeletal survey which showed a marked increase in the bone density with lack of definition of cortex and medulla. There was lack of modelling at the ends of the long bones and in their metaphyses (Fig. 13.5). Other investigations showed Hb F 14 per cent (normal for the age), reticulocytes 11 per cent, blast cells 800/mm³, normoblasts 22 per 100 WBC, normal urinary hydroxyproline, alkaline phosphatase of 28 K.A. units/100 ml, calcium of 3·3 m Eq/l, phosphorus 3·0 mg/100 ml and elevated acid phosphatase 23 K.A. units/100 ml (tartrate-stable form 18·5 K.A. units).

Her Hb fell to 4·0 g/100 ml at the age of 18 months and she was given her first transfusion of 180 ml packed cells. Thereafter the Hb fell progressively more rapidly with transfusions being needed at 4-, 3- and finally 2-week intervals by the age of 2 years. Serum iron at this time was 225 μg/100 ml and TIBC 243. Accompanying the high transfusion requirements there was an increasing bleeding tendency due to thrombocytopenia of around 10,000/mm³. The spleen had now increased to 3 fingers and was firm. Splenectomy was performed to reduce transfusion requirements and the thrombocytopenic bleeding. Platelets rose initially to 92,000 then settled to 25,000/mm³. Histology showed extensive extramedullary haemopoiesis throughout the red pulp.

She was started on long-term Penicillin V 125 mg b.d. to reduce the hazard of post-splenectomy overwhelming pneumococcal infection. Early in her course there had been no significant response to a low calcium diet or to short steroid courses.

Unfortunately the parents did not accept genetic counselling and a subsequent baby is similarly affected.

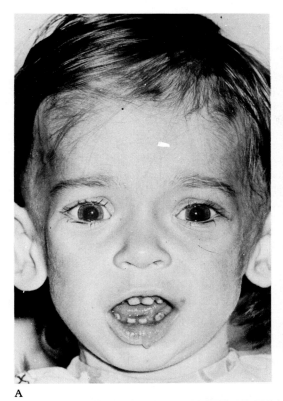
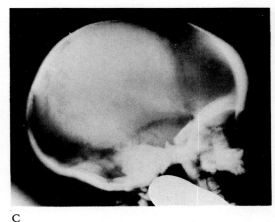
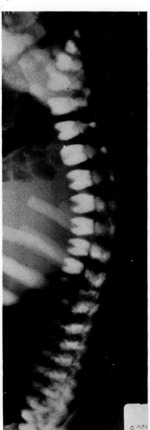
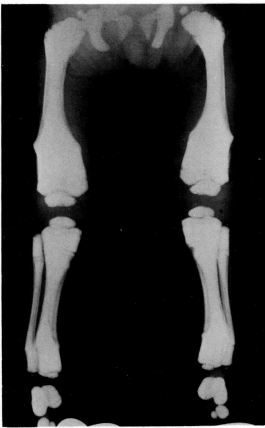

Fig. 13.5 Marble bone disease. Clinical and radiological features of Case 9.

SIDEROBLASTIC ANAEMIAS

A Prussian blue iron stain on a normal marrow smear shows that up to 50 per cent of the erythroblasts contain one or two minute greenish dots at the edge of the nucleus. These iron-containing normoblasts are termed sideroblasts. In certain pathological states nearly 100 per cent of the erythroblasts show a great excess of stainable iron arranged as a ring of larger clumps around the periphery of the nucleus ('ring sideroblasts'). Electron microscopy shows that the mitochondria are encrusted by dense clumps of iron (Grasso and Hines, 1965). The cause of this iron accumulation is not clear since *in vitro* studies using radioactive iron gave no evidence of a block in haem synthesis nor deficiency of the enzymatic pathway concerned (Vavra and Poff, 1967). Haematologically the sideroblastic states present as iron-refractory hypochromic anaemias (Mollin, 1965). Some cases respond to large doses of pyridoxine or pyridoxal-5-phosphate, while a minority with evidence of folate deficiency may respond to folic acid in large doses (MacGibbon and Mollin, 1965).

Sideroblastic anaemias are more characteristically seen in the elderly and are rare in childhood, the majority of cases being secondary to myeloproliferative disorders, malignancy, therapy with antituberculous drugs or chronic inflammatory states (Symposium on Sideroblastic Anaemia, 1965; Weatherall, 1969). Paediatric cases, however, are seen secondary to lead poisoning or occasionally as a hereditary sex-linked form (Cooley, 1945; Rundles and Falls, 1946; Mills and Lucia, 1949; Heilmeyer *et al.*, 1958). Mollin (1965) has tabulated the haematological findings in the 6 patients reported in the literature with the hereditary form of sideroblastic anaemia. Their ages were 3–34 years, all were male, there was a family history in 3 patients in whom detailed studies were performed, the Hb ranged from 4·5 to 8·4 g/100 ml,

MCHC 23–29 per cent, MCV 56–80 μm^3 and reticulocytes 0·1 to 5·0 per cent. The blood film showed marked hypochromia with some elongated red cells and dimorphism. Hb F was absent or slightly increased but Hb A$_2$ not increased, distinguishing this from beta thalassaemia. Osmotic fragility was decreased, due to the hypochromia, and ^{51}Cr red cell survival moderately decreased, with haemolysis less marked than in thalassaemia. In most patients the serum iron level was increased and the TIBC saturated. Mild neutropenia and thrombocytopenia are present in nearly half the patients with hereditary or acquired sideroblastic anaemia. In practice the differential diagnosis includes thalassaemia or dyserythropoietic syndromes. A probable case of congenital sideroblastic anaemia is described below (Case 9), perhaps the youngest yet reported.

Case 10. On routine examination at birth this male infant (No. 98757) was found to have hepatosplenomegaly. There was no lymphadenopathy or jaundice. Neonatal leukaemia was suspected and the infant was transferred to the R.H.S.C. Hb was 16 g/100 ml with normal white cell picture and platelets but with numerous target cells on the blood film. The parents' blood films were normal and haemoglobin analysis excluded any haemoglobinopathy.

At the age of 7 weeks his Hb level had fallen to 5 g/100 ml and he was transfused. At 9 weeks the Hb was again falling and a population of *hypochromic* red cells started appearing in the peripheral blood. A marrow examination at this time showed that virtually all the late normoblasts stained with ferrocyanide as ring sideroblasts. The serum iron at this time was 211 μg/100 ml. Red cell levels of porphyrines and their precursors were normal.

Subsequently this boy has shown persistent slight splenomegaly and anaemia (6–8 g/100 ml) with sideroblasts in the marrow over the subsequent 9 years. He has not shown a convincing haematological response to pyridoxine and has required 3 transfusions over this period.

No other members of the family have anaemia but a sex-linked inheritance cannot be excluded from the family tree. An elder sibling was unaffected.

REFERENCES

Adams, E. B. & Mayet, F. G. H. (1966) Hypochromic anaemia in chronic infections. *S. African Med. J.*, **20**, 738.

Adamson, J. W., Esbach, J. & Finch, C. A. (1968) The kidney and erythropoiesis. *Amer. J. Med.*, **44**, 725.

Aherne, W. A. (1957) The 'burr' red cell and azotemia. *J. Clin. Path.*, **10**, 252.

Al-Rashid, R. A. & Spangler, J. (1971) Neonatal copper deficiency. *New Eng. J. Med.*, **285**, 841.

Axelrod, A. R. & Berman, L. (1951) The bone marrow in hyperthyroidism and hypothyroidism. *Blood*, **6**, 436.

Baty, J. M. (1947) Classification of anemia in infants and children. *J. Am. Med. Assoc.*, **134**, 1002.

Besselman, D. M. (1966) Splenectomy in the management of anemia and thrombocytopenia of ostepetrosis (Marble bone disease). *J. Pediat.*, **69**, 455.

Beresford, C. H., Neale, R. J. & Brooks, O. G. (1971) Iron absorption and pyrexia. *Lancet*, **1**, 268.

Bomford, R. (1938) Anaemia in myxoedema: and the role of the thyroid gland in erythropoiesis. *Quarterly J. Med.*. **7**, 495.

Brain, M. C., Dacie, J. V. & Hourihane, D. O'B. (1962) Microangiopathic haemolytic anaemia: the possible role of vascular lesions in pathogenesis. *Brit. J. Haemat.*, **8**, 358.

Brewer, E. J. (1970) *Juvenile Rheumatoid Arthritis*. Philadelphia: Saunders.

Brown, R. (1965) Plasma erythropoietin in chronic uremia. *Brit. med. J.*, **ii**, 1036.

Brown, R. (1966) Erythropoiesis in chronic renal disease. *Lancet*, **ii**, 319.

Bush, J. A., Ashenbrucker, H., Cartwright, G. E. & Wintrobe, M. M. (1956) The anemia of infection. XX. The kinetics of iron metabolism in the anemia associated with chronic infection. *J. Clin. Invest.*, **35**, 89.

Cartwright, G. E. (1966) The anemia of chronic disorders. *Seminars in Hematology*, **3**, 351.

Cartwright, G. E. & Wintrobe, M. M. (1952) The anaemia of infection. XVII. A Review. *Asvan. Intern. Med.*, **5**, 165,

Cartwright, G. E. & Lee, G. R. (1971) The anaemia of chronic disorders. *Brit. J. Haemat.*, **21**, 147.

Clifford, G. O. (1966) The clinical significance of leucoerythroblastic anaemia. *Medical Clinics of N. Amer.*, **50**, 779.

Cocchi, U. (1952) Erbschaden mit knochenveränderungen. In *Lehrbuch der Röntgendiagnostik*. Edited by Schinz *et al.* Stuttgart: Thieme.

Contreras, E., Ellis, L. D. & Lee, R. E. (1972) Value of the bone marrow in the diagnosis of metastatic carcinoma. *Cancer*, **29**, 778.

Cook, C. D., Wedgewood, R. J. P., Craig, J. M., Hartmann, J. R. & Janeway, C. A. (1960) Systemic lupus erythematosus. Description of 37 cases in children and a discussion of endocrine therapy in 32 of the cases. *Pediat.*, **26**, 570.

Cooley, T. B. (1945) A severe type of hereditary anaemia with elliptocytosis. Interesting sequence of splenectomy. *Amer. J. med. Sci.*, **209**, 561.

Crowther, D. & Bateman, C. J. J. (1972) Malignant disease. *Clinics in Haematology*, **1**, 447.

Dallman, P. R. (1974) Iron, vitamin E and folate in the preterm infant. *J. Pediat.*, **85**, 742.

Desforges, J. F. (1970) Anemia in uremia. *Arch. Int. Med.*, **126**, 808.

Deiss, A., Lee, G. R. & Cartwright, G. E. (1970) Hemolytic anemia in Wilson's disease. *Ann. Int. Med.*, **73**, 413.

Esbach, J. W., Funk, D., Adamson, J., Kuhn, I., Scribner, B. H. & Finch, C. A. (1967) Erythropoiesis in patients with renal failure undergoing chronic dialysis. *New Eng. J. Med.*, **276**, 653.

Freireich, E. J., Ross, J. F., Bayles, T. B., Emerson, C. P. & Finch, S. C. (1957) Radioactive iron metabolism and erythrocyte survival studies of the mechanism of the anemia associated with rheumatoid arthritis. *J. Clin. Invest.*, **36**, 1043.

Gamsu, H., Lorber, J. & Rendle-Short, J. (1961) Haemolytic anaemia in osteopetrosis—a report of two cases. *Arch. Dis. Childh.*, **36**, 494.

Gill, F. M. & Schwartz, E. (1972) Anemia in early infancy. *Pediat. Clin. N. Amer.*, **19**, 841.

Giordano, C. Santo, N. G. de, Rinaldi, S., Acone, D., Esposito, R. & Gallo, B. (1973) Histidine for treatment of uraemic anaemia. *Brit. med. J.*, **4**, 714.

Gorten, M. K. & Cross, E. R. (1964) Iron metabolism in premature infants. II. Prevention of iron deficiency. *J. Pediat.*, **64**, 509.

Grasso, J. A. & Hines, J. D. (1965) A comparative electron microscopic study of refractory and alcoholic sideroblastic anaemia. *Brit. J. Haemat.*, **17**, 35.

Gross, S. & Marymont, J. H. (1963) Extramedullary haemopoiesis and metastatic cancer in the spleen. *Amer. J. Clin. Path.*, **40**, 194.

Gruchy, C. de (1970) *Clinical Haematology in Medical Practice*, p. 204. Oxford: Blackwell Scientific Publications.

Halvorsen, S. (1963) Plasma erythropoietin levels in cord blood and in blood during the first week of life. *Acta Paediat. Scand.*, **52**, 425.

Hampers, C. L., Streiff, R., Nathan, D. G., Snyder, D. & Merrill, J. P. (1967) Megaloblastic hematopoiesis in uremia and in patients on long term dialysis. *New Eng. J. Med.*, **276**, 551.

Heilmeyer, L., Emmrich, J., Hennemann, H. H., Keiderling, W., Lee, M., Bilger, R. & Schubothe, K. (1958) Uber eine chronische hypochrome Anämie bei zwei Geschwistern auf der Grundlage einer Eisenverwertungs-Störung (Anaemia hypochromica sideroachrestica hereditaria). *Folia haemat. N.F.*, **2**, 61.

Hoffbrand, A. V. (1970) Folate deficiency in premature infants. *Arch. Dis. Childh.*, **45**, 441.

Hendler, E. D., Goffinet, J. A., Ross, S., Longnecker, R. E. & Bakovic, V. (1974) Controlled study of androgen therapy in anaemia of patients on maintenance haemodialysis. *New Eng. J. Med.*, **291**, 1046.

Humbert, J. R., Abelson, H., Hathaway, W. E. & Battaglia, F. C. (1969) Polycythemia in small for gestational age infants. *J. Pediat.*, **75**, 812.

Hung, W., Migeon, C. J. & Parrott, R. H. (1963) Possible autoimmune basis for Addison's disease in three siblings, one with idiopathic hypoparathyroidism, pernicious anemia and superficial moniliasis. *New Eng. J. Med.*, **269**. 658.

Jones, S. E., Rosenberg, S. A. & Kaplan, H. S. (1972)—(to be published).

Kelley, V. C. (1960) Rheumatoid disease in childhood. *Pediat. Clin. N. Am.*, **7**, 435.

Kimber, C., Deller, D. J., Ibbotson, R. N. & Lander, H. (1965) The mechanism of anaemia in chronic liver disease. *Quart. J. Med.*, **34**, 33.

Klipstein, F. A. & Lindenbaum, J. (1965) Folate deficiency in chronic liver disease. *Blood*, **25**, 443.

Kneal, E. & Sante, L. P. (1951) Osteopetrosis (marble bones). Report of a case with special reference to early roentgenologic and pathological findings. *Am. J. Dis. Child.*, **81**, 693.

Kurtides, E. S., Rambach, W. A., Alt, H. L. & Del Greco, F. (1964) Effect of hemodialysis on erythrokinetics in anemia of uremia. *J. Lab. Clin. Med.*, **63**, 469.

Lockridge, S., Pass, R. & Cassady, G. (1971) Reticulocyte counts in intrauterine growth retardation. *Pediatrics*, **47**, 919.

McClelland, J. E., Donnegan, C., Thorup, O. A. & Leavell, B. S. (1958) Survival time of the erythrocyte in myxedema and hyperthyroidism. *J. Lab. Clin. Med.*, **51**, 91.

MacGibbon, B. H. & Mollin, D. L. (1965) Sideroblastic anaemia in man: Observations on seventy cases. *Brit. J. Haemat.*, **11**, 59.

McIntyre, N., Clink, H. M., Levi, A. J., Cumings, J. N. & Sherlock, S. (1967) Hemolytic anemia in Wilson's disease. *New Eng. J. Med.*, **276**, 439.

Magid, E. & Hilden, M. (1967) Ferrokinetics in patients suffering from chronic renal disease and anaemia. *Scand. J. Haemat.*, **4**, 33.

Mallick, N. P. & Geary, C. G. (1972) Renal disease. *Clinics in Haematology*, **1**, 553.

Mann, D. L., Sites, M. L., Donati, R. M. & Gallagher, N. I. (1965) Erythropoietin stimulatory activity during the first ninety days of life. *Proc. Soc. Exper. Biol. Med.*, **118**, 212.

Maron, B. J. & Shahidi, N. T. (1970) Refractory hypochromic anaemia in malignant lymphoma. *J. Pediat.*, **77**, 93.

Matoth, Y., Zaizor, R. & Varsano, I. (1971) Postnatal changes in some red cell parameters. *Acta Paediat. Scand.*, **60**, 317.

Mauer, A. M. (1969) *Pediatric Hematology*, p. 398. New York: McGraw-Hill.

Mengel, C. E., Metz, E. & Yancey, W. S. (1967) Anemia during acute infections. *Arch. Int. Med.*, **119**, 287.

Miller, R. P. & Denny, W. F. (1968) Hemolytic anemia during acute renal failure, observations on plasma erythropoietic levels. *Southern Medical Journal*, **61**, 29.

Mills, H. & Lucia, S. P. (1949) Familial hypochromic anemia associated with post-splenectomy erythrocytic inclusion bodies. *Blood*, **4**, 891.

Mitus, W. J. (1966) Anaemias of infection. *Med. Clin. N. Amer.*, **50**, 1703.

Moe, P. J. & Skjaeveland, A. (1969) Therapeutic studies in osteopetrosis—Report of 4 cases. *Acta Paediat. Scand.*, **58**, 593.

Mollin, D. L. (1965) Sideroblasts and sideroblastic anaemia. *Brit. J. Haemat.*, **11**, 41.

Mowat, A. G. (1971) Haematological abnormalities in rheumatoid arthritis. *Seminars in Arthritis and Rheumatism* **1**, 195.

Mowat, A. G. (1972) Connective tissue diseases. *Clinics in Haematology*, **1**, 573.

Mowat, A. G., Hothersall, T. E. & Aitchison, W. R. C. (1969) Nature of anaemia in rheumatoid arthritis XI. Changes in iron metabolism induced by the administration of corticotrophin. *Annals of the Rheumatic Diseases*, **28**, 303.

Murdoch, J. McC. & Smith, C. C. (1972) Infection. *Clinics in Haematology*, **1**, 619.

Nakao, K., Maekawa, T., Shirakura, T. & Yaginuma, M. (1965) Anemia due to hypothyroidism. *Israel J. Med. Sci.*, **1**, 742.

Nunnally, R. M. & Levine, I. (1961) Macronormoblastic hyperplasia of the bone marrow in hepatic cirrhosis. *Amer. J. Med.*, **30**, 972.

O'Brien, R. T. & Pearson, H. A. (1971) Physiologic anemia of the newborn infant. *J. Pediat.*, **79**, 132.

Omer, A. & Mowat, A. G. (1968) Nature of anaemia in rheumatoid arthritis IX. Folate metabolism in patients with rheumatoid arthritis. *Annals of the Rheumatic Diseases*, **27**, 414.

Oski, F. A. & Barness, L. A. (1967) A previously unrecognized cause of hemolytic anemia in the premature infant. *J. Pediat.*, **70**, 211.

Roberts, F. D., Hagedorn, A. B., Slocumb, C. H. & Owen, C. A. (1963) Evaluation of the anemia of rheumatoid arthritis. *Blood*, **21**, 470.

Root, A. W., Iski, F. A., Bongiovanni, A. M. & Eberlein, W. R. (1967) Erythrocyte glucose-6-phosphate dehydrogenase activity in children with hypothyroidism and hypopituitarism. *J. Pediat.*, **70**, 396.

Rosenberg, S. A. (1971) Hodgkin's disease of the bone marrow. *Cancer Research*, **31**, 1733..

Rundles, R. W. & Falls, H. F. (1946) Hereditary (? sex-linked) anaemia. *Amer. J. med. Sci.*, **211**, 641.

Schulman, I. (1959) Anemia of prematurity. *J. Pediat.*, **54**, 663.

Schwartz, E., Baehner, R. L. & Diamond, L. K. (1966) Aplastic anemia following hepatitis. *Pediatrics*, **37**, 681.

Seely, J. R., Humphrey, G. B. & Matter, B. J. (1972) Copper deficiency in a premature infant fed on iron-fortified formula. *New Eng. J. Med.*, **286**, 109.

Seip, M. (1955) The reticulocyte level and erythrocyte production judged from reticulocyte studies in newborn infants during the first week of life. *Acta Paediat. Scand.*, **44**, 355.

Seip, M. & Halvorsen, S. (1956) Erythrocyte production and iron stores in premature infants during the first months of life. The anaemia of prematurity—etiology, pathogenesis, iron requirements. *Acta Paediat. Scand.*, **45**, 600.

Sjölin, S. (1959) Studies on osteopetrosis. II. Investigations concerning the nature of the anaemia. *Acta Paediat. Scand.*, **48**, 529.

Sjölin, S. (1964) Haematologic abnormalities in hepatic cirrhosis in children. *Scand. J. Haemat.*, **1**, 94.

Smith, J. A., Lonergan, E. T. & Sterling, K. (1964) Spur-cell anemia. Hemolytic anemia with red cells resembling acanthocytes in alcoholic cirrhosis. *New Eng. J. Med.*, **271**, 396.

Spector, I. & Metz, J. (1966) Giant myeloid cells in bone marrow of protein malnourished infants: Relationship to folate and vitamin B_{12} nutrition. *Brit. J. Haemat.*, **12**, 737.

Symposium on Sideroblastic Anaemia (1965) *Brit. J. Haemat.*, **11**, 41.

Taylor, J. C. (1972) Haematologic manifestations of systemic disease. *Paed. Clin. N. Amer.*, **19**, 1071.

Tudhope, G. R. & Wilson, G. M. (1960) Anaemia in hypothyroidism. Incidence, pathogenesis and response to treatment. *Quart. J. Med.*, **29**, 513.

Tudhope, G. R. (1972) Endocrine diseases. *Clinics in Haematology*, **1**, 475.

Tullis, J. L., Hinman, J., Sproul, M. T. & Nickerson, R. J. (1970) Incidence of post-transfusion hepatitis in previously frozen blood. *J.A.M.A.*, **214**, 719.

Vaughan, J. M. (1936) Leucoerythroblastic anaemia. *J. Path. Bact.*, **42**, 541.

Vavra, J. D. & Poff, S. A. (1967) Heme and porphyrin synthesis in sideroblastic anemia. *J. Lab. Clin. Med.*, **69**, 904.

Verel, D., Turnbull, A., Tudhope, G. R. & Ross, J. H. (1959) Anaemia in Bright's disease. *Quart. J. Med.*, **28**, 491.

Ward, H. P., Gordon, B. & Pickett, J. C. (1969) Serum levels of erythropoietin in rheumatoid arthritis. *J. Lab. Clin. Med.*, **74**, 93.

Ward, H. P., Kurnick, J. E. & Pisarczyk, M. J. (1971) Serum level of erythropoietin in anaemias associated with chronic infection, malignancy and primary haematopoietic disease. *J. Clin. Invest.*, **50**, 332.

Wardrop, C. & Hutchinson, H. E. (1969) Red-cell shape in hypothyroidism. *Lancet*, **1**, 1243.

Weatherall, D. J. (1969) Hypochromic anaemias not due to iron deficiency: Thalassaemia and sideroblastic anaemia. *J. Roy. Coll. Phycns. Lond.*, **3**, 275.

Weinstein, I. M. (1959) A correlative study of the erythrokinetics and disturbances in iron metabolism associated with the anemia of rheumatoid arthritis. *Blood*, **14**, 950.

Zieve, L. (1966) Hemolytic anemia in liver disease. *Medicine (Baltimore)*, **45**, 497.

14. Polycythaemia

Primary polycythaemia, *Polycythaemia rubra vera, Benign familial polycythaemia (erythrocytosis)* / Secondary polycythaemia, *Cyanotic congenital heart disease, Abnormal haemoglobins, Tumours and renal disease*/Neonatal polycythaemia,

This term implies an increase in circulating red cell mass to above the normal upper limit of 30 ml/kg body weight, the definition thereby excluding haemoconcentration due to dehydration (Murray, 1966). In practice the diagnosis of polycythaemia is considered if the haemoglobin level is chronically greater than 17 g/100 ml during childhood or greater than 22 g/100 ml in the neonatal period. Corresponding upper limits for haematocrits (Hct) are 50 and 65 per cent respectively (Kontras, 1972; Oski and Naiman, 1972). There are a number of different causes of polycythaemia in childhood (Table 14.1). All are rare except cyanotic congenital heart disease.

PRIMARY POLYCYTHAEMIA

Polycythaemia rubra vera

Although relatively common in adult life this disease is excessively rare in childhood. Nevertheless there are a few reports of the disease in children (Marlow and Fairbanks, 1960; Aggeler *et al.*, 1961; Natelson *et al.*, 1971). Presenting symptoms included headaches and episodes of blurred vision. The appearance was plethoric and the spleen palpable. There was no family history of polycythaemia. Haemoglobin levels were in excess of 20 g/100 ml, accompanied by thrombocytosis in one of the patients but with normal white cell counts. Therapy was by means of phlebotomy. The long-term outcome of polycythaemia rubra vera in children is unknown at the present time (Kontras, 1972), but late complications of thrombosis, haemorrhage and perhaps transformation to other myeloproliferative disorders, as occurs in adults, would be expected.

Mauer (1969) points out that this diagnosis should only be made after extensive search for a predisposing cause and 'even then a healthy scepticism would be indicated'.

Benign familial polycythaemia (erythrocytosis)

Although also rare a large number of reports are available in the paediatric literature (Knock and Githens, 1960; Abildgaard *et al.*, 1963; Cassileth and Hymen, 1966; Geary *et al.*, 1967; Kontras and Romshe, 1967). The later workers were able to collect reports of a total of 19 cases in 13 families and added 2 further cases from one family. Inheritance appears to be autosomal with variable penetrance.

Symptoms may be mild including headache, lethargy, dizziness and easy fatigability, or may be absent (Kontras and Romshe, 1967). Clinically there is plethora with conjunctival injection usually without splenomegaly. The onset may occur from 3 years onwards. Diagnosis is made by the finding of an isolated increase in haemoglobin, usually in excess of 20 g/100 ml, due to an absolute increase in circulating red cell mass and without leucocytosis or thrombocytosis. No predisposing cause is present but other members of the family may be similarly affected. Defective control of erythropoietin secretion has been suggested as the cause (Kontras and Romshe, 1967).

The benign course of the disease has been stressed in these reports and it appears that the condition is compatible with a normal life. If symptoms secondary to hyperviscosity develop then phlebotomy or erythrophoresis may be employed (Kontras, 1972).

SECONDARY POLYCYTHAEMIA

In these disorders there is an increase in total circulating red cell mass, but secondary to an identifiable cause. In paediatric practice by far the commonest cause is cyanotic congenital heart disease, viz. associated with a right to left shunt. Other causes of chronically reduced oxygen saturation of arterial blood including residence at high altitude (Treger *et al.*, 1965) or chronic lung disease (Hume, 1968) similarly cause polycythaemia. The mechanism in each case is thought to be through erythropoietin stimulation resulting from

is a corresponding increase in total blood volume. Physiological benefits from the increase in blood volume are twofold; (a) an increase in O_2 carrying capacity of the blood, (b) a rise in cardiac output. At any given Hct the cardiac output is greater with hypervolaemia than with normovolaemia (Rosenthal *et al.*, 1971). The above advantages, however, are offset by the increasing viscosity of the blood as the Hct rises. Kontras *et al.*

Table 14.1   Classification of polycythaemia

I. Relative polycythemia, hemoconcentration

II. Primary polycythemia
   A. Polycythemia vera
   B. Benign familial polycythemia or erythrocytosis

III. Secondary polycythemia
   A. Insufficient oxygen delivery
      1. Low environmental O_2 (high altitude)
      2. Impaired ventilation – pulmonary disease, obesity
      3. Cyanotic congenital heart disease
      4. Abnormal hemoglobins
         a. Methemoglobinemia (congenital, acquired)
         b. Hemoglobin variants
   B. Increases in erythrocyte-stimulating substances (Erythropoietin)
      1. Malignant tissue – renal, cerebellar lesions, hepatic, adrenal
      2. Benign lesions
      3. Exogenous stimulation – chemical and physical agents

IV. Neonatal polycythemia

Reproduced, by permission of the author and publishers, from Kontras (1972), Pediatric Clinics of North America, 19, 920.

the anoxia (Gallo *et al.*, 1964). This aspect has recently been reviewed by Stretton and Lee (1972). Several authors have stressed the importance of investigating pulmonary function in all patients with polycythaemia.

Cyanotic congenital heart disease

In newborn infants with severely cyanotic congenital heart disease (CHD) there is an absence of the normal postnatal fall in haemoglobin, but there is a tendency to relative anaemia from the 3rd and 4th month onwards (Rudolph *et al.*, 1953). Institution of iron therapy causes a rise in haematocrit to 75 per cent or more, sometimes with accentuation of symptoms. Accompanying the rise in Hct in cyanotic CHD there is a progressive and disproportionate increase in circulating red cell mass according to the formula:

Red cell mass/kg $= 26 + 0.056$ (Hct $- 44)^2$

(Rosenthal *et al.*, 1971).

With the rise in circulating red cell mass there

(1970) have shown that above a Hct of 60 per cent small further increments produce large increments in viscosity such that the fluidity of blood in small blood vessels becomes critical above a Hct of 70 per cent. Above this level the benefits of hypervolaemia are outweighed by the increased viscosity. These considerations explain the relationship between degree of polycythaemia and surgical mortality of patients undergoing correction of tetralogy of Fallot reported by Leachman *et al.* (1965)

Hb $< 18 \, \text{g}/100 \, \text{ml}$ prior to correction, mortality 0/9
Hb $> 18 \, \text{g}/100 \, \text{ml}$ prior to correction, mortality 3/5.

Successful reduction of haemoglobin level to less than $18 \, \text{g}/100 \, \text{ml}$ by systemic-pulmonary anastomosis before complete correction greatly reduced the surgical risks.

If attempts are made to reduce the Hct by phlebotomy or erythropheresis in cyanotic CHD it is important that the hypervolaemia should be maintained by exchange infusion of an appropriate volume of plasma or 5 per cent albumen. Rosenthal *et al.* (1970) have shown that acute reduction in the red cell mass without significant alterations of blood volume resulted in decreased peripheral vascular resistance, increased stroke volume, increased systemic blood flow and increased oxygen transport in severe cases. These changes were attributed to a decrease in blood viscosity and associated 'yield shear stress'. The same benefits would not be expected if the blood volume was reduced as occurs with simple phlebotomy. The cardiac conditions associated with severe polycythaemia in the above series were as follows:

Dextraposition of great arteries	8
Laevoposition of great arteries	2
Tetralogy of Fallot	5
Pulmonary stenosis + VSD	4
Tricuspid atresia + Pulmonary stenosis + VSD	2
A — V canal + Pulmonary stenosis	1
	22

Abnormal haemoglobins

Impaired release of oxygen to the tissues due to a haemoglobinopathy exhibiting an altered oxygen dissociation curve with increased O_2 affinity may also cause polycythaemia due to tissue (renal) anoxia. The P_{O_2} is normal. Although rare, the existence of haemoglobinopathies in association with polycythaemia indicates the need for family studies in all such patients, and haemoglobin analysis in suspected cases of familial erythrocytosis (Glynn *et al.*, 1968).

Hb Chesapeake, named after the bay in America where Columbus landed, was the first abnormal Hb in which this association was discovered, but a list of other haemoglobinopathies producing polycythaemia is given in Table 14.2. The mechanism and diagnosis is further discussed in Chapter 9.

Table 14.2 Haemoglobinopathies causing polycythaemia

Haemoglobin variant	Authors
Chesapeake	Charache *et al.*, 1966
Ranier	Adamson *et al.*, 1969
Yakima	Weatherall, 1969
Kempsey	Jenkins *et al.*, 1968
Ypsilanti	Glynn *et al.*, 1968

Tumours and renal disease

A number of tumours are associated with polycythaemia in a proportion of cases (Donati *et al.*, 1963; Crowther and Bateman, 1972) (Table 14.3). In cerebellar haemangioblastoma the incidence of polycythaemia is less than 10 per cent (Cramer

and Kimsey, 1952). In the case of renal tumours polycythaemia is easier to understand. Erythropoietin production has been demonstrated in Wilm's tumours with elevated levels of this hormone in blood and urine (Thurman *et al.*, 1966; Shalet *et al.*, 1967). Benign renal conditions including polycystic disease (Friend *et al.*, 1961) and unilateral hydronephrosis (Jaworski and Wolan, 1963) have also been reported as causing polycythaemia. In general the haemoglobin level returns to normal following resolution of the local tumour or disease.

Table 14.3   Tumours associated with polycythaemia

Cerebellar haemangioblastoma
Renal carcinoma
Nephroblastoma
Hepatoma
Androgen-secreting tumours
Bronchial carcinoma
Phaeochromocytoma

Reproduced, by permission of Professor Crowther and the publishers, from Clinics in Haematology (1972) 1, 459.

Endogenous and exogenous endocrine influences are also capable of raising the red cell mass. These include the chronic administration of testosterone or related steroids (Kennedy and Gilbertson, 1957), the administration of growth hormone in experimental animals (Meineke and Crafts, 1968), adrenal adenoma with primary aldosteronism (Mann *et al.*, 1967), congenital adrenal hyperplasia (Gold and Michael, 1959) and phaeochromocytoma (Sjoerdsman *et al.*, 1966). The clinical impression of polycythaemia in Cushing's syndrome is largely deceptive, being present in only 1 out of 36 patients in a recent series (Mattingly, (1968). In congenital adrenal hyperplasia polycythaemia appears in the neonatal period. The mechanisms by which it is thought that androgens, growth hormone and erythropoietin interact are discussed in a recent review by Tudhope (1972).

NEONATAL POLYCYTHAEMIA

Blood values at birth are usually in the polycythaemic range compared to the normal range in later life. Kontras (1972) regards a venous Hct above 60 per cent as indicative of neonatal polycythaemia and points out that it is above this Hct that viscosity of blood increases exponentially. Oski and Naiman (1972) regard a Hct of over 65 per cent or a haemoglobin level over 22 g/100 ml at any time during the first week of life as evidence of polycythaemia. Normal Hct values for venous blood have been given as 55 ± 6·5 per cent for day 1 and 51 per cent for days 2 and 3 (Sommer and Kontras, 1971).

Causes of neonatal polycythaemia are listed in Table 14.4. Twin to twin transfusion has been

Table 14.4 Neonatal polycythaemia

May be caused by placental hypertransfusion
    Twin to twin transfusion
    Maternal-fetal transfusion
    Delayed cord clamping
        Intentional
        Unassisted home delivery

May be associated with
    Placental insufficiency
        Small for gestational age infants
        Postmaturity
        Toexemia of pregnancy
        Placenta previa

Endocrine and metabolic disorders
    Congenital adrenal hyperplasia
    Neonatal thyrotoxicosis
    Maternal diabetes

Miscellaneous
    Down's syndrome
    Hyperplastic visceromegaly (Beckwith's syndrome)

Reproduced, by permission of the authors and publisher, from Oski and Naiman (1972) Hematologic Problems in the Newborn, p. 79. Philadelphia: Saunders.

discussed in Chapter 12 in the context of the anaemic twin. The hazards to the polycythaemic twin include respiratory distress, congestive cardiac failure, convulsions, hyperbilirubinaemia or even intrauterine death (Philip et al., 1969; Gatti et al., 1966; Wood, 1959). A difference in haemoglobin levels of at least 5 g/100 ml between the (monochorial) twins is necessary before the diagnosis is considered. On occasions, however, the haemoglobin in the recipient twin may be as high as 30 g/100 ml and the haematocrit as high as 82 per cent (Kontras, 1972) (Fig. 14.1).

Materno-foetal transfusion was first demonstrated by Michael and Mauer (1961). In three such infants the haemoglobin levels ranged from 21·2 to 24·6 g/100 ml and the haematocrits from 73 to 80 per cent. The evidence for passage of maternal blood into the foetal circulation included not only the presence of large numbers of adult cells in the baby's circulation by the Kleihauer technique but also a Hb F content less than 60 per cent, the presence of red cells bearing maternal blood group antigens in the baby's circulation and IgA in the foetal serum. The recently developed technique of direct identification of exclusively Hb A-containing RBCs in blood films (Kabat, 1974) may be valuable in this context. IgM and IgA are normally absent at birth unless there has been intrauterine infection or materno-foetal haemorrhage. A similar case was described by Walsh et al. (1962) in whom hepatitis may have resulted from incompatible leucocyte transfer from the mother. Andrews and Thompson (1962) found evidence of a materno-foetal transfusion in only 2 out of 207 consecutive deliveries, indicating its relative infrequency.

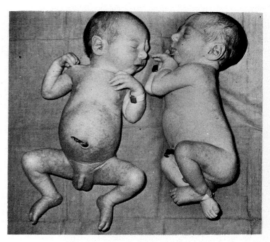

Fig. 14.1 Twin-transfusion syndrome. The infant on the left was born with a Hb of 25·5 g/100 ml, that on the right with a Hb of 12·2 g/100 ml. (*By courtesy of Dr K. M. Goel*).

Intrauterine anoxia and placental insufficiency with small-for-dates infants are also associated with polycythaemia, but in these infants the proportion of foetal haemoglobin is higher than normal rather than lower (Humbert et al., 1969). Polycythaemia in Down's syndrome may be the consequence of myeloproliferative disorder of the marrow function (Weinberger and Oleinick, 1970).

The complications of severe neonatal polycythaemia, whatever the cause, include lethargy, convulsions, respiratory distress, congestive cardiac failure, priapism, jaundice, renal vein thrombosis and tetany (Oski and Naiman, 1972). These are largely the result of hyperviscosity of the blood (Kontras, 1972). Equally the treatment in polycythaemic infants exhibiting these complications is similar and consists of a partial exchange transfusion designed to reduce the venous haematocrit to approximately 60 per cent by using fresh frozen plasma rather than whole blood for the exchange. The following formula has been given by Oski and Naiman (1972):

$$\text{Volume of exchange (ml)} = \frac{\text{Blood volume} \times (\text{Observed PCV} - \text{Desired PCV})}{\text{Observed PCV}}$$

The blood volume in such an infant may be assumed to be approximately 100 ml/kg body weight. The total volume of the exchange may be in the region of 40 ml, and this may be performed in 10 ml increments. Benefit from reduction of blood viscosity by the technique of partial exchange transfusion was first demonstrated by Baum (1966). It is currently an open question whether all infants in whom high haematocrits are found should be treated in this way regardless of the presence of symptoms.

REFERENCES

Abildgaard, C. F., Cornet, J. & Schulman, I. (1963) Primary erythrocytosis. *J. Pediat.*, **63**, 1072.

Adamson, J. W., Parer, J. T. & Stammatoyanopoulos, G. (1969) Erythrocytosis associated with hemoglobin Ranier-oxygen equilibria and marrow regulation. *J. Clin Invest.*, **48**, 1376.

Aggeler, P. M., Pollycone, M., Hoag, S., Donald, W. G. & Lawrence, J. H. (1961) Polycythemia vera in childhood. Studies of iron kinetics with Fe[59] and blood clotting factors. *Blood*, **17**, 345.

Andrews, B. F. & Thompson, J. W. (1962) Materno-fetal transfusion. A common phenomenon. *Pediatrics*, **29**, 500.

Baum, R. (1966) Viscous forces in neonatal polycythemia. *J. Pediat.*, **69**, 975.

Cassileth, P. A. & Hyman, G. A. (1966) Benign familial erythrocytosis. Report of three cases and a review of the literature. *Am. J. Med. Sci.*, **251**, 692.

Charache, S., Weatherall, D. J. & Clegg, J. B. (1966) Polycythemia associated with a hemoglobinopathy. *J. Clin. Invest.*, **45**, 813.

Cramer, F. & Kimsey, W. (1952) Cerebellar haemangioblastomas. Review of 53 cases with special reference to cerebellar cysts and the association of polycythaemia. *Archives of Neurology and Psychiatry*, **67**, 237.

Crowther, D. & Bateman, C. J. T. (1972) Malignant disease. *Clinics in Haematol.*, **1**, 459.

Donati, R. M., McCarthy, J. M., Lange, R. D. & Gallagher, N. I. (1963) Erythrocythemia and neoplastic tumors. *Ann. Intern. Med.*, **58**, 47.

Friend, D. G., Hoskins, R. G. & Kirkin, M. W. (1961) Relative erythrocythemia (polycythemia) and polysystic kidney disease, with uremia. Report of a case, with comments on frequency of occurrence. *New Eng. J. Med.*, **264**, 17.

Gallo, R. C., Fraimow, W., Cathcart, R. T. & Erslev, A. J. (1964) Erythropoietic response in chronic pulmonary disease. *Arch. Internn. Med.*, **113**, 559.

Gatti, R. A., Muster, A. J., Cole, R. B. & Paul, M. H. (1966) Neonatal polycythemia with transient cyanosis and cardiorespiratory abnormalities. *J. Pediat.*, **69**, 1063.

Geary, C. G., Amos, H. E. & McIver, J. E. (1967) Benign familial polycythemia. *J. Clin. Path.*, **20**, 158.

Glynn, K. P., Penner, J. A., Smith, J. R. & Rucknagel, D. L. (1968) Familial erythrocytosis. A description of three families, one with hemoglobin ypsilanti. *Ann. Intern. Med.*, **69**, 769.

Gold, A. P. & Michael, A. F. (1959) Congenital adrenal hyperplasia associated with polycythemia. *Pediatrics*, **23**, 727.

Humbert, J. R., Kurtz, M. L., Hathaway, W. E. & Battaglia, F. C. (1969) Polycythaemia in small for gestational age infants. *J. Pediat.*, **75**, 812.

Hume, R. (1968) Blood volume changes in chronic bronchitis and emphysema. *Brit. J. Haemat.*, **15**, 131.

Jaworski, Z. F. & Wolan, C. T. (1963) Hydronephrosis and polycythemia. A case of erythrocytosis relieved by decompression of unilateral hydronephrosis and cured by nephrectomy. *Am. J. Med.*, **34**, 523.

Jenkins, T., Stevens, K., Gallo, E. & Lehmann, H. (1968) A second family possessing hemoglobin J. Alpha Cape-town. *S. African Med. J.*, **42**, 1151.

Kabat, D. (1974) An elution procedure for visualization of adult hemoglobin in human blood smears. *Blood*, **43**, 239.

Kennedy, B. J. & Gilbertson, A. S. (1957) Increased erythropoeisis induced by androgenic-hormone therapy. *New Eng. J. Med.*, **256**, 719.

Knock, H. L. & Githens, J. H. (1960) Primary erythrocytosis of childhood. *Am. J. Dis. Children*, **100**, 189.

Kontras, S. B. & Romshe, C. (1967) Primary familial erythrocytosis. *Am. J. Dis. Child.*, **113**, 473.

Kontras, S. B., Bodenbender, J. G., Craenen, J. & Hosier, D. M. (1970) Hyperviscosity in congenital heart disease. *J. Pediat.*, **76**, 214.

Kontras, S. B. (1972) Polycythemia and hyperviscosity syndromes in infants and children. *Pediatrics Clinics of N. Amer.*, **19**, 919.

Leachman, R. D., Hallman, G. L. & Cooley, D. A. (1965) Relationship between polycythemia and surgical mortality in patients undergoing total correction for tetralogy of Fallot. *Circulation*, **32**, 65.

Mann, D. L., Gallagher, N. I. & Donati, R. M. (1967) Erythrocytosis and primary aldosteronism. *Annals Intern. Med.*, **66**, 335.

Marlow, A. A. & Fairbanks, V. F. (1960) Polycythemia vera in an eleven-year-old girl. *New Eng. J. Med.*, **263**, 950.

Mattingly, D. (1968) Disorders of the adrenal cortex and pituitary gland. In *Recent Advances in Medicine*, 15th Edition, p. 154. Edited by Baron, D. N., Compston, N. and Dawson, A. M. London: Churchill.

Meineke, H. A. & Crafts, R. C. (1968) Further observations on the mechanism by which androgens and growth hormone influence erythropoiesis. *Annals of the N.Y. Acad. Sci.*, **149**, 298.

Mauer, A. M. (1969) *Pediatric Hematology*, p. 270. New York: McGraw-Hill.

Michael, A. F. & Mauer, A. M. (1961) Materno-fetal transfusion as a cause of plethora in the neonatal period. *Pediatrics*, **28**, 458.

Murray, J. F. (1966) Classification of polycythemia disorders. With comments on the diagnostic value of arterial blood oxygen analysis. *Ann. Intern. Med.*, **64**, 892.

Natelson, E. A., Lynch, E. C., Button, H. A. & Alfrey, C. P. (1971) Polycythemia vera in childhood. *Am. J. Dis. Child.*, **122**, 241.

Oski, F. A. & Naiman, J. L. (1972) *Haematologic Problems in the Newborn*, p. 78. Philadelphia: Saunders.

Philip, A. G., Yee, A. B., Rosy, M., Surti, N., Tsamtsouris, A. & Ingall, D. (1969) Placental transfusion as an intrauterine phenomenon in deliveries complicated by foetal distress. *Brit. med. J.*, **ii**, 11.

Rosenthal, A., Nathan, D. G., Marty, A. T., Button, L. N., Miettinen, O. S. & Nadas, A. S. (1970) Acute hemodynamic effects of red cell volume reduction in polycythemia of cyannotic congenital heart disease. *Circulation*, **42**, 297.

Rosenthal, A., Button, L. N., Nathan, D. G., Miettinen, O. S. & Nadas, A. S. (1971) Blood volume changes in cyanotic congenital heart disease. *Amer. J. Cardiol.*, **27**, 162.

Rudolph, A. M., Nadas, A. S. & Borges, W. H. (1953) Hematologic adjustments to cyanotic congenital heart disease. *Pediat.*, **11**, 454.

Shalet, M. F., Holder, T. M. & Walters, T. R. (1967) Erythropoietin-producing Wilm's tumor. *J. Pediat.*, **70**, 615.

Sjoerdsma, A., Engelman, K., Waldman, T. A., Cooperman, L. H. & Hammond, W. G. (1966) Phaeochromocytoma: current concepts in diagnosis and treatment. *Annals. Intern. Med.*, **65**, 1302.

Sommer, A. & Kontras, S. B. (1971) Studies of blood viscosity in the normal newborn. *Biol. Neon.*, **17**, 441.

Stretton, T. B. & Lee, H. Y. (1972) Respiratory diseases. *Clinics in Haematology*, **1**, 645.

Thurman, W. G., Grabstald, H. & Lieberman, P. H. (1966) Evaluation of erythropoietin levels in association with Wilm's tumor. *Arch. Intern. Med.*, **117**, 280.

Treger, A., Shaw, D. B. & Grover, R. F. (1965) Secondary polycythemia in adolescents at high altitude. *J. Lab. Clin. Med.*, **66**, 304.

Tudhope, G. R. (1972) Endocrine diseases. *Clinics in Haematology*, **1**, 482.

Walsh, R. J., Reye, R. D. K. & Stapleton, T. (1962) Polycythemia and hepatitis in a newborn. *Arch. Dis. Childh.*, **37**, 425.

Weatherall, D. J. (1969) Polycythemia resulting from abnormal hemoglobin. *New Eng. J. Med.*, **280**, 604.

Weinberger, M. M. & Oleinick, A. (1970) Congenital marrow dysfunction in Down's syndrome. *J. Pediat.*, **77**, 273.

Wood, J. L. (1959) Plethora in the newborn infant associated with cyanosis and convulsions: a review of postnatal erythropoiesis. *J. Pediat.*, **54**, 143.

15. Disorders of Granulocytes, Monocytes and Lymphocytes

Neutropenia and agranulocytosis, *Granulocyte kinetics and distribution, Hereditary forms of neutropenia and agranulocytosis, Reticular dysgenesia (congenital aleucocytosis), Chronic benign granulocytopenia of childhood (CG), Ineffective myelopoiesis, Cyclic neutropenia, Lazy-leucocyte syndrome, Neutropenia associated with agammaglobulinaemia and dysglobulinaemia, Neutropenia associated with pancreatic insufficiency, Neutropenia associated with inborn errors of metabolism, Drug-induced neutropenia, Neutropenia secondary to peripheral sequestration, Immunoneutropenias, Other causes of neutropenia* / Disorders of phagocyte function, *Physiology of neutrophil granulocytes, The biochemical defect in CGD and related disorders, Pathology of CGD, Clinical features of CGD and related disorders, Other abnormalities of phagocytic function, Acquired disorders of leucocyte function, Leucocyte changes secondary to infection* / Infectious mononucleosis and related conditions, *Infectious lymphocytosis* / Eosinophilia.

NEUTROPENIA AND AGRANULOCYTOSIS

Granulocyte kinetics and distribution

Mature neutrophil polymorphs emerge from the bone marrow as a result of, firstly, a *proliferative* phase of myelopoiesis, involving approximately four multiplicative divisions between myeloblast and myelocyte; and, secondly, a non-multiplicative *maturation* phase from meta myelocyte to polymorph (Fig. 15.1). Total transit time is 6 to 10 days (Cronkite and Fliedner, 1964) while maturation time from myelocyte to polymorph takes $3\frac{1}{2}$–$5\frac{1}{2}$ days (Killman *et al.*, 1962).

A practical consequence is that the effect of a drug such as cytosine arabinoside which inhibits myelopoiesis by blocking DNA synthesis will not be reflected in the peripheral blood until nearly a week after its administration.

Inspection of a normal marrow smear shows up to 30 per cent of mature neutrophil polymorphs. These cells are the 'reserve' marrow pool from which the circulating granulocytes are derived. This pool size has been estimated as being 20–25 times that of the total circulating granulocytes (Cartwright *et al.*, 1964). Etiocholanolone administration causes release of 'reserve' granulocytes into the circulation (Godwin *et al.*, 1968A) and has been used as a means of assessing marrow reserve prior to cytotoxic therapy (Godwin *et al.*, 1968B). Intravenous injection of bacterial endotoxic produces a 3 to 4-fold rise in absolute granulocyte count between 6 to 12 hours after injection due to mobilization of this marrow reserve (Athens *et al.*, 1961A; Marsh and Perry, 1964). This is

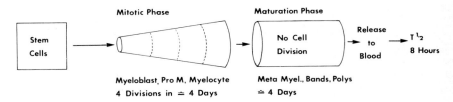

Fig. 15.1 Schematic pipeline of granulocyte production.

preceded by transient neutropenia at 3 hours due to margination of the granulocytes (*vide infra*).

On release from the marrow granulocytes come into equilibrium with a circulating pool, and a similarly sized 'marginating' pool consisting of cells out of circulation residing adjacent to the vessel wall in small veins. The peripheral granulocyte count performed on capillary or venous blood reflects only the circulating pool. The two pools are in continuous equilibrium. An injection of adrenaline (0·1 ml of 1/1,000 SC) causes a rapid and transient shift to the circulating pool, permitting a rough estimation of the size of the marginating pool (Athens et al., 1961B). In prolonged severe neutropenia or agranulocytosis it may be presumed that both circulating and marginating pools are equally depleted.

Circulating granulocytes have a mean half-life of 6·8 hours when measured by DFP^{32} labelling (Mauer et al., 1960; Athens et al., 1961A), showing an exponential disappearance curve indicating random destruction rather than age-dependent senescence. This implies that the circulating granulocytes are being replenished several times each day. The mean turnover rate has been calculated as $1·63 \times 10^9$ cells/kg body wt./day (Cartwright et al., 1964). No granulocytes survive in the circulation beyond about 30 hours (Fliedner et al., 1964). After entering the tissues they migrate upon committed stem cells (Morley and Stohlman, 1970; Rickard et al., 1971). *In vitro* soft agar culture of human marrow yields greater numbers of myeloid colonies, thought to be derived from such stem cells, if granulocyte extracts are added to the medium (Iscove et al., 1971). This suggests a *positive* feed-back mechanism whereby granulocyte utilization or destruction would stimulate production, e.g. as a result of infection. By contrast, King-Smith and Morley (1970) constructed an analogue computer model for granulopoiesis involving two *negative* feed-back loops; one acting at the stem cell level, and therefore containing a time delay; the other controlling the release of mature granulocytes from the marrow to the blood (Fig. 15.2). With this

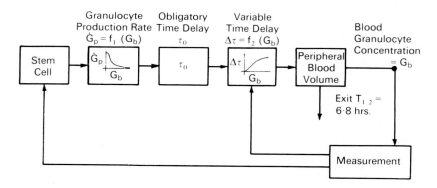

Fig. 15.2 Hypothetical model for granulocyte control. Granulocyte production rate (G_p) and time ($\Delta\rho$) spent by granulocytes in the marrow reserve were each regarded as being controlled by the blood granulocyte concentration (G_b). Obligatory (proliferation + maturation) time = ρ_0; variable storage time = $\Delta\rho$; total delay = $\rho = \rho_0 + \Delta\rho$. (Reproduced from *Blood* (1970), **36**, 254, by permission of Dr Morley and the publishers).

to sites such as buccal mucosa or sites of infection but do not return to the circulation (Craddock et al., 1960). Their accumulation at inflammatory sites may be studied by the Rebuck skin window technique (Rebuck and Crowley, 1955) or by recovery of cells from exudates in special plastic chambers (Senn et al., 1969; Southam and Levin, 1966). Granulocytes are normally the predominant cell in the first 3–6 hours but by 12 hours monocytes become predominant.

Adrenal corticosteroids normally cause a neutrophil leucocytosis in the peripheral blood but this appears to be due to inhibition of the passage of granulocytes from the blood to the tissues, rather than increased marrow release (Boggs et al., 1962). Clearly this effect could be detrimental in a patient with neutropenia.

Regulation of myelopoiesis is imperfectly understood. By analogy with erythropoiesis it is likely that a humoral feed-back mechanism operates model it was found that whether sustained oscillation occurred or not depended upon the degree of responsiveness of the marrow, in terms of granulocyte production, to a fall in blood granulocyte level. If a given fall in granulocyte level resulted in a marked rise in granulocyte production, then sustained oscillation resulted. With lesser degrees of increased production sustained oscillation did not develop. However, in both situations, mild marrow failure of production would produce cyclical neutropenia as has been found in dogs fed a constant dose of marrow-depressant drug (cyclophosphamide) (Morley and Stohlman, 1970). It is questionable if significant cyclical changes occur in the granulocyte level in normal individuals. If so, it is only in a much smaller proportion than originally thought (Morley, 1973). Regulation of granulopoiesis has recently been reviewed by Golde and Cline (1974).

Kauder and Mauer (1966) have classified neutro-

DISORDERS OF GRANULOCYTES, MONOCYTES AND LYMPHOCYTES

Table 15.1 Functional classification of the neutropenias

I. Decreased production
   Drug induced
   Radiation
   Hereditary neutropenia
      Kostmann – autosomal recessive
      Glansslen – autosomal dominant
   deVaal—reticular dysgenesis
   Agammaglobulinemia and dysgammaglobulinemia
   Chronic hypoplastic neutropenia
   Cyclic neutropenia
   Familial neutropenia possibly caused by deficiency of a plasma factor

II. Increased destruction
   Immunoneutropenia
      Neonatal neutropenia
      Drug induced
      Miscellaneous underlying disease
   Splenic neutropenia
   Zuelzer—chronic granulocytopenia in childhood

III. Increased destruction and decreased production
   Mauer and Krill – cirrhosis
   Hong *et al.* – dysgammaglobulinemia
   Cyclic neutropenia
IV. Ineffective myelopoiesis
V. Pseudoneutropenia
VI. Miscellaneous
   Salomonsen—chronic benign neutropenia of childhood
   Shwachman *et al.*—pancreatic insufficiency and bone marrow dysfunction
   Hyperglycinemia

Reproduced from J. Pediat. **69,** *147 (1966) by permission of Dr. A. M. Mauer and the publishers.*

penia in childhood according to decreased production, increased destruction or both wherever data is available on the point (Table 15.1). This is, of course, analogous to the commonly used concepts in anaemia. Ineffective myelopoiesis parallels ineffective erythropoiesis. Pseudoneutropenia refers to the possibility of a disproportionate distribution of granulocytes between circulating and marginating pools. This classification can be used as a cross reference to that used below, thereby indicating the probable pathogenesis of the various clinical syndromes.

Hereditary forms of neutropenia and agranulocytosis

These are rare and appear to be of two types:

(a) Severe agranulocytosis, usually fatal in early childhood and with recessive inheritance, originally described as 'infantile genetic agranulocytosis' by Kostman (1956).

(b) Benign neutropenia with good life expectancy and with dominant inheritance originally described by Glansslen (1941) and by Bousser and Neyde (1947).

Both disorders may be detected in the first weeks of life and can be regarded as examples of congenital neutropenia.

INFANTILE GENETIC AGRANULOCYTOSIS (IGA)

Kostman in 1956 described the onset in early infancy of severe indolent skin infections and fever. Without antibiotic treatment the disease ran a short course with fatal outcome. As in other neutropenic states the skin infections showed erythema and induration but no purulent 'head'. Fourteen children, of both sexes, were described from 9 families with close consanguinity in 5 families, all belonging to the same geographical area in Northern Sweden. Two children had only temporary agranulocytosis and were surviving to $4\frac{1}{2}$ and 5 years at the time of the report.

Blood findings showed an almost complete absence of neutrophil polymorphs (usually less than 1 per cent). The marrow showed a marked retardation or block in maturation of neutrophil myelopoiesis at the promyelocyte and myelocyte stages with virtual absence of band cells or polymorphs. Other cell lines were normal or increased. Some cases showed compensatory monocytosis, eosinophilia and raised serum gamma globulin, as well as raised platelet counts.

Two siblings with severe congenital neutropenia and eosinophilia dying at the ages of 4 and 5 months have been described by Andrews, McClellan and Scott (1960), who likewise suggested a recessive inheritance. Blood and marrow findings were identical with Kostman's. These appear to be the only two reports where more than one member of the family have been affected. However, a number of *isolated* cases have been described (Table 15.2) where the age, haematological findings and early fatal outcome have been similar to Kostman's cases and where a genetic

monocytosis). Strangely one case actually transformed terminally into acute monoblastic leukaemia after surviving to young adulthood (Gilman *et al.*, 1970).

Blood neutrophils have usually been below $300/mm^3$ with an associated monocytosis and eosinophilia causing the total white cell count to approach the normal range (Baehner, 1972). The marrow was hypocellular in Kostman's patients, but has been of normal cellularity in other cases. There is a preponderance of promyelocytes with prominent azurophilic (red) granules, and virtual

Table 15.2 Reports of severe congenital neutropenia

Author	Title of disease	No. of cases	Familial occurrence	Outcome
Kostman (1956)	Infantile genetic agranulocytosis	14	+	All but 2 died in infancy
Kniker and Panos (1957)	Infantile agranulocytosis	1	0	Fatal
Luhby *et al* (1957)	Congenital genetic agranulocytosis	1	0	Fatal
Hedenberg (1959)	Infantile agranulocytosis	1	0	Fatal at $13\frac{1}{2}$ months
Andrews *et al.* (1960)	Congenital neutropenia	2	+	Fatal at 4 and 5 months
Aarskog *et al.* (1961)	Infantile congenital aneutrocytosis	1	0	Fatal at 5 months
Page (1962)	Neutropenia in infancy	1	0	Fatal at 8 months
MacGillivray *et al.* (1964)	Congenital neutropenia	5	0	3 died in infancy
Lang and Cutting (1965)	Infantile genetic agranulocytosis	1	0	Surviving to over $4\frac{1}{2}$ years
Krill and Mauer (1966)	Congenital agranulocytosis	1	0	Fatal at 7 weeks
Miller *et al.* (1968)	Congenital neutropenia	1	0	Fatal
Barak *et al.* (1971)	Infantile genetic agranulocytosis	1	0	Surviving to over $3\frac{1}{2}$ years
Wriedt *et al.* (1970)	Congenital neutropenia	2	0	1 died at 20 years
	Total no. of cases	32		7 Surviving

cause has commonly been suggested but without certain evidence. Many of these authors presumed they were seeing the same disease. Known consanguinity of the parents was only recorded in Kostman's series.

Clinical features which emerge from the above reports include the frequency of chronic and recurrent skin infections, sometimes inflammatory without a 'head' of pus but sometimes showing abscess formation, gum hypertrophy and bleeding, peridontal infection, aphthous ulcers, inflamed nasal and pharyngeal mucosae, otitis media, mastoiditis, generalized lymphadenopathy and terminal lung 'abscesses', consolidation and cavitation, the cellular infiltrate consists mainly of plasma cells (MacGillivray *et al.*, 1964). Viral diseases including mumps and chickenpox have been handled without complication (Wriedt *et al.*, 1970). The spleen has seldom been palpable. Moderate anaemia has been recorded, probably secondary to infection (Lang and Cutting, 1965). The initial clinical and haematological findings have sometimes falsely suggested a diagnosis of monocytic leukaemia (e.g. gum hypertrophy and

absence of neutrophil metamyelocytes, band cells or polymorphs. These features distinguish the disorder from chronic benign granulocytopenia of childhood where the marrow is normal apart from the absence of mature polymorphs, and band cells predominate. Eosinophils, monocytes, histiocytes and plasma cells may be increased (Lang and Cutting, 1965).

Investigations into the pathogenesis of the disease have demonstrated defective proliferation as measured by ^{3}H-thymidine incorporation into myeloid precursors (Wriedt *et al.*, 1970). When marrow fragments were cultured *in vitro* there was a failure to form polymorphs in one case and a delay in a second case. Barak *et al.* (1971) have shown that when such marrow is cultured in soft agar containing an extract of human spleen a normal number of granulocyte colonies with normal maturation are formed. This suggests that the granulocyte precursors are capable of normal proliferation and that a necessary factor present in normal cells is perhaps deficient in this disease. No inhibition was found with the patient's serum and no stimulation with normal serum. Earlier work had suggested that normal serum could stimulate myeloid proliferation *in vitro* and *in vivo* in at least one variety of chronic familial neutropenia (Bjure *et al.*, 1962).

Cellular and humoral immunity is normal. Monocyte function is fortunately unimpaired with respect to phagocytic and bactericidal activity. Transfused granulocytes survive normally (Wriedt *et al.*, 1970).

Therapy has been unsuccessful in altering the course of the disease. Energetic use of antibiotics to treat established infections undoubtedly prolongs life. Corticosteroids and haematinics have been ineffective, except in the somewhat milder form of hereditary neutropenia in siblings reported by Rossman and Hummer (1960) where a response to steroids was claimed. Androgens have not been tried. Prophylactic antibiotics are, in general, contraindicated. Since fatal infections can occur in patients who have survived as long as 20 years spontaneous improvement does not appear to be a feature of this variety of neutropenia.

FAMILIAL BENIGN CHRONIC NEUTROPENIA

A less severe form of neutropenia with survival into adult life and an apparently dominant pattern of inheritance, distinguishing it from IGA, was first described by Glansslen (1941) and subsequently by a number of other authors (Bousser and Neyde, 1947; Levine, 1959; Bjure *et al.*, 1962; Cutting and Lang, 1964). The disorder may be discovered fortuitously. Infections are less troublesome but peridontal lesions may occur.

Neutropenia has been seen from early infancy. The bone marrow has normal cellularity but with a decrease in myeloid precursors beyond the myelocyte stage (i.e. decreased metamyelocytes, band cells and polymorphs).

A possibly unique family has been described by Hitzig (1959) with dominant inheritance, virtual absence of polymorphs (84 and 0/mm³) yet relatively benign clinical course with survival of all affected children until the present time.

Reticular dysgenesia (congenital aleucocytosis)

There are two reports in the literature of congenital absence not only of granulocytes but also absence or great paucity of other leucocytes. They appear to represent the unexpected deficiency of granulocyte and lymphocyte formation with preservation of erythroid and megakaryocyte elements. This pattern is at variance with the usual assumption that lymphoid stem cells are distinct from the stem cell line responsible for myeloid, erythroid and megakaryocyte development. De Vaal and Seynhaeve (1959) described twin male infants with total absence of all leucocytes from birth and suggested the term reticular dysgenesia. Red cells and platelets were unaffected. Both infants died of infection in the neonatal period. Post-mortem histology showed that the bone marrow was devoid of myeloid elements and the thymus and spleen were devoid of lymphocytes. Gitlin, Vawter and Craig (1964) described a very similar infant with a total white cell count between 200 and 600/mm³. The haemoglobin was also low, 10 g/100 ml at 36 hours. Multiple infections developed and this infant also died in the neonatal period. No granulocyte precursors were present in the marrow. The thymus was atrophic and contained few lymphocytes. In lymph nodes lymphocytes were replaced by reticulum cells.

Chronic benign granulocytopenia of childhood (CG)

This entity was comprehensively described by Zuelzer and Bajoghli in 1964 (Table 15.3). Symptoms may date from the neonatal period but diagnosis has more usually been made around the latter part of the first year of life. In earlier reports of what was probably the same disease diagnoses were made at 8 months (Stahlie, 1956) and 9½ months (Salomonsen, 1948). No familial tendency is present.

Bacterial infections in this disease are milder and seldom life-threatening. Zuelzer and Bajoghli mention paronychiae, impetigo, gingivitis, ulcerations about the genitalia and subcutaneous abscesses in various sites. The respiratory tract was also frequently involved. Infections tend to remain localized and are adequately controlled by antibiotic therapy and appropriate local measures. The chronic susceptibility to infections remains, however, with variable lengths of freedom from actual infection. Regional lymphadenopathy may be present and transient splenomegaly has been recorded.

Spontaneous recovery from the neutropenia eventually occurred in 13 out of the 16 cases collected from the literature by Stahlie (1956). Salomonsen's case had a spontaneous remission at 2½ years of age. In Zuelzer's series 3 recovered spontaneously, with a gradual return to normal of the blood picture, at between 27 and 38 months from diagnosis, but 1 still had neutropenia after 5 years. This feature of the natural history appears to distinguish CG from IGA or its milder dominant variant.

228　PAEDIATRIC HAEMATOLOGY

Table 15.3　Summary of data in 5 cases of chronic benign granulocytopenia

Case	Sex	Race	Age at time of diagnosis (mo.)	History prior to diagnosis	Clinical course	Total Leukocytes /mm^3		Absolute PMN /mm^3		Mono-cytes %	Dura-tion (mo.)	Outcome
						Range	Average	Range	Average			
1	F	W	15	history of impetigo, mouth ulcer, and abscess of vulva of 1 month duration	episodes of severe diarrhea, impetigo, paronychiae, and upper respratory infection in interval, doing well	4000–10,000	5000	100–2000	1000	1–10	42	recovered
2	M	W	6½	abscess of right buttock of 1 week duration	episodes of abscesses and one episode of septicemia frequent ear infection	2500–8000	4000	0–400	250	6–31	38	recovered
3	M	W	6	frequent respiratory infection since birth	frequent 'colds'	3000–8000	4000	0–500	200	2–13	27	recovered
4	M	W	10	series of 'colds' and mouth ulcers, of 3 months' duration treated with penicilmide, and chloramphenicol	episodes of paronychiae, cellulitis, mouth ulcers, and tonsillitis several attacks of otitis and lower respiratory infection	3000–8000	5500	100–200	300	10–24	38	under observation
5	F	W	12	recurrent paronychiae, and one episode of gingivitis	paronychiae, and fever of unknown origin	2100–3000	2500	40–600	250	5–10	9	under observation

*Reproduced from Blood (1964), **23**, 359–374 by permission of Dr. W. W. Zuelzer and the publishers.*

Haematologically the isolated neutropenia is less profound than in IGA (Table 15.3). The granulocytes that are present are almost exclusively band forms with mature polymorphs virtually absent. Some increase in granulocyte count occurs at times of abscess formation or surgical stress, although the response is subnormal. At such times band forms, metamyelocytes and myelocytes form the bulk of the circulating granulocytes. Monocytosis is present as in other chronic neutropenias. Haemoglobin and platelet levels are normal.

Marrow examination shows normal or moderately increased cellularity with an increase in lymphocytes and essentially normal myeloid: erythroid ratio (4:1 to 2:1). The striking abnormality is the virtual absence of fully mature segmented neutrophil leukocytes which normally account for approximately one third of the granulocyte series constituting the marrow storage pool (Zuelzer and Bajoghli, 1964). Unlike IGA myelocytes and band cells are plentiful, as are earlier myeloid cells. Proliferative granulopoiesis pools were in some cases increased in proportion to maturation pools. The overall picture suggests normal or increased production at least up to the band form stage and this interpretation was supported by *in vitro* culture experiments in which the ratio of mature to young granulocytes sharply increased after 8–12 hours' incubation. No evidence of humoral inhibition could be found.

The above considerations led Zuelzer and Bajoghli to suggest that increased peripheral destruction or sequestration is the primary cause although, as pointed out by Mauer (1969), it would be interesting to test this hypothesis by *in vivo* ^{32}DFP leucocyte survival studies. It was further speculatively suggested that this phenomenon was an exaggeration of the normal tendency to relative neutropenia and lymphocytosis observed over the first few years of life. The fact that CG is a disease of early life, remitting spontaneously after a few years, is consistent with this suggestion.

Kyle and Linman (1968) have described a more chronic form of idiopathic neutropenia without marrow hypoplasia, splenomegaly or increased frequency of infection. It did not respond to coricosteroids and appears similar to CG.

Ineffective myelopoiesis

A 10-year-old girl has been described with chronic neutropenia yet the ability to respond with a neutrophil leucocytosis at times of infection (Fig. 15.3). Repeated infections had occurred since

released from the marrow and the half-life of those granulocytes entering the blood was very short (Krill *et al.*, 1964). The fundamental defect appears to be intramedullary death of neutrophils or, by analogy with erythropoiesis, 'ineffective myelopoiesis', but the cause is unknown. Zuelzer termed it 'myelokathexis'. Splenectomy, corticosteroids or infusion of fresh plasma did not influence the course of the disease. The same case was separately described by Zuelzer and by Krill *et al.*

Cyclic neutropenia

This is likewise a disorder that can very easily be missed by the normal timing of white cell counts in relation to clinical events. By the time a patient is admitted for investigation of neutropenia or infection observed as an outpatient the neutropenia will have disappeared since this lasts for only a few days in each 21-day cycle (Fig. 15.4). It has been recognized as an entity from early in the present century but more recent case reports and reviews include those of Vahlquist (1946).

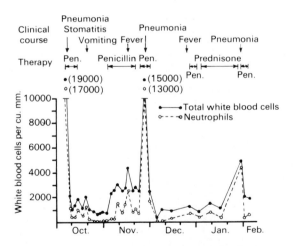
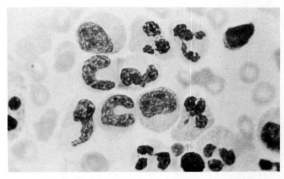

Fig. 15.3 Neutropenia except at times of infection, attributed to 'ineffective myelopoiesis' in a girl of 10 years. (Reproduced from the *New England Journal of Medicine* (1964), **270**, 973, by permission of Dr A. M. Mauer and the publishers).

infancy. Difficulty in appreciating the underlying neutropenia arose from the fact that this was usually absent at the time of hospital admission for infection. Marrow examination showed a 'shift to the right' among the granulocytic series, the predominant cell resembling degenerating polymorphs, with dense pycnotic chromatin (Zuelzer, 1964). DFP^{32}-labelling methods of investigation showed that few granulocytes were

Reiman and de Berardinis (1949), and Page and Good (1957). The latter authors described 7 cases. Malaise, arthralgia and fever occurred before each neutropenic phase. Buccal ulceration occurred at the height of neutropenia. The disorder may be recognized in early infancy and one patient was followed for as long as 34 years until his death from pneumonia (Thompson, 1934). Familial, with dominant transmission, cases have been described (Torrioli-Riggio, 1958), including transmission from a father to a daughter (Hahneman and Alt, 1958). Page (1974) also has a father and daughter with cyclic neutropenia, the daughter now having a female infant with probable cyclic neutropenia.

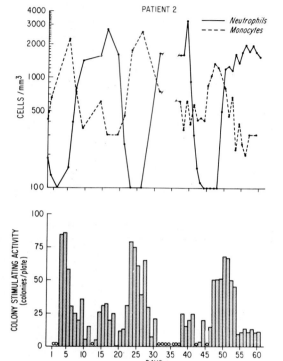

Fig. 15.4 Cyclic neutropenia. The daily neutrophil, monocyte and colony-stimulating factor levels for patient 2. The histogram represents data from two separate periods. ...., days with no data. Neutrophil and monocyte counts of 100 or less are graphed as 100. (Reproduced from *Blood* (1974), **44**, 257, by permission of Dr D. C. Dale and the publishers).

Haematologically the defect predominantly affects the neutrophil granulocytes, with a compensatory monocytosis occurring during the neutropenic phase, and minor cyclic changes in the lymphocytes, eosinophils, reticulocytes and platelets (Guerry et al., 1974). Anaemia can occur secondary to infection. Marrow changes are out of phase with the blood changes, viz. there is an absence of late myeloid precursors just before the development of neutropenia, but by the time neutropenia has occurred the marrow has returned to normal or shows myeloid hyperplasia in anticipation of the impending rise in the neutrophil count. Occasional cases have been associated with agammaglobulinaemia (Good and Zak, 1956) or dysgammaglobulinaemia, with increased 7S and decreased 19S globulins (Kauder and Mauer, 1966).

Corticosteroids, folic acid and pyridoxine have no effect on the occurrence of neutropenia (Page and Good, 1957). Large doses of testosterone enanthate (I.M.), given to an adult with cyclic neutropenia, raised the baseline level of the polymorph curve but did not abolish the periodicity (Brodsky et al., 1965). Improvement after splenectomy has also been recorded (Fullerton and Duguid, 1949). Neither of these therapeutic measures have, however, become widely adopted in this disease and chief reliance is upon adequate antibiotic therapy for established infections which do not resolve between neutropenic phases.

Case 10. A boy of 3 years (No. 86153) presented at the Orthopaedic Department with osteitis of femur and ribs plus septic lesions of scalp. He was severely anaemic and leukaemia or widespread malignant disease was suspected. Marrow examination showed megaloblastic change. There was a history that, while attending another hospital, blood counts performed at an outpatient attendance had, on more than one occasion, showed severe neutropenia, and admission for investigation of this was arranged. But when he was admitted the blood white cell count was normal each time! As serial blood counts were performed in relation to his anaemia and osteitis it gradually became apparent that cyclical episodes of virtual agranulocytosis were recurring at approximately 21-day intervals, with neutrophil peaks of 3,000 to 5,000 between these times. A marrow examination performed at the time of the lowest neutrophil counts showed striking myelocytic hyperplasia (in anticipation of the ensuing leucocytosis), and a marrow performed at the height of the neutrophil count showed almost total myelocytic suppression (in anticipation of the ensuing agranulocytosis). The anaemia must have largely been due to the associated chronic infection, but folate depletion from the same cause plus poor home conditions were responsible for the megaloblastic features. The osteitis slowly responded to appropriate antibiotic therapy and orthopaedic measures.

Over the ensuing years the main clinical problems have been aphthous ulceration (a well-known feature of cyclic neutropenia), gingivitis, dental sepsis and occasional infections of the skin and low grade fever. At different times prophylactic antibiotics and corticosteroids have been tried without clinical or haematological benefit. He leads a virtually normal life and is making good progress at school, now being aged 10 years.

Recent work has shown that moderate marrow depression with a constant oral dose of cyclophosphamide in dogs results in cyclic neutropenia (Morley and Stohlman, 1970). This was predicted from a computer model of granulopoiesis embodying two feed-back loops. These authors suggest that cyclic neutropenia is not necessarily a single entity. Even more recent work has shown that the urinary excretion of colony-stimulating factor increased during the neutropenic period, concomitantly with the maximum monocyte count (Fig. 15.4) (Guerry *et al.*, 1974). The monocyte has been shown to be an important source of colony-stimulating factor (Chervenick and Lo Buglio, 1972).

Lazy-leucocyte syndrome

A new syndrome has recently been described by Miller, Oski and Harris (1971) in which severe peripheral neutropenia results from impaired mobility of neutrophils impeding their egress from the marrow and migration to sites of infection. A girl of 2 years and a boy of nearly 5 years had absolute granulocyte counts of 135 and 170/mm³ respectively with normal bone marrow findings. They suffered from recurrent stomatitis, otitis, gingivitis and low grade fevers. A poor response to bacterial pyrogen injection (Pyromen) indicated impaired marrow release of 'storage' polymorphs. *In vitro* tests disclosed poor random mobility and non-random (chemotactic) mobility of neutrophil granulocytes. Phagocytic and bactericidal activity was normal. It is thought, therefore, that this represents a previously unreported primary defect of neutrophil function, perhaps due to a membrane defect of the polymorphs.

Neutropenia associated with agammaglobulinaemia and dysglobulinaemia

One normally considers neutropenia and agammaglobulinaemia as alternative possible causes of recurrent infection in young children. In fact both abnormalities may occur together (Lonsdale *et al.*, 1967). Among 8 patients with congenital agammaglobulinaemia reported by Good and Zak (1956) persistent neutropenia was present in 2, transient neutropenia in 3 and cyclic neutropenia in one. The marrows showed hypoplasia of myeloid precursors. Infants have also been described where neutropenia was associated with a dysgammaglobulinaemia manifested by reduced 7S and increased 19S globulins. In one case the previous episodes of neutropenia ceased while monthly injections of gamma globulin were given (Ackerman, 1964). In the other case there was evidence of shortened neutrophil survival in the circulation (Hong *et al.*, 1962). Chronic neutropenia has also been seen in association with abnormal cell-mediated immunity (Lux *et al.*, 1970). It is possible that impaired immunity results in increased neutrophil utiliza-

tion, for which the marrow cannot compensate in certain individuals. Hypergammaglobulinaemia has, of course, often been seen as a secondary feature in many of the types of chronic neutropenia discussed above.

Granulocytopenia associated with a defect of cell mediated immunity has been recorded in ataxia telangiectasia (Feigin *et al.*, 1970).

Neutropenia associated with pancreatic insufficiency

Six children with a syndrome of exocrine pancreatic insufficiency, neutropenia, growth retardation with inconstant anaemia, thrombocytopenia and galactosuria were described by Schwachman, Diamond, Oski and Khaw (1964). They presented with diarrhoea, failure to thrive in infancy. Infections including otitis media or pneumonia were present at diagnosis in 3. The first three cases were attending a cystic fibrosis clinic, but had atypical features such as normal sweat electrolyte tests and absence of pulmonary disease.

Investigations showed absence of pancreatic trypsin, lipase, amylase and chymotrypsin. All had neutropenia with 0 to 25 per cent polymorphs, 4 had anaemia and 2 thrombocytopenia. The anaemia could appear as early as 4–6 months of age, and had developed in an older child in spite of folic acid and B_{12} supplements. Serum iron and TIBC were normal. The marrow was hypocellular with reduced numbers of megakaryocytes in one of the patients with thrombocytopenia (89,000/mm³). Elevated levels of Hb F were present, suggesting a fundamental disorder of erythropoiesis from birth. A subnormal total white cell count (3,670/mm³) was recorded in one case on the first day of life, also suggesting that the haematological manifestations may date from birth. Since 3 of these patients were in one family the disorder was thought to be genetically determined.

Similar cases were described by Bodian *et al.* (1964) and Burke *et al.* (1967). Nine of the 36 cases now reported have died from infection in infancy or early childhood (Scmerling *et al.*, 1969).

Treatment is unsatisfactory and has been discussed by Baehner (1972). Administration of pancreatic preparations may improve gastrointestinal symptoms and growth but does not affect the neutropenia. Orthopaedic management may be needed if metaphyseal dysostosis of the hip is present. Vigorous antibiotic therapy is needed at times of infection since this is the major cause of death.

The condition should be suspected in infants

who fail to gain weight, have abnormal stools and neutropenia, as well as in children thought to have cystic fibrosis but with normal sweat electrolytes (Schwachman *et al.*, 1964). At times of infection the neutropenia may be temporarily masked by a normal or even increased number of circulating neutrophils. The diagnosis can be missed if white cell counts are restricted to these times (Mauer, 1969).

Neutropenia associated with inborn errors of metabolism

Three different metabolic disorders have been described in association with neutropenia, viz. idiopathic hyperglycinaemia (Childs *et al.*, 1961), isovaleric acidaemia (Allen *et al.*, 1969) and methylmalonic acidaemia (Morrow *et al.*, 1969). The presenting clinical features in all three conditions are lethargy, vomiting, ketosis and dehydration in the neonatal period, failure to thrive and growth retardation. The marrow is hypoplastic in all three conditions with decreased numbers of myeloid precursors.

The child with hyperglycinaemia had repeated infections due to the neutropenia and periodic purpura due to thrombocytopenia. In addition there was hypogammaglobulinaemia. Treatment with a low protein diet plus sodium benzoate, to conjugate with glycine, was followed by a rise in polymorph count (Childs *et al.*, 1961).

The child with methylmalonic acidaemia similarly had both neutropenia and thrombocytopenia. Osteoporosis was also present. Some such cases respond to massive doses of vitamin B_{12}. Inheritance is autosomal recessive (Morrow *et al.*, 1969). In the case of isovaleric acidaemia the haematological abnormality was corrected by a diet low in leucine (Oski and Naiman, 1972). This disorder is characterized by the additional feature of a 'sweaty foot' odour to the skin.

Drug-induced neutropenia

Three types of mechanism are involved in neutropenia due to drugs:

1. Idiosyncratic suppression of myeloid production affecting a small proportion of exposed individuals (Huguley, 1964), e.g. sulphonamides.
2. Regularly occurring, dose-dependent myeloid depression from cytotoxic drugs or antimetabolites, e.g. 6-MP or radiotherapy involving the bone marrow, e.g. the spine. The neutropenic nadir from antimetabolites occurs approximately 7 days after exposure to the drug; that

from alkylating agents at 10–14 days, or at 3–4 weeks in the case of BCNU.
3. Drug haptene disease, whereby an individual produces antibodies to the complex of drug plus leucocyte resulting in demonstrable *in vitro* leukoagglutinins (Moeschlin, 1958) and in-

Table 15.4 Commoner drugs causing neutropenia

Group I.   Individual idiosyncrasy
Antibiotics
Novobiocin
Ristocetin
Fumagillin
Methicillin
Sulphonamides
Acetazolamide
Sulphaguanidine
Sulphamethoxygyridazine
Anticoagulants
Phenindione
Antidiabetics
Tolbutamide
Chlorpropamide
Antihistamines
Thenaidine
Antihypertensives
Chlorothiazide
Hydrochlorothiazide
Aldomet
Antithyroids
Propylthiouracil
Methimazole
Diuretics
Ethacrynic Acid
Anti-inflammatory drugs
Demecolcine
Hydroxychloroquine
Penicillamine
Amodiaquine
Carbimazole
Pronestyl
Phenothiazine Derivatives
Group II.   Regular, dose-dependent effect
Antimetabolites
6-Mercaptopurine
Methotrexate
Cytosine Arabinoside
Alkylating agents
Cyclophosphamide
Nitrogen Mustard
BCNU
Group III.   Drug haptene
Amidopyrine related drugs
Dipyrone
Phenylbutazone
Sulphapyridine
Mercurial Diuretics
Chlorpropamide

Data from Baehner (1972).

DISORDERS OF GRANULOCYTES, MONOCYTES AND LYMPHOCYTES

creased peripheral destruction of leucocytes with myeloid hyperplasia in the marrow, e.g. phenylbutazone.

Table 15.4 lists the drugs most commonly causing neutropenia.

In the newborn neutropenia can result from maternal ingestion of such drugs as thiazide diuretics (Rodriguez et al., 1964) or Dilantin (Pantarotto, 1965). Presumably other drugs could produce the same effect.

Neutropenia secondary to peripheral sequestration

Hypersplenism is a well-recognized cause of peripheral sequestration not only of red cells and platelets but also of granulocytes (Wiseman and Doan, 1942; Crosby, 1962). The marrow in such cases shows myeloid hyperplasia with normal maturation to the polymorph stage. In paediatric practice the commonest cause of hypersplenism is portal hypertension. In one such case, due to mild cirrhosis, there was a demonstrably shorter half-disappearance time of DFP^{32}-labelled granulocytes (Mauer and Krill, 1964). Splenectomy resulted in cure of the neutropenia and a return to normal of his neutrophil kinetics. Splenomegaly due to thalassaemia, reticuloses or storage diseases may also produce hypersplenism in childhood.

Acute sequestration of polymorphs in the pulmonary vasculature, accompanied by transient profound neutropenia, occurs after intravenous injection of endotoxin, histamine, nicotinic acid, granulocytes or granulocyte products. A similar pulmonary sequestration appears to be the mechanism of the transient neutropenia seen at the beginning of a haemodialysis run in uraemic patients (Kaplow et al., 1968; Toren et al., 1970). The maximum neutropenia occurs at 15 minutes and rebound to leucocytosis levels is seen by 3 hours, presumably due to return of the sequestered cells to the circulation.

Immunoneutropenias

Paediatric interest in immune-induced neutropenias centres upon the occurrence of neonatal neutropenia due to maternal antileucocyte antibodies. These are of two types; *isoimmune*, being due to immunization to foreign antigens on the foetal leucocytes analogous to Rh isoimmunization; and *autoimmune*, occurring in infants born to mothers with neutropenia and possessing antileukocyte antibodies. The marrow in these condi-

tions shows a depletion of mature neutrophils, indicating exhaustion of the reserve pool.

Isoimmunization of a mother to her baby's leucocytes is thought to occur as a result of passage of foetal leucocytes into the mother's circulation (Jensen, 1962). Up to a quarter of pregnant women develop such leukoagglutinins and, being 7S antibodies, they frequently cross the placenta. In the vast majority of instances, however, the transfer of such antibodies fails to cause neutropenia in the infant (Payne, 1964; Abildgaard and Jensen, 1964). It appears that foetal neutropenia results only when the antibody is exclusively reactive to the neutrophils, rather than broadly reactive to all leucocytes, platelets and other tissues. In the latter case absorption onto these other cells could reduce its effect upon neutrophils. Lalezari and Bernard (1966) reported 2 unrelated families where such monospecific antibodies were present in the maternal sera. Two successive infants had suffered from neonatal neutropenia in these families, providing good evidence of a pathogenic role of the maternal antibodies. Neonatal neutropenia persisted for 60–70 days. In another report a third child presented at the age of two weeks with pyodermia of 5 days' duration. Neutropenia persisted for 28 days (Boxer et al., 1972). Earlier instances of the association of neonatal neutropenia and infection with maternal leucoagglutinins were reported by Hitzig and Gitzelmann (1959), Lalezari et al. (1960), Braun et al. (1960), Jensen (1960) and Rossi and Brandt (1960).

The alternative situation of maternal neutropenia and secondary foetal neutropenia was first described by Stefanini et al. (1958) in three infants, two being siblings, born to mothers with chronic neutropenia. Transplacental passage of a neutropenic factor was suggested. A search for maternal neutropenia must therefore be included in the investigation of neonatal neutropenia. Chlorothiazide can produce neutropenia in both mother and newborn baby due to passive transfer of maternal antibody (Baehner, 1972).

Neonatal neutropenia has also been seen when the mother had neutropenia due to DLE (Seip, 1960). The neutropenia secondary to this disease, rheumatoid arthritis, infectious mononucleosis and certain cases of lymphoma have sometimes been associated with leucoagglutinins (Tullis, 1958).

Other causes of neutropenia

Acute leukaemia, aplastic anaemia and various types of marrow infiltration or replacement such as by secondary neuroblastoma or osteopetrosis (marble bone disease) may present with neutropenia, as a component of the ensuing pancytopenia associated with these disorders.

Neutropenia also occurs in some cases of the Chédiak-Higashi syndrome, where defective granulocyte regulation has been suggested (Blume et al., 1968).

Neutropenia is also the earliest and most constant manifestation of copper deficiency in marasmic infants (Cordano et al., 1966). Anaemia may also be present. The marrow shows arrest of myeloid maturation and erythroid hypoplasia. There is a rapid response to oral copper with rise in polymorphs within 36 hours (Cordano et al., 1964). Megaloblastic changes and vacuolization of the erythroblasts have been reported in one such 3-month-old Indian infant with severe anaemia (Hb 4·3 g/100 ml) and neutropenia (120/mm^3) (Al-Rashid and Spangler, 1971). Epiphyseal and periosteal abnormalities with renal glycosuria can also occur (Seely et al., 1972).

DISORDERS OF PHAGOCYTE FUNCTION

Although primarily concerned with granulocyte function much of this section similarly applies to monocytes.

Physiology of neutrophil granulocytes

This has recently been reviewed succinctly by Clein (1972). The characteristic granules by which cells of this series are identified in Romanowsky-stained smears are membrane-bound organelles containing 30 or more different hydrolytic enzymes, thus falling within the general category of lysosomes (Cohn and Hirsh, 1960). The different enzymes in these granules are capable of cleaving almost all known chemical bonds present in biological material. It is likely that different types of granule have different lytic capabilities.

An acute inflammatory response involves local vascular dilatation with margination of the neutrophils, adherence to the vascular endothelium, migration to the tissues by penetration between the endothelial cells. Thereafter the neutrophil is attracted to the site of inflammation by chemotaxis in response to substances released from bacteria, from damaged tissues including leucocytes and from the activation of complement. Thus phagocytosis and subsequent killing of invading microorganisms is possible. Eosinophils and monocytes also have phagocytic and bactericidal ability but these are less effective than neutrophils (Baehner and Johnston, 1971 and 1972). Nevertheless monocytopenia, as well as neutropenia may contribute to risk of infection in aplastic anaemia (Twomey et al., 1973). In patients with severe neutropenia monocytes appear to play a vital role in preventing infection, accumulating normally in the Rebuck skin window technique even in the absence of neutrophils (Dale and Wolf, 1971).

Opsonization, involving exposure of the microorganism to serum, enhances phagocytosis by facilitating surface attachment to the neutrophil. The serum components include type-specific IgG antibodies (e.g. to the pneumococcal capsule), complement-binding IgM antibodies (e.g. to gram negative bacteria) and the first four components of complement (Michael and Rosen, 1963; Rabinovitch, 1968; Johnston et al., 1969). The C3 component of complement is a necessary prerequisite for normal NBT reduction in neutrophils (Mimbs, 1972). The clinical significance of the opsonin system has recently been reviewed by Winkelstein (1973).

The events following phagocytosis have recently attracted renewed interest in view of their rele-relevance to the defect in chronic granulomatous disease (CGD) and related disorders of neutrophil function. Pseudopodia surround and engulf the particle, usually bacterial, which becomes enclosed within a phagocytic vacuole. Following this phase-contrast examination shows 'degranulation' of the cytoplasm. Electron microscopy has shown that this process is due to emptying of the enzymatic contents of the lysosomal granules into the phago-

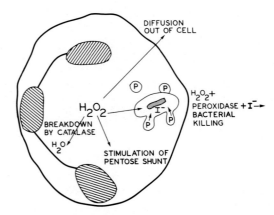

Fig. 15.5 Schematic representation of the metabolic activities of hydrogen peroxide (H_2O_2) within a normal neutrophil. The H_2O_2 contributes to a potent intra-phagocytic bactericidal system in combination with granular myeloperoxidase (P) and iodide ion (I^-). (Reproduced from *Pediatrics* (1971), **48**, 732, by permission of Professor R. L. Baehner and the publishers).

cytic vacuole, with fusion of their respective membranes. This process is followed in normal leucocytes by rapid killing of the ingested bacteria. The main mechanism responsible for this bactericidal effect is probably mediated through the generation of H_2O_2 in the phagocytic vacuole. This in turn results in oxidative iodination of the bacteria, with iodide ion as the substrate and leucocyte myeloperoxidase as the enzyme (Fig. 15.5).

It appears that this H_2O_2-myeloperoxidase-iodide system constitutes the final step in the whole sequence of events leading to intracellular killing of bacteria by the neutrophil polymorphs (Klebanoff and White, 1969). There is a close parallel between the degree of ^{125}I fixation and intracellular bactericidal activity *in vitro*, both being depressed in chronic granulomatous dissease (CGD) and related defects of granulocyte function (Pincus and Klebanoff, 1971). Certain bacteria, the non-catalase producing organisms, effectively generate their own H_2O_2 and may therefore still be killed by CGD neutrophils. These include the *Pneumococcus*, beta haemolytic *streptococcus* and *Haemophilus influenzae*. Such organisms do not cause infections in patients with CGD (Johnston and Baehner, 1971). Catalase-producing bacteria, however, do not effectively produce H_2O_2 and although phagocytosed by CGD neutrophils they are not killed. These bacteria include *Staph. aureus*, *E. coli*, *Klebsiella*, *Pseudomonas*, *Proteus* and *Salmonella*, constituting the organisms that have been recorded as causing infections in CGD (Table 15.5).

Generation of H_2O_2 by the phagocytic cell is a key factor in the bactericidal phase following phagocytosis. It appears to result from a 'burst' of oxidative metabolism with stimulation of both glycolytic and pentose shunt pathways. NADH (reduced DPN) is formed during glycolysis and its oxidation by O_2, catalysed by NADH oxidase, results in H_2O_2 generation:

A

$$\text{Triose} \rightharpoondown \underset{\text{NADH}}{\overset{\text{NAD}}{\rightleftharpoons}} \rightharpoondown \underset{O_2}{\overset{H_2O_2}{\rightleftharpoons}}$$
$$\text{Pyruvate} \qquad\qquad\qquad \text{(or NBT)}$$

Triose phosphate   NAD oxidase
dehydrogenase

This is thought to be the reaction responsible for the increased O_2 consumption by normal neutrophils during phagocytosis (Baehner *et al.*, 1970). It is also thought that the H_2O_2 generated by this reaction may be the initial trigger stimulating the pentose shunt pathway, one function of which is 'detoxication' of H_2O_2 via glutathione peroxidase

B

$$H_2O_2 \rightharpoondown \underset{\text{GSSG}}{\overset{\text{GSH}}{\rightleftharpoons}} \qquad \underset{\text{NADP.H}}{\overset{\text{NADP}}{\rightleftharpoons}} \rightharpoondown \underset{\text{6PG}}{\overset{\text{G.6.P}}{\rightleftharpoons}}$$
$$H_2O$$

Glutathione   Glutathione
peroxidase   reductase   G.6.PD

Once this pathway is stimulated the further metabolism of 6-phosphogluconate (6PG) will result in the formation of an excess of reduced NADP. Oxidation of this NADP.H by NADP oxidase plus O_2 will generate more H_2O_2. Amino acid oxidase is a further possible source (Johnston and Baehner, 1971).

The biochemical defect in CGD and related disorders

Neutrophils from children with CGD show normal phagocytosis but defective killing of (catalase-positive) ingested bacteria (Holmes *et al.*, 1966; Quie *et al.*, 1967). Accompanying this there is an absence of the normal 'oxidative burst' as measured by glucose $1-^{14}C$ oxidation and O_2 consumption following phagocytosis, and there is a marked reduction in H_2O_2 generation and pentose shunt metabolism (Holmes *et al.*, 1967; Baehner and Nathan, 1967). As a consequence of reduced H_2O_2 generation in the phagocytic vacuole there is reduced iodination of the ingested bacteria as

Table 15.5 Frequency of signs and symptoms in 92 patients with chronic granulomatous disease

Finding	Number patients involved
Marked lymphadenopathy	87
Pneumonitis	80
Male sex	80
Suppuration of nodes	79
Hepatomegaly	77
Dermatitis	77
Onset by 1 year	72
Splenomegaly	68
Hepatic-perihepatic abscess	41
Death before 7 years old	34
Osteomyelitis	30
Onset with dermatitis	28
Onset with lymphadenitis	28
Persistent rhinitis	23
Facial periorificial dermatitis	22
Conjunctivitis	21
Death from pneumonitis	21
Persistent diarrhea	20
Perianal abscess	17
Ulcerative stomatis	15

Reproduced from Pediatrics (1971), 48, 732 by permission of Professor R. L. Baehner and the publishers.

measured by ^{125}I binding (Klebanoff and White, 1969). The biochemical events relating to NBT reduction by human phagocytes have recently been reviewed by Nathan (1974). Yellow NBT dye replaces O_2 in reaction A and is reduced to the insoluble blue formazan in the process.

The fundamental biochemical lesion in the majority of cases of CGD is thought to be a deficiency of NADH oxidase (Baehner et al., 1970). Variants of CGD have shown deficiencies of *glutathione peroxidase* in two females with this disease (Holmes et al., 1970). In rare instances of Caucasian G-6-PD deficiency with unusually low levels of neutrophil G-6-PD (less than 1 per cent of normal) a similar defective bactericidal activity has been found (Cooper et al., 1972). It can be seen from reaction B above that both glutathione peroxidase and G-6-PD are necessary for H_2O_2 to act as a trigger in the stimulation of the pentose shunt pathway.

Myeloperoxidase deficiency has also been found in association with defective bactericidal and fungicidal neutrophil activity (Lehrer and Cline, 1969). Here there was normal glucose oxidation and it appears that only the final iodination step was impaired. A simple cytochemical stain for this enzyme is available (Kaplow, 1965).

A delay in intracellular killing of both catalase-producing and non-catalase-producing bacteria by the neutrophils in Chédiak-Higashi disease has also recently been described (Clawson et al., 1971; Root et al., 1973). This appears to be due to delayed emptying of the abnormal lysosomes, characteristic of this disease, into the phagocytic vacuole (Stossel et al., 1972).

NBT TEST IN DIAGNOSIS OF CGD AND RELATED CONDITIONS

Nitroblue tetrazolium dye (NBT) can replace O_2 in the oxidase reactions responsible for H_2O_2 formation, such as in reaction A above. It is reduced thereby to the dark blue insoluble formazan which may then be estimated colourimetrically (Baehner and Nathan, 1968) or cytochemically (Park et al., 1968). In CGD there is virtually no reduction of NBT after stimulation of the neutrophils by phagocytosis of latex microspheres in the quantitative, colourimetric test. This test or one of its qualitative modifications (Johnston, 1969; Gifford and Malawista, 1970) is the recommended screening test for CGD in clinical practice (Johnston and Baehner, 1971). Cytochemical slide tests can be performed on capillary samples of blood with or without added endotoxin (to produce stimulation) plus NBT solution, and are adequate

screening tests for CGD (Park and Good, 1970; Ochs and Igo, 1973). NBT reduction will be impaired not only in the typical type of CGD due to NADH oxidase deficiency but also in those variants due to deficiencies of glutathione reductase or G-6-PD. Intermediate results occur in cases of mild severity (Thompson and Soothill, 1970). In cases with myeloperoxidase deficiency, however, NBT reduction will be normal since H_2O_2 generation remains intact. The defect could still be detected by impaired leucocyte iodination, since this depends upon the myeloperoxidase; or by direct cytochemical staining for the enzyme (Kaplow, 1965; Lehrer and Cline, 1969).

Pathology of CGD

The ingested bacteria or fungi remain viable within the phagocytes where indeed the parasite may be protected from host humoral immunity and from antibiotics which fail to penetrate the cell. Mobility of phagocytes leads to generalized seeding of the reticuloendothelial system (RES) with live microorganisms which eventually overcome their original captors. Unfortunately the same bactericidal defect is probably present in the phagocytic cells of the RES, resulting in the formation of generalized, chronic granulomatous lesions. Johnston and Baehner (1971) have pointed out that this situation is analogous to the granuloma formation well known in association with prolonged intracellular survival of bacteria such as *Listeria* or tubercle bacilli.

Histology of autopsy or biopsy material shows the almost invariable presence of multiple granulomas in the RES. In addition approximately half of such patients show the presence of histiocytes containing yellow or brown lipid material of uncertain origin. This appearance led to the term 'familial lipochrome histiocytosis' being originally applied to relatively mild examples of the disease before the identity with CGD was established (Landing and Shirkey, 1957; Rodey et al., 1970).

Clinical features of CGD and related disorders

In a review of 92 cases of CGD reported in the literature Johnston and Baehner (1971) found 8 where the onset of the disease occurred within the first 2 days of life. Almost all cases had developed their first symptom by the age of 2 years. The male: female ratio was approximately 7:1 with the girls tending to have a milder form of the disease. The usual form in males shows a sex-linked recessive pattern of inheritance.

The frequency of different signs and symptoms among this collected series of patients is shown in Table 15.5. Involvement of the reticuloendothelial system is the commonest site of infection for the reasons given above. In particular, lymphadenopathy is usually present and in most instances the glands are suppurative and drain pus. Hepatosplenomegaly was present in almost all those patients reaching the age of 6 years. Another group of symptoms was related to impaired defences at the site of entry of infection, viz. pneumonitis, subcutaneous abscesses and furunculoid or impetiginous rashes contrasting with the absence of suppuration in skin lesions occurring in the neutropenic states. Osteomyelitis in this disease tends to involve the small bones of the hands and feet with marked bone destruction on X-rays but only mild clinical signs (Wolfson et al., 1969).

Approximately one third of the collected series died before the age of 7, and 40 per cent by 12 years, pulmonary infection being the commonest cause of death. Several female patients, however, are known to have survived into their late twenties or thirties. Haematological features include an appropriate neutrophil leucocytosis, chronic hypergammaglobulinaemia, and often an anaemia due to infection. Treatment is unsatisfactory. When antibiotics are needed consideration should be given to use of those known to penetrate the leucocyte such as co-trimoxazole (Septrin) or Rifampicin (Ezer and Soothill, 1974). Marrow transplantation is being considered as an experimental approach. Granulocyte transfusions might give short-term benefit at times of crisis. A recent report describes enhanced bactericidal activity of the phagocytes in CGD in the presence of sulphisoxazole and attributes the apparent clinical benefit of long-term suphonamide therapy to this effect (Johnston et al., 1975).

INHERITANCE OF CGD

The apparent sex-linked mode of inheritance in the majority of these patients is supported by the quantitative NBT test in so far as an intermediate degree of impairment is found in the mothers of affected boys, and a normal result in the fathers (Windhurst et al., 1968). The Lyon hypothesis in this context implies that the female carriers will have a double population of normal and defective phagocytes and there is cytochemical evidence in support of this in CGD (Windhurst et al., 1967).

The occurrence of a disease with similar clinical and laboratory features but in three female Black siblings suggested an autosomal inheritance with recessive or dominant variable expression in these particular patients (Azimi et al., 1968). Further evidence of an autosomal recessive pattern has come from the finding of impaired neutrophil function in both parents of patients with CGD (Chandra et al., 1959). It is probable, therefore, that both types of inheritance can occur in this disease. Alternatively some cases with an atypical form of inheritance may be suffering from a separate enzyme defect (Douglas et al., 1969). For instance, deficiency of glutathione peroxidase has recently been reported as causing CGD in females (Holmes et al., 1970).

Other abnormalities of phagocytic function

Some of these have already been mentioned as producing a similar biochemical lesion to that seen in typical CGD.

MYELOPEROXIDASE DEFICIENCY

Five patients have been described with an isolated deficiency of this enzyme affecting their neutrophils, but not their eosinophils. Inheritance appears to be autosomal recessive. One of these patients suffered from systemic candidiasis. The others were in normal health although their leucocytes had decreased fungicidal and bactericidal activity (Lehrer and Cline, 1969; Salmon et al., 1970; Klebanoff and Pincus, 1971). This disorder is less severe than CGD. The NBT test and glucose metabolism are normal, but iodination, cytochemical peroxidase staining (Kaplow, 1965) and bactericidal tests abnormal.

JOB'S SYNDROME

'So went Satan forth from the presence of the Lord, and smote Job with sore boils from the sole of his foot unto his crown'. Job II, 7 (quoted by Davis et al., 1966).

Also less severe than CGD is a syndrome seen in light-skinned, red-haired females who are prone to recurrent 'cold' staphylococcal abscesses (Davis et al., 1966). Some of these patients appear to be merely mild forms of CGD (Bannatyne et al., 1969). The 3 patients described in these two reports were surviving at 5, 6 and 9 years, but had suffered from recurrent infection from the age of a few weeks. A selective inability to kill staphylococci has also been described in a young man with manifestations similar to CGD since birth (Davis et al., 1968). Defective granulocyte chemotaxis and very high serum—IgE levels have also been reported in 4 females (Hill et al., 1974).

LEUCOCYTE GLUTATHIONE PEROXIDASE DEFICIENCY

Since this enzyme is on the pathway by which H_2O_2 stimulates pentose shunt metabolism B a defect at this point can impair the normal oxidative 'burst' following phagocytosis. The NBT test will therefore give a similar result as in CGD. Two female patients have been described with a form of chronic granulomatous disease in whom special enzyme assays showed a significant deficiency of this enzyme in their leucocytes, thereby distinguishing them from the more usual type of CGD (Holmes et al., 1970). Phagocytosis was normal but intracellular killing of Staph. aureus was impaired. The enzyme was absent in neutrophils and monocytes, but present normally in monocytes (Salmon et al., 1970). Marked impairment of intracellular killing of Candida albicans was present in Salmon's patient, who suffered from systemic candidiasis. Inheritance is probably autosomal recessive.

G-6-PD DEFICIENCY IN LEUCOCYTES

In some cases of Caucasian G-6-PD deficiency the enzyme is depressed also in the neutrophils. In exceptional instances the level is less than 1 per cent of normal. This would be expected to impair the response of the pentose pathway to H_2O_2 stimulation and to limit the postphagocytic bactericidal potential. An inability of such leucocytes to generate H_2O_2 has been reported in association with a fatal disease due to persistent bacterial infection (Cooper et al., 1972). A further 3 male siblings in a Canadian family have recently been described where a variable liability to recurrent granulomatous infection was accompanied by chronic mild haemolysis (Gray et al., 1973).

CHÉDIAK-HIGASHI DISEASE

A fatal familial syndrome of repeated pyogenic infections, photophobia, pale optic fundi, albinism, excessive sweating, with terminal hepatosplenomegaly, generalized lymphadenopathy and pancytopenia was described by Chédiak in 1952 and independently by Higashi in 1953. The inheritance is autosomal recessive. The striking haematological feature is the presence of giant refractile granules in the neutrophils which stain greenish-grey with Romanowsky's stains and which are peroxidase positive. Good photomicrographs, including colour, are shown in the papers of Donohue and Bain (1957), Page et al. (1962) and Blume et al. (1968).

The inclusions must be distinguished from the Döhle bodies seen in the neutrophils in the benign May–Hegglin anomaly with thrombocytopenia and giant platelets. Comparative photomicrographs are shown in the paper of Oski et al. (1962).

The natural course of the disease includes a high incidence of lymphoma with progression to pancytopenia and histiocytic proliferation (Dent et al., 1966). The increased susceptibility to recurrent infections is thought to be related to defective release of lysosomal enzymes into the phagocytic vacuole (Stossel et al., 1972). Diminished capacity for intracellular bacterial killing has recently been demonstrated (Clawson et al., 1971). Neutropenia may also develop during the course of the disease (Blume et al., 1968), further contributing to lowered bacterial resistance. Impaired cell-mediated immunity with frequent viral infections has also been described, with apparent improvement after treatment with transfer factor (Khan et al., 1973).

CONGENITAL ABNORMALITY OF SPECIFIC GRANULE FORMATION

A boy of 14 has been described who had recurrent staphylococcal respiratory and skin infections since infancy. A morphological abnormality of his circulating neutrophils was present consisting of an almost complete absence of specific granules (Wright–Giemsa stain) together with bilobed nuclei. Neutrophil alkaline phosphatase activity was absent. Ultra-structure studies on marrow cells showed delayed appearance and abnormal structure of the specific granules. In vitro bactericidal function was impaired for staphylococci (Strauss et al., 1974).

Acquired disorders of leucocyte function

Impaired granulocyte migration in response to inflammation has been found in untreated acute myeloblastic, but not lymphoblastic, leukaemia (Holland et al., 1971), and impaired chemotaxis in diabetes mellitus (Mowat and Baum, 1971). Partial leucocyte dysfunction against staphylococci has been found in 7 out of 17 children with untreated acute lymphoblastic leukaemia and in 10 out of 63 children with Down's syndrome (Gregory et al., 1972). Drugs used in the treatment of leukaemia may also impair neutrophil function. Steroids cause a modest depression of NBT reduction and intracellular killing, apparently by inhibiting NADH oxidase, the same enzyme that is thought to be deficient in CGD (Mandell et al., 1970; Matula and Paterson, 1971B). One of the vinca alkaloids, vinkaleukoblastine, impairs neutrophil degranulation, probably by inhibiting microtubule formation by the same mechanism as colchicine (Malawista, 1971). Granulocyte adherence, an important component of the inflammatory reaction, is inhibited after ingestion 40 mg prednisone, 1·2 g aspirin or an intoxicating level of alcohol (MacGregor et al., 1974). Monocyte bactericidal and candicidal activity is similarly impaired by prednisone, 100–200 mg/day (Rinehart et al., 1975). Parenteral hyperalimentation with hypertonic amino acids and glucose has been reported as impairing chemotaxis, phagocytosis and bactericidal activity secondary to hypophosphataemia interfering with ATP function (Craddock et al., 1974).

Reversible defects of neutrophil NBT reduction have been described (Anderson and Soonattrakul, 1973; Rubinstein and Pelet, 1973), including that in association with ataxia telangiectasia (Kretschmer et al., 1972). In some of these a plasma factor may be involved (De La Vega et al., 1973).

To the extent that efficient phagocytosis is dependent upon prior opsonization of the microorganism temporary defects of humoral immunity may be included as indirect causes of impaired phagocytic function. The increased liability of the newborn to gram negative infections attributed to the normal neonatal deficiency of IgM antibodies, is of this type (Michael and Rosen, 1963). A reversible bactericidal defect of neutrophils has been seen in association with macroglobulinaemia (Douglas et al., 1970). Defective phagocytosis and chemotaxis due to deficiency of the C5 component of complement has been described in a child by Miller et al. (1968). Clinical improvement followed the infusion of fresh frozen plasma. Defective chemotaxis and consequent impaired NBT reduction due to an inhibitor in the serum has been described in two siblings by Ward and Schlegel (1969). An abnormal Rebuck skin window response has recently been found in children with kwashiorkor (Freyre et al., 1973). Recent reviews on defects of leukocyte function include those of Klebanoff (1971), Park (1971) and Baehner (1972). 'The molecular basis for functional disorders of phagocytes' have been reviewed by Baehner (1974). Phagocytosis has been reviewed by Lynch (1973) (1973) and Stossel (1974).

Leucocyte changes secondary to infection

Quantitative changes in the peripheral blood leucocytes secondary to specific infections are tabulated below. For the significance of a differential white count in children to be appreciated it is necessary to relate it to the child's age. In the first 4 days of life there is a preponderance of neutrophil polymorphs and usually an absolute neutrophil leucocytosis. From the first week of life until around 4 years of age there is a preponderance of lymphocytes over neutrophils, but beyond this age the adult proportions are regained. During the first few months of life even a pyogenic infection may evoke more of a lymphoid response than the expected polymorph response. The presence of Türk cells with a strongly basophilic cytoplasm ('viracytes') are strongly suggestive of a virus infection at any age and are a useful diagnostic pointer in practice. They are particularly characteristic of measles and rubella.

Qualitative changes include the heavily-staining 'toxic granulations' accompanied by bluish areas of the cytoplasm, Döhle bodies, seen in neutrophils at times of severe bacterial infection, e.g. subphrenic abscess, gram negative septicaemia, anaerobic infections. When toxic granulations and Döhle bodies are accompanied by neutropenia rather than the expected neutrophil leucocytosis the significance is particularly serious and should be interpreted as suggesting overwhelming bacterial infection with inadequate marrow response.

A cytochemical modification of the NBT test (Park et al., 1968) has proved to be a particularly useful screening test for the early detection of acute bacterial infection before there has been time for a neutrophil leucocytosis to develop, and to distinguish between bacterial infections on the one hand, and viral infections or reactive leucocytosis from non-infective conditions on the other. In the original test 0·1 ml of heparinized venous blood was mixed with an equal volume of 0·2 per cent NBT in buffered saline and incubated at 37° C for 15 minutes in a moist chamber. Coverslip smears were prepared, the proportion and absolute number of neutrophil polymorphs containing large black formazan (reduced NBT) deposits being enumerated. The hypothesis was that the NBT reduction within individual neutrophils (and monocytes) without further in vitro challenge might be triggered by actual in vivo phagocytosis of bacteria. In healthy controls the mean percentage of NBT +ve neutrophils was 8·5 (range 3 to 10) and the absolute number 411 per mm^3 (range 145 to 720).

Normal results were found in patients with fever, leucocytosis and leukaemoid reaction associated with rheumatoid arthritis, SLE or a variety of viral infections including measles, chicken-pox, mumps or mumps meningoencephalitis. In primary tuberculosis the results were also normal. By contrast the percentage and absolute numbers of NBT +ve neutrophils were strikingly increased in patients with bacterial meningitis (*Pneumococcal, Haemophilus, Meningococcal, Streptococcal* and *Coliform*) as well as in a variety of other acute bacterial infections (ruptured appendix, empyema, gingival abscess, osteomyelitis) and in 4 patients with *Candida albicans* septicaemia. Positive results are also found in military TB (Mimbs, 1972), malaria (Andersen, 1971), other fungal infections and certain parasitic diseases (Chretien and Garagusi, 1971). Normal results have been found in children with viral or tuberculous meningitis, distinguishing them from pyogenic meningitis. These observations have amply been confirmed (Douwer, 1972) and the value of the test in the management of an acutely febrile young child is self evident. It has been recommended that this should be a routinely available laboratory test (*Lancet*, 1971; Humbert *et al.*, 1971; Park, 1971).

Reservations regarding its clinical usefulness have centred upon the occurrence of false negative results in the presence of bacterial infection. A major limitation is the rapid conversion to normal after effective antimicrobial therapy even before defervescence of fever (Matula and Paterson, 1971A). The test is also normal in bacterial infections that remain superficially localized. False negative tests could also occur because of defective neutrophil function such as in CGD (Park *et al.*, 1969) or due to extraneous factors such as high dose corticosteroids (Matula and Paterson, 1971B), low complement (C3) levels (DeMeo and Andersen, 1972) and perhaps high antibiotic blood levels (Rubinstein and Pelet, 1973). In order to detect this source of error Park and Good (1970) have introduced a 'stimulated NBT test' whereby a control is set up in which 10 μg of bacterial endotoxin per 0·5 ml of blood is added to the system. After 5–10 min incubation at RT approximately half the neutrophils become NBT +ve in normals. Bacterial suspensions or IgM/ anti IgM antibody complexes may be used in place of endotoxin (Rubinstein and Pelet, 1973), over 90 per cent of the cells becoming NBT +ve. In addition to increasing the reliability of the test for active bacterial infection this modification incidentally also provides a good screening test for the detection of patients with innately defective neutrophil function such as CGD (Park and Good, 1970). A further modification in which granulocytes are allowed to migrate and adhere to endotoxin-coated coverslips, followed by incubation with NBT solution has been described by Ochs and Igo (1973). It provides a simple screening test for CGD and shows female carriers of CGD to posses a double population of normal and abnormal

granulocytes, confirming the Lyon hypothesis in this disease.

False positive results may also occur: In the newborn infant and during the first 3 weeks of life an increased proportion of the circulating neutrophils are NBT positive even in the absence of infection (Park, 1971). In premature infants this increase is less marked (Vowels and Goel, 1974). High NBT results are also found in osteogenesis imperfecta (Douwer, 1972). The use of the NBT in clinical paediatrics has recently been reviewed by Baehner (1974).

Whereas the alkaline phosphatase cytochemical reaction distinguishes between the neutrophil leucocytosis of chronic myeloid leukaemia (in which it is negative) and a leukaemoid reaction of inflammatory or infective origin, when it is strongly positive; the NBT test will be positive only when the leukaemoid reaction is due to a bacterial or fungal infection.

The quantitative changes in numbers of circulating neutrophils, monocytes, lymphocytes and eosinophils usually seen in childhood infections and certain inflammatory conditions are shown in Tables 15.6–9. It should be emphasized that the expected leucocyte response is less dependable in the early months of life than in later childhood since even pyogenic infections may cause a lymphocytosis. Mauer (1969) points out that in severe infections such as purulent meningitis the expected neutrophil leucocytosis is absent in about one in five children (Groover *et al.*, 1961). Similarly in appendicitis the leucocyte count can be normal in approximately one fifth of patients (Meagher *et al.*, 1954). In intestinal infections such as shigellosis (Donald and Winkler, 1960) and also in typhoid (Earle, 1954) either neutrophil leucocytosis or neutropenia are possible in different cases, irrespective of the severity. In septicaemias and severe infections such as subphrenic abscess neutropenia may be present, but with a 'shift to the left' (i.e. a high proportion of unsegmented band cells), toxic granulation and Döhle bodies; the latter features indicate the presence of severe pyogenic infection even although neutrophil leucocytosis may be absent. It is this variability in leucocytic response in bacterial infections that constitutes the justification of the NBT test of Park *et al.* (1968). Three additional useful pointers to the diagnosis of septicaemia are thrombocytopenia, decreased serum inorganic phosphate and vacuolation of the granulocytes (Riedler, 1972). Thrombocytopenia was present in 80 per cent of gram −ve and in 60 per cent of gram +ve infections, being more

Table 15.6 Bacterial infections

	Neutrophils	Monocytes	Lymphocytes	Eosinophils	Other features
Pyogenic infections					
(Gm +ve cocci, Gm −ve bacilli)	↑ (↓ if severe)	↑	↑ in infants	(↑ in convalescence)	Over 10 per cent of neutrophils NBT +ve, toxic gran. and Döhle bodies if severe. Thrombocytopenia if septicaemic
Pertussis	↓ usually		↑ up to −80,000		Mature lymphocytes
Meningococcaemia	N				± DIC
Brucellosis	↓	↑ ±		↓ ±	± Leukaemoid reaction
Tularaemia	↑				
Typhoid	↑			↑ late	
Diphtheria	↑ (↓ if severe)				
Clostridial	↑				Intravascular haemolysis Toxic gran.
Weil's disease	↑		↑ late		
Tuberculosis Miliary	↓				± Leukaemoid or Leukoerythroblastic picture
Septic	↑	↑			

Table 15.7 Viral infections

Normal childhood values: per mm³ (beyond first 6 months)	Neutrophils 1,500–7,500	Monocytes 0–800	Lymphocytes 1,500–8,500	Eosinophils 30–800	Other features
Influenza	↓ usual, (↑ if pneumonia)		↑ (relative)	↓ if severe	
Rubella	↓ , ↑ late		↓ ↑ by 5th day		Turk cells persisting for many weeks ± thrombocytopenia
Measles	↑ early, then ↓		↓	↑ at 1 week	± Thrombocytopenia
Mumps	↓ (↑ if orchitis)	± ↑	↑		Rare lympho leukaemoid reaction
Varicella	↑ early,		↑	↑ in convalescence	Rare lymphocytic laukaemoid reaction
Cytomegalovirus	↓	Atypical Monos.	↑ ±		Rising CMV titres
Infectious mononucleosis	↑ early, ↓ late	Atypical Monos.	↑ ↑	↑ occasional	+ve Paul-Bunnell Rising EBV antibodies Rare thrombocytopenia
Infectious lymphocytosis			↑		
Infectious hepatitis	↓ early	Atypical Monos.	↑ ±		Atypical Monos. ±thrombocytopenia occ. aplasia
Poliomyelitis	Mod. ↑ early				
Aseptic meningitis	↓ usual		↑ usual		
Mycoplasma pneumonia	↑				High cold aggs. and MG agglutinins ± Cold AHA
Rickettsia (Q-fever)		Atypical Monos.	↑		
Adenovirus type 12			↑		

242 PAEDIATRIC HAEMATOLOGY

Table 15.8 Fungal and protozoal infections

	Neutrophils	Monocytes	Lymphocytes	Eosinophils	Other features
Actinomycosis	↑				
Coccidioidomycosis	↑			↑	
Histoplasmosis	↑				Anaemia
Candida albicans	↑ ⎰ If pt. capable				
Aspergillus	↑ ⎱ of responding			↑	
Malaria	↓	↑ ±		↑ ±	Anaemia
Trypanosomiasis		↑			Anaemia
Kala-azar	↓		↑ (relative)		Anaemia ± DIC
Trichiniasis	↑			↑	
Filariasis	↑			↑	
Pneumocystis carinii	↑ ±		↓	↑ ±	± ↓ Immunoglobulins
Toxoplasmosis		Atypical	↑		± Thrombocytopenia

Table 15.9 Non-infective causes of leucocyte changes

	Neutrophils	Monocytes	Lymphocytes	Eosinophils
Polyarteritis nodosa	↑			↑ ±
Rheumatoid arthritis	↑			
Burns	↑			
Diabetic acidosis	↑			
Haemorrhage	↑			
Intestinal parasites				↑
Toxocara canis				↑
Hodgkin's disease			↓ ±	↑ ±
Diphenylhydantoin toxicity		Atypical	↑	
Corticosteroid therapy	↑	↑	↓	↓

severe in the gram —ve. Decreased serum phosphate was present in 70 and 20 per cent respectively. All cases showed a 'shift to the left' of the neutrophils; toxic granulations were present in 65 per cent and vacuolation, as originally described by Zieve *et al.* (1966) in 43 per cent of a series of 141 patients. In severe bacterial infections the development of a leucocytosis indicates a better prognosis than neutropenia and lymphopenia. The haematological changes occurring in all the common infections have recently been well reviewed by Murdoch and Smith (1972).

Türk cells are particularly characteristic of viral infections, but may also be seen in bacterial infections. These cells are the circulating equivalent of the tissue plasma cell and, concerned with antibody production, are a valuable diagnostic pointer in paediatric haematology. They have to be distinguished from the 'atypical mononuclear' cell (Plate C) characteristic of infectious mononucleosis but should never cause serious confusion with leukaemic blast cells (Plate D). However, a lymphoid 'leukaemoid reaction' with lymphocyte counts of 100,000/mm³ or more may occur with certain virus infections, and in pertussis. Thrombo-

cytopenia is a relatively frequent accompaniment of the specific viral infections or may follow the infection, running a course indistinguishable from idiopathic thrombocytopenic purpura (ITP). The mechanism of thrombocytopenia during viral infections is not clear (Clancy *et al.*, 1971). It is only occasionally indicative of DIC.

INFECTIOUS MONONUCLEOSIS AND RELATED CONDITIONS

The association of atypical mononucleosis in the peripheral blood with fever, pharyngitis and lymphadenopathy especially of the posterior cervical group form, the well-known syndrome of 'glandular fever' or infectious mononucleosis. Although usually considered a disease of young adults it has also been well recognized in children since its earliest descriptions at the end of the last century (Pfeiffer, 1889). Twenty-five certain cases plus thirty probable cases were seen by one paediatric haematology service over a period of five years (Starling and Fernbach, 1968); 105 cases over 1½ years by another (Baehner and Shuler, 1967). In the series of 105 children presenting clinical features included pharyngitis in 47, lethargy in 25, lymphadenopathy in 19, pyrexia of unknown origin in 9 and symptoms of hepatitis in 5 (Baehner and Shuler, 1967). Other symptoms may include transient rashes, myalgia, arthralgia, facial and periorbital oedema (Fernbach and Starling, 1972). Rare forms of presentation include hepatitis (Marx, 1970), haemorrhage due to thrombocytopenia (Goldstein and Porter, 1969), haemolytic anaemia (Einzig and Neerhout, 1969), the Guillain-Barré syndrome (Ben-Asher et al., 1970), convulsions (Bonforte, 1967), encephalitis (Walsh et al., 1954) acute cerebellar syndrome (Lascelles et al., 1973), facial paralysis (Taylor and Parsons-Smith, 1969) and Reye's syndrome (Rahal and Henle, 1970). The wide range of complications have been summarized by Evans (1967). Alterations in hepatic transminases are so frequent that it has recently been suggested that they should be included among the criteria for diagnosis.

Fever, ranging from 101° to 103° F, may persist for several weeks. Lymphadenopathy is present in virtually all patients and usually involves posterior cervical as well as anterior cervical groups (Table 15.10), thereby distinguishing the condition from

Table 15.10 Physical findings in 105 children with infectious mononucleosis (aged 16 years or under)

Lymphadenopathy		87
Generalized	36	
Anterior + Posterior cervical	25	
Posterior cervical only	16	
Anterior cervical only	7	
Inguinal	3	
Splenomegaly		49
Exudative tonsillitis		30
Hepatomegaly		29
Rash		8

Reproduced from Clinical Pediatrics (1967), 6, 393 by permission of Professor R. L. Baehner and the publishers.

simple regional lymphadenitis secondary to the pharyngitis and membranous tonsillitis that is frequently present. Purpuric petechiae on the soft palate are seen in a quarter (Hoagland, 1960) and splenomegaly in over half of the patients (Baehner and Shuler, 1967).

Haematological criteria for diagnosis include a lymphocyte preponderance of at least 50 per cent with the presence of atypical mononuclear cells (Bender, 1958). Most patients with infectious mononucleosis have 25 per cent or more atypical mononuclear cells during the second or third week of the disease. In other virus infections the percentage is usually less than 10–15. These are large cells with abundant basophilic cytoplasm with Romanowsky stains (Plate C). A few red ('azurophilic') granules may be present and there is often a fine linear division between the darkly basophilic peripheral cytoplasm and a paler perinuclear zone. Nuclei are large, may contain nucleoli, and are sometimes indented, very similar in appearance to monocyte nuclei. Downey's (1923) classical paper illustrating these cells classified them into 3 types. The most characteristic cell, as described above, corresponds most closely to the Downey's Type III. Since, however, some Type I and II cells may be found present in the same film this classification probably now has only historical interest. The traditional discussion as to whether these cells are of lymphocytic or monocytic origin appears to be in process of resolution. Pearmain and Lycette (1963) pointed out that atypical mononuclear cells closely resembled PHA-transformed lymphocytes in terms of morphology. More recently it has been shown that these cells are almost certainly derived from T-lymphocytes of thymic origin (Sheldon et al., 1973). Since the EB virus appears to grow exclusively in the B-lymphocytes it has been suggested that it is EBV associated antigens acquired by these infected cells which trigger the 'transformation' of T-cells into atypical mononuclear cells (Pattengale et al., 1973). The platelet count and haemoglobin levels are usually normal, but thrombocytopenia or direct Coombs positive haemolytic anaemia may occasionally occur as mentioned above. A transient neutrophil leucocytosis may occur in the prodromal phase, but severe neutropenia may develop later (Penman, 1968).

Serological diagnosis has depended upon the Paul-Bunnell (1932) test whereby heterophile agglutinins to sheep red cells are present to a titre of 1:56 or more, being unabsorbed by previous incubation with guinea pig kidney cells but absorbed by beef red cells (Davidsohn et al., 1951). 'Spot tests' have also been developed capable of giving a rapid presumptive result (Galloway, 1969; Hoff and Bauer, 1965). It has been recognized for many years, however, that the Paul-Bunnell test is often negative in young children apparently suffering from this disease (Vahlquist et al., 1958). More recently it has been discovered that an attack of infectious mononucleosis, as judged by the above clinical, haematological and serological criteria, (a) only occurs in the absence of pre-existing antibodies to the Epstein-Bar virus (EBV), and (b) is regularly followed by sero-conversion with the development of antibodies to

EBV (University Health Physicians and P.H.L.S. Laboratories, 1971; Evans, 1972). The virus has been isolated from peripheral blood leucocytes in this disease by Diehl *et al.* (1968). Consistent with the widely held belief that the disease is spread by kissing it is of great interest that Miller *et al.* (1973) have recently presented evidence that EBV can be recovered from oropharyngeal washings in infectious mononucleosis. Positive results were found in 23 out of 25 patients not only in the acute stage but for up to 16 months after the onset. The new criteria that have emerged from this incrimination of EBV as the causative agent in infectious

Käämänen, 1965; Rifkind, 1968) and has particularly been incriminated in those cases of mononucleosis following the massive blood transfusions used in open-heart surgery (Foster and Jack, 1969; Riemenschneider and Moss, 1966; Stevens and Pry, 1971). Acquired glandular toxoplasmosis is also known to cause mononucleosis with a negative Paul-Bunnell test.

The present situation has been summarized by Evans (1972) as follows: Both EBV and CMV can cause typical heterophile antibody-negative infectious mononucleosis, and adenovirus, rubella, herpes simplex and toxoplasmosis are also candi-

Table 15.11 Causes of moderate eosinophilia

Parasitic infections
  Helminthic: Trichinosis, ascariasis, hookworm disease, strongyloidiasis
  Protozoal: Malaria
  Eosinophilic pneumonia
  Tropical eosinophilia

Allergic disorders
  Asthma, seasonal pollinosis, urticaria, eczema

Drug exposure

Primary hematologic disorders
  Hodgkin's disease
  Fanconi's anemia, thrombocytopenia with absent radius
  Congenital immune deficiency syndromes
  Chronic myeloproliferative states
  Post-splenectomy

Miscellaneous disorders
  Periarteritis nodosa
  Cirrhosis
  Malignant neoplasms
  Dermatitis herpetiformis
  Radiation therapy
Peritoneal dialysis
  Congenital heart disease
  Hereditary eosinophilia

Reproduced from Pediat. Clinics of N. America (1972), 19, 969 by permission of Professor J. N. Lukens and the publishers.

mononucleosis consist of: (a) either a positive differential heterophile *or* a positive EBV titre, in association with (b) typical clinical features, (c) lymphocytosis with atypical lymphocytes and (d) abnormality of liver function tests (Fernbach and Starling, 1972). The significance of oral excretion of EBV in infectious mononucleosis has recently been reviewed (*Lancet*, 1973).

Cases with mononucleosis but a negative heterophile antibody test (Paul-Bunnell —ve) have failed to show antibodies to EBV but have developed antibodies to CMV instead (University Health Physicians and P.H.L.S. Laboratories 1971). CMV had previously been recognized as one of the possible aetiological agents of Paul-Bunnell negative infectious mononucleosis (Klemola and

date agents for causing other 'mono-like conditions'. It is clear from this statement that Paul-Bunnell negative cases should be screened serologically for the above mentioned infections and EBV antibodies, or isolation from throat washings attempted if these virological facilities are available.

Symptomatic treatment is all that is usually needed in true infectious mononucleosis since it is a self-limiting disorder although sometimes running a protracted course. Penicillin is given if beta haemolytic streptococci are cultured from the throat. Corticosteroids are occasionally needed in the most severe examples, facial or pharyngeal oedema or with the rare complications of thrombocytopenic purpura or autoimmune haemolytic anaemia. Specific antimicrobial therapy may have to be considered in protracted infections due to the CMV or toxoplasmosis.

Infectious lymphocytosis

Clinically much milder than infectious mononucleosis, this condition may be discovered fortuitously from the blood count. Outbreaks may occur in closed communities such as boarding schools. Symptoms may include those of a mild upper respiratory tract infection with or without slight fever. A minor degree of lymphadenopathy and splenomegaly may be present. The white cell count rises over several weeks to 50,000 or even 100,000/mm³, the cells being mature lymphocytes. Atypical mononuclear cells may also be present and an absolute eosinophilia. Anaemia and thrombocytopenia do not occur. Only symptomatic treatment is needed. Representative reports include those of Smith (1941), Arneil and Riley (1952) and Ryder (1965).

EOSINOPHILIA

The causes of eosinophilia in childhood do not differ significantly from those in adult life. In association with iron deficiency they suggest intestinal parasites, and constitute a common finding in slum children from industrial cities. Table 15.11 from a review of eosinophilia in children by Lukens (1972) lists the causes of moderate eosinophilia. Exaggerated eosinophilia with total white cell counts of 30,000 to 100,000/mm³ and 50 to 90 per cent of the cells eosinophils tends to be caused by visceral *Larva migrans* due to dog or cat *Toxacara* (Huntley *et al.*, 1965), idiopathic hyper-eosinophilic syndrome, related to Loeffler's syndrome (Hardy and Anderson, 1968) or the extremely rare eosinophilic leukaemia, discussed in Chapter 20. Occasionally a marked eosinophilia can also occur with diseases more usually associated with only moderate eosinophilia, including Hodgkin's, polyarteritis nodosa, drug hypersensitivity and parasitic infections.

REFERENCES

Aarskog, D. (1961) Infantile congenital aneutrocytosis. *Arch. Dis. Childh.*, **36**, 511.

Abildgaard, H. & Jensen, K. G. (1964) The influence of maternal leucocyte antibodies on infants. *Scand. J. Haemat.*, **1**, 47.

Ackerman, B. D. (1964) Dysgammaglobulinemia: Report of a case with a family history of congenital gamma globulin disorder. *Pediatrics*, **34**, 211.

Allen, D. M., Necheles, T. F., Rieker, R. & Senior, B. (1969) Reversible neonatal pancytopenia due to isovaleric acidemia. *Abstracts Soc. Pediat. Res. Atlantic City,* May, 156.

Al-Rashid, R. A. & Spangler, J. (1971) Neonatal copper deficiency. *New Eng. J. Med.,* **285**, 841.

Andersen, B. R. (1971) NBT test in malaria. *Lancet*, **ii**, 317.

Andersen, B. R. & Soonattrakul, W. (1973) Neutrophilic reduction of NBT dye: acquired defect. *Ann. Intern. Med.*, **78**, 301.

Andrews, J. P., McClellan, J. T. & Scott, C. H. (1960) Lethal congenital neutropenia with eosinophilia occurring in two siblings. *Am. J. Med.,* **29**, 359.

Arneil, G. C. & Riley, I. D. (1952) Acute infectious lymphocytosis. *Quart. J. Med.,* **21**, 285.

Athens, J. W., Haab, O. P., Raab, S. O., Mauer, A. M., Ashenbrucker, H., Cartwright, G. E. & Wintrobe, M. M. (1961A) Leukokinetic studies. IV. The total blood, circulating and marginal granulocyte pools and the granulocyte turnover rate in normal subjects. *J. Clin. Invest.,* **40**, 989.

Athens, J. W., Raab, S. O., Haab, O. P., Mauer, A. M., Ashenbrucker, H., Cartwright, G. E. & Wintrobe, M. M. (1961B) Leukokinetic studies. III. The distribution of granulocytes in the blood of normal subjects. *J. Clin. Invest.,* **40**, 159.

Azimi, P. H., Bodenbender, J. G., Hintz, R. L. & Kontras, S. B. (1968) Chronic granulomatous disease in three female siblings. *Journal of the American Medical Association,* **206**, 2865.

Baehner, R. L. (1972) Disorders of leukocytes leading to recurrent infection. *Ped. Clin. N. Amer.,* **19**, 935.

Baehner, R. L. & Nathan, D. G. (1967) Leukocyte oxydase: Defective activity in chronic granulomatous disease. *Science,* **155**, 853.

Baehner, R. L. & Shuler, S. E. (1967) Infectious mononucleosis in childhood. Clinical expressions, serologic findings, complications, prognosis. *Clin. Pediat.,* **6**, 393.

Baehner, R. L. & Nathan, D. G. (1968) Quantitative nitroblue tetrazolium test in chronic granulomatous disease. *New Eng. J. Med.,* **278**, 971.

Baehner, R. L., Nathan, D. G. & Karnovsky, M. L. (1970) Correction of metabolic deficiencies in the leukocytes of patients with chronic granulomatous disease. *J. Clin. Invest.,* **49**, 865.

Baehner, R. L., Gilman, N. & Karnovsky, M. L. (1970) Respiration and glucose oxidation in human and guinea pig leukocytes. *J. Clin. Invest.,* **49**, 692.

Baehner, R. L. & Johnston, R. B. (1971) Metabolic and bactericidal activity of human eosinophils. *Brit. J. Haemat.,* **20**, 277.

Baehner, R. L. & Johnston, R. B. (1972) Monocyte function in children with neutropenia and chronic infections. *Blood*, **40**, 431.

Baehner, R. L. (1974) Molecular basis for functional disorders of phagocytes. *J. Pediat.*, **84**, 317.

Baehner, R. L. (1974) Use of the nitro-blue tetrazolium test in clinical pediatrics. *Am. J. Dis. Child.*, **128**, 449.

Bannatyne, R. M., Skowron, P. N. & Weber, J. L. (1969) Job's syndrome—a variant of chronic granulomatous disease. *J. Pediat.*, **75**, 236.

Barak, Y., Paran, M., Levin, S. & Sachs, L. (1971) *In vitro* induction of myeloid proliferation and maturation in infantile genetic agranulocytosis. *Blood*, **38**, 74.

Ben-Asher, M., Chokshi, D. & Feldman, M. (1970) Infectious mononucleosis presented as Guillain-Barré syndrome. *Arizona Med.*, **27**, 88.

Bender, C. E. (1958) Interpretation of hematologic and serologic findings in the diagnosis of infectious mononucleosis. *Ann. Intern. Med.*, **49**, 852.

Bjure, J., Nilsson, L. R. & Plum, C. M. (1962) Familial neutropenia caused by deficiency of a plasma factor. *Acta Paediat.*, **51**, 497.

Blume, R. S., Bennett, J. M., Yankee, R. A. & Wolff, S. M. (1968) Defective granulocyte regulation in the Chediak-Higashi syndrome. *New Eng. J. Med.*, **279**, 1009.

Bodian, M., Sheldon, W. & Lightwood, R. (1964) Congenital hypoplasia of the exocrine pancreas. *Acta Paediat.*, **53**, 282.

Boggs, D. R., Athens, J. W., Haab, O. d., Raab, S. O., Ashenbrucker, K. & Cartwright, G. E. (1962) The influence of adrenal corticosteroids upon the luekocyte composition of inflammatory exudates in man. *Clin. Res.*, **10**, 107.

Bonforte, R. J. (1967) Convulsion as a presenting sign of infectious mononucleosis. *Amer. J. Dis. Child.*, **114**. 429.

Bousser, J. & Neyde, R. (1947) La neutropénie familiale. *Sang.*, **18**, 521.

Boxer, L. A., Yokoyama, M. & Lalezari, P. (1972) Isoimmune neonatal neutropenia. *J. Pediat*, **80**, 783.

Braun, E. H., Buckwold, A. E., Emson, H. E. & Russell, A. V. (1960) Familial neonatal neutropenia with maternal leucocyte antibodies. *Blood*, **16**, 1745.

Brodsky, I., Reimann, H. A. & Dennis, L. H. (1965) Treatment of cyclic neutropenia with testosterone. *Am. J. Med.*, **38**, 802.

Burke, V., Colebatch, J. H., Anderson, C. M. & Simons, M. J. (1967) Association of pancreatic insufficiency and chronic neutropenia of childhood. *Arch. Dis. Childh.*, **42**, 147.

Cartwright, G. E., Athens, J. W. & Wintrobe, M. M. (1964) The kinetics of granulopoiesis in normal man. *Blood*, **24**, 780.

Chandra, R. W., Cope, W. A. & Soothill, J. F. (1969) Chronic granulomatous disease. Evidence for an autosomal mode of inheritance. *Lancet*, **2**, 71.

Chediak, M. (1952) Nouvelle anomalie leucocytaire et caractère constitutionel et familial. *Rev. Hemat.*, **7**, 362.

Chervenick, P. A. & Lo Buglio, A. F. (1972) Human blood monocytes: Stimulators of granulocyte and mononuclear colony formation *in vitro*. *Science*, **178**, 164.

Childs, B., Nyhan, W. L., Borden, M., Bard, L. & Cooke, R. E. (1961) Idiopathic hyperglycinemia and hyperglycinuria: A new disorder of amino acid metabolism. *Pediatrics*, **27**, 522.

Chretien, J. H. & Garagusi, V. F. (1971) NBT test in parasitic disease. *Lancet*, **ii**, 549.

Clancy, R., Jenkins, E. & Firkin, B. (1971) Platelet defect of infectious mononucleosis. *Brit. med. J.*, **4**, 646.

Clawson, C. C., Repine, J. E. & White, J. G. (1971) Chediak-Higashi syndrome: Quantitative defect in bacterial capacity. *Blood*, **38**, 82.

Clein, G. P. (1972) The neutrophil granulocyte. *Brit. J. Hosp. Med.*, **8**, 83.

Cohn, Z. A. & Hirsh, J. G. (1960) The isolation and properties of the specific cytoplasmic granules of rabbit polymorphonuclear leucocytes. *J. Exp. Med.*, **112**, 983.

Cooper, M. R., Chatelet, L. R. de, Lavia, M. F., McCall, C. E., Spurr, C. L. & Baehner, R. L. (1972) Complete deficiency of leukocyte G-6-PD with defective bactericidal activity. *J. Clin. Invest.*, **51**, 769.

Cordano, A., Baertl, J. M. & Graham, G. G. (1964) Copper deficiency in infancy. *Pediatrics*, **34**, 324.

Cordano, A., Placko, R. P. & Graham, G. G. (1966) Hypocupremia and neutropenia in copper deficiency. *Blood*, **28**, 280.

Craddock, C. G., Perry, S. & Lawrence, J. S. (1960) Dynamics of leukopenia and leukocytosis. *Ann. Intern. Med.*, **52**, 281.

Craddock, P. R., Yawata, Y., Santen, L. Van, Gilberstadt, S., Silvis, S. & Jacob, H. S. (1974) Acquired phagocyte dysfunction resulting from parenteral hyperalimentation. *New Eng. J. Med.*, **290**, 1403.

Cronkite, E. P. & Fliedner, T. M. (1964) Granulocytopoiesis. *New Eng. J. Med.*, **270**, 1347.

Crosby, W. H. (1962) Hypersplenism. *Ann. Rev. Med.*, **13**, 126.

Cutting, H. O. & Lang, J. E. (1964) Familial benign chronic neutropenia. *Ann. Intern. Med.*, **61**, 876.

Dale, D. C. & Wolff, S. M. (1971) Skin window studies of the acute inflammatory responses of neutropenic patients. *Blood*, **38**, 138.

Davidsohn, I., Stern, K. & Kashiwagi, C. (1951) The differential test for infectious mononucleosis. *Am. J. Clin. Path.*, **21**, 1101.

Davis, S. D., Schaller, J. & Wedgwood, R. J. (1966) Job's syndrome: Recurrent 'cold' staphylococcal abscesses. *Lancet*, **1**, 1013.

Davis, W. C., Douglas, S. D. & Fudenberg, H. H. (1968) A selective neutrophil dysfunction syndrome: Impaired killing of staphylococci. *Ann. Intern. Med.*, **69**, 1237.

Dent, P. B., Fish, L. A., White, J. C. & Good, R. A. (1966) Chediak-Higashi syndrome: Observations on the nature of the associated malignancy. *J. Lab. Invest.*, **15**, 1634.

Diehl, V., Henle, G., Henle, W. & Kohn, G. (1968) Demonstration of a herpes group virus in cultures of peripheral leukocytes from patients with infectious mononucleosis. *J. Virol.*, **2**, 663.

Donald, W. D. & Winkler, C. H. (1960) The leukocyte response in patients with shigellosis. *J. Pediat.*, **56**, 61.

Donohue, W. L. & Bain, H. W. (1957) Chediak-Higashi syndrome. A lethal familial disease with anomalous inclusions in the leukocytes and constitutional stigmata: Report of a case with necropsy. *Pediatrics*, **20**, 416.

Douglas, S. D., Davis, W. C. & Fudenberg, H. H. (1969) Granulocytopathies: Pleomorphism of neutrophil dysfunction. *Amer. J. Med.*, **46**, 901.

Douglas, S. D., Lahav, M. & Fudenberg, H. (1970) A reversible neutrophil bactericidal defect associated with mixed cryoglobulin. *Am. J. Med.*, **49**, 274.

Douwer, F. R. (1972) Clinical value of NBT test. *New Eng. J. Med.*, **287**, 822.

Downey, H. & McKinlay, C. (1923) Acute lymphadenosis compared with acute lymphatic leukemia. *Arch. Intern. Med.*, **32**, 82.

Earle, A. M. (1954) Some clinical aspects of typhoid fever in infancy. *J. Pediat.*, **44**, 681.

Einzig, M. & Neerhout, R. (1969) Hemolytic anemia in infectious mononucleosis. *Clinical Pediatrics*, **8**, 171.

Evans, A. (1967) Complications of infectious mononucleosis: Recognition and management. *Hospital Med.*, **3**, 24.

Evans, A. S. (1972) Infectious mononucleosis and other mono-like syndromes. *New Eng. J. Med.*, **286**, 836.

Ezer, G. & Soothill, J. F. (1974) Intracellular bactericidal effects of rifampicin in both normal and chronic granulomatous disease polymorphs. *Arch. Dis. Childh.*, **49**, 463.

Feigin, R. D., Vietti, T. J., Wyatt, R. G., Kaufmann, D. G. & Smith, C. H. (1970) Ataxia telangiectasia with granulocytopenia. *J. Pediat.*, **77**, 431.

Fernbach, D. J. & Starling, K. A. (1972) Infectious mononucleosis. *Pediat. Clinics. N. Amer.*, **19**, 957.

Fikrig, S. M., Berkovich, S., Emmet, S. M. & Gordon, C. (1973) Nitroblue tetrazolium dye test and differential diagnosis of meningitis. *J. Pediat.*, **82**, 855.

Fliedner, T. M., Cronkite, E. P. & Robertson, J. S. (1964) Granulocytopoiesis. I. Senescence and random loss of neutrophilic granuloctyes in human beings. *Blood*, **24**, 402.

Foster, K. & Jack, I. (1969) A prospective study of the role of cytomegalovirus in post-transfusion mononucleosis. *New Eng. J. Med.*, **280**, 1311.

Freyre, E. A., Chabes, A., Poémape, O. & Chabes, A. (1973) Abnormal rebuck skin window response in kwashiorkor. *J. Pediat.*, **82**, 523.

Fullerton, H. W. & Duguid, H. L. D. (1949) A case of cyclical agranulocytosis with marked improvement after splenectomy. *Blood*, **4**, 267.

Galloway, E. (1969) Comparison of three slide tests for infectious mononucleosis with Davidson's presumptive and differential heterophile test. *Canad. J. Med.*, **31**, 197.

Gifford, R. H. & Malawista, S. E. (1970) A simple rapid micromethod for detecting chronic granulomatous disease of childhood. *J. Lab. Clin. Med.*, **75**, 511.

Gilman, P. A., Jackson, D. P. & Guild, H. G. (1970) Congenital agranulocytosis: prolonged survival and terminal acute leukemia. *Blood*, **36**, 576.

Gitlin, D., Vawter, G. & Craig, J. M. (1964) Thymic alymphoplasia and congenital aleukocytosis. *Pediatrics*, **33**, 184.

Glansslen, M. (1941) Konsitutionelle familiare Leukopenie (Neutropenie). *Klin. Wchnschr.*, **20**, 922.

Godwin, H. A., Zimmerman, T. S., Kimball, H. R., Wolff, S. M., Perry, S. (1968A) The effect of etiocholanolone on the entry of granulocytes into the peripheral blood. *Blood*, **31**, 461.

Godwin, H. A., Zimmerman, T. S., Kimball, H. R., Wolff, S. M. & Perry, S. (1968B) Correlation of granulocyte mobilization with etiocholanolone and the subsequent development of myelosuppression in patients with acute leukemia receiving therapy. *Blood*, **31**, 580.

Golde, D. W. & Cline, M. J. (1974) Regulation of granulopoiesis. *New Eng. J. Med.*, **291**, 1388.

Goldstein, E. & Porter, D. (1969) Fatal thrombocytopenia with cerebral haemorrhage in mononucleosis. *Arch. Neurol.*, **20**, 533.

Good, R. A. & Zak, S. J. (1956) Disturbances in gamma globulin synthesis as 'experiments of nature'. *Pediatrics*, **18**, 109.

Graham, G. G. (1971) Human copper deficiency. *New Eng. J. Med.*, **285**, 857.

Gray, G. R., Klebanoff, S. J., Stamatoyannopoulos, G., Austin, T., Naiman, S. C., Yoshida, A., Kliman, M. R. & Robinson, G. C. F. (1973) Neutrophil dysfunction, chronic granulomatous disease, and non-spherocytic haemolytic anaemia caused by complete deficiency of glucose-6-phosphate dehydrogenase. *Lancet*, ii, 530.

Gregory, L., Williams, R. & Thompson, E. (1972) Leucocyte function in Down's syndrome and acute leukaemia. *Lancet*, **1**, 1359.

Groover, R. V., Sutherland, J. M. & Landing, B. H. (1961) Purulent meningitis of newborn infants. Eleven-year experience in the antibiotic era. *New Eng. J. Med.*, **264**, 1115.

Guerry, D., Adamson, J. W., Dale, D. C. & Wolff, S. M. (1974) Human cyclic neutropenia: Urinary colony-stimulating factor and erythropoietin levels. *Blood*, **44**, 257.

Hanneman, B. M. & Alt, H. L. (1958) Cyclic neutropenia in a father and daughter. *J.A.M.A.*, **168**, 270.

Hardy, W. R. & Anderson, R. W. (1968) The hypereosinophilic syndromes. *Ann. Intern. Med.*, **68**, 1220.

Hedenberg, F. (1959) Infantile agranulocytosis of probable congenital orogin. *Acta Paediat.*, **48**, 77.

Higashi, O. (1953) Congenital abnormality of peroxidase granules. A case of 'congenital gigantism of peroxidase granules', preliminary report. *Tohuku J. Exper. Med.*, **58**, 246.

Hill, H. R., Ochs, H. D., Quie, P. G., Clark, R. A., Pabst, H. F., Klebanoff, S. J. & Wedgwood, R. J. (1974) Defect in neutrophil granulocyte chemotaxis in Job's syndrome of recurrent 'cold' staphylococcal abscesses. *Lancet*, ii, 617.

Hitzig, W. H. (1959) Familiäre Neutropenie mit dominanten Erbgang und Hypergammaglobulinämie. *Helv. Med. Acta.*, **26**, 779.

Hitzig, W. H. & Gitzelmann, R. (1959) Transplacental transfer of leukoctye agglutinins. *Vox Sang.*, **4**, 445.

Hoagland, R. (1960) The clinical manifestations of infectious mononucleosis: A report of two hundred cases. *Amer. J. Med. Sci.*, **240**, 21.

Hoff, G. & Bauer, S. (1965) A new rapid slide test for infectious mononucleosis. *J.A.M.A.*, **194**, 119.

Holland, J. F., Senn, H. & Banerjee, T. (1971) Quantitative studies of localised leukocyte mobilization in acute leukemia. *Blood*, **37**, 499.

Holmes, B., Quie, P. G., Windhurst, D. B. & Good, R. A. (1966) Fatal granulomatous disease of childhood: an inborn abnormality of phagocytic function. *Lancet*, **1**, 1225.

Holmes, B., Page, A. R. & Good, R. A. (1967) Studies of the metabolic activity of leukocytes from patients with a genetic abnormality of phagocytic function. *J. Clin. Invest.*, **46**, 1422.

Holmes, B., Park, B. H., Malawista, S. E., Quie, P. G., Nelson, D. L. & Good, R. A. (1970) Chronic granulomatous disease in females—a deficiency of leukocyte glutathione peroxidase. *New Eng. J. Med.*, **283**, 217.

Hong, R., Schubert, W. K., Perrin, E. V. & West, C. D. (1962) Antibody deficiency syndrome with beta-2 macroglobulinemia. *J. Pediat.*, **61**, 831.

Huguley, C. M. (1964) Drug-induced blood dyscrasias. II. Agranulocytosis. *J.A.M.A.*, **188**, 817.

Humbert, J. R., Marks, M. I., Hathaway, W. E. & Thoren, C. H. (1971) The histochemical nitroblue tetrazolium reduction test in the differential diagnosis of acute infections. *Pediatrics*, **48**, 259.

Huntly, C. C., Costas, M. C. & Lyerly, A. (1965) Visceral larva migrans syndrome; Clinical characteristics and immunologic studies in 41 patients. *Pediatrics*, **36**, 523.

Iscove, N. N., Senn, J. S., Tell, J. D. & McCulloch, E. A. (1971) Colony formation by normal and leukemic human marrow cells in culture: effect of conditioned medium from human leukocytes. *Blood*, **37**, 1.

Jensen, K. G. (1960) Transplacental passage of leucocyte agglutinins occurring on account of pregnancy. *Dan. Med. Bull.*, **7**, 55.

Jensen, K. G. (1962) Leucocyte antibodies in serums of pregnant women. *Vox Sang*, **7**, 454.

Johnston, R. B. (1969) Screening test for the diagnosis of chronic granulomatous disease. *Pediatrics*, **43**, 122.

Johnston, R. B., Klemperer, M. R., Alper, C. A. & Rosen, R. S. (1969) The enhancement of bacterial phagocytosis by serum. The role of complement components and two cofactors. *J. Exper. Med.*, **129**, 1275.

Johnston, R. B. Jr. & Baehner, R. L. (1971) Chronic granulomatous disease: correlation between pathogenesis and clinical findings. *Pediatrics*, **48**, 730.

Johnston, R. B., Wilfert, C. M., Buckley, R. H., Webb, L. S., DeChatelet, L. R. & McCall, C. E. (1975) Enhanced bactericidal activity of phagocytes from patients with chronic granulomatous disease in the presence of sulphisoxazole. *Lancet*, **i**, 824.

Kaplow, L. S. (1965) Simplified myeloperoxidase stain using benzidine dihydrochloride. *Blood*, **26**, 215.

Kaplow, L. S. & Goffinet, J. A. (1968) Profound neutropenia during early phase of hemodialysis. *J.A.M.A.*, **203**, 133.

Kauder, E. & Mayer, A. M. Neutropenias of childhood. *J. Pediat.*, **69**, 147.

Hhan, A., Hill, J. M., Loeb, E., MacLellan, A. & Hill, N. O. (1973) Management of Chédiak-Higashi syndrome with transfer factor. *Am. J. Dis. Child.*, **126**, 797.

Killman, S. A., Cronkite, E. P., Fliedner, T. M. & Bond, V. P. (1962) Mitotic indices of human bone marrow cells. I. Number and cytological distribution of mitoses. *Blood*, **19**, 743.

King-Smith, E. A. & Morley, A. A. (1970) Computer simulation of granulopoiesis: normal and impaired granulopoiesis. *Blood*, **36**, 254.

Klebanoff, S. J. (1971) Intraleukocytic microbicidal defects. *Ann. Rev. Med.*, **22**, 39.

Klebanoff, S. J. & White, L. R. (1969) Iodinating defect in the leukocytes of a patient with a chronic granulomatous disease of childhood. *New Eng. J. Med.*, **280**, 460.

Klebanoff, S. J. & Pincus, S. H. (1971) Hydrogen peroxide utilization in myeloperoxidase deficient leukocytes: a possible microbicidal control mechanism. *J. Clin. Invest.*, **50**, 2226.

Klemola, E. & Käämänen, L. (1965) Cytomegalovirus as a possible cause of a disease resembling infectious mononucleosis. *Brit. med. J.*, **2**, 1099.

Kniker, W. T. & Panos, T. C. (1957) Idiopathic infantile agranulocytosis with hypergammaglobulinemia. *Amer. J. Dis. Child.*, **74**, 549.

Kostman, R. (1956) Infantile genetic agranulocytosis (agranulocytosis infantilis hereditaria). A new recessive lethal disease in man. *Acta Paediat.*, **45**, 309.

Kretschmer, R. R., Osuna, M. L. & Valenzuela, R. H. (1972) Reversible neutrophil defect in ataxia telangiectasia. *Pediatrics*, **50**, 147.

Krill, C. E., Smith, H. D. & Mauer, A. M. (1964) Chronic idiopathic granulocytopenia. *New Eng. J. Med.*, **270**, 973.

Krill, C. E. Jr. & Mauer, A. M. (1966) Congenital agranulocytosis. *The Journal of Pediatrics*, **68**, 361.

Kyle, R. A. & Linman, J. W. (1968) Chronic idiopathic neutropenia. A newly recognised entity? *New Eng. J. Med.*, **279**, 1015.

Lalezari, P., Nussbaum, M., Gelman, S. & Spaet, T. H. (1960) Neonatal neutropenia due to maternal isoimmunization. *Blood*, **15**, 238.

Lalezari, P. & Bernard, G. E. (1966) An isologous antigen-antibody reaction with human neutrophils related to neonatal neutropenia. *J. Clin. Invest.*, **45**, 1741.

Lancet (1971) Editorial: Nitroblue tetrazolium: a routine test? *Lancet*, **ii**, 909.

Lancet (1973) Editorial: Oral excretion of E.B. virus. *Lancet*, **i**, 811.

Landing, B. H. & Shirkey, H. S. (1957) A syndrome of recurrent infections and infiltration of viscera by pigmented lipid histiocytes. *Pediatrics*, **20**, 431.

Lang, J. E. & Cutting, H. O. (1965) Infantile genetic agranulocytosis. *Pediatrics*, **35**, 596.

Lascelles, R. G., Longson, M., Johnson, P. J. & Chiang, A. (1973) Infectious mononucleosis presenting as acute cerebellar syndrome. *Lancet*, **ii**, 707.

Lehrer, R. I. & Cline, M. J. (1969) Leukocyte myeloperoxidase deficiency and disseminated candidiasis: The role of myeloperoxidase in resistance to *Candida* infection. *J. Clin. Invest.*, **48**, 1478.

Levine, S. (1959) Chronic familial neutropenia with marked peridontal lesions. *Oral Surg.*, **12**, 310.

Lonsdale, D., Deodhar, S. D. & Mercer, R. D. (1967) Familial granulocytopenia associated with immunoglobulin abnormality. *J. Pediat.*, **71**, 760.

Luhby, A. L., Speer, F. D., Lee, R. & Shapiro, A. D. (1957) Congenital genetic agranulocytosis. *Amer. J. Dis. Child.*, **94**, 552.

Lukens, J. N. (1972) Eosinophilia in children. *Pediat. Clinics N. Amer.*, **19**, 969.

Lux, S. D., Johnston, R. B., August, C. S., Say, B., Penchaszadeh, V. B., Rosen, F. S. & McKusick, V. A. (1970) Chronic neutropenia and abnormal cellular immunity in cartilage-hair hypoplasia. *New Eng. J. Med.*, **282**, 231.

Lynch, M. J. (1973) Mechanisms and defect of the phagocytic systems of defence against infection. *Perspectives in Pediatric Pathology*, **1**, 33.

MacGillivray, J. B., Dacie, J. V., Henry, J. R. K., Sacker, L. S. & Tizard, J. P. M. (1964) Congenital neutropenia: A report of five cases. *Acta Paediatrica*, **53**, 188.

MacGregor, R. R., Spagnuolo, P. J. & Lentnek, A. L. (1974) Inhibition of granulocyte adherence by ethanol, prednisone and aspirin. *New Eng. J. Med.*, **291**, 642.

Malawista, S. E. (1971) Vinblastine: colchicine-like effects on human blood leukocytes during phagocytosis. *Blood*, **37**, 519.

Mandell, G. L., Rubin, W. & Hook, E. W. (1970) The effect of an NADH oxidase inhibitor (hydrocortisone) on polymorphonuclear leukocyte bactericidal activity. *J. Clin. Invest.*, **49**, 1381.

Marsh, J. C. & Perry, S. (1964) The granulocyte response to endotoxin in patients with hematologic disorders. *Blood*, **23**, 581.

Marx, G. (1970) Unsuspected preoperative hepatic dysfunction. *Int. Anest. Clin.*, **8**, 369.

Matula, G. & Paterson, P. Y. (1971A) Spontaneous *in vitro* reduction of nitroblue tetrazolium by neutrophils of adult patients with bacterial infection. *New Eng. J. Med.*, **285**, 311.

Matula, G. & Paterson, P. Y. (1971B) NBT tests in a patient on steroids. *Lancet*, **i**, 803.

Mauer, A. M., Athens, J. W., Ashenbrucker, H., Cartwright, G. E. & Wintrobe, M. M. (1960) A method for labelling granulocytes *in vitro* with radioactive di isopropylfluorophosphate (DFP^{32}). *J. Clin. Invest.*, **39**, 1481.

Mauer, A. M. & Krill, C. E. (1964) A study of the mechanisms for granulocytopenia. *Ann. N.Y. Acad. Sci.*, **113**, 1003.

Mauer, A. M. (1969) *Blood Leucocytes in Systemic Diseases*, p. 289. New York: McGraw-Hill.

Meagher, S. W., Crandon, J. H. & Campbell, A. J. A. (1954) Appendicitis in children. *New Eng. J. Med.*, **250**, 895.

Meo, A. N. De & Anderson, B. R. (1972) Defective chemotaxis associated with a serum inhibitor in cirrhotic patients. *New Eng. J. Med.*, **286**, 735.

Michael, J. G. & Rosen, F. S. (1963) Association of 'natural' antibodies to gram negative bacteria with the γ_1-macroglobulins. *J. Exper. Med.*, **118**, 619.

Miller, D. R., Freed, B. A. & Lapey, J. D. (1968) Congenital neutropenia: Report of a fatal case in a negro infant with leukocyte function studies. *Am. J. Dis. Child.*, **115**, 337.

Miller, M. E., Seals, J., Kaye, R. & Levitsky, L. C. (1968) A familial, plasma-associated defect of phagocytosis. A new cause of recurrent bacterial infections. *Lancet*, **ii**, 60.

Miller, M. E., Oski, F. A. & Harris, M. B. (1971) Lazy-leucocyte syndrome. A new disorder of neutrophil function. *Lancet*, **1**, 665.

Miller, G., Niederman, J. C. & Andrews, L. L. (1973) Prolonged oropharyngeal excretion of Epstein-Barr virus after infectious mononucleosis. *New Eng. J. Med.*, **288**, 229.

Mimbs, J. W. (1972) Mechanisms of NBT test. *New Eng. J. Med.*, **287**, 49.

Moeschlin, S. (1958) Leucocyte-auto-antibodies. *Acta Haemat.*, **20**, 167.

Morley, A. (1973) Letter to the Editor. *Blood*, **41**, 329.

Morley, A. & Stohlman, F. (1970) Cyclophosphamide-induced cyclical neutropenia. An animal model of a human periodic disease. *New Eng. J. Med.*, **282**, 643.

Morley, A. & Stohlman, F. (1970) Studies on the regulation of granulopoiesis. I. The response to neutropenia. *Blood*, **35**, 312.

Morrow, G., Barness, L. A., Auerbach, V. H., George, A. M. Di, Ando, T. & Nyhan, W. L. (1969) Observations on the coexistence of methylmalonic acidemia and glycinemia. *J. Pediat.*, **74**, 680.

Mowat, A. G. & Baum, J. (1971) Chemotaxis of polymorphonuclear leukocytes from patients with diabetes mellitus. *New Eng. J. Med.*, **284**, 621.

Murdoch, J. McC. & Smith, C. C. (1972) Infection. *Clinics in Haematology*, **1**, 619.

Nathan, D. G. (1974) NBT reduction by human phagocytes. *New Eng. J. Med.*, **290**, 280.

Ochs, H. & Igo, R. P. (1973) The NBT slide test: A simple screening method for detecting chronic granulomatous disease and female carriers. *J. Pediat.*, **83**, 77.

Oski, F. A., Naiman, L., Allen, D. M. & Diamond, L. K. (1962) Leukocytic inclusions—Dohle bodies—associated with platelet abnormality (the May-Hegglin anomaly). *Blood*, **20**, 657.

Oski, F. A. & Naiman, L. (1972) *Hematologic Problems in the Newborns*, 2nd edn., p. 328. Philadelphia: Saunders.

Page, A. R. (1962) Neutropenia in infancy and childhood. *Lancet*, **82**, 439.

Page, A. R. (1974) Personal Communication.

Page, A. R. & Good, R. A. (1957) Studies on cyclic neutropenia: a clinical and experimental investigation. *A.M. A.J. Dis. Child.*, **94**, 623.

Page, A. R., Berendes, H. ,Warner, J. & Good, R. (1962) The Chédiak-Higashi syndrome. *Blood*, **20**, 330.

Pantarotto, M. F. (1965) Un caso di aplasia midollare transitoria in neonato da farmaci anticonvulsivanti somministrati alla madre durante tutta la gravidänza. *Clima Ostet. Ginec.*, **67**, 343.

Park, B. H., Fikrig, S. M. & Smithwick, E. M. (1968) Infection and nitroblue-tetrazolium reduction by neutrophils: A diagnostic aid. *Lancet*, **ii**, 532.

Park, B. H., Holmes, B. M., Rodey, G. E. & Good, R. A. (1969) Nitroblue-tetrazolium test in children with fatal granulomatous disease and newborn infants. *Lancet*, **i**, 157.

Park, B. H. & Good, R. A. (1970) N.B.T. test stimulated. *Lancet*, **ii**, 616.

Park, B. H. (1971) The use and limitations of the nitroblue tetrazolium test as a diagnostic aid. *J. Pediat.*, **78**, 376.

Pattengale, P. K., Smith, R. W. & Gerber, P. (1973) Selective transformation of B lymphocytes by E.B. virus. *Lancet*, **ii**, 93.

Paul, J. & Bunnell, W. (1932) The presence of heterophile antibodies in infectious mononucleosis. *Amer. J. Med. Sci.*, **183**, 90.

Payne, R. (1964) Neonatal neutropenia and leukoagglutinins. *Pediatrics*, **33**, 194.

Pearmain, G. E. & Lycette, R. R. (1963) Spontaneous mitoses of glandular fever cells in short-term peripheral blood cultures. *Lancet*, **ii**, 1072.

Penman, H. (1968) Extreme neutropenia in glandular fever. *J. Clin. Path.*, **21**, 48.

Pfeiffer, E. (1889) Drusenfieber. *Jahrb. Kinderh.*, **29**, 257.

Pincus, S. H. & Klebanoff, S. J. (1971) Quantitative leukocyte iodination. *New Eng. J. Med.*, **284**, 744.

Quie, P. G., White, J. G., Holmes, B. & Good, R. A. (1967) In vitro bactericidal capacity of human polymorphonuclear leukocytes: Diminished activity in chronic granulomatous disease of childhood. *J. Clin. Invest.*, **46**, 668.

Rabinovitch, M. (1968) Phagocytosis: The engulfment stage. *Sem. Hemat.*, **5**, 134.

Rahal, J. & Henle, G. (1970) Infectious mononucleosis and Reye's syndrome: A fatal case with studies for Epstein-Barr virus. *Pediatrics*, **46**, 776.

Rebuck, J. W. & Crowley, J. H. (1955) A method of studying leukocyte function *in vivo*. *N.Y. Acad. Sci.*, **59**, 757.

Reiman, H. A. & Berardinis, C. T. de (1949) Periodic (cyclic) neutropenia, an entity. *Blood*, **4**, 1109.

Rickard, K. A., Morley, A., Howard, D. & Stohlman, F. (1971) The *in vitro* colony-forming cell and the response to neutropenia. *Blood*, **37**, 6.

Riedler, G. F. (1972) Platelet counts, white blood picture and inorganic phosphates: Three useful pointers to the diagnosis of septicemia. *Schweiz Med. Wochenschr.*, **102**, 497.

Riemenschneider, T. & Moss, A. (1966) Postperfusion syndrome. *J. Pediat.*, **69**, 546.

Rifkind, D. (1968) Cytomegalovirus mononucleosis. *Ann. Intern. Med.*, **69**, 842.

Rinehart, J. J., Sagone, A. L., Balcerzak, S. P., Ackerman, G. A. & Lo Buglio, A. F. (1975) Effects of corticosteroid therapy on human monocyte function. *New Eng. J. Med.*, **292**, 236.

Rodey, G. E., Park, B. H., Ford, D. K., Gray, B. H. & Good, R. A. (1970) Defective bactericidal activity of peripheral blood leukocytes in lipochrome histiocytosis. *Amer. J. Med.*, **49**, 322.

Rodriguez, S., Leikin, S. & Hiller, M. (1964) Neonatal thrombocytopoenia associated with ante-partum administration of thiazide drugs. *New Eng. J. Med.*, **270**, 881.

Root, R. K., Rosenthal, A. S., Balestra, D. J. & Wolff, S. M. (1972) Abnormal bactericidal, metabolic and lysosomal functions in Chédiak-Higashi syndrome leukocytes. *J. Clin. Invest.*, **51**, 649.

Rossi, J. P. & Brandt, I. K. (1960) Transient granulocytopenia of the newborn associated with sepsis due to shigella alkalescens and maternal leukocyte agglutinins. *J. Pediat.*, **56**, 639.

Rossman, Ph. L. & Hummer, G. J. (1960) Chronic neutropenia in siblings: The effect of steroids. *Ann. Intern. Med.*, **52**, 242.

Rubinstein, A. & Pelet, B. (1973) False negative NBT test due to transient malfunction of neutrophils. *Lancet*, **i**, 382.

Ryder, R. J. W. (1965) Acute infectious lymphocytosis. *Am. J. Dis. Child.*, **110**, 299.

Salmon, S. E., Cline, M. J., Schultz, J. & Lehrer, R. I. (1970) Myeloperoxidase deficiency. Immunologic study of a genetic leukocyte defect. *New Eng. J. Med.*, **282**, 250.

Salomonsen, L. (1948) Granulocytopenia in children. *Acta Paediat.*, **35**, 189.

Schwachman, H., Diamond, L. K., Oski, F. A. & Khaw, K-T. (1964) The syndrome of pancreatic insufficiency and bone marrow dysfunction. *J. Pediat.*, **65**, 645.

Scmerling, D. H., Prader, A., Hitzig, W. H., Giedion, A., Hadorn, B. & Kuhni, M. (1969) The syndrome of pancreatic insufficiency, neutropenia, metaphyseal dysostosis and dwarfism. *Helv. Paed. Acta.*, **24**, 547.

Seely, J. R., Humphrey, G. B. & Matter, B. J. (1972) Copper deficiency in a premature infant fed on iron-fortified formula. *New Eng. J. Med.*, **286**, 109.

Seip, M. (1960) Systemic lupus erythematosus in pregnancy with haemolytic anaemia, leucopenia and thrombocytopenia in the mother and her newborn infant. *Arch. Dis. Childh.*, **35**, 364.

Senn, H., Holland, J. F. & Banerjee, T. (1969) Kinetic and comparative studies on localised leukocyte mobilization in normal man. *J. Lab. Clin. Med.*, **74**, 742.

Sheldon, P. J., Papamichail, M., Hemsted, E. H. & Holborow, E. J. (1973) Thymic origin of atypical lymphoid cells in infectious mononucleosis. *Lancet*, **i**, 1153.

Smith, C. H. (1941) Infectious lymphocytosis. *Am. J. Dis. Child.*, **62**, 231.

Southam, C. M. & Levin, A. G. (1966) A quantitative Rebuck technique. *Blood,* **27,** 734.

Stahlie, T. O. V. (1956) Chronic benign neutropenia in infancy and early childhood. *J. Pediat.,* **48,** 710.

Starling, K. & Fernbach, D. (1968) Infectious mononucleosis in the preschool child. *J.A.M.A.,* **203,** 294.

Stefanini, M., Mele, R. H. & Skinner, D. (1958) Transitory congenital neutropenia: a new syndrome. *Am. J. Med.,* **25,** 749.

Stevens, D. & Pry, T. (1971) EB-virus antibodies in post-transfusion mononucleosis and cardiopulmonary by-pass. *J. Med. Microbiol.,* **4,** 13.

Strauss, R. G., Bove, K. E., Jones, J. F., Mauer, A. M. & Fulginiti, V. A. (1974) An anomaly of neutrophil morphology with impaired function. *New Eng. J. Med.,* **290,** 478.

Stossel, T. P., Root, R. K. & Vaughan, M. (1972) Phagocytosis in chronic granulomatous disease and the Chédiak-Higashi syndrome. *New Eng. J. Med.,* **286,** 120.

Stossel, T. P. (1974) Phagocytosis, Pts. 1, 2 and 3. *New Eng. J. Med.,* **290,** 717, 774, 833.

Taylor, L. & Parsons-Smith, G. (1969) Infectious mononucleosis, deafness and facial paralysis. *J. Laryng. Otol.,* **83,** 613.

Thompson, E. N. & Soothill, J. F. (1970) Chronic granulomatous disease. Quantitative clinicopathological relationships. *Arch. Dis. Childh.,* **45,** 24.

Thompson, W. P. (1934) Observations on a possible relation between agranulocytosis and menstruation with further studies on a case of cyclic neutropenia. *New Eng. J. Med.,* **210,** 176.

Toren, M., Goffinet, J. A. & Kaplow, L. S. (1970) Pulmonary bed sequestration of neutrophils during hemodialysis. *Blood,* **36,** 337.

Torrioli-Riggio, G. (1958) Considerazioni su una famiglia di granulopenici. *Acta Genet. Med. (Roma),* **7,** 237.

Tullis, J. L. (1958) Prevalence, nature and identification of leukocyte antibodies. *New Eng. J. Med.,* **258,** 569.

Twomey, J. J., Douglass, C. C. & Sharkey, O. (1973) The monocytopenia of aplastic anemia. *Blood,* **41,** 187.

University Health Physicians & P.H.L.S. Laboratories (1971) Infectious mononucleosis and its relationship to E.B. virus antibody. *Brit. med. J.,* **4,** 643.

Vaal, O. M. de & Seynhaeve, V. (1959) Reticular dysgenesia. *Lancet,* **ii,** 1123.

Vahlquist, B. (1946) Cyclic agranulocytosis: Report of a case with a short survey of the disease. *Acta Med. Scand. Suppl.* **170.**

Vahlquist, B., Ekelund, H. & Tveteras, E. (1958) Infectious mononucleosis and pseudo-mononucleosis in children. *Acta Paediat. Scand.,* **47,** 120.

Vega, G. de la, Freyre-Horta, R. & Benitez-Bibriesca, L. (1973) Plasma factor affecting the NBT reducing capacity of neutrophils. *New Eng. J. Med.,* **289,** 271.

Vowels, M. R. & Goel, K. M. (1974) Leucocyte function in normal and preterm infants. *Acta Paediat. Scand.,* **63,** 122.

Walsh, F. C., Poser, C. M. & Carter, S. (1954) Infectious mononucleosis encephalitis. *Pediatrics,* **13,** 538.

Ward, P. A. & Schlegel, R. J. (1969) Impaired leucotactic responsiveness in a child with recurrent infections. *Lancet,* **ii,** 344.

Windhurst, D. B., Holmes, B. & Good, R. A. (1967) A newly defined X-linked trait in man with demonstration of the Lyon effect in carrier females. *Lancet,* **1,** 737.

Windhurst, D. B., Page, A. R., Holmes, B., Quie, P. G. & Good, R. A. (1968) The pattern of genetic transmission of the leucocyte defect in fatal granulomatous disease of childhood. *J. Clin. Invest.,* **47,** 1026.

Winkelstein, J. (1973) Opsonins: Their function, identity and clinical significance. *J. Pediat.,* **82,** 747.

Wiseman, B. K., & Doan, C. A. (1942) Primary splenic neutropenia. A newly recognized syndrome closely related to congenital hemolytic icterus and essential thrombocytopenic purpura. *Ann. intern. Med.,* **16,** 1097.

Wolfson, J. J., Kane, W. J., Laxdal, S. D., Good, R. A. & Quie, P. G. (1969) Bone findings in chronic granulomatous disease of childhood. *J. Bone Joint Surg.,* **51,** 1573.

Wriedt, K., Kauder, E. & Mauer, A. M. (1970) Defective myelopoiesis in congenital neutropenia. *New Eng. J. Med.,* **283,** 1072.

Zieve, P. D., Haghshenass, M., Blanks, M. & Krevans, J. R. (1966) Vacuolization of the neutrophil. An aid in the diagnosis of septicemia. *Arch. Intern. Med.,* **118,** 356.

Zuelzer, W. W. (1964) Myelokathexis—a new form of chronic granulocytopenia. *New Eng. J. Med.,* **270,** 699.

Zuelzer, W. W. & Bajoghli, M. (1964) Chronic granulocytopenia in childhood. *Blood,* **23,** 359.

16. Thrombocytopenia

The platelet count, Normal platelet life span and sequestration, Kinetics of thrombopoiesis, Morphological aspects of thrombopoiesis, Platelet size as a measure of thrombopoiesis / Classification of thrombocytopenias / Idiopathic thrombocytopenic purpura (ITP), *Nature of ITP, Difficulty in consistent demonstration of autoantibody, Site of platelet destruction in vivo, Course of ITP in children, Management of childhood ITP* / Thrombocytopenia in the neonatal period, *1. Secondary to maternal ITP, 2. Isoimmune neonatal purpura, 3. Secondary to maternal drug ingestion, 4. Intrauterine or neonatal infection, 5. Other causes of platelet consumption, 6. Congenital megakaryocytic hypoplasia, 7. Hereditary thrombocytopenias, 8. Metabolic causes of neonatal thrombocytopenia, 9. Congenital leukaemia* / Drug-induced thrombocytopenia, *Mechanism of drug-haptene disease* / Post transfusion thrombocytopenic purpura / Thrombopoietin deficiency / Cyclical thrombocytopenia / Hypersplenism / *MAHA and DIC, Marrow Encroachment, Thrombocytosis.*

The platelet count

The normal platelet count in children and adults is 150,000 to 400,000/mm³, with a mean of 250,000/mm³. Slightly wider normal ranges occur in newborn infants. Platelet counts of 117,000 to 450,000/mm³, with a median of 263,000/mm³, were found in 88 term infants in the first two days by Aballi *et al.* (1968). Similarly a range of 111,000 to 390,000/mm³, with 8 out of 29 falling below 150,000/mm³, was found in a personally observed series of newborn healthy full term infants at the Queen Mother's Hospital, Glasgow. Counts below 100,000/mm³ do not therefore occur in healthy full term newborn babies.

In the case of premature infants there has been more debate as to whether platelet counts below 100,000/mm³ should be considered pathological or not (Pearson, 1968). Serial counts in a group of predominantly black premature infants reported by Medoff (1964) showed a fall to below 50,000/mm³ at the age of 10 to 20 days in most of the smaller infants with a birth weight of less than 1·7 kg, several being below 25,000/mm³. These low counts were not seen in the larger premature infants with birth weights of over 1·7 kg. Subsequent reports suggest that platelet counts below 100,000/mm³ are quite rare in healthy premature babies. Fogel *et al.* (1968) found that only 4 out of 38 with birth weights less than 1·7 kg fell below 100,000/mm³ between 10 and 20 days of life, and none of 35 with higher birth weight. In one exceptionally low birth weight (0·62 kg) infant the platelets fell to 14,000, but the lowest counts in the other three were 69,000, 71,000 and 83,000/mm³. In a large series Aballi *et al.* (1968) found counts below 100,000/mm³ in only 4 out of 273 premature infants during the first two days of life; in 7 out of 194 at the age of two weeks; and in 2 out of 112 at four weeks. Although slightly lower counts were seen in premature infants than in full term infants, these authors concluded that counts below 100,000/mm³ should be considered pathological, and below 50,000/mm³ as distinctly abnormal, regardless of the infant's weight and gestational age. This conclusion is in line with a more recent investigation by Sell and Corrigan (1973), who found that the platelet count in healthy newborn infants from a gestational age of 27 weeks onwards was the same as for older children and adults. It has been suggested that the high incidence of thrombocytopenia recorded by Medoff may have been due to an unrecognized infectious or toxic agent in the unit at the time (Oski and Naiman, 1972A).

A technical consideration in the performance of platelet counts in young children is that imperfectly performed venepunctures can result in spurious thrombocytopenia in the resulting blood samples. Capillary blood sampling, using the first issuing drops of blood collected into ammonium citrate solution by the technique of Brecher and Cronkite (1950), with phase microscopy for the actual count, are recommended both in the interests of practicality and numerical accuracy in young children. This was also the precise technique used by Aballi *et al.* (1968). Should venepuncture be used siliconized 'Butterfly' needles size 21, (e.g. Abbott Ltd) should be employed, with careful mixing of the blood with EDTA (Sequestrine) anticoagulant and counting without delay. Any difficulty in obtaining the blood will invalidate the platelet count, constituting a major problem in paediatric haematology unless recognized.

Normal platelet life span and sequestration

Platelet kinetics can be studied by labelling a patient's or donor platelets *in vitro* with ^{51}Cr (Aas and Gardner, 1958) or ^{32}P DFP (Bithell et al., 1967). Alternatively *in vivo* labelling can be achieved by the injection of ^{32}P DFP (Leeksma and Cohen, 1956) or ^{45}Se selenomethionine (Najean et al., 1969). With *in vitro* labelling the manipulation inevitably causes some membrane damage which results in sequestration of around 30 per cent in the spleen (Aster, 1966). In the presence of splenomegaly this sequestration is greater and in the absence of the spleen it is less (Fig. 16.1). *In vivo* injection of label is followed by incorporation into a whole cohort of circulating platelets. However, there are problems due to early elution and late reutilization of the label, the latter causing an artificial prolongation of the 'tail' of the curve. These and other aspects of the techniques involved have recently been well reviewed by Gardner (1972), who considers ^{51}Cr the most acceptable label for clinical studies at the present time. The use of such radioisotope methods is seldom justified for routine diagnosis in children. A simple non-radioisotopic method dependent upon inhibition of adrenalin-induced platelet lipid peroxidation in a cohort of platelets after a dose of aspirin has recently been described by Stuart, Murphy and Oski (1975). This should have considerable application in paediatrics.

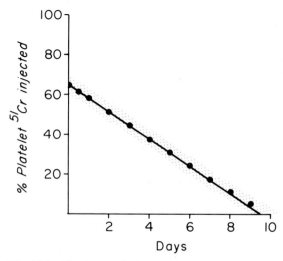

Fig. 16.2 Platelet survival *in vivo*. A composite platelet disappearance curve based on studies in 15 normal subjects. The immediate recovery was 64·6 per cent ± 4·1 and was determined by extrapolating the platelet-^{51}Cr activity in circulation to zero time and dividing this value by the platelet-^{51}Cr activity injected. In order to depict platelet disappearance only, the zero time platelet-^{51}Cr activities of the subjects were equated. The solid bar represents 1 s.d. from the mean, and the range of values is indicated by the shaded area. (Reproduced from Harker and Finch, *Journal of Clinical Investigation* (1969), **48**, 963, by permission of the author and publishers).

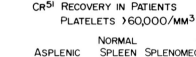
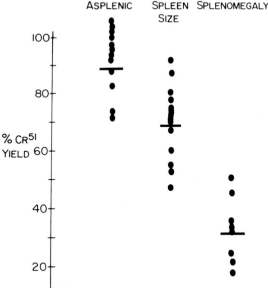

Fig. 16.1 Platelet sequestration related to splenic function. The recovery of ^{51}Cr-labelled platelets (yield) in patients with > 60,000/mm.^{3} The marked decrease in the percentage of circulating platelets in patients with splenomegaly is associated with normal life span. The mean of each group is denoted by a wide bar. (Reproduced from Gardner, *Clinics in Haematology* (1972), **1**, 312, by permission of the author and the publishers).

The normal life span of platelets in the circulation has been shown by these techniques to be 9–11 days, and the decline is linear in normal individuals indicating loss by senescence rather than random destruction (Fig. 16.2). In the steady state platelet production equals platelet destruction permitting the *platelet turnover* to be calculated. This is defined as the platelet count divided by the survival time, and was found by Harker and Finch (1969) to be 35,000 platelets/mm³ per day ± 4,300.

Kinetics of thrombopoiesis

An understanding of the quantitative aspects of thrombopoiesis in both normal and pathological states has largely sprung from the investigations of Harker and Finch (1969). From histological marrow sections they were able to derive estimates of the total number of megakaryocytes in the body, their volume (total Mega K mass) and their number of nuclei. Simultaneous measurement of ^{51}Cr platelet survival curves showed that platelet turnover was directly proportional to the total megakaryocyte mass.

determined not only in normals but also in patients with a wide variety of thrombocytopenic disorders. This permitted classification into those with impaired production (marrow hypoplasia or replacement), increased destruction (ITP, immune thrombocytopenia, consumptive coagulopathy) or disorders of distribution (hypersplenism).

Peripheral thrombocytopenia normally resulted in a thrombopoietic stimulus recognized by increased numbers and volume of megakaryocytes and an increase in the number of nuclei per cell. The rate of platelet production per nuclear unit was constant except in those patients with megaloblastosis, when it was reduced. This pattern was thought to represent 'ineffective thrombopoiesis'.

Thrombocytosis could be classified as 'reactive',

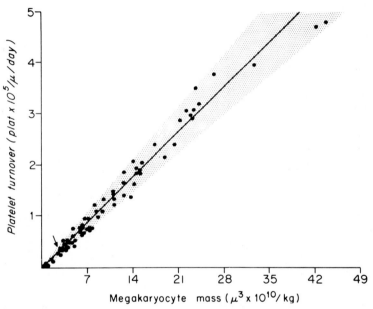

Fig. 16.3 Two measurements of platelet production were compared by plotting megakaryocyte mass against platelet turnover. The correlation indicates that these are equivalent measurements. The normal mean value ± 1 s.d. is represented by the black square (arrow). The 15 per cent confidence limits (± 1 s.d.) are shown in the shaded area. In eight patients (o) marked disparity was seen between platelet turnover and megakaryocyte mass, a finding indicating significant ineffective thrombopoiesis. (Reproduced from Harker and Finch, *Journal of Clinical Investigation* (1969), **48**, 963, by permission of the authors and publishers).

Megakaryocyte volume (or mass) was, in turn, directly related to the number of nuclei present from endomitosis, 2, 4, 8, 16 or 32 (Harker, 1968). Harker and Finch termed these nuclei *megakaryocyte production units* and showed that the number of platelets formed was normally constant at approximately 50 platelets per nuclear unit per day (Fig. 16.3). These parameters of platelet production and destruction, as well as platelet distribution (i.e. splenic sequestration), were

with appropriate reduction in megakaryocyte size and number of nuclei although the total number of megakaryocytes was increased; and 'autonomous', with increased megakaryocyte volume and nuclear volume, indicating an absence of negative feed-back control, as in polycythaemia rubra vera.

It appears that platelet production is normally regulated by a humoral stimulator thrombopoietin (Schulman *et al.*, 1960A) which increases not only the number of megakaryocytes, but also the number of intracellular mitoses and the rate of cytoplasmic maturation and platelet release (Odell et al., 1969; Harker, 1970A).

Current concepts of platelet production have recently been reviewed by Harker (1970B), and platelet sequestration studies in man by Aster (1972).

Morphological aspects of thrombopoiesis

The precursor or stem cell of the megakaryocyte series cannot be identified morphologically although its existence can be deduced from ^{3}H-thymidine labelling studies (Ebbe and Stohlman, 1965). The feature which permits the recognition in marrow smears of the earliest representatives of the megakaryocyte series is the large size of their nuclei compared to other haemic cells. Bessis (1956) classified human megakaryocytes series into the following:

Megakaryoblasts with 2–8 nuclei and dark blue cytoplasm
Promegakaryocytes with 4–16 nuclei and more acidophilic cytoplasm
Mature Megakaryocytes with up to 32 nuclei and granular cytoplasm.

In normal marrow around 10 per cent of the megakaryocytes have 4 nuclei, 65 per cent have 8 nuclei and 25 per cent 16 nuclei, all being diploid (Harker, 1970B).

Electron microscopy shows that following granule formation the cytoplasm is subdivided by 'demarcation membranes' of smooth-surfaced endoplasmic reticulin destined to form the outer membranes of individual platelets after release (French, 1967).

Liberation of platelets finally occurs by disruption of the cytoplasm with phagocytosis of the effete nuclear material by the reticuloendothelial system. Each megakaryocyte is therefore an 'end cell', and the only way that platelet production per cell can be increased is by additional intracytoplasmic nuclear mitotic division, since the number of platelets produced is approximately 50 per nuclear unit (*vide supra*).

Some degree of morphological assessment of 'stimulated' thrombopoiesis is possible, e.g. with excessive peripheral platelet destruction as in ITP. The size and number of nuclei of the individual megakaryocyte is approximately doubled and the number of these cells is increased three-to four-fold. Also a shortened cytoplasmic maturation time is indicated by a relative decrease in the number of mature megakaryocytes (Harker, 1970B). In order to facilitate estimation of the number of megakaryocyte nuclei for this purpose this author suggests using a Papanicolaou stain for marrow smears or examining squash preparations by phase contrast.

Platelet size as a measure of thrombopoiesis

Kinetic data in rabbits suggested that young platelets were larger and heavier than average, and that they progressed with age to smaller, lighter platelets (Karpatkin, 1969). Increased thrombopoiesis after injection of anti-platelet antibody in rats (McDonald et al., 1964), or after acute haemorrhage in dogs (Minter and Ingram, 1967) resulted in release of larger platelets than normal. Defining a large platelet or megathrombocyte as one with a diameter of more than 2·5 μm, Garg, Amorosi and Karpatkin (1971) have shown that the percentage of megathrombocytes in the blood may be used to assess thrombopoiesis in the same way as percentage of reticulocytes can be used to assess erythropoiesis. There was a good correlation between the percentage of megathrombocytes in the blood and the number of megakaryocytes in the marrow in a number of thrombocytopenic and non-thrombocytopenic disorders. The normal percentage was $10·8 \pm 3·1$ and this was regularly increased, in parallel with the numbers of megakaryocytes in the marrow (assessed from smears), in disorders of increased platelet destruction (Table 16.1). A compensated thrombocytolytic state was postulated in certain patients with chronic ITP in remission, SLE and 'easy bruising' because of normal platelet counts with increased percentage of megathrombocytes and megakaryocytes. In thrombocytosis the absolute number of megathrombocytes, rather than the percentage, correlated with the number of megakaryocytes. Only in megaloblastic anaemia was there a lack of correlation.

Murphy et al. (1972) have confirmed the general validity of Karpatkin's work in acquired thrombocytopenia and added the observation that platelets in the Wiskott-Aldrich syndrome are smaller than normal. In two other hereditary forms of thrombocytopenia, however, divergent results were obtained. One family had thrombocytopenia with increased platelet size, yet the autologous platelet life-span was normal. Another family with a disorder resembling Wiskott-Aldrich syndrome had small platelet size but a shortened platelet life-span. These authors caution, therefore, that 'in hereditary disease platelet size is determined

CLASSIFICATION OF THROMBOCYTOPENIAS

From a consideration of platelet survival, immediate recovery of injected labelled platelets, total megakaryocyte mass, platelet production and percentage of megathrombocytes, as discussed in the preceding sections, it is possible to classify most causes of thrombocytopenia into either (a) impaired production, (b) maldistribution or (c) increased destruction (Table 16.1). Such a classification clarifies considerations regarding pathogenesis and treatment. In practice the diagnostic distinction between these groups can usually be made more simply by determining whether megakaryocytes in the marrow are diminished (as in (a)) or present in normal or increased numbers (as in (b) or (c)). Prominent splenomegaly is a prerequisite for (b). Other findings in the marrow, associated clinical features or the history frequently narrow down the diagnosis further. In practice the thrombokinetic data, which have been so valuable in increasing our understanding of these disorders, are seldom necessary in establishing a clinical diagnosis unless this is a new or imperfectly understood disorder.

IDIOPATHIC THROMBOCYTOPENIC PURPURA (ITP)

This is one of the commoner haematological disorders of childhood. It can be defined as a generalized haemorrhagic state in which the platelet count is low but the megakaryocytes are present in normal or increased numbers, and there is no splenomegaly or underlying disease. Frequently it is preceded by a virus infection 1–3 weeks earlier.

Nature of ITP

There has been accumulating evidence that the underlying disorder is immunological in origin. Harrington first proved the existence of a circulating thrombocytopenic factor by infusing plasma from an ITP patient into himself and demonstrating a marked fall in his platelet count (Harrington *et al.*, 1951). This phenomenon has subsequently been verified on many occasions (Harrington *et al.*, 1953; Shulman *et al.*, 1965). This experiment is also paralleled by the occurrence of thrombocytopenia in the newborn babies of mothers with ITP, again suggesting the existence of a humoral anti-platelet factor in this disease. Further studies, summarized by Baldini (1972), indicate that this factor is an immunoglobulin active against the patient's own platelets (Table 16.2).

Table 16.1   Classification of thrombocytopenias (after Harker and Finch, 1969)

	Platelet survival	Immediate platelet recovery	Megakaryocyte mass	Pl. production nucleus	Per cent. of megathrombocytes
Disorders of production					
Hypoplasia Aplastic anaemia (constitutional or acquired)	N	N	↓	N	N
Marrow replacement (leukaemia, neuroblastoma)					
Marrow encroachment (marble bone disease, myelofibrosis)					
Congenital amegakaryocytic					
Ineffective thrombopoiesis Megaloblastic anaemia (folate or B_{12} defic.)	N	N	↓	↓	↑
Erythroleukaemia					
Certain familial thrombocytopenias					
Disorders of distribution					
Hypersplenism (portal hypertension, thalassaemia, Hodgkin's lymphoma, storage disease, myelofibrosis)	↓	↓	↑	N	↑
Disorders of destruction					
Immune ITP or post-infective drug haptene, DLE, neonatal	↓	N	↑	N	↑
Platelet consumption Consumptive coagulopathy (septicaemia, HUS)					
Vascular (giant haemangioma, cyanotic CHD)					

Table 16.2 The ITP Factor: Evidence for autoimmunity in ITP

1. The plasma factor causes thrombocytopenia in normal recipients.
2. It can be adsorbed to normal human platelets.
3. It can be transferred across the placenta.
4. It is a 7S gamma globulin.
5. It is species specific.
6. It is active against isologous as well as autologous platelets.
7. With autologous platelets it causes lymphocyte transformation *in vitro* (Piessens *et al.*, 1970).
8. It is produced *in vitro* by spleen cells in culture (McMillan *et al.*, 1972).

From Baldini (1972) with permission.

At the present time one hypothesis is that an antigen-antibody complex attacks platelets non-specifically; the platelets being passive targets or 'innocent bystanders' (Baldini, 1972). Perhaps the antigen is a viral fragment arising after resolution of the virus infection which so commonly precedes onset of the disease. The onset of purpura coincides with the time of the highest viral antibody titre, at least in post-rubella thrombocytopenia (Morse *et al.*, 1966; Lokietz and Reynolds, 1966). Recent experimental work on the interaction between platelets, viruses and antibodies supports such a hypothesis (Myllyla *et al.*, 1969). Alternative hypotheses are that the initiating event may be a change in platelet antigenicity by adsorption of an exogenous haptene, or alternatively the differentiation of a lymphoid clone that no longer recognizes the patient's normal platelets as 'self'. By emphasizing the immunological nature of this platelet destruction one is specifically excluding those non-immune forms of platelet destruction such as occur in disseminated intravascular coagulation (DIC), microangiopathic haemolytic anaemia, giant haemangioma, hypersplenism, ristocetin toxicity, certain qualitative platelet defects (e.g. Wiskott-Aldrich syndrome) and in bacterial or viral septicaemias (Handin and Smith, 1972; Wybran and Fudenberg, 1972). Thrombocytopenia due to viraemia occurs at the height of the infection, rather than following its resolution as in ITP (Baldini, 1972). Its cause may be direct adsorption of the virus on to the platelet causing clumping and lysis (Terada *et al.*, 1966) or alternately DIC due to the viraemia (McKay and Margaretten, 1967).

Once an immunological basis for idiopathic thrombocytopenic purpura is accepted the disease is seen to have similarities with certain other immunological forms of thrombocytopenia but which are secondary (or symptomatic) to an identifiable cause. Baldini (1966) suggested that this wider group of immune thrombocytopenia could be included within the 'ITP syndrome' (Table 16.3).

Table 16.3 Immune thrombocytopenic syndromes

Idiopathic	Symptomatic
Acute	Drug induced
Chronic	Isoimmune; neonatal
	Post-transfusion
	DLE and Evan's syndrome
	Lymphoproliferative disorders

After Baldini (1966)

In the case of purpura of the drug haptene type (e.g. Sedormid purpura) there is a close analogy with postviral ITP since, again, it is interaction of antibody with antigen on the surface of the platelet which causes platelet destruction (Ackroyd, 1949). But the antigen is drug + platelet rather than viral particle as in the above stated hypothesis.

Clinically it is still useful to separate the 'idiopathic' forms of immune purpura from the secondary or 'symptomatic' forms, and the latter will be described separately. Whereas splenomegaly is very rare in idiopathic cases it is relatively common in some of the diseases causing secondary immunological thrombocytopenia. Their subsequent clinical course and prognosis also differ.

Difficulty in consistent demonstration of autoantibody

While accepting the immunological basis of ITP and related syndromes one must admit that there is still no 'practical, sensitive and well-proved serological test for ITP' (Baldini, 1972). With hindsight it can be seen that early tests depending upon agglutination of platelets by serum suffered from the obvious defects of liability to platelet aggregation by traces of residual thrombin, and accentuation from liberated ADP. Antibodies to foreign platelet antigens, acquired following blood transfusion, were also liable to give false positive results in many of the techniques. In addition most of these methods have given positive results in only about two thirds of patients with ITP (Table 16.4). Many of these methods are

THROMBOCYTOPENIA 259

Table 16.4 *In vitro* methods for detecting platelet autoantibodies in ITP

| | Incidence of +ve results | | |
Principle	Absolute	Per cent	Author
Antiglobulin consumption	46/93	49	Dauset *et al.*, 1966
Two-stage agglutination	11/21	52	Hanna and Nelken, 1970
Immunoglobulin assoc. with platelets	4/7	57	McMillan *et al.*, 1971
Platelet ^{14}C-serotonin release	24/40	60	Hirschman and Shulman, 1973
Immunofluorescent reaction of megakaryocytes	10/16	62	Pizzi *et al.*, 1966
Dextran-enhanced agglutination	17/26	65 ⎫	
Platelet factor-3 release	19/26	73 ⎬ Karpatkin and Siskind, 1969	
Either Dextran agglutination or PF-3 release	22/26	85 ⎭	
Lymphocyte stimulation by autologous platelets			
Chronic ITP	6/7	86	Clancy, 1972
Severe ITP	7/8	87	Wybran and Fudenberg, 1972
Mild ITP	3/6	50	,, ,, ,, ,,
Spleen eluates tested for PF-3 release	11/13	85	Karpatkin *et al.*, 1972
Splenic cultures tested for platelet-binding IgG	19/20	95	McMillan *et al.*, 1974
Surface platelet IgG > 0·4 pg	17/17	100	Dixon *et al.*, 1975

research tools and too complex for widespread diagnostic application. Two of the more recent techniques that show promise of both applicability and sensitivity include detection of antibody-induced platelet injury by measuring release of platelet factor 3 (PF-3), and also Dextran-enhanced platelet agglutination. The design of this test is such as to exclude the possibility of thrombin being responsible. One or other of these two tests was positive in 22 of 26 (85 per cent) of patients with ITP (Karpatkin and Siskind, 1969). A similar proportion of positive tests was also found in DLE. More recently these authors have shown that the PF-3 release activity in serum fell after splenectomy in 7 out of 8 patients with ITP and that the same antiplatelet antibody could be shown to be synthesized during *in vitro* incubation of splenic tissue derived from ITP patients (Karpatkin *et al.*, 1972). Similar splenic antibody synthesis in this disease has been independently reported by McMillan *et al.* (1972, 1974).

A recently described sensitive test for measuring platelet-bound IgG (by inhibition of anti-IgG-induced lysis of IgG-coated sheep erythrocytes) showed that normal platelets had less than 0·4 pg of surface IgG, but that all of 17 patients with ITP had greater than this amount (Dixon *et al.*, 1975). Surface levels greater than 1·1 pg correlated with failure to respond to prednisone.

Site of platelet destruction *in vivo*

A series of elegant clinical experiments by Shulman and coworkers (1965) using the infusion of ITP plasma into healthy individuals as their model suggested the following conclusions: (a) ITP factor sensitizes platelets leading to their sequestration in the reticuloendothelial system (RES), especially the spleen. (b) The severity is proportional to the titre of circulating ITP factor. (c) Steroids inhibit splenic sequestration and response therefore reflects, to some extent, that which will be obtained by splenectomy. (d) Heavily sensitized platelets are sequestrated to a greater extent throughout the RES, including the liver, and this is less inhibited by steroids or splenectomy. To this statement should probably be added, however, the more recent evidence that the spleen is an important site of synthesis of ITP factor, leading to a second benefit from splenectomy (Handin and Smith, 1972; McMillan *et al.*, 1974).

Studies by Aster and Keene (1969) with ^{51}Cr-labelled platelets and external scintillation scanning have confirmed Shulman's work showing that in 16 ITP patients with platelet counts greater than 5,000/mm^3 the platelets were predominantly destroyed in the spleen; but that in 4 patients with lower platelet counts and extremely short half-disappearance times (2–9 min) there was significant hepatic sequestration. Najean and Ardaillou (1971), using similar techniques in a large series of 575 patients with ITP found a good correlation between site of sequestration and results of splenectomy: success in more than 90 per cent of cases with splenic sequestration but complete failure in 70 per cent with hepatic sequestration. They describe also a 'diffuse' type of sequestration seen in severe cases, which cannot be taken as an indication for or against splenectomy. It has been known for many years that platelet survival is restored to normal after a splenectomy-induced remission (Cohen *et al.*, 1961).

Course of ITP in children

The disease may run an acute self-limiting course or a chronic, unremitting course. In adults the chronic form is more usual, but in children the reverse is true, 85 per cent of those with acute ITP were under 8 years of age in one large series (Doan et al., 1960).

In a 10-year follow-up of 152 children Lammi and Lovric (1973) found that 70 per cent recovered spontaneously by 6 months, others taking up to $3\frac{1}{2}$ years for recovery, at which time only 5/152 (3·3 per cent) remained thrombocytopenic. Shulman (1964) stated that 'approximately 20 per cent of cases will persist longer than 6 months and are then usually designated as chronic'. Defining 'chronicity' as persistence or recurrence of purpura after 1 year from onset Lusher and Zuelzer (1966) found only 12 out of 141 such children (8·5 per cent) became chronic. Other series have shown a slightly higher incidence of chronic cases.

There is some debate as to whether the acute and chronic forms are the same disease. Differences include: a 3:1 preponderance of females: males in the chronic form, but an equal sex ratio in the acute form (Baldini, 1966); an incidence of preceding infection in over 80 per cent of acute cases, but not in chronic cases (Baldini, 1972); an insidious onset in those patients destined to have protracted disease (Lammi and Lovric, 1973). Probably more relevant to the disease as seen in children is the fact that most cases have an acute onset, usually following an infection, with 90 per cent proving self-limiting. There is no certain way of determining at presentation which of these patients is destined to remit and which to become chronic (Baldini, 1966). In particular there is no correlation between severity of clinical manifestations or thrombocytopenia with long-term outcome. The transition from acute to chronic forms of ITP argues in favour of their common pathogenesis. The minority of children such as described by Lammi and Lovric (1973) as presenting with an insidious onset and/or an absence of preceding infection, and prone to an unremitting course, must be regarded as having the chronic form throughout. This, by contrast, is the common situation in adult ITP.

A *recurrent* form of ITP has also been described (Dameshek et al., 1963). Acute self-limiting episodes appear to follow intercurrent viral infections such as colds or influenza. Its importance lies in an appreciation of this possibility when giving long-term advice to parents at the time of final discharge. Also a single recurrence of purpura does not necessarily mean that the patient has the unremitting disease.

CLINICAL FEATURES

ITP may occur at any age, but the peak incidence in children is at the age of 3 years, with a seasonal predilection for the springtime (Luscher and Zuelzer, 1966).

The history reveals the occurrence of an acute infection, usually viral, within the preceding 3 weeks in over 80 per cent of childhood cases, as mentioned already. In many instances these can only be classified as upper respiratory tract infections but in a significant proportion, one quarter in one series, a specific viral infection could be identified. Such specific infections include measles (Hudson et al., 1956), chicken-pox (Welch, 1956), mumps (Fama et al., 1964), and infectious mononucleosis (Radel and Schorr, 1963). Rubella must be mentioned separately since there is a quite disproportionate tendency for purpura and thrombocytopenia to occur in association with this infection (Ackroyd, 1949). Ferguson (1960) in a review of the literature found 172 cases of childhood ITP preceded by various infections of which 19 were rubella. The rubella rash preceded the onset of purpura by 2–8 days, with a peak interval of 3 days. Smallpox vaccination (Meindersma and de Vries, 1962) and live measles vaccine (Bachand et al., 1967) have also been recorded as precipitating ITP.

There is striking variation in severity of the haemorrhagic state in different patients at the time of presentation. This may determine the initial management but appears to have little relationship to the length of the subsequent course.

In severe cases the distribution of bruises is widespread with a predilection for the skin over pressure points, particularly around the pelvis and thorax, and natural sites of trauma such as shins, ankles and elbows. Petechiae are more often found where the skin tension is least, such as in the supraclavicular fossae. Mucosal lesions give rise to epistaxis, blood blisters and bleeding from the mouth and gums, haematuria and gastrointestinal blood loss. Deep muscle haematomata, characteristic of coagulation disorders, are not seen except following intramuscular injections. Menorrhagia may occur in older girls.

In the most severe forms of thrombocytopenia, with platelet counts of 5,000/mm³ or less, haemorrhage into solid organs such as the brain, subarachnoid space, spinal cord, retina, or viscera may occur. Intracranial or subarachnoid haemorrhage is rare but constitutes the single most serious hazard of severe ITP. Schulman (1964) estimates its frequency as 2–4 per cent but another large series recorded only 1 instance in 146 cases of childhood ITP, 11 very severe (Lusher and Zuelzer, 1966), and this is more in accord with my own experience. Retinal haemorrhage constitutes another potentially serious complication. The mortality in children has been estimated as less than 1 per cent.

In approximately half the children presenting with ITP the symptoms are mild. Often these patients have only a few bruises on their legs or trunk which could easily be accounted for by normal childhood trauma. The mother may also notice that superficial cuts tend to bleed for a long time or excessively.

Apart from the haemorrhagic manifestations, which are common to all types of severe thrombocytopenia, there are no other particular clinical findings in ITP. The tip of the spleen is just palpable in not more than 10 per cent of cases and the finding of splenomegaly therefore suggests the probability of a different diagnosis such as leukaemia or hypersplenism. A mild throat infection often anticipates the appearance of ITP and slight tender cervical lymphadenopathy is sometimes present from this cause. It is usually easy to distinguish from the more prominent generalized, relatively painless lymphadenopathy of leukaemia.

HAEMATOLOGICAL FINDINGS

The platelet count is usually below 20,000/mm³ in cases with severe, generalized, haemorrhagic manifestations and above this figure in those with milder manifestations.

The peripheral blood findings are usually normal apart from the thrombocytopenia. In particular there are no lymphoblasts, myeloblasts or normoblasts present. Anaemia is only present if there has been substantial blood loss. If active infection is still present there may be a neutrophil leucocytosis, lymphocytosis, Turk cells or atypical mononuclear cells. Approximately 25 per cent of cases of ITP have a mild eosinophilia, perhaps because this is often seen in the convalescent stage of infection.

The marrow is of normal cellularity with normal or increased numbers of megakaryocytes. Specific morphological changes of these megakaryocytes have been described in ITP but are of questionable dependability for diagnostic purposes. Early forms of megakaryocytes are, however, proportionately increased (Dameshek and Miller, 1946). Otherwise the marrow findings are normal apart from an almost invariable increase in eosinophils

and eosinophil myelocytes (Lusher and Zuelzer, 1966). In particular there is no evidence of leukaemia, aplastic anaemia, megaloblastic changes or malignant infiltration.

It must be recognized that the marrow findings are only diagnostic of ITP when related to the presence of a low peripheral platelet count and the clinical exclusion of hypersplenism, drug-induced thrombocytopenia (e.g. Sedormid purpura), DIC, MAHA, DLE or renal failure. In all these conditions there can be increased destruction of platelets peripherally with their normal production in the marrow and the haematological findings can, therefore, be similar. Only in the case of DLE is any real confusion likely to occur and this disease is very rare in childhood.

In common with other diseases of platelet destruction there is a gross shortening of ^{51}Cr-labelled platelet survival from the normal 9·9 days to between 1 and 4 hours (Harker and Finch, 1969), but neither this test nor surface counting are needed in normal paediatric diagnosis or management. The recently described megathrombocyte index (Garg et al., 1971) showed an average of 38·5 per cent large platelets of over 2·5 μm diameter, compared to a normal value of 10·8 $\pm$ 3·1 (SD). Other causes of platelet destruction such as drug-induced purpura, DIC or DLE gave similar abnormal results. It is doubtful if the serological demonstration of anti-platelet antibodies yet constitutes a useful diagnostic tool (Table 16.4). Children with chronic ITP have significantly lowered IgA, unlike children with the more usual acute form (Lusher et al., 1974).

DIAGNOSIS

In paediatric practice the differential diagnosis will usually include aleukaemic acute leukaemia, which may sometimes present without hepatosplenomegaly or lymphadenopathy, and aplastic anaemia that can sometimes closely mimic ITP in the first few days of presentation. Marrow examination immediately distinguishes between these possibilities.

Baldini (1972) describes the diagnosis as being reached in 4 stages as follows:

1. Determining that it is a 'megakaryocytic' form of thrombocytopenia, rather than an 'amegakaryocytic' form such as aplastic anaemia.
2. Excluding the disorders with 'ineffective thrombopoiesis' i.e. megaloblastic anaemias, di Gugland di Guglemo's syndrome and PNH.
3. Excluding the non-immune disorders of platelet destruction such as hypersplenism, septicaemias (bacterial and viral), MAHA, DIC, TTP,

artificial heart valves or giant haemangioma from a consideration of the nature of the case.

4. Finally deciding which type of immune thrombocytopenic purpura it is; e.g. idiopathic or secondary to drug-haptene disease, DLE, isoimmunization or a lymphoproliferative disorder (Table 16.3).

Management of childhood ITP

This is based upon the assumption that most cases of ITP in childhood will prove to be acute self-limiting disorders, and that only a minority will persist to become chronic. Among 325 childhood cases Lusher et al. (1974) found that 90 per cent recovered completely with normal platelet counts within 3 months; a few had recurrent ITP, and the rest chronic ITP.

There is general agreement that the patient with only mild cutaneous manifestations and no overt spontaneous bleeding such as epistaxis requires only restriction of activity to prevent trauma. A brief hospital admission to establish the diagnosis and assess the severity is all that may be needed, with subsequent outpatient visits, initially at weekly intervals, to confirm the gradual return to normal of the platelet count. If bruising or purpura should persist for six months chronicity should be suspected; and if symptoms persist beyond a year splenectomy must be seriously considered. Schulman (1964) has pointed out the difficulty in laying down a specific duration of chronic ITP at which splenectomy should be done. In the absence of serious haemorrhagic symptoms operation can be deferred beyond a year. A minority may still achieve spontaneous remission beyond this time.

In the patient with severe, generalized bruising and purpura, or with spontaneous bleeding from mucosal surfaces, Schulman (1964) advises the administration of steroids since these reduce the bleeding tendency and produce an improvement of the platelet count in 60 per cent of such cases. Steroids tend to 'tide the patient over' the period of hazard of CNS or other life-threatening haemorrhage. Recently Zuelzer and coworkers (Lusher et al., 1974) have questioned the validity of the hazard of intracranial haemorrhage, pointing out that it is extremely rare in true ITP in childhood. McClure (1975), however, saw 3 children with large intracranial haemorrhages over the past 9 years. He points out that there is no certainty that steroids totally protect against this complication.

If the severity of the initial haemorrhagic manifestations is such as to justify the use of steroids than a standard course of 60 mg prednisolone per day in divided doses (40 mg per day for children under 2 years) is given, with stepwise reduction to 40 mg, 20 mg, 10 mg and 5 mg per day at 7 day intervals irrespective of the platelet count. There is no evidence, however, that the use of corticosteroids affects the long-term outcome, viz. the proportion who become chronic (Lusher and Zuelzer, 1966; Lammi and Lovric, 1973). Second courses of steroids may occasionally be justified but I would personally only consider this when the severity of the haemorrhagic state and the severity of thrombocytopenia (usually below 10,000/mm^3) constituted a real hazard in terms of morbidity or mortality, and even then the courses are limited to 4 or 5 weeks as indicated above. Long continued steroid courses are to be avoided. Indeed, instances have been recorded where continuing the steroid therapy appeared to perpetuate the thrombocytopenia, prompt remission following upon cessation of the drug (Cohen and Gardner, 1961; Schulman, 1964). Blood transfusion may be needed at any stage of the disease when significant blood loss has occurred. Platelet transfusions may occasionally be needed to deal with troublesome problems such as persistent epistaxis in severe cases, even although their benefit is short-lived.

For children presenting with intracranial haemorrhage McClure (1975) recommends immediate splenectomy as the surest way to cause a rapid rise in platelet count. If there is no rise in a few minutes he gives steroids and a platelet transfusion. Only after a platelet response are carotid angiograms and neurosurgery performed. All his 3 such cases survived.

In severe ITP, as in the mild cases, one will find a small proportion who fail to remit within 6 months to a year, and in whom splenectomy becomes necessary. Management during this necessary time interval is difficult. A second steroid course is often tried, but usually with only temporary success. When home conditions are good outpatient management is possible, but with emphasis upon restriction of activity so as to avoid trauma as much as possible. School attendance is too great a risk in severe cases. For these reasons splenectomy may be undertaken as early as 6 months in occasional, severe and totally refractory cases.

Preparation for splenectomy includes an attempt to raise the platelet count in the days immediately preceding the operation by instituting corticosteroids at full dosage 5–7 days before the operation is planned. Whole blood is cross-matched and a platelet transfusion may be given immediately before the operation. In spite of the shortened life span of transfused platelets in this disease transitory haemostatic benefit may be obtained. Alternatively platelets may be given after clamping the splenic pedicle (Wilde *et al.*, 1967).

With the present day availability of paediatric surgical units and the above mentioned precautions the operative mortality of elective splenectomy in ITP is less than 1 per cent (Eraklis and Filler, 1972). Anaesthetists make it a 'rule of thumb' to give 100 mg IV hydrocortisone pre-operatively to any patients who have been on steroids in the preceding 3 months.

The haematological response to elective splenectomy in chronic ITP is excellent. At the Royal Hospital for Sick Children 10 out of 12 such patients have shown a complete and permanent cure of ITP, the remaining two showing a partial remission which was clinically worth while. Schulman (1964) states that two thirds recover after splenectomy, Crosby (1972) gives a cure rate of 80 per cent, and Prankerd (1972) a response rate of 90 per cent in patients under 45 years of age. Luscher and Zuelzer (1966) made the interesting observation that 6 out of 7 patients made a complete and long lasting recovery after splenectomy among a group who had previously shown a response to steroids; but that neither of two patients who had failed to respond to steroids benefited from splenectomy. This is consistent with the conclusion reached experimentally by Shulman *et al.* (1965) that steroids inhibit splenic sequestration, and that the response to steroids reflects that which will be obtained by splenectomy. Najean and Ardaillou (1971) have shown a clear relationship between splenic sequestration and long terms of correction of the thrombocytopenia by splenectomy (Table 16.5). Since 90 per cent of those with splenic sequestration showed success but only 30 per cent in those with hepatic sequestration they recommend this investigation prior to splenectomy in adults. Perhaps this recommendation should be applied to children when there is a difficulty in arriving at the decision for splenectomy on other grounds.

The hazards of overwhelming postsplenectomy infection (OPSI) have been fully discussed by Diamond (1969). While there is a distinct hazard of OPSI from rapidly multiplying organisms such as pneumococci (and to a lesser extent meningococci and haemophilus bacilli) in patients with serious systemic diseases such as thalassaemia, Wiskott-Aldrich syndrome or histiocytosis no such fatal infections were found after splenectomy for ITP in a large retrospective survey by Eraklis *et al.* (1967). Splenectomy for hereditary spherocytosis, aplastic anaemia and Gaucher's disease occupied an intermediate group with subsequent OPSI in 1·4 to 3·2 per cent. Horan and Colebatch (1962) similarly recorded a zero incidence of serious infection in 14 ITP patients following splenectomy, although the overall incidence was 11 per cent when this was performed for other diseases. Eraklis *et al.* (1967) also noted that the incidence of OPSI was 2½ times greater in children under 4 years than in older children. This may partly be because the younger child is less able to complain if he has the early symptoms of infection (Diamond, 1969). Early institution of penicillin is recommended in splenectomized children who become febrile, and continuous prophylactic penicillin in the high risk group mentioned above, the pneumococcus never developing resistance to penicillin. Eraklis and Filler (1972) recently reviewed the hazards of splenectomy in 1,413 children confirming that overwhelming infection was an unusual cause of late mortality in older children without underlying systemic disease. The fatality rate was only 2 out of 394 (0·5 per cent) with congenital haemolytic anaemia, 7 out of 262 (2·7 per cent) for those with ITP and 3 out of 342 (1 per cent) for splenectomy following trauma. These 'low risk' groups contrasted with rates of 2/45 (4 per cent) in thalassaemia and 20/32 (6 per cent) in a miscellaneous group including portal hypertension, hypersplenism, histiocytosis, Hodgkin's disease, aplastic anaemia, etc.

Table 16.5 Relation between site of sequestration and response to splenectomy

Site of sequestration pre-operative	Postsplenectomy platelet count and No. of cases			
	No. of cases	Less than 80,000	80,000 200,000	More than 200,000
Splenic	166	11	21	134
Hepato-splenic or diffuse	29	7	11	11
Hepatic	11	8	2	1

*Reproduced by permission from Najean and Ardaillou (1971) Brit. J. Haematol., **21**, 159.*

For the small proportion of children left with serious thrombocytopenia and haemorrhagic symptoms after splenectomy immunosuppressive drug therapy with azothioprine (Imuran), 6-mercaptopurine or cyclophosphamide (Larco and Penner, 1971), with or without steroids, may be tried. Sussman (1967) reported a satisfactory response in 7 out of 8 patients, the youngest being 15 years old. Hilgartner *et al.* (1970) treated five children with refractory ITP with azothioprine for 8 to 27 months at a dose of 2·0 to 3·0 mg/kg/day (usually 2·5 mg). Excellent results were obtained in three, a good result in one and a failure in one. In a survey of the literature up to 1970 Hilgartner and colleagues collected a total of 26 'good' or 'excellent' responses to azathioprine out of 37 patients, 9 of whom were children. In some of these successes a low dose of steroids, e.g. 0·2 mg/kg/day of prednisolone, was given simultaneously. In view of the high success rate and low mortality from splenectomy it is probably the correct policy to reserve immunosuppressive therapy for patients relapsing after splenectomy. Reservations with respect to the use of immunosuppressive drugs in ITP have been expressed by Lo *et al.* (1969).

Vincristine has recently been shown to be of value. Prompt response occurred in 9 of 13 patients refractory to both steroids and splenectomy. Five of these 9 were also refractory to cyclophosphamide or azathioprine or both. For children a course of 3 doses of 1 mg at weekly intervals was suggested (Ahn *et al.*, 1974). Responses were usually seen in about a week. The mechanism of action is not clear but may be immunosuppressive.

The problems of management of childhood ITP are well reviewed by Walker and Walker (1961), Lo *et al.* (1969), Lusher *et al.* (1974) and McClure (1975), while a recent review of ITP in general is that of Prankerd (1972).

THROMBOCYTOPENIA IN THE NEONATAL PERIOD

1 Secondary to maternal ITP

The occurrence of transient neonatal thrombocytopenia when the mother has ITP has already been cited as evidence of the immunological nature of that disease (Harrington *et al.*, 1953). It is surprising and disappointing, however, that the sensitive complement fixation test for antiplatelet antibodies has been consistently negative in these cases (Shulman *et al.*, 1964). Perhaps this is simply a matter of sensitivity of the technique.

The incidence of thrombocytopenia in these infants is approximately 50 per cent when the mother is actually thrombocytopenic at the time of delivery (Goodhue and Evans, 1963; Heyes, 1966). It may also occur at times when the mother's ITP is in remission (Andre *et al.*, 1965), but the incidence is then less. The clinical presentation is with generalized petechiae and bruising, maximal at birth but sometimes with recurring crops of petechiae later. The generalized distribution of these petechiae contrasts with the more localized purpura commonly seen in normal, non-thrombocytopenic infants and confined to the head and upper chest (Poley and Strickler, 1961). Epistaxis, gastrointestinal bleeding, haematuria or bleeding from the cord and needle puncture sites may also occur. The most serious hazard is intracranial haemorrhage. Fortunately this is rare. No mortality or morbidity at all has been recorded in some series (Anthony and Krivit, 1962). In larger series collected from the literature, and before the availability of platelet transfusions, these and other authors have found a mortality rate of approximately 10 per cent in affected infants.

The absence of hepatosplenomegaly in these infants is a distinguishing feature from other causes of neonatal thrombocytopenia such as Rhesus disease, cytomegalovirus, toxoplasmosis and other infections. Jaundice may appear, but usually only *after* 24 hours, and is due to absorption of blood pigment from the petechiae and bruises and a rise in indirect serum bilirubin (Raussen and Diamond, 1961). The baby may show platelet counts as low as 3,000 to 5,000 per mm^3. Anaemia and erythroblastosis are present only in proportion to blood loss except in the rare Evan's syndrome, when an associated Coombs positive haemolytic anaemia may also be present. A routine procedure upon discovering thrombocytopenia in a newborn baby is to check the mother's platelet count. This may bring to light a previously undiagnosed state of mild ITP in the mother (Case 11).

Case 11. A first born male infant (No. 10475) of 39-week maturity showed generalized petechiae after a normal delivery. Otherwise the baby was in good condition, with no hepatosplenomegaly or jaundice. The baby's platelet count was 13,000/mm^3, Hb 17·8 g/100 ml, WBC 12,500/mm^3 and thrombotest 26 per cent. The film showed no increase in normoblasts nor red cell fragmentation. No abnormal leucocytes were present. The maternal platelet count was 35,000/mm^3. On enquiry she had suffered from easy bruising for many years. Blood loss had not been excessive at delivery.

There was no recent maternal exposure to drugs. Marrow findings were those of ITP. LE cell test was negative. The baby's platelet count remained below 15,000/mm³ for a week and then gradually rose to normal at the age of 2 months. He was allowed home when the count reached 66,000/mm³ at the age of 5½ weeks. Subsequent progress was normal. The mother responded to splenectomy.

Because the thrombocytopenic factor is only passively transmitted to the baby its thrombocytopenia is only transient. The time taken for the babies' platelets to rise to 100,000/mm³ or more ranges between 2 to 12 weeks (Anthony and Krivit, 1962), commonly being around 6 weeks (Fig. 16.4). The self-limiting nature of the disorder

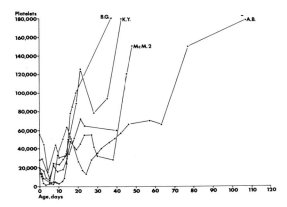

Fig. 16.4 Neonatal thrombocytopenia: secondary to maternal ITP. Sequential platelet counts from birth in five affected infants born in the Queen Mother's Hospital, Glasgow.

discourages active treatment such as steroids, and even more certainly discourages splenectomy. In the event of life threatening haemorrhage or suspected intracranial bleeding Oski and Naiman (1972) suggest giving two units of platelet concentrate and possibly a trial of exchange transfusion. An improvement in the purpura following ET had been reported by Killander (1959) in such an infant, although the platelet count was not improved. 'Washing-out' of the antibody may have been responsible. This would also enhance the value of a platelet transfusion. A trial of steroids would also seem worth while in the face of severe haemorrhage since they have been shown to be beneficial in the closely related neonatal isoimmune purpura (McIntosh et al., 1973). This could be through their non-specific enhancement of the vascular component of haemostasis (Faloon et al., 1952) rather than on antibody levels.

Evan's syndrome in the mother is also capable of causing thrombocytopenia in the newborn infant. Of four surviving infants born to mothers with Evan's syndrome one had thrombocytopenia at birth, and two had a Coombs positive haemolytic anaemia (Oski and Naiman, 1972B).

A similar situation appears to exist in infants born to mothers with DLE. Nathan and Snapper (1958) reported one such infant born with transient thrombocytopenia (30,000/mm³). No haemorrhagic symptoms were present and the platelet count rose to normal by the age of three weeks. In another infant reported by Seip (1960) severe haemolytic anaemia was found together with mild neutropenia and thrombocytopenia. Steroid therapy appeared to be of benefit.

2 Isoimmune neonatal purpura

Key reviews on this subject are those of Pearson et al. (1964) and Pochedley (1971).

Isoimmune thrombocytopenia should be suspected in purpuric infants born to mothers with a normal platelet count, particularly if infants of successive pregnancies are affected. Immunization arises from foeto-maternal passage of platelets, the situation being analagous to Rhesus disease (Desai and Creger, 1963). Maternal antiplatelet antibodies can be found in 1·65 per cent of pregnancies (Klemperer et al., 1966). The incidence of neonatal purpura is, however, very low, being only 1 to 2 per 10,000 births (Shulman et al., 1964). It is therefore encountered much less often than neonatal thrombocytopenia due to maternal ITP or drug administration.

Haemorrhagic manifestations, although variable, tend to be more severe than in neonatal ITP. Generalized petechiae may appear within minutes of birth, and be succeeded by ecchymoses and even cephalhaematomata. Bleeding from umbilicus, skin puncture, gastrointestinal or renal tract may also occur.

Among 55 affected infants collected from the literature by Pearson et al. (1964) intracranial haemorrhage was diagnosed in 8 and suspected in a further 4. Seven of the infants died of haemorrhage during the neonatal period giving an immediate mortality of 12·7 per cent. Two survivors were later found to be mentally retarded. Platelet counts were frequently below 10,000/mm³. Other clinical and haematological features were similar to neonatal ITP but the duration of thrombocytopenia was usually shorter, ranging from 1 week to 4 months. The platelet count remained below 60,000/mm³ for a mean of 21 days. Early jaundice occurred in 20 per cent. Megakaryocytes were present in normal or increased numbers in the marrow of 5 out of the 6 infants with proven isoimmune thrombocytopenia investigated by Pearson et al. (1964). The reduced numbers of megakaryocytes that have sometimes been reported could indicate direct interaction of the antibody with these cells in certain instances, but artefact due to technical difficulties in marrow sampling at this age could alternatively be responsible.

Serological investigation, predominantly utilizing complement fixation or blocking techniques, show the presence of maternal antibodies which react with the father's and the infant's platelets, but not with her own (Shulman et al., 1964; Pearson et al., 1964). Much of our knowledge of platelet antigens springs from study of this disorder. In nearly half the affected families the maternal antibody has specificity to the platelet antigen PL^{A1} (Colombani et al., 1969). The rarity of the disorder may partly be due to the fact that 98 per cent of the population possess this platelet antigen and only 2 per cent, therefore, are capable of forming the antibody. It appears that this particular antigen must be strongly immunogenic compared to other platelet antigens (Pochedly, 1971), in the same way as the 'D' Rhesus antigen is exceptionally immunogenic. Other antigens that have been responsible for neonatal thrombocytopenia include 'Duzo', Ko^a, Pl Gr Ly^{C1}, Fek^a, HLA-5 and HLA-9. Whereas 'Duzo' and Ko^a are antigens unique to platelets, the other named antigens are common to platelets, granulocytes and lymphocytes. In spite of this neutropenia does not occur in neonatal isoimmune thrombocytopenia, perhaps because there are greater reserves in the granulocyte series, as suggested by Pochedly (1971). There are other known platelet antigens (Zw^b, Ko^b, Pe^{E1}) and platelet-leucocyte antigens (Pl Gr Ly^{F2} and HLA 1, 3, 4, 6, 7, 8, 10, 11 and 12) which have not been reported as provoking neonatal thrombocytopenia. Relatively little is known about the factors determining which antibodies cross the placenta and the determinants affecting the development of severe thrombocytopenia in some instances but not in others (Pochedly, 1971).

Half the cases of isoimmune neonatal thrombocytopenia occur in untransfused primipara. In this respect the disorder is more like ABO HD in its occurrence than Rh disease.

Treatment is along similar lines as neonatal ITP but, being more severe, 'a policy of watchful waiting cannot be generally recommended' (Pochedly, 1971). This author emphasized that infants with severe purpura are in danger of intracranial haemorrhage in this condition and that optimal treatment in this group of infants should include exchange transfusion, to remove the antibody, followed by infusion of a platelet concentrate together with corticosteroids to improve haemostasis. Ideally the platelets should be obtained from the mother and suspended in normal plasma (Adner et al., 1969). In this way platelets compatible with possible residual antibody will be infused. If bleeding persists the platelet infusion should be repeated 8 hourly. More recently McIntosh et al. (1973) have reported good results in this disorder by the use of compatible platelets so obtained from the mother or by using exchange transfusion. Corticosteroids also appeared beneficial. Splenectomy is never indicated since the disorder is self-limiting. Pearson et al. (1964) suggested that prenatal administration of corticosteroids to the mother might benefit the baby when severe neonatal thrombocytopenia was anticipated (Fig. 16.5). It should also be mentioned

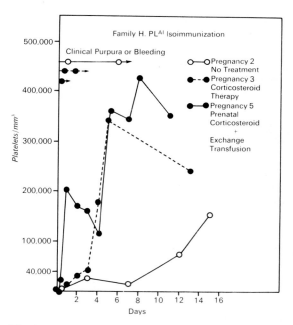

Fig. 16.5 Neonatal isoimmune thrombocytopenia. Comparison of pre-natal and post-natal corticosteroid therapy with natural course of neonatal purpura in three successive pregnancies. (Reproduced from *Blood* (1964), **23**, 158, from a paper by Pearson et al., with permission of the authors).

that such platelet antibodies will be present in breast milk, but that discontinuation of breast feeding has no immediate effect on the platelet count of the affected baby (Jones et al., 1961).

In severe Rhesus disease, thrombocytopenia may be seen and on occasion may have an immunological basis. In one case both mother and infant appeared to have circulating agglutinins active against the infant's platelets (Stephanini and Dameshek, 1962). In other cases it appears to be related to bilirubin level and the effect of this pigment upon platelet aggregation (Suvansri et al., 1969), or to follow upon exchange transfusion (Krevans and Jackson, 1955). Recently intravascular coagulation has been invoked as the cause of thrombocytopenia and haemostatic failure in severe Rh disease (Chessells and Wigglesworth, 1971). Stuart et al. (1973) found thrombocytopenia in 14 of 17 infants with Rh disease, but all had had either an intrauterine or exchange transfusion, and this was thought to account for the thrombocytopenia as the sole defect in 5, or in association with RBC fragmentation in a further 2. In 4 very severely affected infants, however, there were multiple coagulation defects and clinical bleeding in two. These may have had DIC.

3 Secondary to maternal drug ingestion

Neonatal thrombocytopenia may be associated with drug induced thrombocytopenia in the mother or may preferentially affect the infant. In the former situation it is at least theoretically possible that drug-haptene disease is responsible for both maternal and foetal manifestations. Maternal autoantibody would be formed against the drug-platelet complex (Ackroyd, 1949) and the maternal antibody could then cross to the foetal circulation to react against the foetal platelets presumably also requiring the presence of the drug in question to have reached the foetus. Mauer et al. (1957) described one such case where the mother was given quinine just before delivery (in the past this drug was used to induce labour). The drug and the drug-induced antibody both crossed the placenta to produce transient thrombocytopenic purpura in the infant. The mother also suffered an explosive haemorrhagic state. The thrombocytopenia lasted only a few days but the antibody persisted for months. A similar type of neonatal thrombocytopenia could presumably occur with other drugs known to cause drug-haptene disease including sedormid and quinidine.

Thiazide diuretics, used in the treatment of pre-eclampsia, have also been incriminated as causing neonatal thrombocytopenia (Rodriguez et al., 1964), but the mechanism appears to be different since the maternal platelet count is normal and no antibodies have been demonstrated. If the drug exerts a direct toxic effect upon megakaryocytes then foetal thrombopoiesis appears to be preferentially sensitive. The clinical picture in the 7 infants described by Rodriguez et al. was similar to that described above for isoimmune thrombocytopenia. One infant died at 40 hours with subdural and pulmonary haemorrhages. The platelet count ranged from 4,000 to 28,000/mm^3, and was accompanied by neutropenia in 3 out of the 7. Megakaryocytes were reduced in 4 out of 5. Thrombocytopenia persisted for 2 to 12 weeks. A recent prospective study by Merenstein et al. (1970) showed no difference in the platelet counts of 37 infants born to mothers receiving thiazides compared to 47 control infants. This finding now casts doubt on the alleged association.

A similar but less severe degree of transient neonatal thrombocytopenia following maternal ingestion of tolbutamide has been reported by Schiff et al. (1970). It may be expected that other drugs known to produce thrombocytopenia, whether by immunological means or by direct marrow toxicity, will on occasions cause neonatal thrombocytopenia when administered to the mother.

4 Intrauterine or neonatal infection

The same group of infections that have been described in Chapter 12 as causing neonatal haemolytic anaemia may also cause neonatal thrombocytopenia. These infections include toxoplasmosis, cytomegalovirus, rubella, syphilis, listerosis, Coxsackie B and disseminated herpes simplex. The resulting clinical picture may therefore include not only jaundice and hepatosplenomegaly but also purpura and possibly overt bleeding. The blood picture shows the features of haemolytic anaemia with increased normoblasts on the blood film and reticulocytosis plus thrombocytopenia, with platelet counts often as low as 10,000/mm^3. Raised IgM levels in the cord blood are found when the infection occurred before birth. The bone marrow has been reported as showing reduced numbers of megakaryocytes in several of these infections, including rubella, but finding of normal numbers of megakaryocytes in postmortem histology sections (Zinkham et al., 1967) raises the possibility that the paucity of megakaryocytes seen in smears may be related to technical difficulties of marrow aspiration in this age group (Oski and Naiman, 1972C).

The thrombocytopenia in these infections is probably due to platelet destruction. In the case of disseminated herpes infection of the newborn there is good evidence that the platelet consumption is due to disseminated intravascular coagulation (DIC) (Miller *et al.*, 1970; Shershow *et al.*, 1969). DIC could also occur in other virus infections (McKay and Margaretten, 1967), and in severe bacterial infections, especially gram —ve septicaemia (Gotoff and Behrman, 1970), but it is in no way certain that the thrombocytopenia seen in these infants is necessarily due to DIC. It could be simply the consequence of viraemia or bacteraemia without DIC. In the rubella syndrome the thrombocytopenia present at birth usually gradually disappears after a few weeks (Zinkham *et al.*, 1967). It is possible that the same factors are operative here as in the commonly observed thrombocytopenia seen in association with this infection at other ages (Ackroyd, 1949).

5 Other causes of platelet consumption

The association of thrombocytopenic purpura with giant haemangioma is referred to as the Kasabach-Merritt syndrome after the original description by these authors in 1940. Neonatal thrombocytopenia can occur when the haemangioma is apparent in the neonatal period (Case 12).

Case 12. A male infant (No. 144223) was delivered spontaneously at home but was transferred to hospital because the right lower limb was discoloured and was visibly increasing in size in the hours following birth. He had a giant haemolymphangioma affecting the entire lower limb and buttock, with a palpable mass in the right lower abdomen. IVP showed displacement of the ureter and bladder.

At the age of 12 hours the platelet count was 55,000/mm³, Hb 13·2 g/100 ml, WBC 9,900/mm³, with 18 normoblasts per 100 WBC. The thrombocytopenia persisted in the range 35–90,000 until amputation of the extensively involved right leg was performed at the age of a week. The following day the platelet count was 159,000/mm³, and has remained normal since. Because of the danger of haemorrhage into the haemangioma during the period of neonatal hypoprothrombinaemia vitamin K was given on the day of birth. Thrombotest was 100 per cent the following morning. In spite of this steady bleeding occurred from the thigh requiring repeated transfusion before amputation. During amputation and laparotomy total blood loss was approximately 210 ml. Interestingly the serum FDP level was 160–240 μg/ml, before amputation falling to 20, 3 days postoperatively.

Four years later the child is leading a satisfactory life with an artificial limb. He sometimes becomes a little anaemic as a result of bleeding from residual haemangioma in the perianal region. At these times oral iron (Sytron) is given.

Actually it is only very rarely that haemangiomas are large enough to require resection or amputation.

Platelet trapping has been demonstrated in giant haemangiomas (Kontras *et al.*, 1963; Brizel and Raccuglia, 1965), accompanied in some instances by evidence of consumption of coagulation factors (Schneider and Lascari, 1968; Pyesmany *et al.*, 1969) and elevation of fibrin degradation products (FDPs) in the blood draining the tumour (Henriksson *et al.*, 1971). Red cell fragmentation, as in MAHA, can also occur (Propp and Scharfman (1966) due to red cell trauma from contact with intravascular fibrin. The haemangiomas need not necessarily be 'giant'; thrombocytopenia may also occur with smaller haemangiomas (Inglefield *et al.*, 1961; Shim, 1968) or internal haemangiomas of liver (Cooper and Martin, 1962) or spleen (Thatcher *et al.*, 1968) which may not be immediately clinically apparent. Haemangioma on the foetal aspect of the placenta (cholangioma) may also cause a self-limiting thrombocytopenia present at birth (Froelich and Housler, 1971).

Other causes of platelet consumption due to intravascular coagulation in the newborn period include renal vein thrombosis (Jones and Reed, 1965; Renfield and Kraybill, 1973), premature separation of the placenta (abruptio placentae) (Edison *et al.*, 1968), the presence of a dead twin foetus (Moore *et al.*, 1969) and one report of neonatal TTP (Monnens and Retera, 1967).

In all forms of thrombocytopenia due to platelet consumption there are normal or increased numbers of megakaryocytes, the marrow picture being essentially the same as in ITP. Intravascular coagulation is described in greater detail in Chapter 19.

6 Congenital megakaryocytic hypoplasia

This may occur (a) in association with skeletal anomalies, especially bilateral absence of the radii, (b) as part of the pancytopenia of Fanconi's anaemia, and (c) in association with certain trisomy syndromes. The unifying feature in this group of disorders is impaired platelet production with absent or decreased megakaryocytes. There is a familial tendency, probably recessive, in both the syndrome with absent radii and in Fanconi's anaemia. No toxic, infective or immunological agents can be incriminated, although the nature of the associated congenital abnormalities suggests the operation of an environmental factor at an early stage of embryonal development.

(A) BILATERAL ABSENT RADII (TAR) (Fig. 16.6)

This has been reported on a number of occasions and reviewed by Hall *et al.* (1969). Since

20 per cent of affected families have more than one member with the disorder an autosomal recessive inheritance seems probable (Murphy, 1972A). Purpura, epistaxis, gastrointestinal haemorrhage or haematuria have usually appeared within the first week of life with a platelet count as low as 10,000/mm³. In addition there may be a myeloid leukaemoid reaction with grossly elevated total white cell count and myelocytes or myeloblasts in the peripheral blood. The patients with leukaemoid reactions may also have hepatosplenomegaly and lymphadenopathy further mimicking congenital leukaemia. Anaemia develops as a result of blood loss. Marrow examination shows

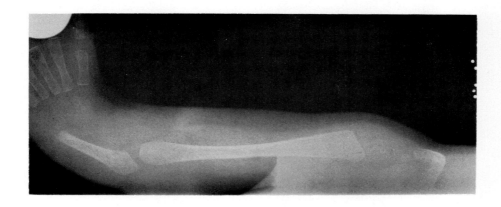

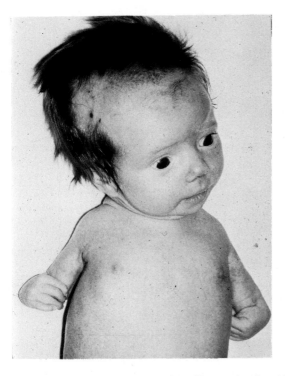

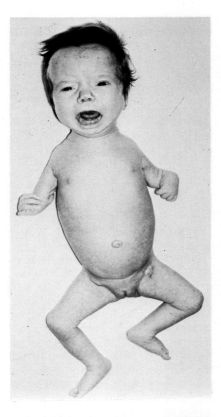

Fig. 16.6 Bilateral absence of radii associated with congenital amegakaryocytic thrombocytopenia (TAR syndrome). There was also congenital heart disease. Marrow smears and trephine showed myelocytic hyperplasia and absence of megakaryocytes. (x 425). (Marrow histology by courtesy of Dr A. A. M. Gibson).

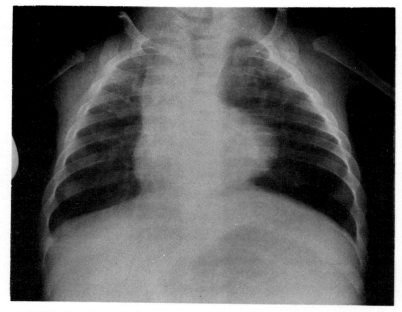

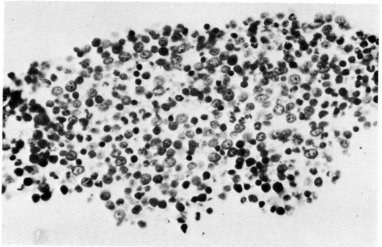

Fig. 16.6 (cont.)

decreased numbers or abnormal morphology of megakaryocytes together with myeloid hyperplasia.

The absence of radii produce shortening of the arms, flexion at the elbows and radial deviation of the wrists. Additional absence of ulnae and occasionally of all long bones of the limbs have been described, producing phocomelia (Dignan et al., 1967). Other associated anomalies that may be present include congenital heart disease, especially Fallot's tetralogy and ASD, dislocation of the hip, micrognathia, defects of the digits, or multiple congenital abnormalities. Amegakaryocytic thrombocytopenia with microcephaly has also been described (Eisenstein, 1966).

Many of the infants die of intracranial haemorrhage in the first few months of life but there is some variation in platelet count with a gradual improvement sometimes occurring with increasing age. Prognosis is good for those surviving a year. Treatment is purely supportive with platelet and blood transfusions as necessary. In the presence of actual haemorrhage two units of platelet concentrate should be given, ideally from donors of similar HL-A type so as to reduce the likelihood of sensitization and subsequent resistance to platelet therapy (Yankee et al., 1973). Steroids have questionable benefit and splenectomy should only be considered if there are some megakaryocytes present, and a modest rise in platelet count is expected to be worth achieving in terms of improved haemostasis. The management has recently been discussed in the review by Pochedly (1971). Cow's milk allergy appears to accentuate the thrombocytopenia, as well as inducing diarrhoea, during the early months of life, and its avoidance may be important in tiding patients over this period (Whitfield and Barr, 1975).

(B) FANCONI'S ANAEMIA

This is associated with a broader range of congenital anomalies than TAR, these including pigmentation, short stature, renal tract abnormalities, deformities of the thumbs and microcephaly. Usually haematological manifestations of pancytopenia do not appear until several years of age but exceptions to this have been recorded with generalized purpura, epistaxis and gastrointestinal bleeding appearing shortly after birth (O'Neill and Varadi, 1963). Also a variant of constitutional aplastic anaemia in males but without congenital anomalies and presenting with isolated thrombocytopenia in the neonatal period has been described (Bloom *et al.*, 1966; O'Gorman Hughes, 1969). Pancytopenia supervenes in later childhood. A good response to combined corticosteroids and androgens was found in two out of the four children described by O'Gorman Hughes and Diamond (1964) as well as in one personally observed case (Case 5, Chapter 4).

(C) TRISOMY SYNDROMES

These have also been associated with amegakaryocytic thrombocytopenia in the newborn. In 3 infants with trisomy 18 (E) and associated radial dysplasia two had thrombocytopenia and oesophageal atresia (Rabinowitz *et al.*, 1967). Another infant with trisomy 18 has been reported with developmental abnormalities of caecum and ascending colon plus fatal thrombocytopenia (Christodoulou and Werner, 1967). Trisomy 13–15 has also been associated with amegakaryocytic thrombocytopenia and multiple congenital anomalies (Mehes and Bata, 1965).

7 Hereditary thrombocytopenias

A familial tendency has been mentioned in the bilateral absent radii syndrome and in Fanconi's anaemia discussed above. A further group of clearly hereditary thrombocytopenias exist with either sex-linked recessive, autosomal dominant or, rarely, autosomal recessive patterns of inheritance. In most of these disorders there is an abundance of megakaryocytes in the marrow, the haematological features therefore superficially resembling ITP. In some of the disorders the fundamental defect is an intrinsic platelet abnormality leading to shortened survival of the patient's platelets; in others it is 'ineffective thrombopoiesis' with increased megakaryocyte mass and normal platelet survival (Murphy, 1972A).

All these disorders are rare by comparison with the hereditary defects of red cells. Certain disorders of platelet function are on occasions associated with thrombocytopenia (e.g. the Bernard-Soulier syndrome). These are described in the following chapter on qualitative defects of platelet function.

(A) WISCOTT-ALDRICH SYNDROME (WAS)

In its complete form WAS usually presents with a thrombocytopenic bleeding tendency in the first weeks or months of life. The subsequent course is punctuated by recurrent pyogenic infections including otitis media, pneumonia and skin infections (Krivit and Good, 1959; Gordon, 1960). There is also lowered resistance to non-bacterial infections including herpes simplex (Geme *et al.*, 1965) and pneumocystis carinii (Weintraub and Wilson, 1964). By the age of two to three months skin lesions resembling ordinary atopic infantile eczema appear, particularly on the head and extremities, sparing the trunk. Fully developed WAS is usually fatal in the first few years of life, mostly from infection, but occasional survival into adult life has been recorded (Mandl, Watson and Rose, 1968). An increased incidence of lymphoreticular malignancy occurs, presumably related to the abnormal immune mechanism (ten Bensel *et al.*, 1960).

Haematological findings include a platelet count around 30,000/mm^3, but sometimes as low as 5,000/mm^3, anaemia if there has been blood loss, and neutrophil leucocytosis if there is infection. Characteristically there is also a lymphopenia and an eosinophilia. Marrow examination shows the megakaryocytes to be present in normal or increased numbers but showing fragmented and karyorrhectic nuclei (Pearson *et al.*, 1966). A striking and possibly unique finding in WAS and closely related disorders is the small size of the platelets (Murphy *et al.*, 1972). This is clearly shown with a Coulter counter model B or electrozone celloscope (Fig. 16.7) but is difficult to appreciate on blood films. The small size of the platelets is especially surprising since platelet survival studies in WAS show that the thrombocytopenia is due to increased destruction (Baldini *et al.*, 1969; Gröttum *et al.*, 1969), and an *increase* in platelet size would normally be expected with increased turnover (Garg *et al.*, 1971). Murphy *et al.* (1972) made the point that 'although in acquired conditions increased platelet size suggests a young platelet population, in hereditary disease platelet size is determined more by the nature of the intrinsic platelet defect than by mean cell age'. Independent evidence of qualitative abnormality of the platelets has been the demonstration of order of antigen processing or recognition (Blaese *et al.*, 1968).

Splenectomy is contraindicated because of the high risk of subsequent overwhelming infection (Eraklis *et al.*, 1967). All 17 patients reported as having splenectomy died with a mean survival of 8 months. Platelet counts increased postoperatively in 10 (Gröttum *et al.*, 1969). Corticosteroids have no effect on the thrombocytopenia but may improve the eczema and the anaemia. Since normal

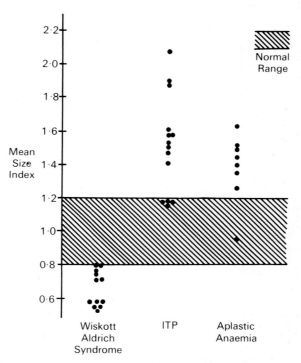

Fig. 16.7 Familial sex-linked thrombocytopenia. (Reproduced from *Acta Paediatrica Scandinavia* (1964), **53**, 365 from a paper by Vestermark and Vestermark, with permission of the authors).

impaired aggregation with ADP and collagen, as well as lack of the normal storage pool of adenine nucleotides in this disease (Gröttum *et al.*, 1969). These authors suggested that these defective platelets are recognized in the reticuloendothelial system as foreign particles. Electron microscopy showed the platelets phagocytosed within macrophages and reticulum cells.

Serological findings typically show absent isohaemagglutinins, reduced IgM and normal or elevated IgG and IgA (Wolf, 1967). Defective cell-mediated immunity has also been demonstrated (Oppenheim *et al.*, 1970). The broad immunological defect involving both humoral and cell-mediated function has been interpreted as a dis-

platelets survive well in these patients platelet transfusion is of value in treating acute haemorrhagic episodes. Experimental lines of treatment include marrow transplantation (Bach *et al.*, 1968), when the immunological deficiency in the patient may favour survival of the graft, and administration of transfer factor (Levin *et al.*, 1970).

(B) SEX-LINKED RECESSIVE THROMBOCYTOPENIA

It appears that thrombocytopenia with this pattern of inheritance can occur either as 'pure' thrombocytopenia or as part of the Wiskott-Aldrich syndrome (WAS). This syndrome is characterized by purpura, recurrent infections and eczema (Wiskott, 1937; Aldrich et al., 1954). Intermediate forms exist, however, and it is possible that most cases of sex-linked thrombocytopenia fall within the broad spectrum of WAS, embracing a wide range of severity (Murphy, 1972A).

Pure thrombocytopenia with inheritance suggesting a sex-linked pattern was first described by Schaar (1963). Four out of 7 sons in the family had apparent 'ITP' from the age of 3 months or less. Two sisters and both parents were normal. Platelet counts as low as 18,000/mm^3 were found in the affected males. Haemorrhagic manifestations included purpura at birth or at a few months, ecchymoses and haematoma of the scalp. Corticosteroids were ineffective but splenectomy was followed by complete correction of the thrombocytopenia in all four patients. No immunological, toxic or infective causative agents could be incriminated and a hereditary aetiology was proposed.

A similar family with 8 thrombocytopenic members was reported by Ata et al. (1965). Although the authors suggested a dominant inheritance with incomplete penetrance in females, a sex-linked pattern was also possible. Seven were males and the one affected female recovered spontaneously. Again there was a poor response to steroids but a complete response to splenectomy in three.

A clear sex-linked inheritance (Fig. 16.8) was shown in a family with thrombocytopenic bleeding

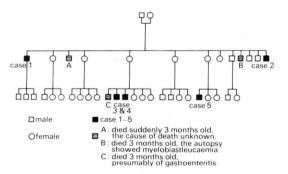

Fig. 16.8 Family tree with platelet counts in autosomal-dominant thrombocytopenia, present in three generations. The propositus (arrow) and his mother were studied in detail. (Reproduced from the *New England Journal of Medicine* (1969), **281**, 857, from a paper by Murphy et al., with permission of the authors.)

and bruising reported by Vestermark and Vestermark (1964). Of 5 affected boys 1 became symptom-free spontaneously at puberty and one responded to splenectomy. The 3 other patients had, in addition to haemorrhagic symptoms, a mild tendency to infection and eczema, suggesting a relationship to WAS. Canales and Mauer (1967) similarly described a family with sex-linked thrombocytopenia but noted that 3 out of the 7 affected males had absent or low isoagglutinins, and a similar number had isolated increases in IgA. These findings led the authors to suggest that the family disorder was a variant of WAS. Another family with sex-linked thrombocytopenia plus mild eczema, but no immunological abnormalities, was included in the study of Murphy et al. (1972) and shown to have a shortened platelet life span and small platelet size; findings identical with and characteristic of WAS. It is these families with features intermediate between 'pure' thrombocytopenia and WAS which have led to the suggestion that all sex-linked recessive forms of thrombocytopenia are part of the same syndrome. As pointed out by Murphy (1972A) these considerations are of more than academic interest. The good platelet response to splenectomy is noteworthy in the reports of Schaar (1963), Vestermark and Vestermark (1964) and Ata et al. (1965). Twelve of Murphy's patients with hereditary thrombocytopenia of various types had splenectomy but in only two did the platelet count become normal. Both the successful cases were in families with a sex-linked recessive inheritance. Whereas it is known that splenectomy is contraindicated in patients with the full-blown immunological defect of WAS because of the serious hazard of subsequent overwhelming infection (Eraklis et al., 1967), it now becomes important to discover if splenectomy is justified in those intermediate cases with minimal or non-existent immunological defect (Murphy, 1972A).

Sex-linked thrombocytopenia with elevated IgA and glomerulonephritis which may or may not be related to WAS has been described by Gutenberger et al. (1970). A syndrome of hereditary thrombocytopenia, nephritis and deafness has also been reported (London et al., 1969).

(C) AUTOSOMAL THROMBOCYTOPENIAS

This is a heterogeneous group of rare disorders including the dominant May-Hegglin anomaly (Hegglin, 1945) and both dominant and recessive forms of pure thrombocytopenia.

The May-Hegglin anomaly is a rare familial disorder with dominant inheritance characterized by giant platelets and inclusions in neutrophils, eosinophils and monocytes but not lymphocytes. These inclusions appear bluish in Romanowsky stained films and are often misleadingly referred to as Döhle bodies (Cawley and Hayhoe, 1972). True Döhle bodies are small basophilic areas of the cytoplasm seen more commonly in patients with severe sepsis or burns (Chapter 15). They consist largely of RNA (Wassmuth et al., 1963). Cawley and Hayhoe (1972) have shown that May-Hegglin inclusions have characteristic electron microscopy features consisting of electron-dense rods plus small particles, probably ribosomes. By contrast true Döhle bodies are smaller and less discrete by light microscopy, only occurring in neutrophils, and on EM consist of rough endoplasmic reticulum as seen in myelocytes. Döhle bodies may reflect increased turnover of neutrophils with a rapid passage through the myelocyte stage (Cawley and Hayhoe, 1972).

The majority of May-Hegglin patients are asymptomatic with only a minority showing haemorrhagic manifestations (Najean et al., 1966), and these not in the neonatal period. The bleeding is due to thrombocytopenia which has occurred in over one third of such patients (Oski et al., 1962; Buchanan et al., 1964; Easton and Fessas, 1966). Megakaryocytes are present in normal numbers in the marrow (Davis and Wilson, 1966). These authors also found shortened platelet survival, but a more recent investigation by Godwin and Ginsberg (1971) showed normal platelet survival, leading to the suggestion that thrombocytopenia in this disorder is due to defective megakaryocyte fragmentation.

Autosomal dominant thrombocytopenia. Wooley in 1956 briefly reported what appeared to be 'familial ITP'. A boy of 5 had a platelet count of 5,000/mm^3 and purpura with increased megakaryocytes in the marrow. He showed an excellent response to splenectomy. The father had 74,000 platelets with a bleeding tendency since childhood, and the boy's sister was mildly affected. Seip in 1963, in a more extensive investigation, reported a mother and two sons with moderate thrombocytopenia. Megakaryocytes were normal or increased and the ^{51}Cr platelet survival was normal. An extensive family study by Bithell et al. (1965) showed mild thrombocytopenia in 11 members over 3 generations. Inheritance appeared to be autosomal dominant. A similar family (Fig. 16.9) was investigated by Murphy et al. (1969). The clinical and haematological picture was quite similar to ITP but thrombokinetic studies clearly distinguished between the two disorders. Survival of the patients' platelets was shortened both in the patients themselves and in normal volunteers. Platelets from healthy individuals showed normal survival if transfused into the patients, whereas

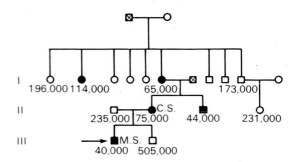

Fig. 16.9 Family tree, with platelet counts. Thrombocytopenia was present in three generations. The propositus (arrow) and his mother were studied in detail. Reproduced, with permission, from Murphy et al. (1969), N.E.J.M., **281**, 257.

this is not the case in ITP (Abrahamsen, 1970). Murphy et al. (1969) interpreted these results as indicating accelerated platelet destruction resulting from an intrinsic platelet defect, rather than from one extrinsic to the platelet. Splenectomy in two patients was followed by improvement in the thrombocytopenia but platelet survival remained short. Stavem et al. (1969) found the opposite pattern of platelet survival in a family with a similar pattern of inheritance. The patient's platelets had a shortened survival in their own circulation, but survived normally in healthy recipients. Some factor or mechanism operating in the patient's blood or vascular system which shortened the life span of autologous or transfused platelets was postulated, making this a unique disease. Another unusual feature was a disproportionately prolonged Ivy bleeding time (e.g. over 30 minutes when the platelet count was 98,000/mm^3). The authors pointed out, however, that a number of other reports show this feature. It is certainly to be expected in those patients with associated qualitative and quantitative platelet defects such as the Bernard Soulier syndrome, discussed in a later section.

Autosomal recessive thrombocytopenia has only rarely been described. Roberts and Smith (1950) reported a family where 4 children, 1 boy and 3 girls, died of a haemorrhagic diathesis at ages between 3½ and 9 years. In three the platelet counts were determined and found to be low (15,000–30,000/mm^3). Post-mortem histology showed normal numbers of megakaryocytes. Splenectomy was performed in one child without benefit. Both parents and all 4 grandparents, as well as 6 other children, were normal suggesting an autosomal recessive inheritance. One further family with this type of inheritance has been reported (Murphy, 1972B).

Murphy *et al.* (1972) have proposed a more detailed classification of hereditary thrombocytopenia based upon (a) platelet size, (b) platelet life span, and (c) inheritance pattern. Harker (1970) studied three such families having normal platelet survival and found a three-fold increase in megakaryocyte mass. This was interpreted as indicating *ineffective thrombopoiesis* as the basic cause of the thrombocytopenia in these particular patients.

8 Metabolic causes of neonatal thrombocytopenia

Hyperglycinaemia with ketosis and the closely related metabolic disorder of methylmalonic acidaemia may cause periodic thrombocytopenia during infancy, as well as the neutropenia already discussed (Morrow *et al.*, 1969). Infants with these metabolic disorders present with lethargy, vomiting and ketosis in the neonatal period. A similar disorder, isovaleric acidaemia, is associated with a general marrow hypoplasia causing both thrombocytopenia and neutropenia (Allen *et al.*, 1969). The haematological abnormalities were corrected by a low leucine diet in the one infant in which this was tried. Oski and Naiman (1972D) suggest that the factor of severe acidosis common to each of these disorders may play a role in the mechanism of the haematological defects.

Neonatal thrombocytopenic purpura has also been reported in three successive infants born to a hyperthyroid mother (Zaidi and Mortimer, 1965). Other clinical features included jaundice, hepatosplenomegaly and respiratory distress. The mechanism of the thrombocytopenia is unknown.

9 Congenital leukaemia

These infants may present with thrombocytopenic purpura, ecchymoses and a characteristic nodular skin infiltration (Fortina and Petrocini, 1953). Hepatosplenomegaly is usually present. The peripheral blood commonly shows a gross leucocytosis of up to 500,000/mm^3. In about 90 per cent of cases the cytological diagnosis is myeloblastic in contrast to the more usual lymphoblastic leukaemia seen in older children (Pochedly, 1971). Other aspects of this disease are discussed in Chapter 20. Leukaemoid reactions are also common in the newborn with Down's syndrome (mongolism). In translocation mongolism thrombocytopenia has been found in association with myeloid metaplasia and haemolysis (Behrman *et al.*, 1966). It has been my own experience that most bizarre blood pictures showing all these features may occur during the newborn period in mongols, especially of the translocation variety.

DRUG-INDUCED THROMBOCYTOPENIA

Although relatively rare in childhood this enters into the differential diagnosis of acute acquired thrombocytopenic purpura such as ITP or the thrombocytopenia associated with infections. Drugs can cause thrombocytopenia by two different mechanisms: marrow depression or increased platelet destruction. Table 16.6 lists some of the drugs known to cause thrombocytopenia.

The drugs that can cause thrombocytopenia by marrow depression are essentially the same as those that can cause pancytopenia and aplastic anaemia. Instead of affecting all three cell lines they may, in some patients, selectively depress the megakaryocytes. As in the case of drug-induced aplastic anaemia it is useful to distinguish between drugs which will invariably produce marrow depression if given in large enough doses (e.g. anti-leukaemic drugs such as 6-MP, methotrexate, cyclophosphamide, cytosine arabinoside) and those which do so only when an idiosyncrasy to the particular drug exists (e.g. to chloramphenicol).

Of the drugs causing excessive platelet destruction the majority do so by virtue of an immune mechanism (Table 16.7), drug-haptene disease, but Ristocetin differs in this respect, exerting a direct effect upon platelet function (Gangarosa *et al.*, 1960).

A marrow examination will distinguish between thrombocytopenia due to toxic depression, when the megakaryocytes are scanty or absent, and thrombocytopenia due to peripheral destruction, when they will be normal or increased. It will also exclude marrow infiltration by tumour or leukaemia, which might enter into the differential diagnosis. *In vivo* and *in vitro* tests are available which can detect drug-haptene disease (Table 16.8).

Mechanism of drug-haptene disease

This was first elucidated for Sedormid purpura by Ackroyd (1949). Drugs of M.Wt. 500–1,000 which are unable to initiate immunity themselves but may do so when attached to proteins are termed haptenes. The resulting antibody will then

276 PAEDIATRIC HAEMATOLOGY

Table 16.6 Drugs known to cause thrombocytopenia

Type	Specific drug	
Antimitotic drugs	All*	
Antibiotics	Sulphonamides Penicillin Chloramphenicol* Streptomycin	Tetracyclines PAS INAH Ristocetin
Diuretics	Acetazolamide Chlorothiazide*	
Antidiabetics	Chlorpropamide Tolbutamide	
Hypnotics etc.	Phenobarbitone Prochlorperazine Meprobamate Chlorpromazine	Phenytoin Troxidone* Methoin* Promazine
Analgesics	Phenylbutazone* Salicylates	Amidopyrine Indomethacin
Metals	Gold* Mercury Bismuth Organic arsenicals*	
Various	Digitoxin Quinine Quinidine Ergot Potassium perchlorate Antazoline	Methyldopa Thiouracil Dinitrophenol Oestrogens Penicillamine Phenindione

*Drugs particularly prone to cause thrombocytopenia.
Reproduced, by permission, from Prankard (1972), Clinics in Haematology,
1, *330.*

Table 16.7 Drugs associated with induction of immunothrombocytopenia

Sedatives	Meprobamate, phenobarbital, allylisopropylbarbituric acid, allylisopropylbarbituric acid, allylisopropyl-acetylurea (Sedormid)
Cinchona alkaloids	Quinine and quinidine
Antibiotics	Oxytetracycline, chloramphenicol, streptomycin, ristocetin, para-aminosalicylic acid
Antibacterial sulfonamides	Sulfasoxazole (Gantrisin), sulfadiazine, sulfamethoxypiridadine (Kynex), sulfadimidine, sulfamethazine
Other sulfonamide derivatives	Tolbutamide (Orinase), chloro-thiazide (Diuril), acetazolamide (Diamox), chlorpropamide (Diabinese), diazoxide
Other agents	Dinitrophenol, gold, mercurials, bismuth compounds, arsenicals, potassium iodide, digitoxin, estrogens, ergotrate, thiourea, carbamezepine

Reproduced, by permission, from Pochedly and Ente (1972), Pediatric Clinics of
North America, **19,** *1101.*

Table 16.8 Tests for demonstration of specific antibody in drug-induced immunothrombocytopenia

In vitro tests
1. Direct microscopic demonstration of agglutination or lysis of patient's platelets in the presence of patient's serum and the drug
2. Complement fixation tests for detection of drug-induced platelet antibody
3. Indirect demonstration of alteration of platelet function or behavior in the presence of sensitized serum and the drug
   (a) Inhibition of clot retraction
   (b) Increased liberation of platelet factor 3 by damaged platelets
   (c) Increased amino acid generation by damaged platelets
   (d) Increased platelet sedimentation rate
4. Precipitate formation by the drug on gel diffusion

In vivo tests (cutaneous)
1. Patch testing
2. Intradermal injection
3. Passive transfer reaction

Reproduced, by permission, from Pochedly and Ente (1972), *Pediatric Clinics of North America*, **19**, 1102.

interact only with original drug-protein complex; not with the drug or protein separately.

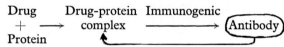

In the case of drug-haptene thrombocytopenia it was thought that the protein concerned was a platelet component, and that the antibody was specific to the drug-platelet complex. The clinical consequence was recurrent thrombocytopenic purpura *whenever the drug was taken, but not at other times*, differing thereby from ITP. Drugs capable of producing drug-haptene purpura are shown in Table 16.7.

More recently it has been demonstrated that it may be a metabolic product of the drug, rather than the drug itself, which is the haptene. This was shown in a patient who developed gross purpura with a platelet count of 4,000/mm³ while taking an analgesic mixture containing aspirin, caffeine, salicylamide and n-acetyl-p-aminophenol (NAPA, also known as acetaminophenol). His plasma was found to contain antibody only to a metabolite of NAPA, the sulphate conjugate of the drug (Eisner and Shahidi, 1972). Shulman (1972) has pointed out that most drugs are not chemically reactive enough to form the irreversible complexes with proteins necessary for sensitization, but the metabolic or oxidative products of drugs are often more reactive (i.e. polar) and so able to form immunogenic complexes. A practical consequence of this is that a common metabolite from two closely related drugs might result in an individual being apparently sensitive to both. Shulman quotes work to suggest that this is the case with quinine and quinidine which are both oxidized to the more reactive quininone. Antibodies reacting with quininone are present in 20 per cent of patients sensitized to quinine or quinidine.

The mechanism of interaction of antibody with platelets may also differ slightly from that originally proposed by Ackroyd. More recent experimental evidence suggests that drug-antibody complexes are absorbed to the surface of the platelet, rather than that antibodies react against drug-platelet complexes (Shulman, 1972). Karpatkin (1971) has suggested that platelets actually phagocytose the antigen-antibody complexes, triggering irreversible platelet aggregation *in vivo*.

1. Antibody + drug or metabolite ⟶ Antigen-antibody complex
2. Antigen-antibody complex —Cell→ Antigen-antibody cell complex

This *final* reaction is similar to that currently postulated in the pathogenesis of ITP, where the antigen may be a viral fragment.

Clinical features of drug-induced thrombocytopenia include purpura and haemorrhage from mucous membranes which may be severe and fulminating. The onset may be accompanied by fever and shock. Fatal intracranial haemorrhage has been recorded (Weisfuse *et al.*, 1954). Blood and marrow findings are similar to those in ITP. Only the history of drug ingestion gives an initial clue to the diagnosis. On stopping the drug the haemorrhagic symptoms and thrombocytopenia resolve in a few days. Steroid therapy is of no benefit and confuses the diagnostic situation since it is then difficult to know whether the improvement is due to a response to the steroids (as in ITP) or to cessation of the drug (Crosby and Kaufman, 1964).

Confirmation that a particular drug was responsible should be made when the platelet count has returned to normal. Attempts to incriminate a drug by giving a further, small provocative dose are to be condemned on the grounds that this is not without danger. *In vitro* tests should be attempted first, followed by *in vivo* cutaneous tests if these prove inconclusive. Available tests are shown in Table 16.8. The two simplest tests are inhibition of clot retraction by a 0·02 mg/ml solution of the drug *in vitro* (Weintraub *et al.*, 1962; Young *et al.*, 1966) and a patch test using a saturated solution of the drug in propylene glycol (Ackroyd, 1949). Many tests, however, may fail if indeed it is a metabolite rather than the drug itself which is responsible. Perhaps the most sensitive and comprehensive test in this respect was that used by Eisner and Shahidi (1972). In this test plasma from a normal volunteer who had taken the drug contained enough of the metabolite to cause complement fixation and platelet factor 3 release in mixtures of normal platelets plus the patient's serum.

It is important to identify the offending drug so that correct advice is given concerning its absolute avoidance in future. This subject has been well reviewed by Horowitz and Nachman (1965), Karpatkin (1971) and by Pochedly and Ente (1972).

Post-transfusion thrombocytopenic purpura

Sudden onset of severe thrombocytopenic purpura approximately one week following a blood transfusion was first described by Shulman et al. in 1961. A further 9 cases have now been reported and in every one it has been shown that the patient's platelets lacked the antigen Pl^{A1} and that anti-Pl^{A1} had developed after the transfusion. Ninety seven per cent of individuals are Pl^{A1} +ve. The mystery was how an antibody to the foreign platelets could cause profound thrombocytopenia in the patient, sometimes lasting up to a month. It has been suggested (Cimo and Aster, 1972; Gockerman and Shulman, 1973) that antigen-antibody complexes are produced by interaction of the transfused incompatible platelets (or their fragments) and the antibody. These antigen-antibody complexes may become adsorbed on to the patient's own (compatible) platelets causing thrombocytopenia *by the same mechanism* as described above for drug-haptene disease and for ITP. Herein lies the main justification for discussion of the syndrome here. It has not been described in childhood, all cases having been middle aged or elderly women with a history of previous pregnancies. The implication is that primary immunization of Pl^{A1}—ve mothers originated from their Pl^{A1}+ve babies, and that subsequent blood transfusion caused a secondary immune response. In the report by Cima and Aster (1972) it appeared that a plasma transfusion containing platelet fragments, was the precipitating event rather than a whole blood transfusion. These authors also describe the successful treatment of the condition by a 70 per cent exchange transfusion, and suggest that this success was as much

due to removal of the antigen as of the antibody. There was no response to steroids. A fatality due to intracranial haemorrhage has occurred (Gockerman and Shulman, 1973). A recent report by Abramson, Eisenberg and Aster (1974) describes a patient with both anti-Pl^{A1} and anti-HLa anti-platelet antibodies who showed a rapid rise in platelet count following plasmapheresis.

Thrombopoietin deficiency

One patient has been described with chronic thrombocytopenia and numerous immature megakaryocytes in the marrow, but refractory to splenectomy, and in whom infusion of normal plasma was followed by a rise in a platelet count to normal with apparent maturation of the megakaryocytes (Schulman et al., 1960A). The effect was transient but repeatable. The authors suggested that their patient had a congenital deficiency of thrombopoietin. Subsequent investigation (Schulman et al., 1960B) showed that plasma from ITP patients produced the same response, confirming that ITP is not due to deficiency of thrombopoietin. Nevertheless the possibility was considered that the numerous immature megakaryocytes present in ITP might be further stimulated to platelet production by normal plasma infusions. Fresh frozen plasma (10 to 30 ml/kg) was given to 7 children with ITP and a significant rise in platelet count was found in 4. In 3 of these the rise was transitory. Berglund (1962) reported similar findings in 6 children with ITP. These observations should not be construed as indicating that true ITP is due to thrombopoietin deficiency, nor are they of practical therapeutic value except perhaps on rare occasions. They could be relevant, however, to interpretation of changes of platelet count related to transfusion in ITP patients.

Cyclical thrombocytopenia

Thrombocytopenia at intervals of 10 to 25 days has been seen in children with cyanotic congenital heart disease (Goldschmidt and Fonio, 1972). These authors found high thrombopoietin levels in the plasma at times of thrombocytopenia and low levels when the platelet count was normal. When the thrombopoietin level was high there was a 'shift to the left' in the megakaryocytes, which was interpreted as evidence of homeostatic stimulation. De Gabrielle and Pennington (1967) found that platelets adsorbed thrombopoietin from plasma thereby producing a very simple form of 'feed-back' mechanism.

Hypersplenism

As well as causing neutropenia and mild anaemia this quite consistently causes thrombocytopenia in the 50,000 to 80,000/mm³ range. The marrow shows normal numbers of megakaryocytes. In paediatric practice the commonest cause of hypersplenism is chronic portal hypertension. Other causes include thalassaemia major and hepatic fibrosis due to transfusion haemosiderosis in longstanding erythrogenesis imperfecta. The gradual appearance of thrombocytopenia in this disease is otherwise mystifying. In the case of Gaucher disease the fate of the sequestrated platelets has been traced to ingestion by the actual Gaucher cells themselves (Green *et al.*, 1971). Electron microscopy studies showed the presence of platelets as well as red cells and granulocytes within the Gaucher cells. It is, however, probably the red cells and granulocytes that contribute most to the accumulation of cerebroside in these cells since the platelet content of cerebroside is very low.

Although the platelet count is lowered in hypersplenism this is seldom sufficiently marked to produce a haemostatic defect. The Ivy bleeding time is usually normal and this may be because the increased platelet turnover results in most of the circulating platelets being 'young' and with full haemostatic activity. This is of practical importance when screening for a haemorrhagic state in such patients prior to percutaneous portosplenograms. It is my practice to take the Ivy bleeding time into consideration in evaluating the significance of moderate thrombocytopenia (e.g. 70,000/mm³) in this context. A further complication arises, however, when the prothrombin complex is lowered due to associated liver disease, and this may need correction independently of the thrombocytopenia since a double defect is of more serious haemostatic significance. In patients with hypersplenism undergoing splenectomy (e.g. as part of a lienorenal shunt procedure) it is a useful practice to administer a platelet transfusion immediately after the splenic pedicle has been clamped. Splenectomy is never indicated purely to correct the thrombocytopenia of hypersplenism.

Microangiopathic haemolytic anaemia (MAHA) and disseminated intravascular coagulation (DIC)

Thrombocytopenia is a usual, but not obligatory, component of MAHA. A list of the main causes of MAHA in childhood is given in Table 9.1. Considerable debate exists as to which of these diseases where platelets are consumed or trapped in the microvasculature are accompanied by disseminated (or even localized) intravascular coagulation. Resolution of these problems depends upon demonstration of lowered levels or shortened *in vivo* survival of the consumable coagulation factors (fibrinogen, Factor V, prothrombin and Factor VIII) and raised levels of fibrin degradation products (FDPs). This aspect is discussed in the later chapter on acquired coagulation disorders. When actual DIC is occurring there is a rapid fall in platelet count, and other consumable coagulation components, but the significance of the level at a particular time depends upon knowledge of the preceding, normal level for that individual (Deykin, 1970). DIC can therefore not be fully excluded upon a single platelet count, and it is my practice to perform platelet counts at least twice daily in ill children in whom DIC is suspected.

The prime importance of thrombocytopenia in MAHA and DIC is in drawing attention to the diagnosis. It also serves as an index of successful correction of the underlying process. The marrow shows normal or increased numbers of megakaryocytes, the thrombocytopenia being due to shortened platelet survival. Steroids are ineffective and splenectomy is not indicated. The mechanisms and sites of platelet destruction or sequestration in the various syndromes of MAHA or DIC are discussed in Chapter 19.

Marrow encroachment

Amegakaryocytic thrombocytopenia due to impaired platelet production occurs secondary to marrow infiltration in leukaemia, tumour (particularly neuroblastoma) or reticulosis; due to encroachment upon the marrow cavity in marble bone disease (osteopetrosis) and in aplastic anaemia. These disorders are discussed more fully in other sections of the book. A leuco-erythroblastic blood picture is usual in all these conditions with the exception of aplastic anaemia.

THROMBOCYTOSIS

A platelet count in excess of 500,000/mm³ is sometimes seen in association with chronic inflammatory disease (Morowitz *et al.*, 1968) or malignancy (Levin and Conley, 1964). An inexplicable association has also been found in half the reported cases of infantile cortical hyperostosis

PAEDIATRIC HAEMATOLOGY

(Pickering and Cuddigan, 1969). Primary thrombocythaemia associated with myocardial infarction and widespread thromboses have rarely been described in infants (Sanyal *et al.*, 1966) and children (Spach *et al.*, 1963). The adult disorder haemorrhagic thrombocythaemia has only occasionally been seen in late childhood (Ozer *et al.*, 1960).

Postsplenectomy thrombocytosis with counts in the region of 1,000,000/mm³, are common in the immediate postsplenectomy period for diseases such as hereditary spherocytosis (Lipson *et al.*, 1959). No report of thromboembolism from this cause has, however, been reported in a collection of data from 1413 splenectomies in childhood (Eraklis *et al.*, 1972) and postoperative anticoagulation is not indicated.

Gross, Keefer and Newman (1964) also found thrombocytosis (up to 750,000/mm³) accompanying moderate iron deficiency anaemia in children between 8 and 24 months. They suggested stimulation of platelet production 'in a manner analagous to the erythropoietin increase seen in many anaemic states'. In the most severely anaemic children with Hb levels less than 5 g/100 ml, however, the platelet count was 100,000/mm³ or less, with some as low as 50,000/mm³. Iron therapy was followed by a rise in platelet count coinciding with the reticulocyte peak with parenteral iron or following it with oral iron.

In a succinct recent review of thrombocytosis in infants and children Addiego, Mentzer and Dallman (1974) list the conditions associated with thrombocytosis as shown in Table 16.9 below.

Table 16.9 Conditions associated with thrombocytosis in infants and children

Hereditary
  Asplenia★
  Myeloproliferative disorder in Down's syndrome
Nutritional
  Iron deficiency★
Megaloblastic anaemia
  Vitamin E deficiency★
Metabolic
  Hyperadrenalism
Immune
  Graft vs host reaction
  nephrotic syndrome
Infectious
  Viral
  Bacterial
  Mycobacterial
Drug response
  Vinca alkaloids★
  Citrovorum factor
  Corticosteroid therapy
Neoplastic
  Chronic (adult) myeloid leukaemia★
  Histiocytosis
  Carcinoma
  Lymphoma
  Megakaryocytic leukaemia
Traumatic
  Surgery★
  Fractures
  Haemorrhage★
Miscellaneous
  Splenectomy★
  Caffey's disease
  Inflammatory bowel disease
  Pulmonary embolism
  Thrombophlebitis
  Cerebrovascular accident
  Sracoidosis
  Idiopathic

★Conditions in which thrombocytosis is common.
Data reproduced by permission of the authors and publishers from Addiego et al., (1974), J. Pediat., 85, 805.

REFERENCES

Aas, K. A. & Gardner, F. H. (1958) Survival of blood platelets labelled with chromium. *J. Clin. Invest.*, **37**, 1257.

Aballi, A. J., Puapondh, Y. & Desposito, F. (1968) Platelet counts in thriving premature infants. *Pediat.*, **42**, 685.

Abrahamsen, A. R. (1970) Survival of ⁵¹Cr-labelled autologous and isologous platelets as differential diagnostic aid in thrombocytopenic states. *Scand. J. Haematol.*, **7**, 525.

Abramson, N., Eisenberg, P. D. & Aster, R. H. (1974) Post-transfusion purpura: Immunologic aspects and therapy. *New Eng. J. Med.*, **291**, 1163.

Ackroyd, J. F. (1949) The pathogenesis of thrombocytopenic purpura due to hypersensitivity to Sedormid. *Clinical Science*, **7**, 249.

Ackroyd, J. F. (1949) Three cases of thrombocytopenic purpura occurring after rubella, with review of purpura associated with infections. *Quart. Med. J.*, **18**, 299.

Addiego, J. E., Mentzer, W. C. & Dallman, P. R. (1974) Thrombocytosis in infants and children. *J. Pediat.*, **85**, 805.

Adner, M. M., Fisch, G. R., Starobin, S. G. & Aster, R. H. (1969) Use of 'compatible' platelet transfusions in the treatment of congenital isoimmune thrombocytopenic purpura. *New Eng. J. Med.*, **280**, 244.

Ahn, Y. S., Harrington, W. J., Seelman, R. C. & Eytel, C. S. (1974) Vincristine therapy of idoipathic and secondary thrombocytopenias. *New Eng. J. Med.*, **291**, 376.

Aldrich, R. A., Steinberg, A. G. & Campbell, D. C. (1954) Pedigree demonstrating a sex-linked recessive condition characterized by draining ears, eczematoid dermatitis and bloody diarrhoea. *Pediatrics*, **13**, 133.

Allen, D. M., Necheles, T. F., Rieker, R. & Senior, B. (1969) Reversible neonatal pancytopenia due to isovaleric acidemia. *Abstract Soc. Pediat. Res. (Atlantic City)*, 156.

Andre, R., Ducas, P., Vergoz, D. & Mayer, M. (1965) Purpura thrombocytopenique neonatal thrombopenie maternelle cliniquement latente. *Arch. Franç. de Pediat.*, **22**, 167.

Anthony, B. & Krivit, W. (1962) Neonatal thrombocytopenic purpura. *Pediatrics*, **30**, 776.

Aster, R. H. (1966) Pooling of platelets in the spleen: role in the pathogenesis of 'hypersplenic' thrombocytopenia. *J. Clin. Invest.*, **45**, 645.

Aster, R. H. & Keene, W. R. (1969) Sites of platelet destruction in idiopathic thrombocytopenic purpura. *Brit. J. Haemat.*, **16**, 61.

Aster, R. H. (1972) Platelet sequestration studies in man. *Brit. J. Haemat.*, **22**, 259.

Ata, M., Fisher, O. D. & Holman, C. A. (1965) Inherited thrombocytopenia. *Lancet*, **1**, 119.

Bach, F. H., Albertini, R. J., Joo, P., Anderson, J. L. & Bortin, M. M. (1968) Bone-marrow transplantation in a patient with the Wiskott-Aldrich syndrome. *Lancet*, **ii**, 1364.

Bachand, A. J., Rubenstein, J. & Morrison, A. N. (1967) Thrombocytopenic purpura following live measles vaccine. *Am. J. Dis. Child.*, **113**, 283.

Baldini, M. (1966) Idiopathic thrombocytopenic purpura. *New Eng. J. Med.*, **274**, 1245.

Baldini, M. G. (1972) Idiopathic thrombocytopenic purpura and the ITP syndrome. *Med. Clin. N. Amer.*, **56**, 47.

Baldini, M., Kim, B., Steiner, M., Kuramoto, A., Okuma, M. & Otridge, B. W. (1969) Metabolic platelet defect in Wiskott-Aldrich syndrome. *Pediat. Res.*, **3**, 377.

Behrman, R. E., Sigler, A. T. & Patcheesky, A. S. (1966) Abnormal haematopoiesis in 2 of 3 siblings with mongolism. *J. Pediat.*, **68**, 569.

Bensel, R. W. ten, Stadlan, E. M. & Krivit, W. (1960) The development of malignancy in the course of the Aldrich syndrome. *J. Pediat.*, **68**, 761.

Berglund, G. (1962) Plasma transfusion treatment of six children with idiopathic thrombocytopenic purpura. *Acta Paed.*, **51**, 523.

Bessis, M. (1956) *Cytology of the Blood Forming Organs*. New York: Grune & Stratton.

Bithell, T. C., Didisheim, P., Cartwright, G. E. & Wintrobe, M. M. (1965) Thrombocytopenia inherited as an autosomal dominant trait. *Blood*, **25**, 231.

Bithell, T. C., Athens, J. W., Cartwright, G. E. & Wintrobe, M. M. (1967) Radioactive diisopropyl fluorophosphate as a platelet label: an evaluation of *in vitro* and *in vivo* technics. *Blood*, **29**, 354.

Blaese, R. M., Strober, W., Brown, R. S. & Waldmann, T. A. (1968) The Wiskott-Aldrich syndrome: A disorder with a possible defect in antigen processing or recognition. *Lancet*, **ii**, 1056.

Bloom, G. E., Warner, S., Gerald, P. S. & Diamond, L. K. (1966) Chromosome abnormalities in constitutional aplastic anemia. *New Eng. J. Med.*, **274**, 8.

Brecher, G. & Cronkite, E. P. (1950) Morphology and enumeration of human blood platelets. *J. Appl. Phys.*, **3**, 365.

Brizel, H. & Raccuglia, G. (1965) Giant hemangioma with thrombocytopenia: Radioisotopic demonstration of platelet sequestration. *Blood*, **26**, 751.

Buchanan, J., Pearce, L. & Wetherley-Mein, G. (1964) The May-Hegglin anomaly: a family report and chromosome study. *Brit. J. Haemat.*, **10**, 508.

Canales, L. & Mauer, A. M. (1967) Sex-linked hereditary thrombocytopenia as a variant of Wiskott-Aldrich syndrome. *New Eng. J. Med.*, **277**, 899.

Cawley, J. C. & Hayhoe, F. G. J. (1972) The inclusions of the May-Hegglin anomaly and Döhle bodies of infection: An ultrastructural comparison. *Brit. J. Haemat.*, **22**, 491.

Chessels, J. M. & Wigglesworth, J. S. (1971) Haemostatic failure in babies with Rhesus isoimmunization. *Arch. Dis. Childh.*, **46**, 38.

Christodoulou, C. & Werner, B. (1967) A girl with 18-trisomy and thrombocytopenia. *Acta Genet. (Basel)*, **17**, 77.

Cimo, P. L. & Aster, R. H. (1972) Post-transfusion purpura. Successful treatment by exchange transfusion. *New Eng. J. Med.*, **287**, 290.

Clancy, R. (1972) Cellular immunity to autologous platelets and serum-blocking factors in idiopathic thrombocytopenic purpura. *Lancet*, **1**, 6.

Cohen, P., Gardner, F. H. & Barnett, G. O. (1961) Reclassification of the thrombocytopenias by Cr^{51}-labelling method for measuring platelet life span. *New Eng. J. Med.*, **264**, 1294.

Cohen, P. & Gardner, F. H. (1961) The thrombocytopenic effect of sustained high-dose prednisone therapy in thrombocytopenic purpura. *New Eng. J. Med.*, **265**, 611.

Colombani, J. & Dausset, J. (1969) Thrombopénies néo-natales immunologiques. *Rev. Med. Suisse Rom.*, **89**, 2.

Cooper, W. & Martin, J. (1962) Hemangioma of the liver with thrombocytopenia. *Roentgenol.*, **88**, 751.

Crosby, W. H. & Kaufman, R. M. (1964) Drug-induced blood dyscrasias. IV. Thrombocytopenia. *J.A.M.A.*, **189**, 417.

Crosby, W. H. (1972) splenectomy in hematologic disorders. *New Eng. J. Med.*, **286**, 1252.

Dameshek, W. & Miller, E. B. (1946) The megakaryocytes in idiopathic thrombocytopenic purpura. a form of hypersplenism. *Blood*, **1**, 27.

Dameshek, W., Ebbe, S., Greenberg, L. & Baldini, M. (1963) Recurrent idiopathic thrombocytopenic purpura. *New Eng. J. Med.*, **269**, 647.

Dauset, J., Colombani, J. & Colombani, M. (1969) Studies of leukopenias and thrombocytopenias by the direct antiglobulin consumption test on leucocytes and/or platelets. *Blood*, **18**, 672.

Davis, J. W. & Wilson, S. J. (1966) Platelet survival in the May-Hegglin anomaly. *Brit. J. Haemat.*, **12**, 61.

Desai, R. & Creger, W. (1963) Maternofetal passage of leucocytes and platelets in man. *Blood*, **21**, 665.

Deykin, D. (1970) The clinical challenge of disseminated intravascular coagulation. *New Eng. J. Med.*, **283**, 636.

Diamond, L. K. (1969) Splenectomy in childhood and the hazard of overwhelming infection. *Pediatrics*, **43**, 886.

Dignan, P. St. J., Mauer, A. M. & Frantz, C. (1967) Phocomelia with congenital hypoplastic thrombocytopenia and myeloid leukaemoid reactions. *J. Pediat.*, **70**, 561.

Dixon, R., Rosse, W. & Ebbert, L. (1975) Quantitative determination of antibody in idiopathic thrombocytopenic purpura: Correlation of serum and platelet-bound antibody with clinical response. *New Eng. J. Med.*, **292**, 230.

Doan, C. A., Bouroncle, B. A. & Wiseman, B. K. (1960) Idiopathic and secondary thrombocytopenic purpura: clinical study and evaluation of 381 cases over a period of 28 years. *Ann. Intern. Med.*, **53**, 861.

Easton, J. & Fessas, C. (1966) The incidence of Döhle bodies in various diseases and their association with thrombocytopenia. *Brit. J. Haemat.*, **12**, 54.

Ebbe, S. & Stohlman, F. J. (1965) Megakaryopoiesis in the rat. *Blood*, **26**, 20.

Edison, J., Blaese, R., White, J. & Krivet, W. (1968) Defibrination syndrome in an infant born after abruptio placentae. *J. Pediat.*, **72**, 342.

Eisenstein, E. M. (1966) Congenital amegakaryocytic thrombocytopenic purpura. *Clin. Pediat.*, **5**, 143.

Eisner, E. V. & Shahidi, N. T. (1972) Immune thrombocytopenia due to a drug metabolite. *New Eng. J. Med.*, **297**, 376.

Ekert, H. & Mathew, R. Y. (1967) Platelet counts and plasma fibrinogen levels in erythroblastosis foetalis. *Med. J. Austr.*, **2**, 844.

Eraklis, A. J., Kevy, S. V., Diamond, L. K. & Gross, R. E. (1967) Hazard of overwhelming infection after splenectomy in childhood. *New Eng. J. Med.*, **276**, 1225.

Eraklis, A. J. & Filler, R. M. (1972) Splenectomy in childhood: A review of 1413 cases. *J. Pediatric Surgery*, **7**, 382.

Faloon, W. W., Greene, R. W. & Lozer, E. L. (1952) Hemostatic defect in thrombocytopenia as studied by the use of ACTH and cortisone. *Am. J. Med.*, **13**, 12.

Fama, P. G., Paton, W. B. & Bostock, M. I. (1964) Thrombocytopenic purpura complicating mumps. *Brit. med. J.*, **11**, 1244.

Ferguson, A. W. (1960 Rubella as a cause of thrombocytopenic purpura. *Pediatrics*, **25**, 400.

Fogel, B. J., Amias, D. & Kung, F. (1968) Platelet counts in healthy premature infants. *J. Pediat.*, **73**, 108.

Fortina, A. & Petrocini, S. (1953) Contributo alto studio della manifestazoni cutanee nelle leucemie dell' infanzia. *Pediatrica*, **61**, 199.

French, J. E. (1967) Blood platelets: morphological studies on their properties and life cycle. *Brit. J. Haemat.*, **13**, 595.

Froehlich, L. A. & Housler, M. (1971) Neonatal thrombocytopenia and chorangioma. *J. Pediat.*, **78**, 516.

Gabrielle, G. de & Penington, D. G. (1967) Regulation of platelet production: Thrombopoietin. *Brit. J. Haemat.*, **13**, 210.

Gangarosa, E. J., Johnson, B. S. & Ramos, H. S. (1960) Ristocetin-induced thrombocytopenia: Site and mechanism of action. *Arch. Intern. Med.*, **105**, 84.

Gardner, F. H. (1972) Platelet kinetics and life span. *Clinics in Hematology*, **1**, 307.

Garg, S. K., Amorosi, E. L. & Karpatkin, S. (1971) Use of the megathrombocyte as an index of megakaryocyte number. *New Eng. J. Med.*, **284**, 11.

Geme, J. W. St., Prince, J. T., Burke, B. A., Good, R. A. & Krivit, W. (1965) Impaired cellular resistance to herpes simplex virus in Wiskott-Aldrich syndrome. *New Eng. J. Med.*, **273**, 229.

Gockerman, J. P. & Shulman, N. R. (1973) Isoantibody specificity in post-transfusion purpura. *Blood*, **41**, 817.

Godwin, H. A. & Ginsberg, A. D. (1971) May-Hegglin anomaly: ? Defect in megakaryocyte fragmentation. Abstract No. 279, 14th Annual Meeting of the American Soc. Hematol. New York: Grunn & Stratton.

Goldschmidt, B. & Fonio, R. (1972) Cyclic fluctuations in platelet count, megakaryocyte maturation and thrombopoietin activity in cyanotic congenital heart disease. *Acta Paediat. Scand.*, **61**, 310.

Goodhue, P. A. & Evans, T. S. (1963) Idiopathic thrombocytopenic purpura in pregnancy. *Obst. Gynec. Surv.*, **18**, 671.

Gordon, R. R. (1960) Aldrich's syndrome: Familial thrombocytopenia, eczema and infection. *Arch. Dis. Childh.*, **35**, 362.

Gotoff, S. & Behrman, R. (1970) Neonatal septicaemia. *J. Pediat.*, **76**, 142.

Green, D., Battifora, H. A., Smith, R. T. & Rossi, E. C. (1971) Thrombocytopenia in Gaucher's disease. *Ann. Int. Med.*, **74**, 727.

Gross, S., Keefer, V. & Newman, A. J. (1964) The platelets in iron-deficiency anemia. I. The response to oral and parental iron. *Pediatrics*, **34**, 315.

Gröttum, K. A., Hovig, T., Holmsen, H., Abrahamsen, A. F., Jeremic, M. & Seip, M. (1969) Wiskott-Aldrich syndrome: Qualitative platelet defects and short platelet survival. *Brit. J. Haemat.*, **17**, 373.

Gutenberger, J., Trygstad, C. W., Stiehm, E. R., Opitz, J. M., Thatcher, L. G. & Bloodworth, J. M. B. (1970) Familial thrombocytopenia, elevated serum IgA levels and renal disease—A report of a kindred. *Amer. J. Med.*, **49**, 729.

Hall, J. G., Levin, J., Kuhn, J. P., Ottenheimer, E. J., Berkum, K. A. P. van & McKusick, V. A. (1969) Thrombocytopenia with absent radius. *Medicine*, **48**, 411.

Handin, R. & Smith, A. L. (1972) Editorial: Immunoidiopathic or immunogenic thrombocytopenic purpura. *New Eng. J. Med.*, **286**, 720.

Hanna, N. & Nelken, D. (1970) A two-stage agglutination test for the detection of antithrombocyte antibodies. *Vox Sang.*, **18**, 342.

Harker, L. A. (1968) Kinetics of thrombopoiesis. *J. Clin. Invest.*, **47**, 458.

Harker, L. A. (1970) Platelet kinetics in hereditary thrombocytopenia. 13th Annual Meeting of the American Soc. Hematol. Abstract 261. New York: Grunn & Stratton.

Harker, L. A. (1970A) The regulation of thrombopoiesis. *Amer. J. Physiol.*, **218**, 1376.

Harker, L. A. (1970B) Current concepts. Platelet production. *New Eng. J. Med.*, **282**, 492.

Harker, L. A. & Finch, C. A. (1969) Thrombokinetics in man. *J. Clin. Invest.*, **48**, 963.

Harrington, W. J., Minnich, V., Hollingsworth, J. & Moore, C. V. (1951) Demonstration of thrombocytopenic factor in blood of patients with thrombocytopenic purpura. *J. Lab. & Clin. Med.*, **38**, 1.

Harrington, W. J., Sprague, C. C., Minnich, V., Moore, C. V., Aulvin, R. C. & Dubach, R. (1963) Immunologic mechanisms in idiopathic and neonatal thrombocytopenic purpura. *Ann. Int. Med.*, **38**, 433.

Hegglin, V. R. (1945) Gleichzeitige Konstitutionelle veranderungen an Neutrophilen und Thrombozyten. *Helv. Medica Acta.*, **4**, 439.

Henriksson, P., Nilsson, I. M., Bergentz, S.-E., Ljungqvist, U. & Rosengren, B. (1971) Case report: Giant haemangioma with a disorder of coagulation. *Acta Paediat. Scand.*, **60**, 227.

Heys, R. F. (1966) Steroid therapy for idiopathic thrombocytopenic purpura during pregnancy. *Obst. Gynec.*, **28**, 532.

Hilgartner, M. W., Lanzkowsky, P. & Smith, C. H. (1970) The use of azathioprine in refractory idiopathic thrombocytopenic purpura in children. *Acta Paediat. Scand.*, **59**, 409.

Hirschman, R. J. & Shulman, N. R. (1973) The use of platelet serotonin release as a sensitive method for detecting anti-platelet antibodies and a plasma anti-platelet factor in patients with idiopathic thrombocytopenic purpura. *Brit. J. Haemat.*, **24**, 793.

Horan, M. & Colebatch, J. H. (1962) Relation between splenectomy and subsequent infection. *Arch. Dis. Childh.*, **37**, 398.

Horowitz, H. & Nachman, R. (1965) Drug purpura. *Sem. Hemat.*, **2**, 287.

Hudson, J. B., Weinstein, L. & Chang, T.-W (1956) Thrombocytopenic purpura in measles. *J. Pediat.*, **48**, 48.

Inglefield, J., Tisdale, P. & Fairchild, J. (1961) A case of hemangioma with thrombocytopenia in a newborn infant treated by total excision. *J. Pediat.*, **59**, 238.

Jones, T., Goldsmith, K. & Anderson, I. (1961) Maternal and neonatal platelet antibodies in a case of congenital thrombocytopenia. *Lancet*, **ii**, 1008.

Jones, J. & Reed, J. (1965) Renal vein thrombosis and thrombocytopenia in a newborn infant. *J. Pediat.*, **67**, 681.

Karpatkin, S. (1969) Heterogeneity of human platelets. I. Metabolic and kinetic evidence suggestive of young and old platelets. *J. Clin. Invest.*, **48**, 1073.

Karpatkin, S. & Siskind, G. W. (1969) *In vitro* detection of platelet antibody in patients with ITP and SLE. *Blood*, **33**, 795.

Karpatkin, S. (1971) Drug induced thrombocytopenia. *Amer. J. Med. Sci.*, **262**, 68.

Karpatkin, S., Strick, N. & Siskind, G. W. (1972) Detection of splenic anti-platelet antibody synthesis in idiopathic autoimmune thrombocytopenic purpura. *Brit. J. Haemat.*, **23**, 167.

Kasabach, H. H. & Merritt, K. K. (1940) Capillary hemangioma with extensive purpura. Report of a case. *Am. J. Dis. Child.*, **59**, 1063.

Killander, A. (1959) On the use of exchange transfusion in neonatal thrombocytopenic purpura. *Acta Paediat.*, **48**, 29.

Klemperer, M. R., Osthold, M., Vasquez, D. & Diamond, L. K. (1966) The incidence of complete complement-fixing platelet antibodies in pregnant women. *Vox Sang.*, **11**, 124.

Kontras, S. B., Green, O. C., King, L. & Duran, R. J. (1963) Giant hemangioma with thrombocytopenia: case report with survival and sequestration studies of platelets labelled with chromium 51. *Amer. J. Dis. Child.*, **105**, 188.

Krevans, J. & Jackson, D. (1955) Hemorrhagic disorder following massive whole blood transfusion. *J.A.M.A.*, **159**, 171.

Krivit, W. & Good, R. A. (1959) Aldrich's syndrome (thrombocytopenia, eczema and infection in infants). *Am. J. Dis. Child.*, **97**, 137.

Lammi, A. T. & Lovric, V. A. (1973) Idiopathic thrombocytopenic purpura: An epidemiological study. *J. Pediat.*, **83**, 31.

Larco, R. K. & Penner, J. A. (1971) Refractory thrombocytopenic purpura treated successfully with cyclophosphamide. *J.A.M.A.*, **215**, 445.

Leeksma, C. H. W. & Cohen, J. A. (1956) Determination of the life span of human blood platelets using labelled diisopropylfuorophosphonate. *J. Clin. Invest.*, **35**, 964.

Levin, J. & Conley, C. L. (1964) Thrombocytosis associated with malignant disease. *Arch. Intern. Med.*, **114**, 497.

Levin, A. S., Spitler, L. E., Stites, D. P. & Fudenberg, H. H. (1970) Wiskott-Aldrich syndrome, a genetically determined cellular immunologic deficiency: Clinical and laboratory response to therapy with transfer factor. *Proc. Nat. Acad. Sci.*, **67**, 821.

Lipson, R. L., Bayrd, E. D. & Watkins, C. H. (1959) The postsplenectomy blood picture. *Am. J. Clin. Pathol.*, **32**, 526.

Lo, S. S., Hitzig, W. H. & Sigg, P. (1969) Management of chronic idiopathic thrombocytopenic purpura in children with particular reference to immunosuppressive therapy. *Acta Haematologica*, **41**, 1.

Lokietz, H. & Reynolds, F. A. (1966) Post-rubella thrombocytopenic purpura. *Lancet*, **88**, 226.

London, I. L., Epstein, C. J., Sahud, M., Goodman, J., Piel, C. & Bernfield, M. (1969) A new syndrome of hereditary thrombocytopenia, nephritis and deafness. *Clinical Research*, **17**, 315.

Lusher, J. M. & Zuelzer, W. W. (1966) Idiopathic thrombocytopenic purpura in childhood. *J. Pediat.*, **68**, 971.

Lusher, J. M., Iyer, R., Khalifa, A. S. & Zuelzer, W. W. (1974) Idiopathic thrombocytopenic purpura in childhood. *Blood*, **44**, 932.

McClure, P. D. (1975) Idiopathic thrombocytopenic purpura in children: Diagnosis and management. *Pediatrics*, **55**, 68.

McDonald, T. P., Odell, T. T. & Gosslee, D. G. (1964) Platelet size in relation to platelet age. *Proc. Soc. Exp. Biol. Med.*, **115**, 684.

McIntosh, S., O'Brien, R. T., Schwartz, A. D. & Pearson, H. A. (1973) Neonatal isoimmune purpura: Response to platelet infusions. *J. Pediat.*, **82**, 1020.

McKay, D. G. & Margaretten, W. (1967) Disseminated intravascular coagulation in virus diseases. *Arch. Int. Med.*, **120**, 129.

McMillan, R., Smith, R. S., Longmire, R. L., Yelenosky, R., Reid, R. T. & Craddock, C. G. (1971) Immunoglobulin associated with human platelets. *Blood*, **37**, 316.

McMillan, R., Longmire, R. L., Yelenosky, R., Smith, R. S. & Craddock, C. G. (1972) Immunoglobulin synthesis *in vitro* by splenic tissue in idiopathic thrombocytopenic purpura. *New Eng. J. Med.*, **286**, 681.

McMillan, R., Longmire, R. L., Yelenosky, R., Donnell, R. L. & Armstrong, S. (1974) Quantitation of platelet-binding IgG produced *in vitro* by spleens from patients with idiopathic thrombocytopenic purpura. *New Eng. J. Med.*, **291**, 812.

Mandl, M. A. J., Watson, J. I. & Rose, B. (1968) The Wiskott-Aldrich syndrome. Immunopathologic mechanisms and a long-term survival. *Annals of Internal Med.*, **68**, 1050.

Mauer, A. M., Vaux, L. O. De & Lahey, M. E. (1957) Neonatal and maternal thrombocytopenic purpura due to quinine. *Pediatrics*, **19**, 84.

Medoff, H. S. (1964) Platelet counts in premature infants. *J. Pediat.*, **64**, 287.

Mehes, K. & Bata, G. (1965) Congenital thrombocytopenia in 13-15 trisomy. *Lancet*, **i**, 1279.

Meindersma, T. E. & Vries, S. I. de (1962) Thrombocytopenic purpura after smallpox vaccination. *Brit. med. J.*, **1**, 266.

Merenstein, G. B., O'Loughlin, E. P. & Plunket, D. C. (1970) Effects of maternal thiazides on platelet counts of newborn infants. *J. Pediat.*, **76**, 766.

Miller, D. R., Hanshaw, J. B. O'Leary, D. S. & Hnilicka, J. V. (1970) Fatal disseminated herpes simplex virus infection and hemorrhage in the neonate. *J. Pediat.*, **76**, 409.

Minter, N. & Ingram, M. (1967) Density distribution of platelets. *Blood*, **30**, 551.

Monnens, L. A. H. & Retera, R. J. M. (1967) Thrombotic thrombocytopenic purpura in a neonatal infant. *J. Pediat.*, **71**, 118.

Moore, C. M., McAdams, A. J. & Sutherland, J. M. (1969) Intrauterine disseminated intravascular coagulation. A syndrome of multiple pregnancy with a dead twin fetus. *J. Pediat.*, **74**, 523.

Morowitz, D. A., Allen, L. W. & Kirsner, J. B. (1968) Thrombocytosis in chronic inflammatory bowel disease. *Ann. Intern. Med.*, **68**, 1013.

Morrow, G., Barness, L. A., Auerbach, V. H., DiGeorge, A. M., Ando, T. & Nyhan, W. L. (1969) Observations on the coexistence of methylmalonic acidemia and glycinemia. *J. Pediat.*, **74**, 680.

Morse, E. E., Zinkham, W. H. & Jackson, D. P. (1966) Thrombocytopenic purpura following rubella infection in children. *Arch. Intern. Med.*, **117**, 573.

Murphy, S. Oski, F. A. & Gardner, F. H. (1969) Hereditary thrombocytopenia with an intrinsic platelet defect. *New Eng. J. Med.*, **281**, 857.

Murphy, S., Oski, F. A., Naiman, J. L., Lusch, C. J., Goldberg, S. & Gardner, F. H. (1972) Platelet size and kinetics in hereditary and acquired thrombocytopenia. *New Eng. J. Med.*, **286**, 499.

Murphy, S. (1972A) Hereditary thrombocytopenia. *Clinics in Haematology*, **1**, 359.

Murphy, S. (1972B) Intrinsic platelet defects in heriditary thrombocytopenia. *Annals N.Y. Acad. Sci.* (in Press).

Myllyla, G., Vaheri, A., Vesikari, T. & Pettinen, K. (1969) Interaction between human blood platelets, viruses and antibodies. *Clin. Exper. Immunol.*, **4**, 323.

Najean, Y., Schaison, G., Binet, J-L., Dresch, C. & Bernard, J. (1966) Le syndrome de May-Hegglin. *La Presse Medicale*, **74**, 1649.

Najean, Y., Ardaillou, N. & Dresch, C. (1969) Platelet lifespan. *Ann. Review of Medicine*, **20**, 47.

Najean, Y. & Ardaillou, N. (1971) The sequestration site of platelets in idiopathic thrombocytopenic purpura: its correlation with the results of splenectomy. *Brit. J. Haemat.*, **21**, 153.

Nathan, D. L. & Snapper, I. (1958) Simultaneous placental transfer of factors responsible for L.E. cell formation and thrombocytopenia. *Am. J. Med.*, **25**, 647.

Odell, T. T., Jackson, C. W., Friday, T. J. & Charsh, D. E. (1969) Effects of thrombocytopenia on megakaryocytopoiesis. *Brit. J. Haemat.*, **17**, 91.

O'Gorman Hughes, D. W. & Diamond, L. K. (1964) A new type of constitutional aplastic anemia without congenital anomalies presenting as thrombocytopenia in infancy. *J. Pediat.*, **65**, 1060.

O'Gorman Hughes, D. W. (1969) Aplastic anaemia in childhood: a reappraisal. I. Classification and assessment. *Med. J. Aust.*, **1**, 1059.

O'Neill, E. & Varadi, S. (1963) Neonatal aplastic anaemia and Fanconi's anaemia. *Arch. Dis. Childh.*, **38**, 92.

Oppenheim, J. J., Blaese, R. M. & Waldman, T. A. (1970) Defective lymphocyte transformation and delayed hypersensitivity in Wiskott-Aldrich syndrome. *J. Immnuol.*, **104**, 835.

Oski, F. A., Naiman, J. L., Allen, D. M. & Diamond, L. K. (1962) Leukocytic inclusions—Döhle bodies—associated with platelet abnormality (the May-Hegglin anomaly). Report of a family and review of the literature. *Blood*, **20**, 657.

Oski, F. A. & Naiman, J. L. (1972A) *Hematologic Problems in the Newborn*, p. 277. Philadelphia: Saunders.

Oski, F. A. & Naiman, J. L. (1972B) *Hematologic Problems in the Newborn*, p. 281. Philadelphia: Saunders.

Oski, F. A. & Naiman, J. L. (1972C) *Hematologic Problems in the Newborn*, p. 301. Philadelphia: Saunders.

Oski, F. A. & Naiman, J. L. (1972D) *Hematologic Problems in the Newborn*, p. 309. Philadelphia: Saunders.

Ozer, F. L., Truax, W. E., Miesch, D. C. & Levin, W. C. (1960) Primary hemorrhagic thrombocythemia. *Am. J. Med.*, **28**, 807.

Pearson, H. A., Shulman, N. R., Marder, V. J. & Cone, T. E. (1964) Isoimmune neonatal thrombocytopenic purpura. Clinical and therapeutic considerations. *Blood*, **23**, 154.

Pearson, H. A., Shulman, N. R., Oski, F. A. & Eitzman, D. V. (1966) Platelet survival in Wiskott-Aldrich syndrome. *J. Pediat.*, **68**, 754.

Pearson, H. A. (1968) Editorial: Thrombocytopenia in premature infants—physiological or pathological. *J. Pediat.*, **73**, 160.

Pickering, D. & Cuddigan, B. (1969) Infantile cortical hyperostosis associated with thrombocythaemia. *Lancet*, **ii**, 464.

Piessens, W. F., Wybran, F., Manaster, J. & Strijckmans, P. A. (1970) Lymphocyte transformation induced by autologous platelets in a case of thrombocytopenic purpura. *Blood*, **36**, 421.

Pizzi, F., Cona, P. M. & Aldeghi, A. (1966) Immunofluorescence of megakaryocytes in the thrombocytopenic purpuras. *Blood*, **27**, 521.

Pochedly, G. (1971) Thrombocytopenic purpura of the newborn. *Obst. Gynec. Survey*, **26**, 63.

Pochedly, C. & Ente, G. (1972) Adverse hematologic effects of drugs. *Pediatric Clin. N. Amer.*, **19**, 1095.

Poley, J. R. & Strickler, G. B. (1961) Petechiae in the newborn infant. *Am. J. Dis. Child.*, **102**, 365.

Prankerd, T. A. J. (1972) Idiopathic thrombocytopenic purpura. *Clinics in Haematology*, **1**, 327.

Propp, R. & Scharfman, W. (1966) Hemangioma-thrombocytopenia syndrome associated with microangiopathic hemolytic anemia. *Blood*, **28**, 623.

Pyesmany, A., Ekert, H., Williams, K. & Hittle, R. (1969) Intravascular coagulation secondary to cavernous hemangioma in infancy: Response to radiotherapy. *Canad. Med. Ass. J.*, **100**, 1053.

Rabinowitz, J. G., Moseley, J. E., Mitty, H. A. & Hirschhorn, K. (1967) Trisomy 18, oesophageal atresia, anomalies of the radius, and congenital hypoplastic thrombocytopenia. *Radiology*, **89**, 488.

Radel, E. G. & Schorr, J. B. (1963) Thrombocytopenic purpura with infectious mononucleosis: Report of 2 cases and a review of the literature. *J. Pediat.*, **63**, 46.

Raussen, A. R. & Diamond, L. K. (1961) Enclosed hemorrhage and neonatal jaundice. *Am. J. Dis. Child.*, **101**, 164.

Renfield, M. L. & Kraybill, E. N. (1973) Consumptive coagulopathy with renal vein thrombosis. *J. Pediat.*, **82**, 1054.

Roberts, M. H. & Smith, M. H. (1950) Thrombocytopenic purpura. *Amer. J. Dis. Child.*, **79**, 820.

Rodriguez, S., Leikin, S. & Hillier, M. (1964) Neonatal thrombocytopenia associated with antepartum administration of thiazide drugs. *New Eng. J. Med.*, **270**, 881.

Sanyal, S. K., Yules, R. B., Eidelman, A. I. & Talner, N. S. (1966) Thrombocytosis, central nervous system disease, and myocardial infarction pattern in infancy. *Pediat.*, **38**, 629.

Schaar, F. E. (1963) Familial idiopathic thrombocytopenic purpura. *J. Pediat.*, **62**, 546.

Schiff, D., Aranda, J. V. & Stern, L. (1970) Neonatal thrombocytopenia and congenital malformations associated with administration of tolbutamide to the mother. *J. Pediat.*, **77**, 457.

Schneider, H. J. & Lascari, A. D. (1968) Consumption coagulopathy in an infant with Kasabach-Merritt syndrome. *Helv. Paediat. Acta.*, **23**, 674.

Schulman, I., Pierce, M., Lukens, A. & Currimbhoy, Z. (1960A) Studies on thrombopoiesis I. A factor in normal human plasma required for platelet production; chronic thrombocytopenia due to its deficiency. *Blood*, **16**, 943.

Schulman, I., Currimbhoy, Z., Fort, E. & Alcade, V. (1960B) Platelet stimulating properties of human plasma. *Amer. J. Dis. Child.*, **100**, 747.

Schulman, I. (1964) Diagnosis and treatment: Management of idiopathic thrombocytopenic purpura. *Pediatrics*, **33**, 979.

Seip, M. (1960) Systemic lupus erythematosus in pregnancy with haemolytic anaemia, leucopenia and thrombocytopenia in the mother and her newborn infant. *Arch. Dis. Childh.*, **35**, 364.

Seip, M. (1963) Hereditary hypoplastic thrombocytopenia. *Acta Paediatrica*, **52**, 370.

Sell, E. J. & Corrigan, J. J. (1973) Platelet counts, fibrinogen concentrations, and factor V and factor VIII levels in healthy infants according to gestational age. *J. Pediat.*, **82**, 1028.

Shershow, L. W., Ekert, H., Swanson, V. L., Wright, H. T. & Gilchrist, G. S. (1969) Intravascular coagulation in generalized herpes simplex infection of the newborn. *Acta Paediat. Scand.*, **58**, 535.

Shim, W. (1968) Hemangiomas of infancy complicated by thrombocytopenia. *Amer. J. Surg.*, **116**, 896.

Shulman, N. R., Aster, R. K., Leitner, A. & Hiller, M. C. (1961) Immunoreactions involving platelets. V. Post-transfusion purpura due to a complement-fixing antibody against a genetically controlled platelet antigen. A proposed mechanism for thrombocytopenia and its relevance in 'autoimmunity'. *J. Clin. Invest.*, **40**, 1597.

Shulman, N. R., Marder, V. J., Hiller, M. C. & Collier, E. M. (1964) Platelet and leucocyte isoantigens and their antibodies: serologic, physiologic and clinical studies. *Prog. Hemat.*, **4**, 222.

Shulman, N. R., Weinrach, R. S., Libre, E. P. & Andrews, H. (1965) Role of reticuloendothelial system in pathogenesis of idiopathic and thrombocytopenic purpura. *Trans. Assoc. Amer. Phys.*, **78**, 374.

Shulman, N. R. (1972) Immunologic reactions to drugs. *New Eng. J. Med.*, **287**, 408.

Spach, M. S., Howell, D. A. & Harris, J. S. (1963) Myocardial infarction and multiple thromboses in a child with primary thrombocytosis. *Pediatrics*, **31**, 268.

Stavem, P., Jeremic, M., Hjort, P. F., Wislöff, F., Vogt, E., Öyen, R., Abrahamsen, A. F. & Sövde, A. (1969) Hereditary thrombocytopenia with excessively prolonged bleeding time. *Scand. J. Haematology*, **6**, 250.

Stephanini, M. & Dameshek, W. (1962) *The Hemarrhagic Disorders*, p. 193. New York: Grune & Stratton.

Stuart, J., Picken, A. M., Breeze, G. R. & Wood, B. S. B. (1973) Capillary-blood coagulation profile in the newborn. *Lancet*, **2**, 1467.

Stuart, M. J., Murphy, S. & Oski, F. A. (1975) Simple nonradioisotope technic for the determination of platelet life-span. *New Eng. J. Med.*, **292**, 1310.

Sussman, L. N. (1967) Azathioprine in refractory idiopathic thrombocytopenic purpura. *J.A.M.A.*, **202**, 259.

Suvansri, U., Cheung, W. H. & Sawitsky, A. (1969) The effect of bilirubin on the human platelet. *J. Pediat.*, **74**, 240.

Tereda, H., Baldini, M., Ebbe, S. & Madoff, M. (1966) Interaction of influenza virus with blood platelets. *Blood*, **28**, 213.

Thatcher, L., Clatanoff, D. & Stiehm, E. (1968) Splenic hemangioma with thrombocytopenia and afibrinogenemia. *J. Pediat.*, **73**, 345.

Vestermark, B. & Vestermark, S. (1964) Familial sex-linked thrombocytopenia. *Acta Paediat.*, **53**, 365.

Walker, J. & Walker, W. (1961) Idiopathic thrombocytopenic purpura in childhood. *Arch. Dis. Childh.*, **36**, 649.

Wassmuth, D. R., Hamilton, H. E. & Sheets, R. F. (1963) May-Hegglin anomaly. *J.A.M.A.*, **183**, 737.

Weintraub, R. M., Pechet, L. & Alexander, B. (1962) Rapid diagnosis of drug-induced thrombocytopenic purpura: Report of three cases due to quinine, quinidine, and dilantin. *J.A.M.A.*, **180**, 528.

Weintraub, H. D. & Wilson, W. J. (1964) Pneumocystis carinii pneumonia in Wiskott-Aldrich syndrome. *Am. J. Dis. Child.*, **108**, 198.

Weisfuse, L., Spear, P. W. & Sass, M. (1954) Quinidine-induced thrombocytopenic purpura. Report of a 14th case and review of clinical and experimental studies. *Amer. J. Med.*, **17**, 414.

Welch, R. G. (1956) Thrombocytopenic purpura and chickenpox. *Arch. Dis. Childh.*, **31**, 38.

Whitfield, M. F. & Barr, D. G. D. (1975) Cow's milk allergy in the syndrome of thrombocytopenia with absent radius. *Arch. Dis. Childh.*, **51**, 337.

Wilde, R. C., Ellis, L. D. & Cooper, W. M. (1967) Splenectomy for chronic idiopathic thrombocytopenic purpura. *Arch. Surg.*, **95**, 344.

Wiskott, A. (1937) Familiärer angeborener morbus werlhofii? *Mischr. Kinderheilk.*, **68**, 212.

Wolf, J. A. (1967) Wiskott-Aldrich syndrome: clinical, immunologic and pathologic observations. *J. Pediat.*, **70**, 221.

Woolley, E. J. S. (1956) Familial idiopathic thrombocytopenic purpura. *Brit. med. J.* **1**, 440.

Wybran, J. & Fudenberg, H. H. (1972) Cellular immunity to platelets in idiopathic thrombocytopenic purpura. *Blood*, **40**, 856.

Yankee, R. A., Graff, K. S., Dowling, R. & Henderson, E. S. (1973) Selection of unrelated compatible platelet donors by lymphocyte HL-A matching. *New Eng. J. Med.*, **288**, 760.

Young, R., Nachman, R. & Horowitz, H. (1966) Thrombocytopenia due to digitoxin: Demonstration of antibody and mechanism of action. *Amer. J. Med.*, **41**, 605.

Zaidi, Z. H. & Mortimer, P. E. (1965) Congenital thyrotoxicosis with hepatosplenomegaly and thrombocytopenia, associated with aniridia and dislocated lenses. *Proc. Roy. Soc. Med.*, **58**, 390.

Zinkham, W. H., Medearis, D. N. & Osborn, J. E. (1967) Blood and bone marrow findings in congenital rubella. *J. Pediat.*, **71**, 512.

17. Defects of Platelet and Capillary Function

Normal platelet function / Tests of platelet function, *Bleeding time, Platelet size and morphology, Platelet aggregation and ADP release in virto, Platelet adhesion to glass beads, Clot retraction, Platelet-factor 3 (PF-3) availability* / Inherited disorders of platelet function, *Glanzmann's thrombasthenia, Thrombopathia (or defects of ADP release), Bernard-Soulier syndrome, May-Hegglin anomaly, Von Willebrand's disease, Congenital afibrinogenaemia* / Acquired defects of platelet function, *Drug ingestion, Platelet function in the newborn, Uraemia, Liver disease, dysproteinaemia* / Platelet transfusion / Non-thrombocytopenic purpura, *Anaphylactoid purpura (Henoch-Schönlein syndrome), Scurvy, Drugs, food and infections* / Inherited vascular and connective tissue disorders, *Hereditary-haemorrhagic telangiectasia (Rendu-Osler-Weber disease), Ehler-Danlos syndrome, Pseudoxanthoma elasticum and osteogenesis imperfecta.*

NORMAL PLATELET FUNCTION

The first reaction to vascular trauma is local vasoconstriction, but this is insufficient to achieve complete arrest of bleeding (Hughes, 1966). The initial phase of haemostasis in capillaries and other small blood vessels is largely dependent upon platelets. They do not adhere to intact vascular endothelium but when the vessels are torn or punctured a break in endothelial continuity allows platelets to come into contact with subendothelial collagen. Electron microscopy shows that adherence between collagen fibres and platelets is followed *in vivo* by platelet aggregation and the formation of a haemostatic platelet plug (French *et al.*, 1964). Subsequently this plug becomes 'consolidated' by the appearance of fibrin around and among the mass of platelets (Marcus, 1969A).

In vitro studies have shown that this sequence of events is triggered by a specific biochemical interaction between the platelet membrane and free amino groups in the triple helix of native collagen (Wilner *et al.*, 1968A). The platelet aggregation that follows this contact with collagen is thought to be mediated through release of ADP (Spaet and Zucker, 1964). The sequence of events can diagrammatically be represented as in Fig. 17.1. A finite delay occurs between exposure to collagen and release of ADP. Transmission of this 'message' between platelet membrane and ADP pool may be mediated by a fall in cyclic AMP concentration (Salzman, 1972). When directly exposed to ADP there is no such delay in aggregation.

It is the release of ADP into the surrounding medium which causes actual platelet aggregation although the precise mechanism is uncertain. It can be simulated *in vitro* by the addition of ADP to platelet-rich citrated plasma and recording the change in optical density, which progressively decreases as more platelet aggregates are formed. There is normally a 'storage pool' of ADP in platelets concentrated within their granules. During interaction with collagen these granules disappear accompanying release not only of ADP,

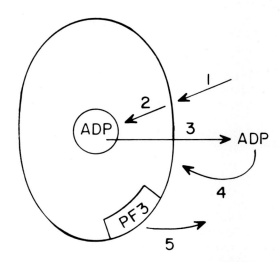

Fig. 17.1 Sequence of events following contact of platelet with collagen. 1, Adhesion to collagen; 2, 'intracellular transmission', dependent partly on glycolysis and the adenyl cyclase—cyclic AMP system; 3, release of ADP from storage granules; 4, action of ADP leading to cohesion or aggregation; 5, availability of PF3. (Reproduced from *Pediatric Clinics of North America* (1972), **19**, 1048, by permission of the author Professor Gilchrist and the publishers).

but also of adrenaline, serotonin and platelet factor 4 (heparin-neutralizing factor) (Marcus *et al.*, 1966). This 'release reaction' is also accompanied by an alteration in the platelet membrane which renders its phospholipid (PF-3) available for activation of the plasma coagulation factors leading to thrombin generation and fibrin formation (Horowitz and Papayoanou, 1968). Since the products of the 'release reaction', viz. ADP, adrenaline, serotonin, and thrombin are also active in *inducing* platelet aggregation, the process becomes self-perpetuating (Salzman,1972), which is clearly advantageous in haemostasis. Thus when a low dose of ADP (0·5 μg/ml) is added to a platelet suspension *in vitro* there is transient aggregation followed by disaggregation, but when stronger aggregation is induced by a higher ADP concentration (10 μg/ml) or by adrenaline (1·0 μg/ml) or thrombin (1 unit/ml) then the further liberation of endogenous ADP results in a second wave of aggregation that is irreversible (Fig. 17.1). It has also been pointed out that ADP is released from damaged red cells and that this may occur in the vicinity of platelet or fibrin plugs and would accentuate the process (Rorvik *et al.*, 1968). This could occur in MAHA where red cells are fragmented while being forced through intravascular fibrin deposits. In understanding the sequence of changes in haemostasis it is of note that collagen, exposed in traumatized vessels, also activates Hageman factor, the first of the coagulation factors concerned in initiation of the 'contact phase' of the blood coagulation (Wilner *et al.*, 1968B). The liberation of platelet factor 3 (PF-3) thus merely accelerates the coagulation process that is already in progress. Although initiated by platelet activity the final integrity of the fibrin-containing haemostatic plug is dependent upon an intact system of coagulation factors, including ultimately the fibrin-stabilizing factor XIII. If a defect of these coagulation factors exists this second phase of haemostasis is impaired, and delayed bleeding occurs following initial haemostasis. Finally contraction of the fibrin-platelet plug occurs, further consolidating haemostasis, through the action of a contractile protein 'thrombasthenin' normally present on the platelet membrane (Nachman *et al.*, 1967; Booyse *et al.*, 1972).

It has been found by Karpatkin (1969A and 1969B) that metabolically and functionally there is a double population of circulating platelets with the 'young' cells larger and releasing more ADP after exposure to adrenaline or thrombin than do the 'older' and smaller platelets. There is also evidence that newly formed platelets have greater haemostatic effect as judged by the bleeding time (Harker and Slichter, 1972).

A number of drugs have been found to inhibit platelet aggregation including anti-inflammatory agents (O'Brien, 1968), particularly acetyl salicylic acid (Evans *et al.*, 1968; Weiss *et al.*, 1968), dipyridamole (Emmons *et al.*, 1965), and prostaglandins (Kloeze, 1969). Fibrin degradation products (FDPs), especially the 'early' fractions, also produce inhibition (Kowalski, 1968). In general these agents impair the release of ADP, and therefore aggregation, after exposure to collagen, thrombin or adrenaline, as well as impairing adhesiveness of the platelets to glass or collagen. These changes can be accompanied by a haemostatic defect *in vivo*. Platelets in the newborn are unduly sensitive to this drug effect (Corby and Schulman, 1971), already possessing diminished aggregating activity in normal infants (Mull and Hathaway, 1970).

TESTS OF PLATELET FUNCTION

The following tests are of practical use in the diagnosis of platelet dysfunction:
1. Bleeding time;
2. Platelet size and morphology;
3. Platelet aggregation and ADP release *in vitro*;
4. Platelet adhesion to glass beads;
5. Clot retraction;
6. Release of PF-3.

Hess's tourniquet test could be included, but it adds little to the information gained by the bleeding time and gives far less consistent results. In recent years I have omitted this test from routine use. Additional tests that are more useful in research than in practical diagnosis include the *in vivo* platelet consumption during bleeding from skin punctures (Borchgrevink, 1960), and the closely related measurement of platelet adhesiveness to collagen *in vitro* either by enumeration (Weiss *et al.*, 1968), or optical density changes (Spaet and Lejnieks, 1969).

Bleeding time

A prolonged bleeding time in the presence of a normal platelet count is presumptive evidence of platelet dysfunction and is the single most valuable screening test for this group of disorders. The Ivy method, using skin lancets set to a depth of 3 mm and a sphygmomanometer cuff inflated to 40 mm Hg, (Ivy *et al.*, 1941) is the preferred method (*M.R.C.*, 1955; Biggs and Macfarlane, 1962; Hardisty and Ingram, 1965). The standardized punctures and moderate degree of back pressure in the postcapillary venules renders this a more reproducible and more sensitive test of haemostasis than the Duke's bleeding time, performed by stabbing the ear lobe. The duration of bleeding is determined by blotting the three punctures at quarter minute intervals with a large circular filter paper. None of the punctures normally bleed for longer than 6 minutes, and this is taken as the approximate upper limit of normal. The *rate* of blood loss may also be visualized by the size of the blots or may be measured by elution (Willoughby and Allington, 1961). A prolonged bleeding time is often accompanied by an initial high rate of blood loss from all punctures, such patients colloquially being referred to as 'big blobbers'. On occasions the rate of blood loss may be obviously increased when the bleeding time is normal or borderline, and this feature may be helpful or confirmatory in diagnosis (Willoughby and Crouch; 1961; Mielke *et al.*, 1969). Recently an automated technique for measuring the rate of blood loss has been described (Sutor *et al.*, 1971).

Refinements in the Ivy bleeding time have been described when used for research purposes. These include the use of a 'template' which allows standardized linear skin incisions of 1 mm depth and 9 mm length to be made (Mielke *et al.*, 1969). This technique carries a hazard of causing keloid scars and is not suitable for children. The original Ivy method is entirely acceptable from the age of 3–6 months onwards providing paediatric sphygmomanometer cuffs are used.

By the 'template' technique a clear cut relationship between the bleeding time and the platelet count has been elegantly demonstrated. When platelet function is normal the bleeding time is $4\frac{1}{2} \pm 1\frac{1}{2}$ minutes (i.e. up to 6 minutes) with platelet counts of 100,000/mm³ or over (Harker and Slichter, 1972). Below this level there is a progressive linear increase in the bleeding time. Platelet dysfunction, as in uraemia, von Willebrand's disease or aspirin exposure, caused distinct prolongation of the bleeding time in spite of a platelet count of over 100,000/mm³. In Wiskott-Aldrich syndrome the bleeding time is disproportionately prolonged relative to the platelet count, but the platelets are of small size in this disease, and when a correction is applied for 'platelet mass' the relationship becomes normal. Rather surprisingly the 'young' and large platelets present during the early stages of response in ITP, or in early marrow regeneration following toxic marrow depression, have better than normal haemostatic function, giving a normal bleeding time when the count was below 50,000/mm³.

The aspirin tolerance test (Quick, 1966) may be used to detect a group of patients with mild bruising tendency and a normal bleeding time but whose platelet function is unduly sensitive to aspirin. Deykin (1974) describes an adaptation performing the template bleeding time before and 2 hours after ingesting 900 mg (3 tablets) of aspirin. In 21 normal volunteers the mean bleeding time was $3\frac{1}{2}$ min before aspirin and $7\frac{1}{2}$ min two hours after aspirin.

Platelet size and morphology

The majority of normal platelets are less than 3 μm in diameter. Up to 5 per cent may exceed 2·5 μm (Howard *et al.*, 1973A).

In addition to the age dependent shrinking of platelet size which is a normal phenomenon (Garg *et al.*, 1971), inherited abnormalities of platelet size and function may occur independently of platelet kinetics (Murphy *et al.*, 1972); for example, the small platelets in Wiskott-Aldrich syndrome. Bernard and Soulier (1948) originally described a congenital type of platelet dysfunction with giant platelets which could not support prothrombin consumption. Thrombocytopenia was sometimes present. A more recent report of similar cases confirms the association with platelet dysfunction and suggests the presence of a platelet membrane defect (Gröttum and Solum, 1969).

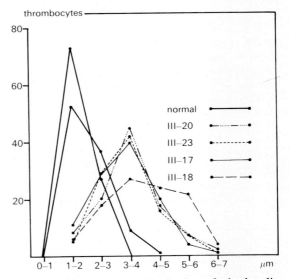

Fig. 17.2 Abnormal size-distribution of platelet diameters in a family with a hereditary thrombopathy. (Roman and arabic symbols refer to patients). (Reproduced from the *British Journal of Haematology* (1968), **15**, 311, by permission of the author Dr R. Kurstjens).

Giant platelets are also part of the May-Hegglin anomaly, with thrombocytopenia in one third of patients. Kurstjens et al. (1968) described a family with an abnormal size distribution of platelets (Fig. 17.2) and decreased or absent alpha granules on electron microscopy which are concerned with the 'release' reaction. Other reports describe a familial haemorrhagic platelet defect with small platelets and impaired ADP release (Maurer et al., 1971).

Platelet size may be determined for these purposes by examination of a stained blood film using a micrometer eyepiece. Alternatively the size may be determined electronically using a Coulter counter (models B, F or S) or an electrozone celloscope. Blood for this purpose should be collected in 1/10th volume of 3·2 per cent sodium citrate rather than EDTA which may cause platelet swelling (Weiss and Rogers, 1972). The size distribution curves can be analysed by computer, if available, or by planimeter, thus determining the absolute number of platelets over $13\,\mu^3$ in size, megathrombocytes (Sanderson, 1975).

Platelet aggregation and ADP release *in vitro*

Great strides in both the understanding and the practical diagnosis of platelet disorders have sprung from the development of turbimetric techniques by O'Brien (1962) and Born (1962) to measure this phenomenon. Aggregation causes a fall in O.D. When ADP in a low final concentration of 0·3 to 1·0 μM (0·15 to 0·5 μg/ml) is mixed with constantly stirred platelet-rich citrated plasma at 37° C there is immediate aggregation. At this 'low' concentration of ADP the initial aggregation is followed by disaggregation, but if a higher ADP concentration of 2 to 5 μM (1 to 2·5 μg/ml) is used the initial wave is followed by a second wave of aggregation which is irreversible (Fig. 17.3). Concentrations in excess of this (e.g. 10 μg/ml) cause such rapid and irreversible aggregation that the biphasic response is masked. Adrenaline (1 μg/ml) (or noradrenaline 20 μM) and thrombin (0·1 unit/ml) similarly produce biphasic aggregation in this system, but with collagen there is a single delayed, irreversible aggregation corresponding to the second wave of the other agents. This second wave in each instance, and the single collagen wave, is due to release of endogenous ADP by the platelets themselves (MacMillan, 1966). In the case of collagen this release is triggered as part of a specific physiological response (Fig. 17.1); in the case of ADP, adrenaline and thrombin, the first wave is due to a direct effect on the platelets and the secondary release of ADP is the consequence of aggregation. As this process is self-perpetuating beyond a certain degree of aggregation the secondary waves are irreversible. Defects of the 'release reaction' show themselves by a lack

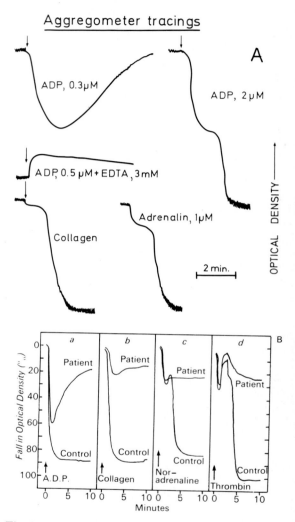

Fig. 17.3 A, Aggregometer tracings on addition of ADP, collagen or adrenaline to normal platelet-rich plasma at 37° in a cuvette. B, Aggregometer tracings in a patient with a defect in ADP release as compared to a normal control. a, Platelet aggregation and disaggregation following addition of ADP to platelet-rich plasma (PRP); b, platelet aggregation following addition of a collagen suspension to PRP; c, platelet aggregation following the addition of noradrenaline to PRP; d, changes following addition to thrombin to PRP. (Reproduced (A) from *Clinics in Haematology* (1972), **1**, 248, by permission of H. Holmsen and the publishers W. B. Saunders; (B) from *Lancet* (1962), **1**, 983, by permission of the authors Hardisty and Hutton).

of this second wave and by an absence of response to collagen. Recent reviews of this subject include those of Marcus (1969A), Holmsen (1972), Salzman (1972) and Weiss (1972). Practical aspects are described by Sanderson (1975).

Diagnostically these techniques are of value since one group of disorders of platelet function (thrombasthenia, Glanzmann's disease) show no aggregation to collagen, adrenaline, thrombin and even 'strong' ADP (i.e. the platelets do not respond to ADP endogenous or exogenous), while another group (thrombopathia, 'storage pool disease', Portsmouth syndrome) essentially show an absence of the secondary wave of aggregation after adrenaline, thrombin and 'strong' ADP, with a total absence of response to collagen (i.e. platelets do not release ADP). A similar pattern is seen after

column, devised by Hellem (1960). In Salzman's technique blood from a clean venepuncture is drawn through a standardized glass bead column by the vacuum in a vacutainer tube. The rate of blood flow through the column was not completely standardized. The percentage of platelets adhering was calculated by comparison of the count in the effluent with that in venous blood obtained from the opposite arm. The validity of the technique in the diagnosis of von Willebrand's disease, in which the adhesiveness is decreased, has repeatedly been confirmed (Strauss and Bloom, 1965; Murphy and Salzman, 1972). Defective adhesiveness is also found in chronic uraemia (Salzman and Neri, 1966), afibrinogenaemia (Weiss and Rodgers, 1971), myeloproliferative syndromes as well as in thrombasthenia (i.e. Glansmann's disease) and

Table 17.1   Inherited disorders of platelet function

Disorder	Frequency	Bleeding time	Platelet size	Aggregation response			Nucleotides	Factor-VIII antigen	Special features
				ADP collagen epinephrine	OX fibrinogen	Ristocetin			
von Willebrand's disease	Common	↑ -N	N	N	N	0-N	N	↓	Hyperresponse to transfusion
Thrombasthenia	Rare	↑	N	0	N (1°)	N	N	N	Poor clot retraction; low platelet fibrinogen
Bernard-Soulier syndrome	Rare	↑	↑	N	0	0	N	N	Thrombocytopenia
Storage-pool disease	Rare	↑	N- ↓	1°	1°	N-1°	↓	N	Occurs in albinos
Mild platelet disorders	Common	N ± ↑	N	1°	1°	N-1°	N	N	May be detected by aspirin tolerance test

Reprinted, by permission, from D. Deykin. (1974) New England Journal of Medicine 290, 149.

taking aspirin. In von Willebrand's disease, a platelet aggregation to these agents is entirely normal in spite of the impaired adhesiveness to glass of platelets in this disease.

Recently the antibiotic ristocetin (1 mg/ml) and bovine fibrinogen (1·7 mg/ml) have been introduced as investigative tools in platelet aggregation (Howard *et al.*, 1973). Abnormal results are obtained with both agents in the Bernard-Soulier syndrome and with ristocetin alone in most cases of von Willebrand's disease (Table 17.1).

Platelet adhesion to glass beads

The application of this measurement to the diagnosis of haemorrhagic states was pioneered by Salzman (1963) using a modification of glass bead

thrombopathia (i.e. defects of ADP release) (Weiss, 1972; Sanderson, 1975). This is therefore a good screening test for platelet dysfunction.

Standardization of the technique is all important. A recent investigation of the variables in this method by Rossi and Green (1972) has shown that consistent results can be obtained if blood from a clean venepuncture is drawn into a plastic syringe and subsequently ejected through the column at a steady rate of 1 ml per 10 seconds, being collected in successive 2 ml aliquots anticoagulated with sodium EDTA (4·5 mg). There is a progressive fall in the platelet count over the first three of these 2 ml aliquots, indicating increasing adhesion, but beyond 6 ml the count rises due to platelets becoming eluted from the glass. The greatest discrimination between normals and patients with

PAEDIATRIC HAEMATOLOGY

Table 17.2 Per cent platelet adhesiveness in normal subjects, von Willebrand's disease and chronic uraemia

	Aliquot 1	Aliquot 2	Aliquot 3	Aliquot 4
Normals (54)★	47 ± 15	88 ± 10	82 ± 23	50 ± 52
	(range 9 to 77)	(range 52 to 100)	(range 8 to 100)	(range −85 to 100)
Von Willebrand's disease (4)†	16 ± 10	11 ± 6	−5 ± 17	−12 ± 25
	(range 5 to 28)	(range 5 to 17)	(range −11 to 10)	(range −47 to 7)
	$t = 5.6206$	$t = 23.7738$	$t = 9.6375$	$t = 4.3607$
Chronic uraemia (8)	9 ± 8	5 ± 10	8 ± 12	7 ± 9
	(range 0 to 21)	(range −10 to 27)	(range −10 to 27)	(range − 6 to 22)
	$t = 10.5088$	$t = 22.3583$	$t = 13.8748$	$t = 5.6104$

The 't' tests compare the patient groups with the group of normal subjects and yield 'p' values that are all significant at the 0·001 level. However, the 't' values for the second aliquot, in which there was no overlap between the normal and patient groups, are much higher than those observed for the first, third and fourth aliquots.

★The numbers in parentheses refer to the number of subjects studied.

†All four patients with von Willebrand's disease had significant bleeding histories. The platelet adhesiveness, factor-VIII levels and bleeding times on these four patients were:

	Platelet adhesiveness (per cent) (second aliquote)	Factor VIII (per cent) (normal 50–150)	Bleeding time (min) (normal 4–7 min)
Patient 1	7	17	4
Patient 2	17	45	9
Patient 3	5	32	9
Patient 4	15	13	20

Reproduced, by permission of Dr. Rossi and the publishers, from Brit. J. Haemat., (1972), **23,** *51.*

von Willebrand's disease or uraemia was seen in the 2nd and 3rd 2 ml aliquots (Table 17.2). The modification of Salzman's technique used at the Manchester Royal Infirmary is described by Sanderson (1975), giving useful details for making one's own glass bead columns.

Clot retraction

In vitro clot retraction depends upon adequate numbers of platelets and integrity of function of their thrombosthenin—a contractile protein in the platelet membrane. It may be judged visually after incubation of whole blood at 37° C for 1 hr and 24 hr (Corby *et al.*, 1971). The absence of normally extruded serum would be clearly apparent. The same phenomenon may be observed in recalcified citrated platelet-rich plasma. A quantitative measure of clot retraction in whole blood has been described by Macfarlane (1939), using a cork-screw shaped wire within a 10 ml conical test tube and withdrawing the attached clot after 1 hour's incubation. A modification for paediatric work using 1 ml samples has been described by Hardisty *et al.* (1964) with a normal range of 40–60 per cent.

Impaired clot retraction in the presence of a normal platelet count is characteristic of Glanzmann's thrombasthenia (Caen, 1972), although it may also occur artefactually in the presence of a pathologically high haematocrit or in the presence of gross dysproteinaemia.

Platelet factor 3 (PF-3) availability

The participation of platelets in blood coagulation is mediated by PF-3. In the past this was assessed by the ability of the platelets to promote 'prothrombin consumption' in clotting blood or by their ability in the thromboplastin generation test. More recently it has been shown that release of PF-3 is closely related to platelet aggregation and ADP release (Horowitz and Papayoanou, 1968). It is thought that aggregation causes an alteration in the platelet membrane whereby lipoprotein (PF-3) become available for participation in the coagulation 'cascade' accelerating the activation of both Factor VIII (AHG) and prothrombin (Marcus, 1969A). Defects of aggregation also show impaired PF-3 availability (Weiss, 1972). Weiss suggests that it is likely that the earlier case reports in the literature where there was a defect of PF-3 availability would have shown impaired aggregation if tested by modern techniques. It is possible therefore that the test is redundant.

The most widely used technique for measuring PF-3 availability is that described by Hardisty and Hutton (1965). This compares the kaolin clotting time of:

1. Patients platelet-rich plasma + normal platelet-poor plasma
2. Normal platelet-rich plasma + patients platelet-poor plasma.

The plasma coagulation factor content of the two mixtures is identical and the only difference is the source of the platelets. Kaolin activation will make PF-3 available in the system containing normal platelets, giving a clotting time in the region of 30 to 50 seconds. Platelets with defective ADP release generally give clotting times in the range of 50–70 seconds (Weiss and Rodgers, 1972).

INHERITED DISORDERS OF PLATELET FUNCTION

In general these disorders produce only relatively mild bleeding tendencies, commonly brought to light after dental extraction or surgery but perhaps accompanied by a life-long tendency to excessive bruising or epistaxis. The bleeding is usually restricted to mucosae, including the renal tract, and the skin, rather than producing haemarthroses or deep haematomata as seen in haemophilia or Christmas disease. There is a tendency for the bleeding tendency to improve with age and life-threatening haemorrhage is unusual. Treatment, if necessary, is by transfusion of platelet concentrates or platelet-rich plasma. Only in von Willebrand's disease is the therapy fresh frozen plasma or cryoprecipitate.

Glanzmann's thrombasthenia

Named from Glanzmann's observations in 1918 of defective clot retraction in the presence of normal or subnormal platelet counts this disorder is nowadays recognized by the following characteristics (Caen *et al.*, 1966; Hardisty *et al.*, 1964; Corby *et al.*, 1971; Caen, 1972):
1. Mucosal and cutaneous bleeding from early life
2. Autosomal recessive inheritance
3. A prolonged bleeding time
4. Decreased or absent clot retraction in the presence of a normal platelet count
5. Absence of platelet aggregation by ADP, thrombin, adrenalin or collagen
6. Deficient PF-3 availability
7. Platelet adhesiveness to glass beads is diminished
8. On a blood film the platelets remain discrete and unclumped, but are of normal size (Papayannis and Israel, 1970).
Heterozygous carriers can be detected only by the clot retraction measurement.

The fundamental defect appears to be a failure of the platelet membrane to react to ADP. The release reaction of ADP is normal but aggregation does not follow, resulting also in impaired adhesiveness and PF-3 availability. The precise explanation for the characteristically poor clot retraction is not entirely clear. In the majority of patients it can be corrected *in vitro* by Mg++ (Caen, 1972). It could possibly be related to the decreased levels of platelet fibrinogen found in this disease (Marcus, 1969B). Plasma fibrinogen levels are normal. There is conflicting evidence as to whether the contractile actomyosin-like protein thrombosthenin on the platelet surface is reduced or not (Weiss and Kochwa, 1968; Caen, 1972). Hardisty *et al.* (1964) have suggested that there is a lack of orientation in the laying down of fibrin strands in relation to individual platelets rendering them unable to exert their normal contractile influence. Recent data has suggested a defect in the reductive capacity of thrombasthenic platelets due to a deficiency of glutathione peroxidase (Karpatkin and Weiss, 1972), but the significance of this finding remains *sub judice* at present (Beutler, 1972).

From a practical point of view it should be reiterated that platelet transfusion is the definitive treatment at times of severe bleeding. As in aplastic anaemia HLa matching between donor and recipient would be important if repeated platelet transfusions are necessary (Gilchrist, 1972; Yankee *et al.*, 1973). It is fortunate that the bleeding tendency usually becomes less marked as the patient grows older. The main problem is likely to be menorrhagia (Hardisty *et al.*, 1964).

Thrombopathia (or defects of ADP release)

This term has been proposed by Weiss (1967) to define those disorders characterized by a failure of normal ADP release in response to aggregating agents (collagen, adrenaline, thrombin), although the platelets still respond to added ADP (Marcus, 1969B). As there is no secondary wave this initial aggregation is followed by rapid disaggregation, even after exposure to 'strong' ADP (2·5 to 10 μg/ml). More recently the term 'thrombocytopathia' has also been used for this type of abnormality (Weiss and Rodgers, 1972).

Criteria for diagnosis in this group of disorders includes:
1. Mild life-long bruising and bleeding from mucosae, especially after dental extraction or surgery
2. Autosomal dominant inheritance
3. A prolonged bleeding time with normal platelet count
4. Normal clot retraction
5. Aggregation $\rightarrow$ disaggregation with ADP, and absent response to collagen, with defective response to adrenaline and thrombin showing a smaller than usual secondary wave (Weiss and Rodger, 1972)

6. Variable deficiency of PF-3 availability
7. Platelet adhesiveness to glass beads usually diminished
8. Morphologically platelets have been normal, small (Maurer *et al.*, 1971) or large in different reports (Weiss and Rodgers, 1972).

Originally described as a 'new' platelet abnormality (Hardisty and Hutton, 1967; Caen *et al.*, 1968), as the 'Portsmouth syndrome' (O'Brien, 1967) or as 'platelet dysfunction' (Sahud and Aggeler, 1969), perhaps the most definitive title is 'Storage Pool Disease' (Holmsen and Weiss, 1970; Holmsen and Weiss, 1972). This term implies impaired ADP release because of reduced amounts of ADP available. In some patients this has been confirmed by low platelet nucleotide levels. In other cases the nucleotide levels are normal, implying a defect of the *release* mechanism (Holmsen and Weiss, 1972). In one family with small platelets there is also an abnormal phospholipid composition of the platelets (Safrit *et al.*, 1972). Deykin (1974) suggests that failure to release ADP constitutes a common disorder with a usually mild bruising tendency that is sharply accentuated if they take aspirin or other drugs that impair platelet function. The bleeding time may be normal unless challenged by aspirin (Quick, 1966).

A similar defect of ADP storage and release has recently been reported in a proportion of albino children in association with a mild bleeding tendency, prolonged bleeding time and normal platelet count (Logan *et al.*, 1971; Maurer *et al.*, 1972; Hardisty *et al.*, 1972). Electron microscopy shows a lack of the normal dense granules containing ADP and serotonin. The haemostatic defect seems identical to that in thrombopathia. Indeed, the original report of Hardisty and Hutton (1967) on a 'new' platelet abnormality included 2 unrelated albino patients. The association of albinism, mild haemorrhagic state due to platelet dysfunction and accumulation of ceroid-like lipopigment in bone marrow macrophages is referred to as the Hermansky-Pudlak syndrome (Hermansky and Pudlak, 1959). The more recent literature on this syndrome is included in the report by White *et al.* (1973) who also describe unusual inclusions in the circulating leucocytes, studied by electron microscopy.

Other hereditary disorders in which 'release abnormalities' occur in association with a mild haemorrhagic state include Wiskott-Aldrich syndrome (Grottum *et al.*, 1969), glycogen storage disease Type I (Gilchrist *et al.*, 1968; Czapek *et al.*, 1973) and osteogenesis imperfecta (Hathaway *et al.*, 1972). Nilsson and Öckerman (1970) investi-gated 10 patients with glycogen storage diseases Types I, III and VI. High platelet counts with prolonged Ivy bleeding times and impaired platelet adhesiveness were the most common abnormalities, with decreased PF-3 release in Type I. The platelet dysfunction in glycogen storage disease Type I can be reversed when the general metabolic state is restored to normal by intravenous alimentation, suggesting that it is an acquired state superimposed upon an inherited metabolic disorder (Czapek *et al.*, 1973). Recently Hutton (1975) has shown that chronic hypoglycaemia (common in Types I, III and VI) causes a defect of platelet aggregation due to reduced levels of ADP and ATP in the platelet, and that these abnormalities are temporarily restored by continuous IV glucose infusion. The platelet defect in the Wiskott-Aldrich syndrome has been reported as improving after successful marrow transplantation (August *et al.*, 1973). The platelet dysfunction associated with congenital afibrinogenaemia differs from that in the 'release' abnormalities and is described separately below.

Bernard-Soulier syndrome

This is a rare but relatively severe haemorrhagic state originally described by Bernard and Soulier (1948), with similar cases subsequently reported by Cullum *et al.* (1967), Kurstjens *et al.* (1968), Grottum and Solum (1969), Howard *et al.* (1973) and others.

The disorder differs from those described above in that there is usually a mild thrombocytopenia (25,000 to 80,000/mm³). Haemorrhagic symptoms and prolongation of the bleeding time, however, are disproportionately severe relative to the degree of thrombocytopenia. Criteria for diagnosis include:
1. Marked life-long bleeding tendency affecting skin and mucosae, but not producing haemarthroses or deep haematomata
2. The fully expressed disease inherited as autosomal recessive, but incomplete features may be found in the heterozygotes
3. A prolonged bleeding time (disproportionate to mild thrombocytopenia)
4. Large platelets with the majority over $4\,\mu$m in diameter (normally the majority are less than $3\,\mu$m)
5. Normal aggregation by ADP, collagen, adrenaline and thrombin, and normal PF-3 release
6. Normal adhesion to glass beads and collagen
7. Normal Factor VIII and Factor VIII-antigen level

DEFECTS OF PLATELET AND CAPILLARY FUNCTION 295

8. Defective aggregation by ristocetin and bovine fibrinogen.

Normal platelets undergo aggregation when exposed to the antibiotic ristocetin (Howard and Firkin, 1971) but this reaction will only take place if Factor VIII or Factor VIII-antigen is also present. The latter is the von Willebrand's factor, absent in von Willebrand's disease and thought to be essential for normal platelet function and haemostasis. Howard, Hutton and Hardisty (1973A) have shown that the platelets of 3 patients with the Bernard-Soulier syndrome failed to aggregate in response to ristocetin, even if suspended in normal plasma. Their experiments suggest that 'the response to ristocetin depends upon an interaction between a platelet component, defective in (these) patients, and a plasma factor deficient in von Willebrand's disease'. This aspect is further discussed in relation to von Willebrand's disease later in this chapter.

Other observations in this interesting syndrome are that the platelets fail to promote prothrombin consumption (Bernard and Soulier, 1948), that the thrombocytopenia is due to shortened *in vivo* platelet survival (Cullum *et al.*, 1967; Grottum and Solum, 1969), and that the shortened survival may be due to a membrane defect associated with reduced electrostatic repulsive forces, the platelets having reduced electrophoretic mobility and an

May-Hegglin anomaly

Giant platelets associated with a variable degree of thrombocytopenia also occur as part of this autosomal dominant disorder described by Hegglin in 1945, the further characteristic of which is the presence of basophilic inclusions in the cytoplasm of granulocytes in blood and marrow. Diagnosis can be confirmed by finding similar changes in one of the parents or a sibling. Purpura and epistaxes occur in about one quarter of cases (Strauss, 1972). Early studies suggested shortened platelet survival, but recent improved techniques show normal results (Murphy, 1972). Most studies have shown normal platelet function (Lusher *et al.*, 1968). Management of the mild haemorrhagic state is not a major problem and splenectomy has seldom been tried.

Von Willebrand's disease

Unlike the rare disorders described above von Willebrand's disease has an incidence of around 1 per 150,000 of population, making it comparable in frequency with Christmas disease. Even this incidence fails to take account of the fact that many of the milder forms of the disease may escape precise diagnosis unless the newer techniques are employed. It is therefore one of the relatively common causes of excessive bleeding encountered in children.

Table 17.3 Results of Factor VIII assay, Duke bleeding time and modified Ivy bleeding time in 28 patients with von Willebrand's disease

Test	Number studied	Number abnormal	Percentage of abnormal
Factor VIII assay	117	67	59
Duke bleeding time	74	59	79
Ivy bleeding time (modified)	121	101	83

The modification of the Ivy bleeding time was that of Borchgrevink and Waaler (1960) *Acta med. Scand.*, 168, 157.
Reproduced by permission from Abildgaard, C. F. et al. (1968), Von Willebrand's disease: A comparative study of diagnostic tests. J. Pediat., 73, 355–363.

abnormally low content of sialic acid (Grottum and Solum, 1969).

Platelet transfusion is the only dependable therapy for temporary control of severe bleeding. Splenectomy has sometimes moderately raised the platelet count, but without clinical improvement, as would be anticipated in view of the qualitative defect (Grottum and Solum, 1969; Kurstjens *et al.*, 1968). The latter authors also reported a significant rise in platelet count in 2 patients on prednisolone, but do not mention any haemostatic benefit.

Described by von Willebrand (1926) and Minot (1928) as an autosomal dominant inherited haemorrhagic state characterized by a prolonged bleeding time later reports included the additional criteria of lowered plasma Factor VIII (AHG) levels (Singer and Ramot, 1956; Spurling and Sacks, 1959) and reduced adhesiveness of platelets to glass beads (Salzman, 1963; Strauss and Bloom, 1965). Not every patient shows all the above abnormalities all of the time (Weiss, 1968; Papayannis *et al.*, 1971). In particular the Factor VIII level gives variable results (Table 17.3). In

27 patients reported by Abildgaard *et al.* (1968) Factor VIII was consistently below 50 per cent of normal in 10, intermittently below 50 per cent in 13, and consistently above 50 per cent (i.e. in the normal range) in 4. Similarly Papayannis *et al.* (1971) found the Factor VIII subnormal in only 59 per cent of tests. The bleeding time was prolonged on 45 occasions and normal on 10, being prolonged at least once in all their 29 patients. Platelet adhesiveness was always less than 50 per cent, but with some overlap with normals. A strong statistical correlation existed between adhesiveness and bleeding time, between adhesiveness and factor VIII level, but not between bleeding time and factor VIII. The variability of the bleeding time, as well as the haemorrhagic symptoms, from time to time in the same patient has been noted since the report of Minot, and further adds to difficulties in diagnosis. They do not necessarily vary in parallel. Severely affected patients have fairly consistent prolongation of their bleeding time. In mild cases it is more variable (Dormandy, 1969). One should remember that a possible cause of phasic variation in bleeding tendency is aspirin ingestion. To confuse matters the prolonged bleeding time after aspirin ingestion in a normal individual can be corrected by cryo-precipitate infusion (Veltkamp and Oosterom, 1973)!

Advances in knowledge of the pathogenesis of this disorder have led to a more precise set of diagnostic criteria (Murphy and Salzman, 1972; Deykin, 1974), as well as increasing our knowledge of platelet participation in haemostasis (Howard *et al.*, 1973A).

The paradoxical finding that transfusion of normal or even haemophilic platelet-poor plasma to a patient with von Willebrand's disease caused a slowly rising and protracted elevation of their Factor VIII level with correction of their bleeding time (Cornu *et al.*, 1963; Biggs and Matthews, 1963; Lewis, 1964) can now be explained. Cryoprecipitate produces the same effect (Bennett and Dormandy, 1966; Perkins, 1967).

Normal plasma contains a large molecular species (antihaemophilic factor or Factor VIII) which corrects the coagulation defect in haemophilic plasma and assays as Factor VIII. After rigorous purification on a sephadex column it can be used to raise a specific antiserum in rabbits. However, this antiserum is found to react not only with the large molecular Factor VIII present in normal plasma but also with a smaller molecule lacking the coagulation activity of Factor VIII, and present in normal serum and in haemophilic plasma. It is termed 'Factor VIII antigen' and is thought to be a fragment of Factor VIII (Deykin, 1974). In von Willebrand's disease both clotting Factor VIII and Factor VIII antigen are low; in classical haemophilia only clotting Factor VIII is low, Factor VIII antigen being normal or elevated (Zimmerman *et al.*, 1971). A possible explanation of the slow rise in clotting Factor VIII activity in a von Willebrand patient after transfusion of Factor VIII antigen from a haemophilic is that the antigen is a precursor or subunit of the clotting factor. Haemophiliacs are unable to effect this conversion but von Willebrand's patients can. From these considerations it has been suggested that 'the absolute hallmark of von Willebrand's disease is a depression of Factor VIII antigen to below 50 per cent of normal' (Deykin, 1974). A study of heterozygous carriers in a severe recessive form of the disease has also suggested that a low Factor VIII antigen level is more directly related to the gene-product of the von Willebrand locus than the antihaemophilic factor activity (Veltkamp and van Tilburg, 1973). There is evidence that this Factor VIII antigen corrects the defective platelet adhesiveness to glass beads in von Willebrand's disease (Bouma *et al.*, 1972). It is probably also the factor required for normal haemostasis in the bleeding time test, consistent with the normality of both platelet adhesiveness and bleeding time in classical haemophilia (with normal Factor VIII antigen levels) and the abnormality of both tests in typical cases of von Willebrand's disease (with low Factor VIII antigen).

Ristocetin-induced platelet aggregation similarly appears to require the presence of normal Factor VIII or Factor VIII antigen (Howard *et al.*, 1973B), being defective in von Willebrand's disease when the Factor VIII antigen level is below 25 per cent of normal (Deykin, 1974). A qualitative abnormality of Factor VIII antigen, demonstrable by two-dimensional crossed immuno-electrophoresis, has recently been demonstrated in a subgroup of von Willebrand's patients (Thomson *et al.*, 1974; Peake *et al.*, 1974). Although present in detectable amounts (15 to 100 per cent) this abnormal Factor VIII antigen did not support ristocetin aggregation. Von Willebrand's disease may therefore include a spectrum of molecular variants.

Howard *et al.* (1973A) have shown that the response to ristocetin depends upon an interaction between a platelet component, defective in the Bernard-Soulier syndrome, and a plasma factor, probably Factor VIII antigen, lacking in von Willebrand's plasma. This interaction appears to be necessary for capillary haemostasis since significant bleeding symptoms associated with a prolonged bleeding time occur in both these disorders. The pathway involved in this aspect of platelet haemostasis is parallel to and independent of ADP release, normal aggregation by collagen occurring in both diseases (Table 17.1). A second mode of platelet haemostasis may thus have been defined by this series of observations.

Diagnostic criteria of typical von Willebrand's disease may therefore be defined as follows:
1. Life-long bleeding tendency affecting skin and mucosae
2. Autosomal dominant inheritance
3. Prolonged bleeding time on at least some occasions
4. Reduced platelet adhesiveness
5. Factor VIII assay below 50 per cent of normal
6. Factor VIII antigen below 50 per cent of normal (or qualitatively abnormal antigen)
7. Normal platelet aggregation with collagen, ADP, adrenaline and thrombin but defective with ristocetin.

Dormandy and coworkers (Stableforth *et al.*, 1975) have suggested that the term von Willebrand's *disease* should be confined to those patients with reduced Factor VIII antigen and reduced ristocetin aggregation, and that von Willebrand's *syndrome* should be used for the various subgroups that are emerging. The latter would include the patients with qualitatively abnormal Factor VIII antigen described by Thomson *et al.* (1974) and Peak *et al.* (1974). Holmberg and Nilsson (1973) had slightly earlier reported a subdivision of their 77 patients with von Willebrand's disease into two separate genetic groups; 57 patients with low Factor VIII antigen and an autosomal dominant inheritance, and 20 patients with a normal Factor VIII antigen level and an X-linked inheritance. These observations may explain some of the inconstancy in diagnostic findings previously described. A similar subdivision on the basis of ristocetin aggregation has also been proposed (Howard *et al.*, 1973B). Only those patients with zero adhesiveness showed absent ristocetin aggregation. The point has also been made that patients with a combination of mild or moderate X-linked classical haemophilia plus a platelet-release defect may clinically mimic typical von Willebrand's disease until Factor VIII antigen is measured and found to be high, and platelet aggregation with ADP and collagen tested (Pechet *et al.*, 1973). A

haemophiliac taking aspirin poses a similar problem (Veltkamp and Oosterom, 1973).

Case 13. A one-year-old boy (No. 177069) presented to the orthopaedic department with a left swollen knee and a history of easy bruising. There was no known haemorrhagic disorder in the family but the maternal grandmother and paternal grandfather were said to bruise easily. The mother had had appendicectomy and dental extractions without trouble. Asked by the orthopaedic department to exclude haemophilia coagulations tests were performed. (This was a mistake. He should have had the routine set of screening tests to detect a possible haemorrhagic state.) Kaolin clotting time was 110″ (control 60″), thromboplastin generation test showed a defect in the patient's adsorbed plasma, one-stage prothrombin time was normal and Factor VIII assay was 3 per cent of normal. On these findings a confident diagnosis of classical haemophilia, of a fairly severe grade, was made. Treatment of what was now recognized to be haemarthrosis was commenced with cryoprecipitate and the patient made a good clinical response.

As the mother wished to have genetic counselling her level of Factor VIII and Factor VIII antigen was determined. Instead of the disproportionately high Factor VIII antigen expected in a haemophilia carrier she showed a marked reduction in the antigen. This finding raised the possibility that the true diagnosis was von Willebrand's disease, rather than haemophilia. Belatedly a bleeding time was performed on her son. This was in excess of 22 minutes! The parents' bleeding times were normal. Further tests on their son showed platelet adhesiveness (Salzman) of 6 per cent (normal > 60 per cent), normal platelet aggregation by collagen, adrenalin and ADP but defective aggregation by ristocetin. His Factor VIII antigen was very low.

Subsequently he has had episodes of post-traumatic bleeding responding to cryoprecipitate and, on one occasion, to human Factor VIII concentrate.

Clinically the disease may present in infancy and extend into adult life but there is a tendency for the symptoms to become less marked with advancing years. The severity varies considerably from patient to patient and from time to time but is seldom as incapacitating as haemophilia. Bruises are often to be found on the shins and over bony prominences such as the iliac crests, being caused by 'physiological' trauma. Purpura (i.e. true petechiae) occurs in only about a quarter of patients. Spontaneous mucosal bleeding may also occur, including epistaxis, gastrointestinal haemorrhage and menorrhagia after puberty. Protracted haemorrhage will follow dental extraction or operations such as tonsillectomy in undiagnosed, untreated patients, this being a common mode of presentation. I know of one such fatality. Bleeding after surgery or trauma is immediate, rather than delayed, and once stopped by pressure or ligation does not recur as in haemophilia, since the coagulation phase of haemostasis is normal in all but those with very low Factor VIII levels. In these, the most severely affected group, haemarthroses, deep haematomata and haematuria may occur as in haemophilia (Dormandy, 1969) (Case 13).

Management consists of the rapid infusion of cryoprecipitate (2 units per 10 kg body wt) or fresh frozen plasma (15 ml/kg) before surgery or in the event of severe spontaneous or post-traumatic bleeding. Infusions on alternate days are usually adequate. The efficacy of the infusion may be monitored both by a shortening of the bleeding time (inconstant) and by correction of the Factor VIII level. Prophylactic dental care and issue of a card indicating the patient's diagnosis and blood group should be arranged. Clinic visits at 2–3 month intervals are advisable to detect and treat iron deficiency anaemia which is common in the more severely affected children. The mother must be advised never to give aspirin, but to give paracetamol when needed instead. A good discussion of management is included in the article by Dormandy (1969).

Congenital afibrinogenaemia

This is inherited as an autosomal recessive haemorrhagic state. Although it is a coagulation factor which is missing the haemostatic defect is similar in type to that of von Willebrand's disease with a prolonged bleeding time and absent platelet adhesiveness to glass (Weiss and Rodgers, 1971). Fibrinogen may interact with platelets at the same locus as von Willebrand's factor and the missing platelet factor in Bernard-Soulier syndrome (Howard et al., 1973A). Other tests of platelet function are normal including clot retraction, PF-3 release, platelet aggregation and ADP release (Gugler and Lüscher, 1965). Whole blood will not clot, one stage prothrombin times and thrombin times are grossly prolonged. Only traces of fibrinogen can be detected in the plasma.

Clinically the disorder may present by bleeding from the umbilical cord in the neonatal period. Thereafter the patients behave like mild haemophiliacs with excessive bleeding after trauma or dental extractions, and prolonged oozing from venepunctures. With major accidents or surgery it is likely that blood transfusions will have been given and excessive bleeding may not be noted since the transfused fibrinogen corrects the defect. Treatment with plasma or whole blood corrects the bleeding time, platelet adhesiveness and haemorrhagic symptoms (Weiss and Rodgers, 1971), and the clinical improvement persists for

longer than fibrinogen can be measured in the patient's plasma (Marcus, 1969B).

Hereditary dysfibrinogenaemia has also been described (Beck et al., 1965; Blombäch et al., 1968). A structurally abnormal fibrinogen is inherited as an autosomal dominant. The reaction with thrombin is defective, so coagulation investigations suggest afibrinogenaemia; but immunological methods show the presence of normal concentrations of fibrinogen. Haemorrhagic states of variable severity have been reported.

ACQUIRED DEFECTS OF PLATELET FUNCTION

Drug ingestion

In 1968 a number of workers independently discovered that aspirin (acetylsalicylic acid) impaired platelet aggregation in vivo and in vitro, largely by inhibiting the release of ADP (Evans et al., 1968; O'Brien, 1968; Weiss et al., 1968). Salicylates did not produce the same effect. Accompanying the impaired aggregation there was a prolongation of the bleeding time, as originally noted by Quick (1966), both in normals (Weiss et al., 1968) and in patients with severe haemophilia or Christmas disease in whom the bleeding time was previously normal (Kaneshiro et al., 1969). As low a dose as 300 mg may permanently affect the cohort of platelets circulating at the time, so the defect can be detected in decreasing severity over a period of 4 to 7 days after exposure, this being related to the normal platelet life span.

Detailed study of the nature of the defect has shown that the ADP storage pool is of normal size (Holmsen and Weiss, 1972) and that it is only the 'release reaction' that is affected, probably through blocking prostaglandin production by platelets (Smith and Willis, 1971; Hamberg et al., 1974). Sahud and Aggeler (1969) contrasted the pattern of laboratory results in patients on aspirin with those suffering from an intrinsic 'storage pool' type of defect. The main differences were normal adhesiveness to glass after aspirin, and the fact that only the second phase of adrenaline-induced aggregation was impaired after aspirin whereas both phases were absent with the intrinsic defect of ADP release.

The clinical relevance of this work lies in the relationship between aspirin ingestion and excessive post-tonsillectomy bleeding (Singer, 1945), gastrointestinal bleeding even when the drug is given parenterally (Weiss et al., 1968), and the occurrence of purpura in children after taking the drug (Casteels-van Daele and De Gaetano, 1971). Specific enquiry will reveal recent aspirin administration in a high proportion of children referred for investigation of bleeding after dental extraction and in whom a prolonged bleeding time also may be found. Suspicion may be raised by the combination of these findings with an absence of a family history and absence of a past history of a bleeding tendency. A number of patients mislabelled as 'capillary bleeders' or mild von Willebrand's disease in the past may have been due to this cause (Gilchrist, 1972). Repeating the bleeding time after 2 weeks without taking aspirin will help to identify these patients. It is also true that patients with an intrinsic haemostatic defect such as von Willebrand's disease, thrombocytopenia, haemophilia or a hereditary platelet function defect may suffer an exaggeration of their bleeding tendency after taking aspirin. This emphasizes the importance of advising parents against giving even small doses of aspirin to children with haematological disorders or undergoing surgery (Schwartz and Pearson, 1971). A safe alternative analgesic is paracetamol. Acetaminophenol (Tylenol) is similarly recommended in the USA (Mielke and Britten, 1970).

Other drugs commonly used in paediatric practice which have been reported as causing platelet dysfunction include antihistamines, tranquillizers, antidepressants, alpha-adrenergic blocking agents, local anaesthetics and antiinflammatory agents such as phenylbutazone and indomethacin (Gilchrist, 1972). The vasodilator drug dipyridamole has been used deliberately to produce the same effect (Emmons *et al.*, 1965; Zucker and Peterson, 1970). Good reviews on this topic are by Mills (1972) and Pochedly and Ente (1972) at fundamental and clinical levels respectively.

Platelet function in the newborn

Platelets in the newborn show subnormal adhesion to glass (Hrodek, 1966) and delayed or impaired aggregation to collagen and adrenaline indicating a partial defect of the release reaction (Mull and Hathaway, 1970; Corby and Schulman, 1971) (Fig. 17.4). These changes do not seem to be accompanied by a haemorrhagic state in the normal baby and the bleeding time is normal. They may, however, render the platelets of newborns unduly sensitive to maternal ingestion of certain drugs. Increased *in vitro* inhibition of collagen-induced aggregation by both aspirin and promethazine in newborns compared to adults has been clearly shown (Fig. 17.5) by Corby and Schulman (1971). *In vivo* these workers found that when promethazine plus pethidine was administered in the management of labour no effect was demonstrable on the mother's platelets, but in 7 of 10 infants there was markedly impaired platelet aggregation by collagen. When aspirin had been taken by the mothers within a week of delivery, 8 of 10 women

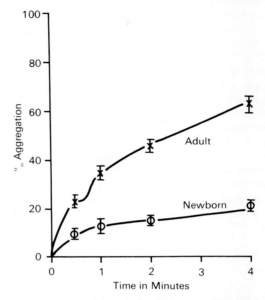

Fig. 17.4 Comparison of platelet aggregation of newborn and adult platelets (no drug exposure) in response to added adrenaline. (Reproduced from The Effect of Antenatal Drug Administration on Aggregation of Platelets of Newborn Infants, in the *Journal of Pediatrics* (1971), **79**, 307, by permission of the authors D. G. Corby and I. Schulman).

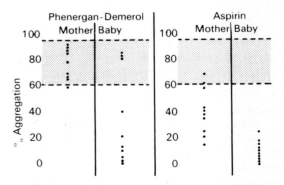

Fig. 17.5 Platelet aggregation in paired maternal-infant platelet suspension, in response to added collagen. (Reproduced from The Effect of Antenatal Drug Administration on Aggregation of Platelets of Newborn Infants, in *Journal of Pediatrics* (1971), **79**, 307, by permission of the authors D. G. Corby and I. Schulman).

showed impaired platelet aggregation and all 10 of their infants had even greater dysfunction (Fig. 17.5). These observations were closely parallel to those of Bleyer and Breckenridge (1970) who similarly found that maternal aspirin ingestion within two weeks of delivery was associated with striking impairment of collagen-induced aggregation of the infants platelets. Bleyer et al. (1970) recorded three haemorrhagic incidents (cephalhaematoma, meleana and periorbital purpura) among 14 infants whose mothers had ingested aspirin. Haslam and Gillam (1974) have reported severe gastrointestinal haemorrhage occurring between 4 and 10 hours after birth in a newborn whose mother had taken Disprin for 3 days before delivery. Platelet aggregation was impaired. These observations indicate the clinical significance of the functional platelet impairement noted in the other reports. It is clear that specific enquiry regarding maternal drug therapy is an essential part of investigation of haemorrhagic states in the newborn. Pochedly and Ente (1972) have listed the drugs that may cause platelet dysfunction in the newborn after administration to the mother (Table 17.4).

from venepunctures ('large vessel haemostasis') has been recognized in advanced uraemia for many years. Thrombocytopenia is present in a minority of patients but more often the platelet count is above 100,000 per mm³. A relationship between defective haemostasis, as judged by the Ivy bleeding time, and platelet dysfunction, as shown by a modification of the prothrombin consumption test, was demonstrated in uraemic patients by Willoughby and Crouch (1961). More recent investigations have shown reduced platelet adhesiveness to glass (Salsman and Neri, 1966) and defective ADP-induced platelet factor 3 activation (Horowitz et al., 1967). Abnormal PF-3 availability was found in three quarters of 55 patients with renal insufficiency by Rabiner and Hrodek (1968), occurring slightly more commonly in those with haemorrhagic symptoms. The platelet dysfunction appears to be caused by guanidino succinic acid, which accumulates in uraemic plasma (Horowitz et al., 1967). This compound is also known to inhibit platelet aggregation by ADP (Jerushalmy et al., 1966). High plasma levels of magnesium ions may also contribute to the platelet dysfunction in uraemic bleeding (Davies

Table 17.4 Drugs which impair platelet function in the newborn

Classification	Trade name	Generic name
Anti-inflammatory nonsteroids	Aspirin	acetylsalicylic acid
	Indocin	indomethacin
	Butazolidin	phenylbutazone
Antihistaminics	Phenergan	promethazine
	Benadryl	diphenhydramine
Tranquilizers	Librium	chlordiazepoxide
	Thorazine	chlorpromazine
	Compazine	prochlorperazine
	Valium	diazepam
	Nisentil	alphaprodine
Antidepressants	Tofranil	imipramine
Cough medicament	several	glyceryl quaiacolate

Reproduced, by permission, from Pochedly and Ente (1972), Pediatric Clinics of North America. **19**, 1095.

Carbenicillin has recently been found to cause a prolonged bleeding time accompanied by impaired ADP-induced aggregation ($2\cdot3\,\mu M$) in healthy volunteers. Three out of 11 volunteers showed gastrointestinal bleeding and 2 out of 5 patients on the drug showed haemorrhagic manifestations (Brown et al., 1974).

Uraemia

A generalized haemorrhagic state affecting skin and mucosae together with a tendency to oozing

et al., 1968). The platelet abnormality and haemorrhagic state respond to dialysis (Stewart and Castaldi, 1967).

Liver disease, dysproteinaemia

In addition to deficiency of coagulation factors of the prothrombin complex in liver disease an abnormality of platelet function has also been described. Thomas et al. (1967) found that platelet aggregation by ADP and thrombin was significantly delayed in patients with cirrhosis and prolonged thrombin times. It was suggested that this was due to the known inhibition of platelet function by fibrinogen degradation products (Kowalski *et al.*, 1964) resulting from excessive fibrinolysis occurring in advanced liver disease. In paediatric practice this situation might be encountered in children with severe portal hypertension or in those with advanced haemosiderosis (e.g. in erythrogenesis imperfecta or thalassaemia major). Although there is usually moderate thrombocytopenia in portal hypertension, due to hypersplenism, the bleeding time is often normal (Hedenberg and Korsan-Bengtsen, 1962). This is presumably because most of the platelets are 'young'.

Platelet aggregation can also be impaired in dysproteinaemia such as Waldenströms macroglobulinaemia (Rozenberg and Dintenfass, 1965) and myelomatosis (Marcus, 1969A), both extremely rare in childhood. The mechanism is 'coating' of the platelet by the pathological plasma protein.

The wide range of acquired and congenital disorders associated with platelet dysfunction in children has recently been reviewed by Hathaway (1971).

PLATELET TRANSFUSION

Platelet transfusion has an important therapeutic role in the control of haemorrhage due to thrombocytopenia or platelet dysfunction. It is clearly in thrombocytopenia caused by failure of production, rather than increased destruction, that most benefit can be expected (Flatow and Freireich, 1966; Grumet and Yankee, 1970). In paediatric practice acute leukaemia is by far the commonest occasion for platelet transfusion (Alvarado *et al.*, 1965), with aplastic anaemia a 'poor second'.

Haemostatically active platelets are rapidly lost in normally banked and stored blood. For effective platelet transfusion the possibilities include freshly collected whole blood, platelet rich plasma or platelet concentrates, plastic bags and siliconized needles being used throughout. Whole blood is the least satisfactory of these since it cannot be given in sufficient volume or at a sufficient rate to achieve the elevation of platelet count desired. Platelet-rich plasma has the advantage that, like whole blood, the platelets have not been sedimented and are therefore unlikely to be clumped. For the child who is actively bleeding I have commonly administered 2–3 units/m^2 of platelet-rich plasma

over $\frac{1}{2}$ hour with rapid resultant haemostasis and negligible hazard of circulatory overload because of the recent blood loss. If hypervolaemia is thought to be a serious hazard IV frusemide can also be given. After haemostasis has been obtained a slow transfusion of packed red cells can be given to restore the haemoglobin level if indicated. Platelet concentrates have the clinical advantage that more units can be given without any problems of hypervolaemia, even in patients without actual blood loss. The centrifugation, sedimentation and resuspension cause inevitable losses, so that the recovery in thrombocytopenic patients ranges between only 25 and 39 per cent with a considerably shortened *in vivo* half life (Cash, 1972). The problems of resuspension in the preparation of platelet concentrates have been greatly reduced by using a buffer which reduces the pH of the platelet-rich plasma to 6·5–6·8 (Aster, 1969). Also it has recently become appreciated that platelets for transfusion are damaged by cooling to 4° C, and are better kept at room temperature (approx. 22° C) until use (Murphy and Gardner, 1969). It has been demonstrated that transfusion of such platelets stored for 24 hours at 22° C corrected platelet aggregation in recipients with impaired aggregation caused by experimental aspirin administration (Handin and Valeri, 1971). The same investigators demonstrated that transfusion of fresh platelets to equal more than 10 per cent of the total immediately shortened the Ivy bleeding time, as well as restoring the platelet aggregation to normal, in aspirin-treated healthy volunteers. Platelets frozen for 24 hours in 6 per cent dimethyl sulphoxide at −80° C have normal *in vivo* survival and haemostatic effectiveness (Valeri, 1974).

The frequency of aspirin self-medication among the general public has occasioned fears that much of the donor blood would contain haemostatically inactive platelets on this account. A careful study by Stuart *et al.* (1972), however, has shown that prolonged bleeding times in thrombocytopenic recipients were corrected when the platelet donor had taken aspirin 36 hours before giving the blood, but not if they had taken aspirin only 12 hours before. Analysis of their data suggested that as long as approximately 20 per cent of the circulating platelets had not been exposed to aspirin the haemostatic function of the platelet pool was maintained.

Clinical indications for platelet transfusion in acute leukaemia are an individual matter partly depending upon such matters as whether the patient is in the initial or terminal stage of the disease. As a general rule they are given *when there is thrombocytopenic bleeding or purpura with a platelet count below 20,000/mm³.* For the average child 4 units of platelet concentrate are adequate, since 1 unit per m² surface area is expected to give a rise of approximately 12,000/mm³ (Cohen, 1971). In older children 6 units could be given, and in infants 2 units. In order to sustain an elevated platelet count transfusion on alternate days will be necessary, but if the need is determined by the reappearance of bleeding longer intervals are often practicable. In the presence of infection, particularly if bacteraemic, the number of units and their frequency will need to be increased (Gardner and Cohen, 1966). A decreased platelet survival has been found and it may prove impossible to elevate the platelet count in such patients (Freireich, 1966). In the presence of severe infection no haemostatic benefit is found. DIC may be a factor in some cases.

In aplastic anaemia the indications are usually similar to those in acute leukaemia, but there is the added problem of long-term immunization with the formation of platelet antibodies and resulting shortened platelet survival. Yankee *et al.* (1973) have shown that, in ideal circumstances, HL-A identical donors should be used since immunization depends primarily upon the HL-A leucocyte system. 3 patients refractory to random donor platelets responded normally to HL-A compatible platelets from unrelated donors. In practice this usually means the use of a suitable sibling, in which there is a 1 in 4 chance of HL-A identity. In the general population such identity is infinitely smaller (Cash, 1972). Large platelet yields can be obtained from single donors by the use of an IBM or AMINCO cell separator (Graw *et al.*, 1971). ABO and Rh incompatibility between donor and recipient are undesirable because small numbers of red cells are inevitably 'carried over' with the platelets, although most investigations have shown that platelet survival *per se* is not affected by the presence of incompatible antibodies to the ABO or Rh antigens present on the donor's red cells (Cash, 1972). Immunization is especially to be avoided, if possible, in patients with aplastic anaemia in whom a subsequent marrow transplant may be needed.

In platelet dysfunction, other than von Willebrand's disease which is primarily due to a plasma defect, there is a clear indication for platelet transfusion at times of severe haemorrhage or as prophylaxis before surgery. A case has also been made for platelet transfusion in postoperative bleeding states of indeterminate origin when the patient has received many units of blood (McGhee and Rapaport, 1968). It is presumed that this transfused blood is deficient in haemostatically active platelets.

In ITP there is a very occasional indication for platelet transfusion, contrary to theory and in the knowledge that all platelets have grossly shortened survival in this disorder. These are patients in whom intracranial haemorrhage is suspected or other severe life-threatening haemorrhage is occurring (Gardner and Cohen, 1966). This can be brought under control for a few hours or even days while other therapeutic approaches are instituted, e.g. steroids or splenectomy. In patients undergoing splenectomy for hypersplenism and thrombocytopenia, I have found it useful giving a platelet transfusion during the operation immediately after splenic pedicle is clamped.

Hazards of platelet transfusion include the transmission of infections including cytomegalovirus, toxoplasmosis and occasionally septicaemia (Buchholz *et al.*, 1971). Since the platelets are used shortly after donation there may not be time to ensure that the donors are free of the Australia antigen before administration. A low grade fever of several hours' duration after transfusion may occur and has been attributed to antileucocyte antibodies in the recipient reacting with contaminating leucocytes in the platelet concentrate (Perry and Yankee, 1971). Acute dyspnoea and cyanosis developing during the platelet transfusion is thought to be caused by pulmonary sequestration of platelet aggregates (Jenevin and Weiss, 1964). In addition the allergic urticarial reactions common to all blood product infusions can be encountered, responding to IV Piriton.

Good recent reviews on platelet transfusion include those of Cash (1972), Becker and Aster (1972) and Buchholz (1974).

NON-THROMBOCYTOPENIC PURPURA

Although not strictly speaking haematological disorders these conditions require brief mention as they enter into the clinical differential diagnosis of purpura due to thrombocytopenia or platelet dysfunction. Purpura occurs in approximately one quarter of patients with von Willebrand's disease, as mentioned above.

Anaphylactoid purpura (Henoch-Schönlein syndrome)

Henoch-Schönlein purpura is the vascular form most commonly encountered in paediatric practice. The purpuric eruption differs greatly from that due to thrombocytopenia in that the lesion is maculopapular, due to oedema and perivascular infiltration initially resembling urticaria, later becoming erythematous with central areas of haemorrhage and finally fading to brown due to denaturation of the extravasated haemoglobin. Initially the lesion is irritative or painful. The rash appears in crops predominantly on the buttocks and the extensor surfaces of the arms and lower legs. Accompanying the rash there are joint or gastrointestinal symptoms in the majority of patients, localized areas of oedema and renal damage with initial haematuria in about one third of patients.

The disease is a manifestation of a hypersensitivity reaction in which the main effect falls upon the capillaries of many tissues, resulting in exudation initially of plasma and later of red cells, together with perivascular infiltration including eosinophils. The platelet count and bleeding time are normal, as is the blood coagulation system, but a positive tourniquet test is found in 25 per cent of patients. Eosinophilia sometimes occurs.

For a recent comprehensive review the reader is referred to the article by Silber (1972). The relation to renal involvement is discussed in the *B.M.J.* (1971).

Scurvy

Although relatively rare nowadays vitamin C deficiency can still occur in undernourished populations and in bottle fed infants if supplements of the vitamin are not given. It presents towards the end of the first year with excessive pain and tenderness of the limbs due to subperiosteal haemorrhages. Epistaxes, haematuria, gastrointestinal bleeding, petechiae and ecchymoses may also appear. A positive tourniquet test is the only demonstrable defect of haemostasis but coagulation studies may show a qualitative abnormality of platelet function (Cetingil *et al.*, 1958).

Drugs, food and infections

Diffuse, benign and self-limiting purpura has been described after exposure to certain drugs, including sulphonamides; food to which the patient is allergic; and infections including, in particular, rubella. Unlike the thrombocytopenic purpura frequently seen after this infection the non-thrombocytopenic form occurs at the height of the illness. Other infections that may present with non-thrombocytopenic purpura include subacute bacterial endocarditis, meningococcal septicaemia, *Coxsackie* and *Echo* viruses (Mauer, 1969). A good review of this group of allergic and vascular purpuras is that by Ackroyd (1953).

INHERITED VASCULAR AND CONNECTIVE TISSUE DISORDERS

Inheritance is the autosomal dominant pattern in this rare group of mild bleeding states, giving little trouble except after trauma, surgery, dental extraction or childbirth. Questionable and ill-defined abnormalities of platelet function have been claimed in Ehler's-Danlos syndrome by Kashiwagi *et al.* (1965) and also in osteogenesis imperfecta, Marfan's syndrome, Hurler's syndrome and Hunter's syndrome by Estes (1968). At present, however, this work is unconfirmed.

Hereditary haemorrhagic telangiectasia
(Rendu-Osler-Weber disease)

Characteristically the lesions appear on the skin of the face, lips, palm or surface of fingers and hands, under the fingernails and on the ears; and on the mucous membranes of the nasal septum, tip and dorsum of the tongue. Internally the gut, lungs, kidneys and brain may be involved. The cutaneous lesions are small, slightly elevated, red to purple, and blanching on pressure (unlike true purpura). The mucosal lesions are similar but appear brighter in colour because of their thinner epithelial covering. Both types of lesion consist of dilated capillaries and venules lacking muscle or connective tissue in their walls and, therefore, incapable of haemostatic contractions. Tests of coagulation and haemostasis are normal unless the bleeding time test fortuitously involves a telangiectatic spot.

The disease is not usually fully developed until adulthood but the first lesions to appear, often in later childhood, are those on the nasal septum. The lesions respond temporarily to cautery.

A good review of this disease is given by Harrison (1963).

Ehler-Danlos syndrome

In this disease there is a deficiency of collagen fibres and an excess of elastic fibres in the skin, resulting in the gradual development of elastic, 'rubbery' scars particularly at the knees and elbows. This is associated with a life-long tendency to excessive bruising and haematoma formation together with increased bleeding and poor wound healing after surgery. There is no coagulation defect and the bleeding time is normal. Recently it has been claimed that the collagen in this disorder is less active than normal collagen in inducing platelet aggregation (Karaca *et al.*, 1972).

304 PAEDIATRIC HAEMATOLOGY

Dissecting aneurysm of aorta, Marfan's syndrome, and other congenital cardiac malformations are known associations. It is thought that an increase in subcutaneous fat may partly protect the subcutaneous blood vessels from trauma. Otherwise there is no specific treatment. For further description of this syndrome see the article by McKusick (1960).

Pseudoxanthoma elasticum and osteogenesis imperfecta

These are other connective tissue disorders in which haemorrhagic manifestations including gastrointestinal, ocular, renal, cutaneous and mucosal haemorrhages can occur in the absence of a demonstrable coagulation or haemostatic defect.

REFERENCES

Abildgaard, C. F., Simone, J. V., Honig, G. R., Forman, E. N., Johnson, C. A. & Seeler, R. A. (1968) Von Willebrand's disease: A comparative study of diagnostic tests. *J. Pediat.*, **73**, 355.

Ackroyd, J. F. (1953) Allergic purpura, including purpura due to food, drugs and infections. *Am. J. Med.*, **14**, 605.

Alvardo, J., Djerassi, I. & Farber, S. (1965) Transfusion of fresh concentrated platelets to children with acute leukemia. *J. Pediat.*, **67**, 13.

Aster, R. H. (1969) Effect of acidification in enhancing viability of platelet concentrates: current status. *Vox Sang.*, **17**, 23.

August, C. S., Hathaway, W. E., Githens, J. H., Pearlman, D. P., McIntosh, K. & Favara, B. (1973) Improved platelet function following bone marrow transplantation in an infant with the Wiskott-Aldrich syndrome. *J. Pediat.*, **82**, 58.

Beck, E. A., Charache, P. & Jackson, D. P. (1965) A new inherited coagulation disorder caused by an abnormal fibrinogen ('Fibrinogen Baltimore'). *Nature*, **208**, 143.

Becker, G. A. & Aster, R. H. (1972) Platelet transfusion therapy. *Med. Clin. N. Amer.*, **56**, 81.

Bennett, E. & Dormandy, K. (1966) Pool's cryoprecipitate and exhausted plasma in the treatment of von Willebrand's disease and Factor-XI deficiency. *Lancet*, **11**, 731.

Bernard, J. & Soulier, J. P. (1948) Sur une nouvelle variété de dystrophie thrombocytaire hémorragipare congénitale. *Sem. Hôp. Paris*, **24**, 3217.

Beutler, E. (1972) Glanzmann's thrombasthenia and reduced glutathione. *New Eng. J. Med.*, **287**, 1094.

Biggs, R. & MacFarlane, R. G. (1962) *Human Blood Coagulation and its Disorders*. 3rd Edn. Oxford: Blackwell Scientific Publications.

Biggs, R. & Matthews, J. M. (1963) The treatment of haemorrhage in von Willebrand's disease and the blood level of Factor VIII (AHG). *Brit. J. Haemat.*, **9**, 203.

Bleyer, W. A. & Breckenridge, R. T. (1970) Studies in the detection of adverse drug reactions in the newborn. II. The effects of prenatal aspirin on newborn hemostasis. *J.A.M.A.*, **213**, 2049.

Bleyer, W. A., Au, W. Y., Lange, W. A. & Raisz, L. G. (1970) Studies on the detection of adverse drug reactions in the newborn. I. Fetal exposure to maternal medication. *J.A.M.A.*, **213**, 2046.

British Medical Journal (1971) Leading article: Henoch-Schönlein purpura and the kidneys. *Brit. med. J.*, **ii**, 352.

Blombäch, M., Blombäch, B., Mammen, E. F. & Prasad, A. S. (1968) Fibrinogen Detroit—a molecular defect in the N-terminal disulphide knot of human fibrinogen. *Nature*, **218**, 134.

Booyse, F. M., Kisieleski, D. & Seeler, R. (1972) Possible thrombosthenin defect in Glanzmann's thrombasthenia. *Blood*, **39**, 377.

Borchgrevnik, C. F. (1960) A method for measuring platelet adhesiveness *in vivo*. *Acta Med. Scand.*, **168**, 157.

Born, G. V. R. (1962) Aggregation of blood platelets by adenosine diphosphate and its reversal. *Nature (London)*, **194**, 927.

Buccholz, D. H., Young, V. M., Friedman, N. R., Reilly, J. A. & Mardiney, M. R. (1971) Bacterial proliferation in platelet products stored at room temperature—transfusion-induced enterobacter sepsis. *New Eng. J. Med.*, **285**, 429.

Bouma, B. N., Wiegerinck, Y., Sixma, J. J., Mourik, J. A. van & Mochtar, I. A. (1972) Immunological characterization of purified antihaemophilic factor A (factor VIII) which corrects abnormal platelet retention in von Willebrand's disease. *Nature*, **236 NB**, 104.

Brown, C. H., Natelson, E. A., Bradshaw, W., Williams, T. W. & Alfrey, C. P. (1974) The hemostatic defect produced by Carbenicillin. *New Eng. J. Med.*, **291**, 265.

Buchholz, D. H. (1974) Blood transfusion: Merits of component therapy. I. The clinical use of red cells, platelets and granulocytes. *J. Pediat.*, **84**, 1.

Caen, J. P., Castaldi, P. A., Leclerc, J. C., Inceman, S., Larrieu, M. J., Probst, M. & Bernard, J. (1966) Congenital bleeding disorders with long bleeding time and normal platelet count: I. Glanzmann's thrombasthenia (report of 15 patients). *Amer. J. Med.*, **41**, 4.

Caen, J. P., Sultan, T. & Larrieu, M. (1968) A new familial platelet disease. *Lancet*, **i**, 203.

Caen, J. (1972) Glanzmann's thromnasthenia. *Clinics in Haematology*, **1**, 383.

Cash, J. D. (1972) Platelet transfusion therapy. *Clinics in Haematology*, **1**, 395.

Casteels-van Daele, M. & Gaetano, G. De (1971) Purpura and acetyl salicylic acid therapy. *Acta Paediat. Scand.*, **60**, 203.

Cetingil, A. I., Ulutin, O. N. & Karaca, M. (1958) A platelet defect in a case of scurvy. *Brit. J. Haemat.*, **4**, 350.

Cohen, E. (1971) Transfusion of platelets and leukocytes. *N.Y. State J. Med.*, **71**, 1522.

Corby, D. G. & Schulman, I. (1971) The effects of antenatal drug administration on aggregation of platelets of newborn infants. *J. Pediat.*, **79**, 307.

Corby, D. G., Zirbel, C. L., Lindley, A. & Schulman, I. (1971) Thrombasthenia. *Am. J. Dis. Child.*, **121**, 140.

Cornu, P., Larrieu, M. J., Caen, J. & Bernard, J. (1963) Transfusion studies in von Willebrand's disease: Effect on bleeding time and factor VIII. *Brit. J. Haemat.*, **9**, 189.

Cullum, C., Cooney, D. P. & Schrier, S. L. (1967) Familial thrombocytopenic thrombocytopathy. *Brit. J. Haemat.*, **13**, 147.

Czapek, E. E., Deykin, D. & Salzman, E. W. (1973) Platelet dysfunction in glycogen storage disease type I. *Blood*, **41**, 235.

Davies, D. T. P., Hughes, A., Lomax, G. D. & Tonks, R. S. (1968) Hypermagnesaemia and platelet function in uraemic bleeding. *Lancet*, **1**, 301.

Deykin, D. (1974) Emerging concepts of platelet function. *New Eng. J. Med.*, **290**, 144.

Dormandy, K. M. (1969) Von Willebrand's disease: pathogenesis and management. *J. Roy. Coll. Phycns. Lond.*, **3**, 211.

Emmons, P. R., Harrison, M. J., Honour, A. J. & Mitchell, J. R. A. (1965) Effect of dipyridamole on human platelet behaviour. *Lancet*, **ii**, 603.

Estes, J. W. (1968) Platelet size and function in the heritable disorders of connective tissue. *Ann. Intern. Med.*, **68**, 1237.

Evans, G., Packham, M. A., Nishizawa, E. E., Mustard, J. F. & Murphy, E. A. (1968) The effect of acetyl salicylic acid on platelet function. *J. Exp. Med.*, **128**, 877.

Flatow, F. A. & Freireich, E. J. (1966) Effect of splenectomy on the response to platelet transfusions in three patients with aplastic anaemia. *New Eng. J. Med.*, **274**, 242.

Freireich, E. J. (1966) Effectiveness of platelet transfusion in leukemia and aplastic anemia. *Transfusion*, **6**, 50.

French, J. E., Macfarlane, R. G. & Sanders, A. G. (1964) Structure of haemostatic plugs and experimental thrombi in small arteries. *J. Exper. Path.*, **45**, 467.

Gardner, F. H. & Cohen, P. (1966) The use of platelet transfusions. *Med. Clinics. N. Amer.*, **50**, 1559.

Garg, S. K., Amorosi, E. L. & Karpatkin, S. (1971) Use of the megathrombocyte as an index of megakaryocyte number. *New Eng. J. Med.*, **284**, 11.

Gilchrist, G. S., Fine, R. N. & Donnell, G. N. (1968) The haemostatic defect in glycogen storage disease, type I. *Acta Paediat. Scand.*, **57**, 205.

Gilchrist, G. S. (1972) Platelet disorders. *Paediat. Clin. N. Amer.*, **19**, 1047.

Glanzmann, E. (1918) Hereditäre hämorrhagische Thrombasthenie. Ein Beitrag zür Pathologie der Blütplättchen. *Jahrbuch fur Kinderheilkunde*, **88**, 113.

Graw, G. R., Herzig, G. P., Eisel, R. J. & Perry, S. (1971) Leukocyte and platelet collection from normal donors with continuous flow blood cell separator. *Transfusion*, **11**, 94.

Gröttum, K. A. & Solum, N. O. (1969) Congenital thrombocytopenia with giant platelets: a defect in the platelet membrane. *Brit. J. Haemat.*, **16**, 277.

Gröttum, K. A., Hovig, T., Holmsen, H., Foss Abrahamsen, A., Jeremic, M. & Seip, A. (1969) Wiskott-Aldrich syndrome: qualitative platelet defects and short platelet survival. *Brit. J. Haemat.*, **17**, 373.

Grumet, F. C. & Yankee, R. A. (1970) Long-term platelet support of patients with aplastic anaemia. *Annals of Internal Med.*, **73**, 1.

Gugler, E. & Lüscher, E. F. (1965) Platelet function in congenital afibrinogenemia. *Thromb. et Disth. Haemorrh.*, **14**, 361.

Hamberg, M., Svensson, J. & Samuelsson, B. (1974) Mechanism of the anti-aggregating effect of aspirin on human platelets. *Lancet*, **ii**, 223.

Handin, R. I. & Valeri, C. R. (1971) Hemostatic effectiveness of platelets stored at 22°C. *New Eng. J. Med.*, **285**, 538.

Hardisty, R. M., Dormandy, K. M. & Hutton, R. A. (1964) Thrombasthenia. Studies on three cases. *Brit. J. Haemat.*, **10**, 371.

Hardisty, R. M. & Hutton, R. A. (1965) The kaolin clotting time of platelet-rich plasma: a test of platelet factor-3 availability. *Brit. J. Haemat.*, **11**, 258.

Hardisty, R. M. & Ingram, G. I. C. (1965) *Bleeding Disorders*. Aylesbury, Bucks.: Hazell Watson & Viney.

Hardisty, R. M. & Hutton, R. A. (1967) Bleeding tendency associated with 'new' abnormality of platelet behaviour. *Lancet*, **1**, 983.

Hardisty, R. M., Mills, D. C. B. & Ketsar-ard, K. (1972) The platelet defect associated with albinism. *Brit. J. Haemat.*, **23**, 679.

Harker, L. A. & Slichter, S. J. (1972) The bleeding time as a screening test for evaluation of platelet function. *New Eng. J. Med.*, **287**, 155.

Harrison, D. F. N. (1963) Familial haemorrhagic telangiectasia. *Quarterly J. Med. (N.S.)*, **33**, 25.

Haslam, R. R. & Gillam, G. L. (1974) Hemorrhage in a neonate possibly due to maternal ingestion of salicylate. *J. Pediatrics*, **84**, 556.

Hathaway, W. H. (1971) Bleeding disorders due to platelet dysfunction. *Amer. J. Dis. Child.*, **121**, 127.

Hathaway, W. E., Solomons, C. C. & Ott, J. E. (1972) Platelet function and pyrophosphates in osteogenesis imperfecta. *Blood*, **39**, 500.

Hedenberg, L. & Korsan-Bengtsen, K. (1962) Clotting tests and other tests of the haemostatic mechanism in cirrhosis of the liver and their diagnostic significance. *Acta med. Scand.*, **172**, 229.

Hegglin, V. R. (1945) Gleichzeitige konstitutionelle Veränderungen an Neutrophilen und Thrombozyten. *Helvetica Medica Acta*, **4**, 439.

Hellem, A. J. (1960) The adhesiveness of human blood platelets *in vitro*. *Scandinavian Journal of Clinical and Laboratory Investigation*, **12**, Suppl. 51.

Hermansky, F. & Pudlak, P. (1959) Albinism associated with hemorrhagic diathesis and unusual pigmented reticular cells in the bone marrow: Report of two cases with histochemical studies. *Blood*, **14**, 162.

Holmberg, L. & Nilsson, I. M. (1973) Two genetic variants of von Willebrand's disease. *New Eng. J. Med.*, **288**, 595.

Holmsen, H. & Weiss, H. J. (1970) Hereditary defect in platelet release reaction caused by a deficiency in the storage pool of platelet adenine nucleotides. *Brit. J. Haemat.*, **19**, 643.

Holmsen, H. (1972) The platelet: Its membrane, physiology and biochemistry. *Clinics in Haematology*, **1**, 235.

Holmsen, H. & Weiss, H. J. (1972) Further evidence for a deficient storage pool of adenine nucleotides in platelets from some patients with thrombocytopathia—storage pool disease. *Blood*, **39**, 197.

Horowitz, H. I., Cohen, B. D., Martinez, P. & Papayoanou, M. F. (1967) Defective ADP-induced platelet factor 3 activation in uremia. *Blood*, **30**, 331.

Horowitz, H. I. & Papayoanou, M. F. (1968) Activation of platelet factor 3 by adenosine 5′diphosphate. *Thromb. Diath. Haemorrh.*, **19**, 18.

Howard, M. A. & Firkin, B. G. (1971) Ristocetin—a new tool in the investigation of platelet aggregation. *Thromb. Diath. Haemorrh.*, **26**, 362.

Howard, M. A., Hutton, R. A. & Hardisty, R. M. (1973A) Hereditary giant platelet syndrome: A disorder of a new aspect of platelet function. *Brit. med. J.*, **2**, 586.

Howard, M. A., Sawers, R. J. & Firkin, B. G. (1973B) Ristocetin: A means of differentiating von Willebrand's disease into two groups. *Blood*, **61**, 687.

Hrodek, O. (1966) Blood platelets in the newborn. *Acta Univ. Carol. Med. Monograph*, **22**.

Hughes, J. (1966) Facteurs locaux du premier temps de l'hémostase. *Acta Haemat.*, **36**, 109.

Hutton, R. A. (1975) Abnormal platelet function in chronic hypoglycaemia. (Also in press in *Archives of Diseases in Childhood.*) *Brit. J. Haemat.*, **30**, 129.

Ivy, A. C., Nelson, D. & Bucher, G. (1941) The standardization of certain factors in the cutaneous 'venostasis' bleeding time technique. *J. Lab. Clin. Med.*, **26**, 1812.

Jenevin, E. P. & Weiss, D. L. (1964) Platelet thromboembolism associated with massive transfusion. *Amer. J. Pathology*, **45**, 313.

Jerushalmy, Z., Skoza, L., Zucker, M. B. & Grant, R. (1966) Inhibition by guanidino compounds of platelet aggregation induced by adenosine diphosphate. *Biochem. Pharmacol.*, **15**, 1791.

Kaneshiro, M. M., Mielke, C. H., Kasper, C. K. & Rapaport, S. I. (1969) Bleeding time after aspirin in disorders of intrinsic clotting. *New Eng. J. Med.*, **281**, 1039.

Karaca, M., Cronberg, L. & Nilsson, I. M. (1972) Abnormal platelet-collagen reaction in Ehlers-Danlos syndrome. *Scand. J. Haematol.*, **9**, 465.

Karpatkin, S. (1969A) Heterogeneity of human platelets. I. Metabolic and kinetic evidence suggestive of young and old platelets. *J. Clin. Invest.*, **48**, 1073.

Karpatkin, S. (1969B) Heterogeneity of human platelets. II. Functional evidence suggestive of young and old platelets. *J. Clin. Invest.*, **48**, 1083.

Karpatkin, S. & Weiss, H. J. (1972) Deficiency of glutathione peroxidase associated with high levels of reduced glutathione in Glanzmann's thrombasthenia. *New Eng. J. Med.*, **287**, 1062.

Kashiwagi, H., Riddle, J. M., Abraham, J. P. & Frame, B. (1965) Function and ultrastructural abnormalities of platelets in Ehler-Danlos syndrome. *Ann. Intern. Med.*, **63**, 249.

Kloeze, J. (1969) Relationship between chemical structure and platelet aggregation activity of prostaglandins. *Biochim. Biophys. Acta*, **187**, 285.

Kowalski, E., Kopéc, M. & Wegrzynowicz, Z. (1964) Influence of fibrinogen degradation products (FDP) on platelet aggregation, adhesiveness and viscous metamorphosis. *Thromb. Diath. Haemorrh.*, **10**, 406.

Kowalski, E. (1968) Fibrinogen derivatives and their biologic activities. *Seminars in Hemat.*, **5**, 45.

Kurstjens, R., Bolt, C., Vossen, M. & Haanen, C. (1968) Familial thrombopathic thrombocytopenia. *Brit. J. Haemat.*, **15**, 305.

Lewis, J. H. (1964) Synthesis of AHF in von Willebrand's disease. *Blood*, **23**, 233.

Logan, L. J., Rapaport, S. I. & Maher, I. (1971) Albinism and abnormal platelet function. *New Eng. J. Med.*, **284**, 1340.

Lusher, J. M., Schneider, J., Mizukami, I. & Evans, R. (1968) The May-Hegglin anomaly: platelet function, ultrastructure and chromosome studies. *Blood*, **32**, 950.

Macfarlane, R. G. (1939) A simple method for measuring clot retraction. *Lancet*, **i**, 1199.

McGhee, W. G. & Rapaport, S. I. (1968) Systemic haemostatic failure in the severely injured patient. *Surgical Clinics of N. Amer.*, **48**, 1247.

McKusick, V. A. (1960) *Heritable Disorders of Connective Tissue*. 2nd Edn., p. 135. St. Louis: Mosby.

Macmillan, D. C. (1966) Secondary clumping effect in human citrated platelet-rich plasma produced by adenosine diphosphate and adrenaline. *Nature (London)*, **211**, 140.

Marcus, A. J., Zucker-Franklin, D., Safier, L. B. & Ullman, H. L. (1966) Studies on human platelet granules and membranes. *J. Clin. Invest.*, **45**, 14.

Marcus, A. J. (1969A) Platelet function. *New Eng. J. Med.*, **280**, 1278.

Marcus, A. J. (1969B) Platelet function. *New Eng. J. Med.*, **280**, 1330.

Mauer, A. M. (1969) *Pediatric Hematology*, p. 429. London & New York: McGraw-Hill.

Maurer, H. M., Still, W. J. S., Caul, J., Valdes, O. S. & Laupus, W. E. (1971) Familial bleeding tendency associated with microcytic platelets and impaired release of platelet adenosine diphosphate. *J. Pediat.*, **78**, 86.

Maurer, H. M., Wolff, J. A., Buckingham, S. & Spielvogel, A. R. (1972) Impotent platelets in albinos with prolonged bleeding times. *Blood*, **39**, 490.

Medical Research Council Memorandum No. 32 (1955) *The Diagnosis and Treatment of Haemophilia and Related Conditions.* London: H.M.S.O.

Mielke, C. H., Kaneshiro, M. M., Maher, I. A., Weiner, J. M. & Rapaport, S. I. (1969) The standardized normal Ivy bleeding time and its prolongation by aspirin. *Blood*, **34**, 204.

Mielke, C. & Britten, A. (1970) Use of aspirin or acetaminophen in hemophilia. *New Eng. J. Med.*, **282**, 1270.

Mills, D. C. B. (1972) Drugs that affect platelet behaviour. *Clinics in Haematology*, **1**, 295.

Minot, G. R. (1928) A familial hemorrhagic condition associated with prolongation of the bleeding time. *Am. J. Med. Sci.*, **3**, 301.

Mull, M. M. & Hathaway, W. E. (1970) Altered platelet function in newborns. *Pediat. Res.*, **4**, 229.

Murphy, S. & Gardner, F. H. (1969) Platelet preservation: effect of storage temperature on maintenance of platelet viability—deleterious effect of refrigerated storage. *New Eng. J. Med.*, **280**, 1094.

Murphy, S. (1972) Hereditary thrombocytopenia. *Clinics in Haematology*, **1**, 359.

Murphy, E. A. & Salzman, E. W. (1972) The diagnosis of von Willebrand's disease. *Blood*, **39**, 284.

Murphy, S., Oski, F. A., Naiman, J. L., Lusch, C. J., Goldberg, S. & Gardner, F. H. (1972) Platelet size and kinetics in hereditary and acquired thrombocytopenia. *New Eng. J. Med.*, **286**, 499.

Nachman R. L., Marcus, A. J. & Safier, L. B. (1967) Platelet thrombosthenin: Subcellular localization and function. *J. Clin. Invest.*, **46**, 1380.

Nilsson, I. M. & Ockerman, P. A. (1970) The bleeding disorder in hepatomegalic forms of glycogen storage disease. *Acta Paediat. Scand.*, **59**, 127.

O'Brien, J. R. (1962) Platelet aggregation. *J. Clin. Path.*, **15**, 446.

O'Brien, J. R. (1967) Platelets: a Portsmouth syndrome. *Lancet*, **ii**, 258.

O'Brien, J. R. (1968) Effects of salicylates on human platelets. *Lancet*, **i**, 779.

O'Brien, J. R. (1968) Effect of anti-inflammatory agents on platelets. *Lancet*, **1**, 894.

Papayannis, A. G. & Israels, M. C. G. (1970) Glanzmann's disease and trait. *Lancet*, **11**, 44.

Papayannis, A. G., Wood, J. K. & Israels, M. C. G. (1971) Factor VIII levels, bleeding times, and platelet adhesiveness in patients with von Willebrand's disease and in their relatives. *Lancet*, **1**, 418.

Peake, I. R., Bloom, A. L. & Giddings, J. C. (1974) Inherited variants of factor VIII-related protein in von Willebrand's disease. *New Eng. J. Med.*, **291**, 113.

Perkins, H. A. (1967) Correction of the hemostatic defects in von Willebrand's disease. *Blood*, **30**, 375.

Pechet, L., Chesney, C. & Colman, R. W. (1973) Variants of von Willebrand's disease. *New Eng. J. Med.*, **288**, 1129.

Perry, S. & Yankee, R. A. (1971) Transfusion and preservation. In *The Circulating Platelet*. Edited by S. A. Johnson. New York and London: Academic Press.

Pochedly, C. & Ente, G. (1972) Adverse hematologic effects of drugs. *Pediat. Clin. N. Amer.*, **19**, 1095.

Quick, A. J. (1966) Salicylates and bleeding: the aspirin tolerance test. *Amer. J. Med. Sci.*, **252**, 265.

Rabiner, S. F. & Hrodek, O. (1968) Platelet factor 3 in normal subjects and patients with renal failure. *J. Clin. Invest.*, **47**, 901.

Rorvik, T. O., Holmsen, I. & Stormorken, H. (1968) Release of ADP from red blood cells. *Thromb. Diath. Haemorrh.*, **19**, 77.

Rossi, E. C. & Green, D. (1972) A study of platelet retension by glass bead columns ('platelet adhesiveness' in normal subjects). *Brit. J. Haemat.*, **23**, 47.

Rosenberg, M. C. & Dintenfass, L. (1965) Platelet aggregation in Waldenström's macroglobulinemia. *Thromb. Diath. Haemorrh.*, **14**, 202.

Safrit, H., Weiss, H. J. & Phillips, G. B. (1972) The phospholipid and fatty acid composition of platelets in patients with primary defects of platelet function. *Lipids*, **7**, 60.

Sahud, M. A. & Aggeler, P. M. (1969) Platelet dysfunction—differentiation of a newly recognized primary type from that produced by aspirin. *New Eng. J. Med.*, **280**, 453.

Salzman, E. W. (1963) Measurement of platelet adhesiveness: a simple *in vitro* technique demonstrating an abnormality in von Willebrand's disease. *J. Lab. Clin. Med.*, **62**, 724.

Salzman, E. W. & Neri, L. L. (1966) Adhesiveness of blood platelets in uremia. *Thromb. Disth. Haemorrh.*, **15**, 84.

Salzman, E. W. (1972) Cyclic AMP and platelet function. *New Eng. J. Med.*, **286**, 358.

Sanderson, J. H. (1975) Platelet function tests. Association of Clinical Pathologists: Broadsheet 83. *J. clin Path.*

Schwartz, A. & Pearson, H. (1971) Aspirin, platelets and bleeding. *J. Pediat.*, **78**, 558.

Silber, D. L. (1972) Henoch-Schönlein syndrome. *Pediat. Clinics N. Amer.*, **19**, 1061.

Singer, R. (1945) Acetylsalicylic acid, a probable cause for secondary post-tonsillectomy hemorrhage. *Arch. Otolaryng.*, **42**, 19.

Singer, K. & Ramot, B. (1956) Pseudohemophilia type B hemorrhagic diathesis characterized by a prolonged bleeding time and decrease in antihemophilic factor. *Am. Med. Assoc. Arch. Intern. Med.*, **97**, 715.

Smith, J. B. & Willis, A. L. (1971) Aspirin selectively inhibits prostaglandin production in human platelets. *Nature*, **231**, 235.

Spaet, T. H. & Zucker, M. B. (1964) Mechanism of platelet plug formation and role of adenosine diphosphate. *Am. J. Physiol.*, **206**, 1267.

Spaet, T. H. & Lejnieks, I. (1969) A technique for estimation of platelet-collagen adhesion. *Proc. Soc. Exp. Biol. Med.*, **132**, 1038.

Spurling, C. L. & Sacks, M. S. (1959) Inherited hemorrhagic disorder with antihemophilic globulin deficiency and prolonged bleeding time (vascular hemophilia). *New Eng. J. Med., 261,* 311.

Stableforth, P., Hughes, J., Wilson, E. & Dormandy, K. M. (1975) The von Willebrand 'syndrome'. *Brit. J. Haemat., 29,* 605.

Stewart, J. H. & Castaldi, P. A. (1967) Uraemic bleeding: reversible platelet defect corrected by dialysis. *Quart. J. Med., 36,* 409.

Strauss, H. S. & Bloom, G. E. (1965) Von Willebrand's disease: use of a platelet-adhesiveness test in diagnosis and family investigation. *New Eng. J. Med., 273,* 171.

Strauss, H. S. (1972) Diagnosis and treatment of inherited bleeding disorders. *Pediatrics Clinics of N. Amer., 19,* 1009.

Stuart, M. J., Murphy, S., Oski, F. A., Evans, A. E., Donaldson, M. H. & Gardner, F. H. (1972) Platelet function in recipients of platelets from donors ingesting apsirin. *New Eng. J. Med., 287,* 1106.

Sutor, A. H., Bowie, E. J. W., Thompson, J. H., Didisheim, P., Mertens, B. F. & Owen, C. A. (1971) Bleeding from standardized skin punctures: automated technic for recording time, intensity and pattern of bleeding. *Am. J. Clin. Path., 55,* 541.

Thomas, D. P., Ream, V. P. & Stuart, R. K. (1967) Platelet aggregation in patients with Laennec's cirrhosis of liver. *New Eng. J. Med., 276,* 1344.

Thomson, C., Forbes, C. D. & Prentice, C. R. M. (1974) Evidence for a qualitative defect in factor-VIII-related antigen in von Willebrand's disease. *Lancet, 1,* 594.

Veltkamp, J. J. & Tilburg, N. H. van (1973) Detection of heterozygotes for recessive von Willebrand's disease by the assay of antihaemophilic-factor-like antigen. *New Eng. J. Med., 289,* 882.

Veltkamp, J. J. & Oosterom, A. T. van (1973) Two genetic variants of von Willebrand's disease. *New Eng. J. Med., 288,* 1411.

Valeri, C. R. (1974) Hemostatic effectiveness of liquid and previously frozen human platelets. *New Eng. J. Med., 290,* 353.

Weiss, H. J. (1968) Analytic review: von Willebrand's disease—diagnostic criteria. *Blood, 32,* 668.

Weiss, H. J. & Kochwa, S. (1968) Studies of platelet function and proteins in 3 patients with Glanzmann's thrombasthenia. *J. Lab. Clin. Med., 71,* 153.

Weiss, H. J., Aledort, L. M. & Kochwa, S. (1968) The effect of salicylates on the hemostatic properties of platelets in man. *J. Clin. Invest., 47,* 2169.

Weiss, H. J. & Rodgers, J. (1971) Fibrinogen and platelets in the primary arrest of bleeding. Studies on two patients with congenital afibrinogenemia. *New Eng. J. Med., 285,* 369.

Weiss, H. J. (1972) Thrombocytopathia. *Clinics in Haematology, 1,* 369.

Weiss, H. J. & Rodgers, J. (1972) Thrombocytopathia due to abnormalities in the platelet release reaction—studies on six unrelated patients. *Blood, 39,* 187.

White, J. G., Witkop, C. J. & Gerritsen, S. M. (1973) The Hermansky-Pudlak syndrome: Inclusions in circulating leucocytes. *Brit. J. Haemat., 24,* 761.

Willebrand, E. A. von (1926) Hereditäre pseudohemofili. *Finska Läk-Sällsk. Handl., 68,* 87.

Willoughby, M. L. N. & Allington, M. J. (1961) The rate of blood loss from skin punctures during the Ivy bleeding time test. *J. Clin. Path., 14,* 381.

Willoughby, M. L. N. & Crouch, S. J. (1961) An investigation of the haemorrhagic tendency in renal failure. *Brit. J. Haemat., 7,* 315.

Wilner, G. D., Nossel, H. L. & LeRoy, E. C. (1958A) Aggregation of platelets by collagen. *J. Clin. Invest., 47,* 2616.

Wilner, G. D., Nossel, H. L. & LeRoy, E. C. (1968B) Activation of Hageman factor by collagen. *J. Clin. Invest., 47,* 2608.

Yankee, R. A., Graff, K. S., Dowling, R. & Henderson, E. S. (1973) Selection of unrelated compatible platelet donors by lymphocyte HL-A matching. *New Eng. J. Med., 288,* 760.

Zimmerman, T. S., Ratnoff, O. D. & Powell, A. E. (1971) Immunological differentiation of classic hemophilia (factor VIII deficiency) and von Willebrand's disease: with observations on combined deficiencies of antihaemophilic factor and proaccelerin (factor V) and on an acquired circulating anticoagulant against antihemophilic factor. *J. Clin. Invest., 50,* 244.

Zucker, M. B. & Peterson, J. (1970) Effect of acetylsalicylic acid, and other non-steroidal antiflammatory agents, and dipyridamole on human blood platelets. *J. Lab. Clin. Med., 76,* 66.

18. Coagulation Disorders. I. Hereditary

Physiology of blood coagulation / Investigation of disorders of coagulation / Hereditary coagulation defects, *Haemophilia, Management of specific problems, Other hereditary coagulation disorders.*

PHYSIOLOGY OF BLOOD COAGULATION

Haemostasis is initiated by platelet adhesion and aggregation but is consolidated by fibrin formation between and around the platelets of the 'haemostatic plug'. In capillaries the combination of vascular constriction and platelet aggregation may be sufficient, but for permanent haemostasis in larger vessels the addition of fibrin is essential. In the presence of a severe coagulation defect such as haemophilia initial arrest of bleeding may occur normally, but after an hour bleeding restarts.

Fibrin formation is the visible and haemostatically significant end result of a large number of preceding biochemical events involving a series of soluble coagulation factors, the first step of which is the activation of Factor XII (Hageman factor) by contact with a foreign surface, such as damaged endothelium. Macfarlane (1964) first suggested that the subsequent chain of events could best be explained by 'a cascade of proenzyme-enzyme transformations, each enzyme activating the next until the final substrate, fibrinogen, is reached (Fig. 18.1). Coagulation factors would normally be circulating in inactive state. Macfarlane pointed out that such a mechanism would act as a 'biochemical amplifier' whereby a small initial stimulus would result in a massive final reaction since each enzyme might activate ten times its own number of proenzymes. Rapid fibrin formation seems to be

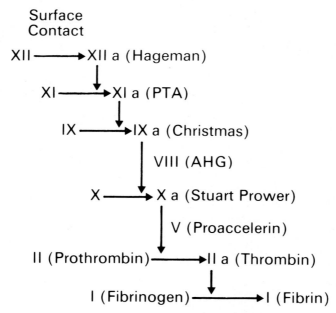

Fig. 18.1 The cascade hypothesis with alternative names of numerical Factors. (After MacFarlane, 1964. Reproduced by permission of Professor MacFarlane and the Editor of *Nature*).

essential for efficient haemostasis. A similar theory was proposed by Davie and Ratnoff (1964). There have been minor modifications since (Macfarlane, 1968; Davie *et al.*, 1969) with evidence suggesting that Factor VIII (antihaemophilic factor; AHG) and Factor V do not function as proenzymes but as cofactors for the action of the enzyme generated in the preceding stage, viz. IXa and Xa respectively.

Platelets participate, by PF3 or phospholipid availability, at the stage of interaction between activated Factor X and Factor V. Calcium ions are necessary for most of the steps.

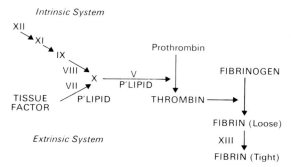

Fig. 18.2 Intrinsic and extrinsic coagulation systems. 'P' Lipid' indicates interaction by platelet phospholipid. (Reproduced from the *New England Journal of Medicine* (1970), **283**, 636, with permission from the author Dr Deykin and the publisher).

The coagulation factors involved in the series of reactions beginning with activation of Factor XII and ending in fibrin formation constitute the *intrinsic coagulation system*, all the components of which are present in, or intrinsic to, the circulating blood. There is also an *extrinsic coagulation system* involving tissue thromboplastin and a further factor (VII) not included in the intrinsic system (Fig. 18.2). Both systems have a final common pathway from Factor X to fibrin formation (Stor-

morken and Owren, 1971). Thrombin cleaves fibrinopeptides A and B from the alpha and beta chains of fibrinogen. The residual peptide chains aggregate by means of loose hydrogen bonds to form *fibrin monomer*. This can be brought back into solution by 5M urea. Under the influence of Factor XIII, itself activated by thrombin, further covalent cross links are formed which convert it into a more permanent, urea insoluble, form of fibrin (Robbins, 1944; Laki and Lorand, 1948).

The fibrinolytic system provides a mechanism for removal of physiologically deposited fibrin (Fig. 18.3). Plasminogen from the circulating

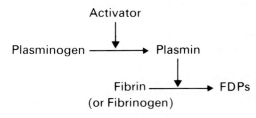

Fig. 18.3 The fibrinolytic system.

plasma is laid down with fibrin during the formation of thrombi. Activator present in the walls of blood vessels is capable of transforming this plasminogen into the free proteolytic enzyme plasmin the natural substrate of which is fibrin. Circulating inhibitors of fibrinolysis, antiplasmins, are present in the circulating plasma but are excluded from the interior of thrombi. Increased fibrinolysis is usually a reaction to intravascular coagulation (secondary fibrinolysis) rather than the initial event (primary fibrinolysis). It may therefore be construed as a beneficial response (Mersky *et al.*, 1964). The products of digestion of fibrin by plasmin are a series of fibrin degradation products (FDPs) (Table 18.1). These may be detected in serum by virtue of their immuno-

Table 18.1 Products of fibrinolysis

	PLASMIN	
FIBRINOGEN or FIBRIN	$\longrightarrow$	FRAGMENT X + Peptides
	PLASMIN	
FRAGMENT X	$\longrightarrow$	FRAGMENTS Y + D
	PLASMIN	
FRAGMENT Y	$\longrightarrow$	FRAGMENTS D + E

X is still slowly clottable by thrombin
Y is the most potent anticoagulant
D inhibits fibrin monomer polymerization
E competitively inhibits thrombin clotting of fibrinogen and aggregation of platelets (Larrieu *et al.*, 1972).

COAGULATION DISORDERS. 1. HEREDITARY   311

logical cross-reaction with antibodies raised in rabbits against human fibrin (Mersky *et al.*, 1966). The detection of raised levels of FDPs in the serum has proved a useful screening test for intravascular coagulation. *In vivo* FDPs exert anticoagulant effects and also impair platelet aggregation (Kowalski, 1968; Deykin, 1970; Larrieu *et al.*, 1972) (Table 18.1).

INVESTIGATION OF DISORDERS OF COAGULATION

From a clinical appraisal it is usually possible to determine whether one is dealing with a life-long or acquired haemorrhagic state, and whether it is primarily a disorder of coagulation on the one hand, or platelet abnormality on the other.

Previous dental extraction or surgical operation without undue bleeding is good evidence against a life-long haemorrhagic disorder. Tonsillectomy is a particularly demanding haemostatic challenge. Mild haemorrhagic states, including the less severe forms of haemophilia, manifest themselves only following surgical or other trauma. More severe defects give rise to apparently spontaneous bruising or bleeding, in reality brought about by 'physiological trauma'.

A family history of bleeding tendency is quite naturally more dependable in the autosomal dominant disorders, such as von Willebrand's disease, hereditary haemorrhagic telangiectasia, and Ehler's Danlos syndrome than in the sex-linked recessive disorders such as haemophilia or Christmas disease or the autosomal recessive coagulation or platelet defects. In haemophilia about one third of newly diagnosed patients have no known family history either because the disease has been transmitted through a long line of female carriers or because it is the result of a new mutation.

In patients with an acquired haemorrhagic state not only will the above features be absent but there may also be a history of recent drug ingestion, such as aspirin, (acetylsalicylic acid), or there may be evidence of a systemic disorder, e.g. renal disease, liver disease, dysproteinaemia or severe sepsis.

A distinction between a platelet disorder or a coagulation defect can often be made from the nature of the bleeding. Whereas platelet or 'capillary' bleeding affects primarily the skin (purpura) and mucous membranes (gum bleeding, epistaxis, gastrointestinal haemorrhage, menorrhagia) coagulation defects are prone to give rise to deep muscle haematomata or haemarthroses. Haematuria, however, can occur with either type

of defect. In haemophilia initial haemostasis is normal and bleeding may only restart some hours later. In thrombocytopenia once arrest of bleeding has been obtained it is likely to be permanent. These considerations may lead the haematologist to focus more attention upon investigation of platelet (Chapter 16 and 17) or coagulation disorders in investigation of the bleeding patient. In the case of disseminated intravascular coagulation or consumptive coagulopathy, however, the situation is complicated by the fact that thrombocytopenia, platelet dysfunction and coagulation defect may develop simultaneously, sometimes associated even with a thrombotic tendency (e.g. bilateral renal vein thrombosis of infancy, *vide infra*).

Laboratory investigations of a patient with alleged bleeding tendency must include at least the following preliminary screening tests:

1. Full blood count including platetet count
2. Ivy bleeding time or some modification thereof
3. A test of liver synthesized coagulation factors (e.g. thrombotest, 'P and P' or Quick's prothrombin time)
4. A test of the intrinsic coagulation system (e.g. kaolin clotting time, partial thromboplastin time or thromboplastin screening test).

The exact choice of coagulation screening tests will largely depend upon whether venous or capillary blood is available, the latter having great practical advantages in infants and young children. Dormandy and Hardisty (1961) devised a simple method of obtaining citrated plasma, diluted approximately 1 in 20 in saline, directly from a free flowing skin prick. Anticoagulant diluting fluid, 1·8 ml, of the following composition is measured into a capped polythene tube (60 × 15 mm):

Trisodium citrate	2 g
Sodium chloride	5·6 g
Barbitone buffer pH 7·35	200 ml
Distilled water	800 ml.

0·2 ml of this fluid is drawn up from the polythene tube into a pipette calibrated to contain 0·2 and 0·4 ml. A well-warmed finger (or heel in the case of an infant) is stabbed with a sharp Hagedorn needle, and, after wiping away the first drop, blood is drawn up under the fluid until the total volume is 0·4 ml. After mixing with the rest of the buffer one has 0·2 ml of whole blood diluted with buffer to 2 ml and, after centrifugation of the red cells, approximately 0·1 ml of plasma in 2 ml (a 1 in 20 dilution). The exact dilution is determined from the haematocrit, obtained by collecting a further drop of blood into a microhaematocrit tube. The resulting diluted citrated plasma can be used for performing the 'P and P' assay for prothrombin +

Factor VII ('proconvertin'), for the thromboplastin screening test (TPST) to detect defects of the 'early' stages of blood coagulation, and for specific assays of Factors VIII (AHG) or IX (Christmas) (Dormandy and Hardisty, 1961).

For purposes of screening patients for defects of either the intrinsic or extrinsic arm of the coagulation system it is necessary to perform two separate tests. Using capillary blood one such pair of tests is the TPST (Macpherson and Hardisty, 1961) and 'P and P' assay (Owren and Ass. 1951) (Fig. 18.4).

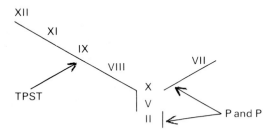

Fig. 18.4 Use of capillary blood for TPST and 'P and P' test.

Powerful inhibitors of thromboplastin formation or of thrombin and fibrin formation may also be detected by these tests, but not a deficiency of fibrinogen. To detect this an additional test such as the fibrinogen titre (Sharp et al., 1958) will need to be done. Plasma with a normal content of fibrinogen can be diluted to 1 in 120 or more and still produce a visible fibrin clot after addition of thrombin. Starting with approximately 1 in 20 citrated plasma obtained by the method of Dormandy and Hardisty above serial dilutions can be made and the visible end-point of fibrin formation after addition of thrombin determined. If significant fibrinogen deficiency is present, as in consumptive coagulopathy, the titre may be less than 1 in 40.

An alternative pair of screening tests applicable to capillary blood sampling are the kaolin clotting time of Margolis (1961) and the thrombotest (Owren, 1959) testing the intrinsic and extrinsic systems respectively (Fig. 18.5).

The kaolin clotting time is performed by collecting 0·1 ml of freely flowing capillary blood into a 0·2 ml pipette already containing 0·1 ml of citrate water, and expelling the contents into citrate water. Lysis of the red cells takes place providing an excess of platelet-like thromboplastin. After standing for 1 hour at R.T. in siliconized tubes the lysate is 'contact activated' by adding kaolin suspension, and the recalcification time determined at 37° C. The normal result is up to 60 seconds and major coagulation defects give results of 2 to 3 minutes. I have found this a useful and dependable screening test in paediatric practice.

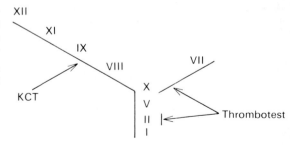

Fig. 18.5 Use of capillary blood for kaolin-clotting tissue and thrombotest.

The thrombotest is also of particular value in neonatal and paediatric practice, having been designed to detect combined deficiencies of the vitamin K dependent factors synthesized in the liver (prothrombin, Factors VII, X and IX). It cannot be wholly relied upon to detect isolated deficiencies of single factors; in particular it cannot detect pure Factor IX deficiency (Christmas disease). However, multiple deficiencies within this group of factors (the prothrombin complex) are far commoner than isolated deficiencies. It is a particularly useful test in detecting haemorrhagic disease of the newborn. It is not markedly depressed in consumptive coagulopathy since only one of the factors measured (prothrombin) is characteristically 'consumed' during coagulation.

When venous blood is readily available, as in older children, then screening tests and assays can be performed upon citrated plasma. The kaolin activated partial thromboplastin time (PTT) (Rodman et al., 1958) and Quick's one-stage prothrombin time (QPT) form a satisfactory pair of tests for the intrinsic and extrinsic system, including fibrinogen (Fig. 18.6). They are also sensitive to inhibitors.

None of the above screening tests will show a deficiency of Factor XIII, fibrin stabilizing factor. For this purpose 0·2 ml of citrated plasma is recalcified by 0·2 ml of M/40 $CaCl_2$ and the resultant clot incubated in 5 M urea at 37° C overnight. Clots from Factor XIII deficient plasma dissolve (Josso et al., 1964).

When disseminated intravascular coagulation (DIC) and its associated consumptive coagulopathy is suspected sequential platelet counts may be of more immediate value, augmented by measurement of fibrin degradation products (FDPs) in serum and the fibrinogen level and thrombin time in plasma (Deykin, 1970). Defects of the earlier stages of coagulation, due to V and VIII consumption, are found in the more severe examples and will be reflected by prolonged TPST, KCT or PTT in the schemes outlined above.

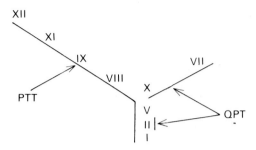

Fig. 18.6 Use of venous blood for partial thromboplastin tissue and Quick's prothrombin tissue.

Fibrinolysis is usually secondary to intravascular coagulation, except in advanced liver disease when the normal hepatic clearance of circulating 'activator' is impaired (Fletcher *et al.*, 1964). Circulating activator may be detected by pipetting 0·03 ml of plasma (kept at 0° C until testing) on to human or bovine fibrin plates and incubating the plates for 18 hr at 37° C (Nilsson *et al.*, 1960). Hyperplasminaemic states, due to explosive hyperfibrinolysis, can be detected by similarly testing plasma on fibrin plates incorporating 10 M epsilon amino caproic acid (EACA) which inhibits activation of plasminogen but not plasmin digestion of fibrin (Fig. 18.3). Marked fibrinolysis will usually be detectable by the simpler procedure of incubating a series of fibrinogen titre tubes. When clinically significant fibrinolysis exists clots which were present earlier will totally disappear after several hours' incubation at 37° C (Sharp and Eggleton, 1963). For research purposes the plasminogen level may be measured, since this is consumed during *in vivo* fibrinolysis, and the euglobulin lysis time may be determined.

It should be emphasized that platelet numbers and function, as well as the bleeding time, must be determined in addition to the coagulation tests mentioned above when investigating a patient with an undetermined haemorrhagic state.

HEREDITARY COAGULATION DEFECTS

Haemophilia

This disease probably existed in antiquity. Duthie *et al.* (1972) suggest that the earliest reference was in the Tractat Jebamoth of the Talmud in which three sons of three sisters are described as dying from circumcision. It became recognized in Europe in the early nineteenth century after Nasse in 1820 emphasized the unusual mode of inheritance with males being affected but with

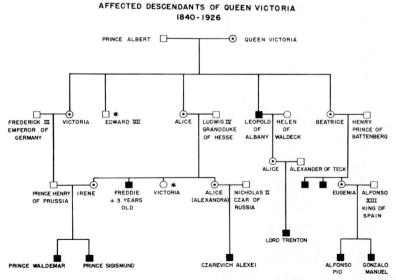

Fig. 18.7 Haemophilia in the descendants of Queen Victoria. ■, Haemophiliac male; ⊙, heterozygous or carrier female. (Reproduced from *Bulletin of the New York Academy of Medicine* (1954), **3**, 325, by permission of Dr Brinkhouse and the New York Academy of Medicine).

transmission through females. Of recent historical interest was the transmission of haemophilia through Queen Victoria to Czarevich Alexei and other European Royalty of the early part of this century (Fig. 18.7). The nature of the disease was not fully understood until knowledge of the coagulation system evolved in the 1930's (Patek and Stetson, 1936).

INCIDENCE

Surveys in Finland have shown an incidence of 1 per 13,000–14,000 males (Ikkala, 1960) and in Denmark of 1 per 7,000 males (Sjolin, 1960). Incidence in the whole population is 3–4 per 100,000 for the relatively severe form, and perhaps as high as 8 per 100,000 if the mildest form, brought to light only after major surgery, is

Table 18.2 Patients with bleeding disorders registered at Oxford Haemophilia Centre (June 1969)

Diagnosis	No. of patients	Percentage
Haemophilia	623	61
Christmas disease	120	12
von Willebrand's disease	183	18
Others:		
Afibrinogenaemia	1	
Circulating anticoagulant	27	
Factor XIII deficiency	1	
Factor V deficiency	3	
Factor VII deficiency	2	
Factor X deficiency	4	9
Factor XII deficiency	2	
Factor IX deficiency	14	
Qualitative platelet defects	37	
Combined clotting factor deficiencies	5	
Total	1022	100

Reproduced by permission of the editor of the B.M.A., and of Dr. Rizza, from Archives of Disease in Childhood (1972), 47, 451.

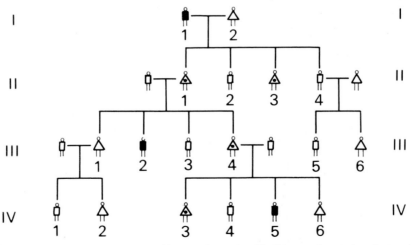

Transmission through an affected male (I, 1) and carrier females (II, 1 and III, 4).

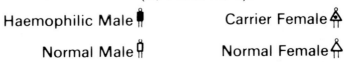

Fig. 18.8 The pattern of hereditary transmission of haemophilia and Christmas disease. (Reproduced from *Archives of Diseases in Childhood* (1972), **47**, 451, by permission of Dr Rizza, and the Editor of the British Medical Association).

included (Duthie et al., 1972). From a collection of world-wide reports Ikkala (1960) found that the ratio of haemophilia to Christmas disease was 85:15. Von Willebrand's disease has a rather similar frequency to Christmas disease. All other life-long haemorrhagic states are relative rareties compared to haemophilia, Christmas disease and von Willebrand's disease (Table 18.2).

INHERITANCE

Both haemophilia and Christmas disease are classic examples of X-linked, or sex-linked recessive, hereditary disorders. All other coagulation deficiencies have autosomal recessive inheritance. The implications of X-linked transmission are that a carrier female will have a 50/50 chance of any of her sons being haemophiliacs and a 50/50 chance of her daughters being carriers like herself (Fig. 18.8). A haemophiliac male cannot transmit the disease to his sons but all his daughters will be carriers. The severity of haemophilia and Christmas disease tends to be constant within one family. In approximately 30 per cent of cases there is no family history of the disease. This can be due either to a new mutation or to fortuitous transmission through a series of female carriers.

The identification of female carriers is important with respect to genetic counselling. Occasional female carriers show mild haemorrhagic manifestations of haemophilia (Bond et al., 1962) or Christmas disease (Hardisty, 1957). The Factor VIII level was 8 per cent and Factor IX level 17 per cent in two recently reported examples (Clark, 1973). This incomplete recessivity is more common in Christmas disease than in haemophilia. Simpson and Biggs (1962) found that 13 per cent of female carriers had Factor IX levels below 28 per cent (i.e. more than 2 standard deviations below the normal mean). Since, however, the great majority of such carriers have factor levels within the normal range, dependable identification by assay alone is not often possible. Rapaport et al. (1960) showed the same to be true in haemophilia carriers. Israels, Lempert and Gilbertson (1951) reported the infinitely less usual occurrence of a homozygous haemophilic female who had inherited the abnormality from both parents (a haemophilic father and a mother with an affected brother). The clinical severity is, of course, much greater in the rare female homozygote than in the symptomatic female carrier. At one time it was supposed that the homozygote would die in utero (Lancet, 1973C).

NEWER KNOWLEDGE REGARDING THE NATURE OF ANTIHAEMOPHILIC FACTOR

Dependable identification of female carriers has recently become possible by a combination of immunological and assay techniques. In haemophilic plasma devoid of clot-promotic Factor VIII activity there is nevertheless a near normal amount of antigenic material which cross-reacts with antiserum to normal Factor VIII (Zimmerman et al., 1971A). Currently it is not known whether this antigenic material is non-functional because it is an incomplete subunit of normal Factor VIII or whether it is a structurally abnormal variant of Factor VIII (Bennett, 1974). This has been the subject of extended recent correspondence and debate (Denson and Ingram, 1973; Hougie and Sargent, 1973; Bennett and Grove, 1973; Kernoff and Rizza, 1973; Bloom et al., 1973) of especial interest since the non-clot-promoting Factor VIII antigen appears to be identical to the 'bleeding time' factor deficient in von Willebrand's disease (see Chapter 17). Whatever the final answer to this question it is nevertheless true that *one of the biological stigmata of haemophilia is the disproportionate synthesis of Factor VIII antigen relative to clot-promoting Factor VIII*. This being so it should follow from the Lyon hypothesis that approximately one half of the cells in a female carrier would produce the abnormal, non-functional but antigenic protein (Bennett, 1974). This has been confirmed to be the case (Fig. 18.9). Forty out of

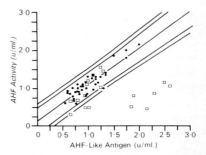

Fig. 18.9 Relation between antihaemophilic-Factor (AHF) clot-promoting activity and AHF-like antigen in normal women (●) and women with a 50 per cent chance of being a carrier of haemophilia (□). The regression line and the 95 and 99 per cent confidence belts for the group of normal women are indicated. (Reproduced from the *New England Journal of Medicine* (1973), **288**, 342, by permission of the publishers and Dr O. Ratnoff).

42 known carriers were found to have a significant excess of antigenic over clot-promotic Factor VIII (Zimmerman et al., 1971B; Bennett and Ratnoff, 1973). This represents a detection rate of over

90 per cent compared to the 25 per cent or so that could be detected by Factor VIII assay alone (Rapaport *et al.*, 1960; Zimmerman *et al.*, 1971B). This constitutes one of the most interesting new developments in haemophilia. Good recent reviews include those of Bennett (1974) and Colman (1973).

Although the great majority of true haemophiliacs conform to the above pattern around 5 per cent differ in that Factor VIII antigen is low or absent (Bennett and Huehns, 1970; Stites *et al.*, 1971).

CLINICAL MANIFESTATIONS

Both haemophilia (Factor VIII deficiencies, haemophilia A) and Christmas disease (Factor IX deficiency, haemophilia B) are characterized by repeated episodes of prolonged bleeding following trauma. Spontaneous haemorrhage occurs only

rhage and to haemarthrosis usually have Factor VIII levels in the 0–2 per cent range. It is clinically convenient and valid to classify this group of patients as 'severe' or 'high-grade' haemophiliacs. Unfortunately the majority of patients with haemophilia fall into this category. The same grading of severity exists in Christmas disease in relation to the Factor IX level. The degree of clinical disability in severe Christmas disease is similar to that in severe haemophilia, but the proportion of patients falling into the severe group is smaller in Christmas disease. This has erroneously given rise to the impression that it is intrinsically a milder disease.

Another misconception is that an affected newborn baby seldom shows manifestations of haemophilia because of passive transfer of maternal Factor VIII. This is not so. Severe deficiency of

Table 18.3   Relation of observed blood levels of Factor VIII to the severity of clinical manifestations of defective haemostasis

Blood level of Factor VIII (per cent of normal)	Level of haemostatic efficiency
50–100	Normal
25–50	Tendency to excessive bleeding after major trauma; often not diagnosed
5–25	Severe bleeding after minor trauma or surgical operations
1–5	Gross bleeding after minor injuries; some haemarthroses and 'spontaneous' bleeding
0	Severe haemophilia; haemarthroses and crippling; deep tissue haemorrhages

Reproduced by permission of the editor of the B.M.A. and of Dr. Rizza, from Archives of Disease in Childhood (1972), **47**, *451.*

in the more severely affected patients, and may in reality be the consequence of physiological trauma to the muscles and joints. The characteristic of haemophilic bleeding, as seen for instance after dental extraction, is continuous slow loss often following a period of initial haemostasis, rather than a massive or exsanguinating haemorrhage. This is the converse of bleeding in thrombocytopenic states where only initial haemostasis is at fault. For this reason local pressure will often achieve permanent haemostasis in thrombocytopenic bleeding but seldom in haemophilia. Superficial cuts often stop bleeding normally and permanently, drying of the crust of blood seeming to be a substitute for normal coagulation. Similar cuts on moist mucosal surfaces such as the tongue do not have this advantage and continue to ooze.

There is a clear relationship between the severity of the clinical course and level of coagulation factor (VIII or IX) in the plasma (Table 18.3). Patients liable to apparently spontaneous haemor-

Factor VIII has been found in the cord blood of affected infants (Didisheim and Lewis, 1958; Baehner and Strauss, 1966). There is no evidence for transplacental passage of this or other coagulation factors (Cade *et al.*, 1969). Although it is true that the majority do not show haemorrhagic manifestations until they begin to crawl at 3 to 4 months earlier bleeding can occur. Circumcision is the particular hazard. Hartmann and Diamond (1957) recorded 2 intracranial and 1 umbilical haemorrhage among 94 infants with haemophilia or Christmas disease, as well as 30 with haemorrhage following circumcision. Baehner and Strauss (1966) found 9 out of 192 such infants with bleeding unrelated to circumcision. Strauss (1965) recorded a high incidence (14/20) of postcircumcision bleeding in infants with less than 1 per cent Factor VIII and a low incidence (2/16) in those with higher Factor VIII levels. Other early manifestations include massive scalp haemorrhage in haemophilia (Kozinn *et al.*, 1963) and fatal intracranial haemorrhage in a 6-week-old infant with Christmas disease (Curran and Wang, 1971). The mother slipped on a staircase while carrying the baby 4 days before, but there was no direct head injury.

By the age of 18 months most haemophiliacs will have shown an abnormal tendency to bruise, often on forehead or limbs, and to subcutaneous haematoma formation. The intramuscular injections of triple vaccine in the first year of life also constitute a haemostatic challenge. Bleeding from lips, gums or tongue may also occur around this period as a result of injury from teeth or toys. Whereas bleeding from superficial cuts in the skin tends to stop in the normal time if undisturbed, much more prolonged oozing occurs when it is a moist mucous membrane such as the mouth which is involved. This is partly because the acts of breathing, chewing, swallowing and talking make immobilization impossible, and partly because coagulation through drying is absent.

From the time that the child learns to walk strains to the joints and muscles lead to the characteristic manifestations of severe haemophilia, viz. haemarthrosis and deep intramuscular haematomata. Hinge joints are particularly vulnerable because of their susceptibility to angular and rotary strain. In older children the knee is the most commonly affected joint, followed by ankle and elbow (Stuart et al., 1966), but in the young child ankles are most commonly affected (Rizza and Matthews, 1972). Bleeding in haemarthroses is usually intracapsular and probably arises from the rich synovial plexus of vessels in the loose areolar tissue. Each episode leads to hypertrophy and increased vascularity, predisposing to further haemorrhage (Lancet, 1973C).

Deep intramuscular haematomata are another characteristic lesion of severe haemophilia. They may seem to be spontaneous or may follow an identifiable strain. If involving the forearm or calf they may cause scarring and subsequent contracture resulting in limb deformity. If large enough intramuscular haematomata may compress blood vessels or nerves causing gangrene or paralysis. Involvement of the femoral nerve in iliopsoas haematoma is particularly characteristic. This lesion can superficially mimic appendicitis but the presence of a mass just within the pelvic brim, ipsolateral femoral nerve compression, falling haemoglobin level and rapid improvement following Factor VIII replacement therapy help to distinguish these diagnoses (Rizza and Matthews, 1972).

Haemorrhages into the tongue require special mention because by tracking posteriorly they can pose a life-threatening hazard. They therefore require prompt replacement therapy and careful observation.

Haemorrhage and haematoma formation can, indeed, occur in any site or organ of the body. Attention must in all cases be paid to the possibility of pressure upon nerves, blood vessels, air passages or other important organ such as the eye, with a view to forestalling serious complication by prompt replacement therapy. Intracranial haemorrhage following minor head injury is a small but constant hazard.

Bleeding from the gut, nose or urinary tract is uncommon in childhood, although haematuria is the third most common form of bleeding in adolescence and adulthood (Rizza and Matthews, 1972). Epistaxis usually follows local injury. Rarely a progressive 'pseudotumour' of bone may arise from intraosseous haemorrhage (Abell and Bailey, 1960).

Milder cases of haemophilia are likely to be brought to light as a result of prolonged bleeding after dental extraction or surgery such as tonsillectomy, which is a particularly severe test of haemostasis.

A study of the incidence of haemorrhagic episodes in this disease showed that in the age group up to 12 years severe cases suffered an average of 7·2 spontaneous and 1·0 post-traumatic such episodes per annum resulting in loss of 66·9 and 8·8 days from school per patient. Joint haemorrhages accounted for 5·66 spontaneous episodes per annum and muscle plus other tissues 1·0 per annum in this age group (Stuart et al., 1966). Details of the frequency of bleeding in adolescent boys with haemophilia, Christmas disease or von Willebrand's disease has been reported from the Treloar College at Alton by Rainsford and Hall (1973). There was no seasonal variation and frequency could not be correlated entirely with Factor VIII levels.

There appears to be a slight alleviation in symptoms as adulthood progresses. Whether this is due to the avoidance of hazards in the light of experience or to the slight increase in level of Factor VIII with increasing years is uncertain.

DIAGNOSIS

The general clinical and laboratory approach to the diagnosis of haemorrhagic states in childhood has already been discussed under 'Investigation of disorders of coagulation'. A diagnosis of haemophilia or Christmas disease is often suggested from the nature of the bleeding tendency and the family history. It should be noted, however, that no positive family history can be elicited in approximately one third of patients. Subdivision into severe or mild haemophilia can usually be made by the age of two years from consideration of the frequency of bleeding and the presence or absence of spontaneous haematomata or haemarthroses. If the subsequent Factor VIII assay is at variance with the clinical grading I would regard the assay as *sub judice* until repeated.

In infants and young children it is preferable that the initial coagulation investigations are performed upon capillary blood samples. This avoids subjecting many infants to the hazards of difficult and unnecessary venepunctures at a point in time when one is ignorant as to whether he has a serious coagulation defect or not. Also, venous blood collected under difficult circumstances may some-

The exact choice of coagulation tests performed, whether on capillary or venous blood, will depend upon the practice in the individual laboratory concerned. As shown in Figs. 18.4, 5 and 6 haemophilia or Christmas disease will give abnormal results in the screening tests of the intrinsic coagulation system. These include the PTT, TPST or kaolin clotting time. Normal results will be found in tests of the extrinsic coagulation system, such as the thrombotest or Quick's one-stage prothrombin time, and of the later stages of blood coagulation, such as the thrombin time or fibrinogen titre. Distinction between haemophilia and Christmas disease is traditionally made by the thromboplastin generation test of Biggs and Douglas (1953) employing mixtures of diluted serum and adsorbed citrated plasma from the patient and a normal control (Table 18.4). This test is not,

Table 18.4   Thromboplastin generation test (TGT)

Adsorbed plasma		Serum	Thromboplastin generation
Contains V, VIII, XI, XII		Contains IX, X, XI, XII	
Patient	+	Normal	Defective in haemophilia or Factor V deficiency
Normal	+	Patient	Defective in Christmas disease or Factor X deficiency
Patient	+	Patient	Defective in XI or XII deficiency or inhibitor of thromboplastin generation

Quick's one-stage prothrombin time is prolonged in Factor V or X deficiency, but not in haemophilia or Christmas disease. The TGT is normal in isolated Factor VII deficiency.

times give erroneous coagulation results, either by consumption of coagulation factors if partial clotting occurs in the syringe, or by spurious shortening of one-stage screening tests such as the PTT due to contamination by tissue fluid activating the coagulation system. If the venepuncture is other than 'clean' this fact should be noted. Unless there are pressing clinical reasons it is best to avoid the immediate neonatal period since multiple coagulation deficiencies are common at that time. Factor IX in particular can be abnormally low in the first weeks of life.

In those infants where the initial capillary coagulation investigations indicate a diagnosis of haemophilia or Christmas disease it is my practice to confirm this at a later date (e.g. at the age of a year) on venous blood obtained under optimum conditions and with due precautions *in the knowledge that one is performing a venepuncture in a haemophiliac.* With a life-long 'label' of such far-reaching consequences the independent confirmation so obtained is well worth while.

however, obligatory if individual assays of Factor VIII and IX are performed, and this is increasingly the practice in many laboratories. These assays should be performed at some time in all new cases both so as to provide an irrefutable diagnosis and to give an indication of the probable clinical severity. The patient, or an appropriately transported plasma sample, may need to be referred to a Haemophilia Centre or Reference Laboratory for this purpose. Where appropriate such a centre would also be able to test for the presence of circulating inhibitors to Factor VIII. Also it could test both the patient and his mother for the level of Factor VIII antigen so as to determine whether the disease arose by mutation or whether the mother was a genetic carrier when this is in doubt. This information may be needed for genetic counselling.

Other laboratory tests that should be performed include an Ivy bleeding time, to exclude von Willebrand's disease with low Factor VIII, a full blood count, to detect iron deficiency due to recurrent blood loss. The blood group should be determined and the serum screened for antibodies that might cause difficulty in cross-matching blood in an emergency. These results, as well as the exact diagnosis, are entered into the haemophilia card that the patient or his parents carry.

For further details of coagulation tests, their interrelation and interpretation the reader is referred to Hardisty and Ingram (1965). A good recent review of clinical and laboratory diagnosis of inherited bleeding disorders in children is that of Strauss (1972).

MANAGEMENT

This is a broad subject including not only the prevention and treatment of haemorrhage and deformity, but also support and explanation of the disease to the parents, and consideration of the patient's education, recreational activities and future employment. Recent articles covering certain aspects of particular relevance to the paediatrician include 'Management of the haemophilic child' (Rizza and Matthews, 1972) and 'Haemophilia: A challenge to social work' (Miller, 1973). The management of musculoskeletal problems is the subject of an outstanding monograph by Duthie, Matthews, Rizza and Steel (1972). Comprehensive accounts of all aspects of management are available in the text books of Hardisty and Ingram (1965) and Biggs and Macfarlane (1966). Shorter recommended reviews include 'Haemophilia today' (Rizza and Biggs, 1971), 'Management of hereditary coagulation disorders' (Mason and Ingram, 1971), 'Diagnosis and treatment of inherited bleeding disorders' (Strauss, 1972) and 'Treatment of haemophilia' (*Lancet*, 1973A).

At initial interview with the mother after diagnosis has been established a Haemophilia Card should be issued and an outline of future problems should be discussed, based upon one's assessment of the severity of the defect in the particular patient. The pattern of inheritance is usually well known to parents at this stage but confirmation of the probabilities of future offspring being affected or carriers may be sought and genetic counselling requested. The mother must not be allowed to feel a social Pariah as a result of the publicity given to genetic counselling concepts. The following points need emphasizing both to parents and to the general practitioner:

1. No intramuscular injections must ever be given to the child by any doctor or nurse. Immunizations can be given using intracutaneous or deep subcutaneous injections (25 size needle)

which, in most instances, is an acceptable alternative.

2. Aspirin should never be given. Paracetamol (Panadol) is a safe alternative.

3. At the first sign of pain or swelling in a joint immediate attendance is necessary at the hospital (day or night) so as to have IV cryoprecipitate, given as an outpatient. This point was forcibly made by Ali, Gandy, Britten and Dormandy in 1967 but is still not widely acted upon.

4. Prophylactic dental care should be instituted, by regularly attending a dental surgeon experienced in the management of haemophilia.

5. The future importance of a good education should be stressed.

Finally, they should be informed of the existence and objects of the Haemophilia Society.

Later, when the boy is going to school, the importance of good attendance and encouragement in school work should be reiterated. This is especially important if there are unavoidable spells in hospital. Intellectual pursuits and hobbies such as music are to be encouraged. Advice as to which sports are suitable will be needed. As with all physical activities the maximum that can be undertaken without the development of bruising or injury should be encouraged. This level of activity can only be determined by each individual patient by trial and error, although reasonable suggestions can be made from a knowledge of the severity of his disease and past performance. If there are difficulties at school the hospital social service can be of great help.

CORRECTION OF THE COAGULATION DEFICIENCY

Infusion replacement therapy of the missing factor is the cornerstone of treatment. Fresh or fresh-frozen plasma is effective in all the congenital coagulation deficiencies; cryoprecipitate in haemophilia and von Willebrand's disease but not in Christmas disease. Appropriate concentrates of Factor VIII, Factor IX and the prothrombin complex (II, VII and X) have also become available in recent years and are of use in particular circumstances.

One unit of Factor VIII or IX is defined as the activity present in 1 ml of fresh pooled normal plasma. A recipient's plasma volume is 40–50 ml per kg body weight. Therefore in haemophilic patients without inhibitors infusion of

1 unit/kg body wt raises Factor VIII approx. 2 per cent.

The same *in vivo* dose response and disappearance rate occurs regardless of the source of Factor VIII (Abildgaard, 1969).

A lower *in vivo* recovery of Factor IX is found after infusion of plasma or concentrate in Christmas disease:

1 unit of Factor IX/kg body wt raises the level 0·5–1·0 per cent

(Gilchrist *et al.*, 1969; Hoag *et al.*, 1969). This is partly because it is distributed in a larger extravascular space averaging 2·7 times the plasma volume.

In the presence of fever, continuing haemorrhage or circulating inhibitors less than the expected recovery is found. Occasional patients show poor recovery without explanation (Abildgaard, 1969).

The disappearance curve of these infused factors in the deficient patient is biphasic. There is a rapid initial fall with a $T\frac{1}{2}$ of around 8 hours compounded both of diffusion into a depleted extravascular compartment and of the catabolic half-life. This is followed by a slower fall with $T\frac{1}{2}$ of approximately 14 hours for Factor VIII and 30 hours for Factor IX, representing the true catabolic rate (Bowie *et al.*, 1967). From these considerations a large loading dose (e.g. 15–16 ml/kg fresh-frozen plasma) should be followed by two thirds of the dose (e.g. 10–11 ml/kg) at 12-hour intervals in haemophilia or 24-hour intervals in Christmas disease. The same is true when using cryoprecipitate or concentrates.

The degree of coagulation correction required depends upon the clinical situation (Strauss, 1972).

Closed soft tissue haemorrhages such as haemarthroses and small haematomata can be controlled by modest elevation of Factor VIII to 10–20 per cent or of Factor IX to 5–10 per cent. Cryoprecipitate is the product of choice in the case of haemophilia, but these levels can be achieved with fresh-frozen plasma in either haemophilia or Christmas disease.

Bleeding from a surface wound such as of tongue, lips or gums, where there is no restraining external pressure require somewhat higher levels, i.e. Factor VIII 20–40 per cent or Factor IX 10–20 per cent. These are difficult to maintain with plasma because of circulatory overload caused by both the volume and high protein content. Cryoprecipitate or concentrates are needed.

During and after surgery the level of Factor VIII must never be allowed to fall below the 30 per cent, nor the Factor IX below 15 per cent. To ensure this the peak levels need to be in the region of 60 and 30 per cent respectively, with 12-hourly doses in haemophilia and daily doses in Christmas disease. These levels are best obtained by the use of concentrates.

Treatment of intracranial haemorrhage in haemophilia requires even higher factor levels, close to 100 per cent throughout, and this can only be achieved by the use of concentrates (Davies *et al.*, 1966).

USE OF PLASMA, CRYOPRECIPITATE AND CONCENTRATES

The activity of all products can be expressed as units (one unit being the activity in 1 ml of normal pooled plasma). As stated above 1 unit/kg body wt raises the level 2 per cent in the case of Factor VIII, 0·5 to 1 per cent in the case of Factor IX. The clinical use of plasma components in the paediatric context has been reviewed by Buchholz (1974).

1. Fresh or fresh-frozen plasma. This should be thawed rapidly in a 37° C water bath immediately before use. At the time of use it contains an average of 0·7 units/ml (Rizza and Matthews, 1972).

A loading dose of 15–16 ml/kg will give a peak Factor VIII level of approximately 20 per cent. By giving further doses of 10–11 ml/kg at 12-hour intervals the level will usually be kept above 10 per cent. Each infusion must be given rapidly over $\frac{1}{2}$–$\frac{3}{4}$ hour. In Christmas disease the resulting Factor IX levels are about half of these figures. Due to slower *in vivo* decay, however, subsequent doses can be given daily rather than 12-hourly. In either disease the levels attained are adequate to control mild spontaneous bleeding or closed soft tissue haematomata including haemarthroses. Single dental extractions may also be covered but not multiple extractions or surgery. Circulatory overload is the limiting factor preventing further increase in dosage.

2. Cryoprecipitate. This method of concentrating most of the Factor VIII activity from 1 bag or bottle of plasma into 10–20 ml was first developed by Judith Pool (Pool and Shannon, 1965). Larger doses of Factor VIII can be given in smaller volumes obviating the problem of circulatory overload. In children the dose can be given by syringe and scalp vein set avoiding the need for setting up a transfusion. The small volume per bag allows rapid thawing in a 37° C water bath.

The average activity per bag has been given as 75 units in the UK (Rizza and Matthews, 1972), while in the US 100 units (Abildgaard, 1969) and 110 units (Strauss, 1972) have been quoted. In practice there is considerable variation from one bag to another since the range of Factor VIII in healthy donors is 50 to 200 per cent of the mean. In children receiving only small numbers of bags per dose this variation can prove troublesome and it is a good practice to *double the calculated dose* to ensure adequate dosage (Dallman and Pool), 1968).

Taking the lower figure of 75 units per average bag a useful guide to therapy is

1 bag of cryo per 10 kg body wt raises the Factor VIII 15 per cent.

Twice this dose is therefore a little more effective than the standard fresh-frozen plasma dose of 15 ml/kg. Since there is no problem from the volume infused higher Factor VIII levels, in the 20–40 per cent range can be maintained allowing control of bleeding from external surfaces or after multiple dental extractions. The clinical use of cryoprecipitate in haemophilia has been well documented (Bennett *et al.*, 1967; Brown *et al.*, 1967; Prentice *et al.*, 1967). It is also highly effective in the correction of both the coagulation defect and the bleeding time in von Willebrand's disease (Bennett and Dormandy, 1966). It is of no value, however, in the treatment of Christmas disease. Factor IX, Factor XI (PTA) and most other coagulation factors remain in the supernatant 'exhausted' plasma during the separation of cryoprecipitate containing Factor VIII and fibrinogen.

Both plasma and cryoprecipitate have an advantage over human concentrates in carrying a low risk of transmitting serum hepatitis since each bag is prepared from a single donor rather than a pool.

3. Concentrates of Factors VIII and IX. Human concentrates are now commercially available of Factor VIII (e.g. Hemofil, Hyland Laboratories) and Factor IX (e.g. Konyne, Cutter Laboratories), similar concentrates also being available from many of the UK Blood Transfusion Centres. These have additional advantages over cryoprecipitate that their precise activity is known, that they can be stored at $4°$ C and can be carried by the patient when travelling, and that a concentrate is available for the treatment of Christmas disease as well as one for haemophilia. They are, of course, expensive (e.g. 10p per unit for Hemofil) and are not entirely free of the hepatitis hazard. Dosage is calculated in units as before, the Hemofil vials containing around 250 units in 10 ml or 800 units in 30 ml. 250 units given to a 10 kg child would raise the Factor VIII level from zero to 50 per cent providing no inhibitor was present. The Factor IX concentrates also contain Factors II (pro-

thrombin), VII and X (Stuart-Prower) and are therefore of value in other clinical situations.

The particular use of concentrates is in the management of surgical operations in haemophilia and Christmas disease, where it is necessary to keep the level of Factor VIII continuously above 30 per cent or the Factor IX continuously above 15 per cent. Because of the short supply or high commercial price some units reserve concentrates for use in children or for adults who are allergic to plasma or cryoprecipitate (Rizza and Matthews, 1972), but the use of concentrates is increasing in the US.

Recent reports on the use of human concentrates include those of Mazza *et al.* (1970) and Johnson *et al.* (1971) for haemophilia and von Willebrand's disease, and of Hoag *et al.* (1969), Gilchrist *et al.* (1969) and Dike *et al.* (1972) for Christmas disease.

Bovine and porcine Factor VIII concentrates have the serious disadvantage that allergy develops within 10 to 20 days of their administration after which that particular species cannot be used again. Thrombocytopenia may also be induced. Animal Factor VIII is now largely reserved for life-threatening haemorrhage or major surgery in patients who have developed antibodies to human Factor VIII (Rizza and Matthews, 1972). Bovine and porcine Factor VIII are usually less susceptible than human Factor VIII to neutralization by these antibodies.

MANAGEMENT OF SPECIFIC PROBLEMS

On admission to hospital a notice should be placed on the patient's bed saying 'No intramuscular injections under any circumstances'. This includes premedication, for which oral atropine can be given.

1. Cuts and lacerations. Superficial cuts tend to stop bleeding in the normal time through drying if left undisturbed. If not this can be achieved by cleaning the wound and applying an absorbable dressing such as surgical or oxidized cellulose with or without the addition of topical thrombin.

Similar cuts in the mouth and tongue give more trouble since drying does not occur and the movements of speaking and eating prevent immobilization. Cotton wool pledgets soaked in topical thrombin often stop the bleeding. Otherwise a single dose of 15 units Factor VIII or IX per kg are needed. Corrigan (1972) has reported the efficacy of combining cryoprecipitate (2 bags/ 10 kg) with oral epsilon amino caproic acid (EACA) 200 mg/kg loading dose followed by 100 mg/kg 6-hourly. Continued cryoprecipitate infusions were obviated. EACA alone was ineffective.

More severe lacerations will inevitably need a similar dose of replacement therapy followed by normal wound hygiene. Local pressure should not be excessive or prolonged. The indications for suturing the wound are the same as in non-haemophilic individuals. In this case replacement therapy must be continued until the wound is healed. Sutures are of no value as an aid to haemostasis. Prevention of infection is doubly important in haemophilia. If blood loss is sufficient to cause anaemia this should be made good by the *slow* transfusion of packed cells in the intervals between the 12- or 24-hourly *rapid* infusions of replacement therapy.

2. Soft tissue bleeding. This is the most common manifestation of severe haemophilia. Subcutaneous haematomata require one or more infusions of 15 units/kg, until symptoms subside. In certain areas such as the pharynx, floor of the mouth or neck it may be life-threatening. In restricted areas such as the limbs it may press on nerves or blood vessels leading to paralysis or contracture. Eye or ear may similarly be threatened. In unrestricted tissue spaces such as the back, thigh or abdominal wall the blood loss may be massive. In the psoas muscle or the retroperitoneal tissues an appendicitis or acute abdomen may be simulated. In all these more serious situations higher and more protracted doses of replacement therapy are needed, aiming to keep the Factor VIII level in the 30–40 per cent range for several days. Immobilization of the involved part in a functional position and physiotherapy after cessation of the bleeding are important adjuncts to the specific treatment (Abildgaard, 1969).

3. Haemarthrosis. Recurrent haemarthrosis is the single most crippling complication of severe haemophilia. Its prevention is the most important contribution to the patient's future life that the physician can make, since a previously affected joint is more prone to recurrent bleeds in future. Unfortunately there is evidence that full use has not been made of replacement therapy in the past (Ali *et al.*, 1967). The correct policy is to encourage parents and patients to attend hospital at the earliest sign of joint swelling so that an injection of replacement therapy can be given, usually without admission to hospital. This procedure will cut short many otherwise damaging periods of inactivity and hospitalization and subsequent atrophy or permanent joint disability (Ali *et al.*, 1967). A single high dose of 20 to 30 units/kg sufficient to raise the Factor VIII level to 40–50 per cent has practical advantages over a more protracted low dose course in hospital (Honig

et al., 1969). Cryoprecipitate 6 bags/10 kg or a Factor VIII concentrate should be given, since the volume of fresh-frozen plasma would be unacceptably large.

More severe haemarthroses, including those following trauma, require hospitalization, temporary immobilization of the joint in the position of maximum comfort and 2–3 days replacement therapy. In a minority of haemarthroses there may be benefit in aspiration under cover of full replacement therapy. Rizza and Matthews (1972) suggest the following criteria: A large, tense and very painful haemarthroses seen within 24 hours of onset in patients without circulating anticoagulants. After 24 hours the blood in the joint has probably clotted. The knee is the joint most frequently aspirated. A trial of replacement therapy (10–20 units/kg) with or without joint aspiration at the Children's Hospital, Cleveland, Ohio showed a reduction in average hospital stay from 4·9 days to 2·8 days in those aspirated (Wanken *et al.*, 1969).

The place of steroids in the management of haemarthroses has also been investigated. A double-blind trial using replacement therapy (25 units/kg) with or without prednisone (1 mg/lb b.wt./day × 1, followed by a half dose for 2 days) showed an increase in response rate from 34 to 89 per cent in the group given steroid (Kisker and Burke, 1970).

Physiotherapy becomes important within 1–2 days when the acute pain has resolved. The initial splint keeping the limb in the position of maximum comfort is removed and intermittent movements encouraged. If continued immobilization is necessary this should now be in a more functional position, accompanied by static muscle exercises. There is a special liability to quadriceps wasting in the case of the knee, which if allowed to occur will leave the joint unstable and liable to recurrence of haemarthroses. Static exercises are followed by straight leg raising and then gradual flexion exercises, prior to partial and finally full weight bearing. In severe haemarthroses replacement therapy can be given daily, just before the physiotherapist's visit, and during the first 2–3 days of weight bearing (Rizza and Matthews, 1972).

Advances in reconstructive elective operations in patients with chronic haemarthropathy are described in the monograph on 'Management of Musculoskeletal Problems in the Haemophilias' by Duthie *et al.* (1972).

4. Nosebleeds. This is less frequent in haemophilia than in von Willebrand's disease, but tends to occur in individual patients. Loose packing with an absorbable dressing is often effective. If not, replacement therapy is indicated, followed by removal of the packing.

5. Haematuria. This is a common site of spontaneous bleeding in haemophilia and does not usually warrant detailed urological investigation. It may prove relatively refractory to normal replacement therapy. In such cases a trial of prednisone is justified, 2 mg/kg/day for 2 days, followed by 1 mg/kg for 2–3 days (Abildgaard *et al.*, 1965; Hartman, 1965). EACA should not be used because of the hazard of producing unlysable fibrin clots in the renal tract (Stark *et al.*, 1965).

6. Gastrointestinal bleeding. Again this is a relatively rare occurrence in haemophilia. As well as 12-hourly replacement therapy until the bleeding has ceased packed red cells will need to be given between Factor VIII infusions so as to restore the haemoglobin level. If recurrent, a radiological search for a local gastric or intestinal lesion is indicated. The development of iron deficiency anaemia must be watched for, as in other patients with haemophilia, and treated with oral iron (e.g. Sytron) if present.

7. CNS bleeding. This should be suspected in any haemophiliac developing lethargy, headache or vomiting, especially if following a blow to the head. Replacement therapy should precede a diagnostic lumbar puncture. If angiography is needed massive replacement therapy should be given beforehand so as to raise the Factor VIII level to normal (Davies *et al.*, 1966). Although a rare site of haemorrhage in haemophilia subdural haemorrhage nevertheless constitutes one of the few causes of death in this disease that I have encountered in the paediatric age group. Management of one such problem is illustrated in Case 14.

Case 14. A boy of 4 (No. 188612) who was known to be a severe grade haemophiliac was transferred to the Royal Hospital for Sick Children for management by the paediatric neurologist. He had developed a persistent headache and was found to have neurological signs suggestive of an intraparietal lobe haemorrhage. There was no history of trauma. Only non-invasive investigative procedures were considered justified and arteriography was deferred. Ultrasonography showed displacement of the central fissure. The prime object of haematological management was to restore the coagulation system to normal 'round the clock' for a week, so as to allow spontaneous resolution of the haemorrhage if possible. His weight was 16 kg. It was therefore calculated that 16 units (1 unit per kg body wt.) should raise the Factor VIII level by approx. 2 per cent, therefore 800 units should be needed to raise it by 100 per cent. Because the available Factor VIII concentrate (Hemofil) contained 230 units per vial we chose to give him 690 units

instead of 800 as a trial dose expected to raise the level by 86 per cent. In fact it was raised from less than 1 per cent to 78 per cent immediately after the dose. The level had fallen to 9 per cent 22 hours later, giving a calculated $T\frac{1}{2}$ of $6\frac{1}{2}$ hours. It was clear that twice-daily injections of Factor VIII would be needed to achieve a sustained level. Twelve hours after a dose of 460 units the level was 32 per cent and a further dose of 930 units (330 units per vial) pushed this up by 108 per cent to a level of 140 per cent (expected level 148 per cent). Twelve hours after this dose the level was 33 per cent (calc. $T\frac{1}{2} = 6$ hr). This was thought to be a reasonably satisfactory minimal haemostatic level. Subsequently it was found that good minimal levels could be maintained with smaller doses given 12-hourly, e.g. 46–55 per cent 12 hours after 620 units. The key point in dose control was to perform assays just before each 12-hourly dose, using the same venepuncture (21 butterfly needle). Piriton (10 mg) was always available while giving the concentrate but no reactions occurred. One possible complication of such a high-dose course as the above is an excessive rise in plasma fibrinogen level since this is a contaminant in such concentrates. In fact there was only a modest rise in fibrinogen level from 295 mg/100 ml before therapy to 463 mg/100 ml at the end of a week's therapy. By the end of the 7-day course the neurological signs had regressed, and the patient made an uneventful recovery.

8. Dental treatment. Prophylactic dental care should be instituted on a regular basis at an early age (Webster *et al.*, 1968). A régime of 4-monthly dental visits, topical fluoride application with a 1 mg daily fluoride supplement, restriction of between meal snacks and regular tooth brushing after meals reduced the rate of dental extraction from 9 per annum to zero in a group of 34 children (Steinle and Kisker, 1970). Extrusion of deciduous teeth often occurs without bleeding providing they are not forcibly loosened. Sometimes local pressure and topical thrombin are needed. A soft or liquid diet is given at such times. Dental fillings or restorations can usually be performed without replacement therapy or hospital admission. If local anaesthesia is required it should be by papillary infiltration. Mandibular or posterosuperior alveolar nerve block must not be used without prior replacement therapy because of the danger of bleeding into the neck and floor of the mouth.

Extraction of permanent teeth requires admission to hospital for 5–7 days. In the past our policy was to give 12-hourly fresh-frozen plasma (15 ml/kg) or cryoprecipitate (2 bags/10 kg) for 3–4 days, commencing immediately before extraction. Following the demonstration by Tavenner (1968) and confirmation by Walsh *et al.* (1971), Corrigan (1972) and Forbes *et al.* (1972) that antifibrinolytic agents EACA or AMCA (tranexamic acid) reduced the need for continuing replacement therapy in both haemophilia and Christmas disease we have changed to this policy. A single preoperative dose of cryoprecipitate is given to raise the Factor VIII level to around 50 per cent (say 4 bags/10 kg). This is followed by an IV dose of EACA 0·1 g/kg and 6-hourly oral EACA postoperatively in the same dose for 7–10 days. Alternatively tranexamic acid (AMCA, Cyclokapron) can be given orally at a dose of 0·5 to 1·0 g 8-hourly for 5 days. The incidence of nausea may be lower after tranexamic acid (Tavenner, 1972). Before commencing either of these antifibrinolytic drugs it is a good practice to formally exclude haematuria by examining the urine for RBCs. It is also my practice to check the haemoglobin level and cross-match one unit of whole blood before extraction, and to give an antiseptic mouth wash such as 0·1 per cent pure Hibitane in the days following extraction.

9. Surgery in haemophilia. In all major surgery the essential principle is to keep the Factor VIII level consistently above 30–40 per cent until healing is complete (Biggs, 1957; Britten and Salzman, 1966). Haemostasis is normal at this level. For this purpose each dose should be aimed to give peak levels of 60–80 per cent. Half these levels are needed in Factor IX deficiency. Concentrates are the preferred source for replacement therapy. If at all possible a test dose should be given to the patient a day before operation aiming to bring the level to 60–80 per cent, with confirmation by assay. This allows a more accurate assessment of the individual patient's requirement than can be made on the basis of weight alone. It is also advisable to exclude the presence of circulating inhibitor since very much higher doses would then be required, perhaps using animal Factor VIII.

Eight-hourly infusions should be given on the day of operation and for the first 3–4 days, with 12-hourly infusions for the next 8–10 days until the wound is healed (Rizza and Matthews, 1972). It is wise to have 4–6 units of blood cross-matched and available before starting the operation and to provide close haematological monitoring throughout the postoperative period. Elective surgery in haemophiliacs should only be performed in hospitals capable of providing accurate assays at frequent intervals (Abildgaard, 1969).

In serious accidents the same situation applies as in major surgery and high initial Factor VIII doses are needed. Management of elective surgery in Christmas disease is illustrated by Case 15.

Case 15. A boy of 8 with mild Christmas disease (No. 38663) required elective surgery for an inguinal hernia. A concentrate of Factor XI prepared by the Blood Transfusion Service was used, which contained 280 units per vial. Six such vials were given (1,680 units) as a test dose. This raised the Factor XI level from 10 to 90 per cent, which was 80 per cent of the expected rise. Just prior to operation several days later he was given a similar dose of 6 vials. There was no problem with haemostasis during the operation. Subsequently it was found that a 24-hourly dose of only 4 vials was sufficient to maintain a minimal level of 32–40 per cent, i.e. just prior to the next dose. The course was continued for 11 days and healing was uneventful.

10. Injections and immunization. Intramuscular injections are prohibited in haemophilia or Christmas disease. Drugs can be given orally or IV where appropriate. This must be remembered in the context of premedication for surgical anaesthesia. Routine childhood immunizations can be given by deep subcutaneous injection with pressure on the site for several minutes.

11. Home transfusion and prophylactic treatment. Rabiner and Telfer (1970) have reported on a programme of home transfusion in a group of selected severe haemophiliacs with previous frequent haemorrhagic episodes. A responsible member of the family was trained in the administration of Factor VIII concentrate, stored at home, after consultation with the centre by telephone. Their preliminary experience has shown a reduction in the number of school or work days lost, an increased consumption of Factor VIII and no instances of anaphylaxis. The patients are clearly spared time-consuming and psychologically undesirable frequent visits to hospital and the Factor VIII will in most instances be given with less delay. This could well be of importance in haemarthroses. Lazerson (1973) analysed utilization in such a programme and found that there was an overall increase in 14 out of 17 patients, but that this increase was not likely to exceed 5 units/kg/per year. Rizza and Matthews (1972) comment favourably upon a similar pilot study in this country. It is reserved for those with very frequent haemorrhage (e.g. at least once every 2 weeks) and is unsuitable for patients with inhibitors. Le Quesne *et al.* (1974) in the UK and Levine (1974) in the US have similarly come to the conclusion that home treatment is highly efficacious in reducing the morbidity of haemophilia and improving the quality of life. No increase in utilization occurred except in patients previously undertreated.

Closely related to this 'early warning' treatment of haemophilia are the recent explorations into prophylaxis for selected severely affected patients with frequent haemorrhagic episodes. Trials of the prophylactic administration of antifibrinolytic drugs have produced conflicting evidence. Gordon et al. (1965) in Glasgow used EACA 3·3 g q.d.s. for six weeks and found a lower, but not statistically significant, incidence of haemorrhagic episodes compared to a placebo group of patients. Bennett et al. (1973) gave tranexamic acid, a more powerful drug, 2 g/day and found minimal effect with no change in incapacity from the disease or in amount of replacement therapy needed. They review the previous trials, and the hypothesis that antifibrinolytic drugs are useful for prophylaxis clearly remains unproven at present. There is no question of any elevation of coagulation factors during antifibrinolytic drugs, but perhaps a 'shift in the balance' between coagulation and fibrinolysis.

Prophylactic administration of Factor VIII or IX in severely affected patients has met with greater success. Clearly this is reserved for patients with quite exceptionally severe and frequent haemorrhages. Kasper et al. (1970) reported their experience in two such adults. Bleeding episodes were reduced to a half by 250 units/day and to a quarter by 500 units/day. When 2,000 units per week were used there was complete freedom from bleeding for the first 48 hours, but a recurrence by mid-week. Hirschman et al. (1970) investigated the effect of cryoprecipitate (6 to 12 bags) upon the incidence of spontaneous haemarthroses in 2 adults with severe haemophilia and two 12-year-old twins with the usual combination of haemophilia plus von Willebrand's disease. Haemarthroses continued to occur but less often. A haemophilic pseudotumour of the iliac crest that had been steadily getting larger showed distinct regression in one of the adults.

The rationale for intermittent prophylactic replacement therapy is that spontaneous haemorrhage is only seen in patients with Factor VIII levels below 1–2 per cent and infusions of concentrates at 36 to 48-hour intervals can keep the concentration above this level for most of the time (Fig. 18.10). Strauss (1972) found that 20 units/kg of Factor VIII every 48 hours kept the level above 1 per cent. In Christmas disease the longer half-life of Factor IX allowed effective prophylaxis from 10 units/kg twice-weekly.

12. Treatment of pain in haemophilia. The lack of effective drugs to control the recurrent episodes of pain suffered by those with established haemophilic arthropathy has been graphically described in a letter to the *Lancet* by an affected patient (Harvey, 1973) and a leading article in the same issue (*Lancet*, 1973B). Since aspirin is prohibited

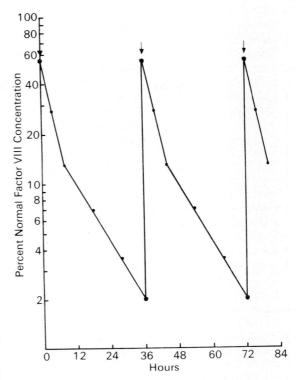

Fig. 18.10 Factor VIII levels in a patient receiving cryoprecipitate derived from 2–4 l of whole blood every 36 h (arrows). ●, measured values; ●, values based on diffusion and decay rates that are uniform in uncomplicated cases of haemophilia. (Reproduced from *Blood* (1970), **35**, 189, by permission of the authors Hirschman et al.).

and chronic administration of phenacetin may cause renal papillary necrosis, only a limited range of drugs including dihydrocodein (DF 118) and pentazocine (Fortral) are left. Pentazocine may give rise to physical dependence as well as causing somnolence and sometimes hallucinations. Stronger drugs such as pethidine are excluded on grounds of liability to addiction. Paracetamol (Panadol, Acetaminophen) is probably the safest analgesic in spite of the theoretical possibility of renal damage, being a metabolite of phenacetin, and of hepatotoxicity after massive overdose. In subsequent correspondence on this subject Dormandy (1973) recommended IV pentazocine plus promazine for severe pain due to acute haemarthroses or muscle haematoma; and 'ringing the changes' between dihydrocodein (DF 118), dextropropoxyphene (Doloxene) and oral pentazocine (Fortral) for constant and severe pain of established arthropathy. She makes a strong plea against the use of addictive drugs in this chronic disease.

13. Treatment of patients who have developed inhibitors. It is well recognized that inhibitors to Factor VIII develop in 10–20 per cent of severe haemophiliacs, i.e. those with Factor VIII levels below 1 per cent at diagnosis. Similar inhibitors to Factor IX can develop in severe Christmas disease. These are IgG antibodies which result from the immunizing effect of transfusions in patients for whom normal Factor VIII or IX are foreign proteins. Their presence should be suspected in any patient failing to respond to adequate doses of replacement therapy, especially if assay or other coagulation tests fail to show the expected rise in factor level. The theoretic considerations concerned with susceptibility to such immunization by replacement therapy in a number of genetically determined diseases, including various coagulation factor deficiencies, have recently been discussed by Boyer *et al.* (1973).

It is not possible to predict which patients will develop inhibitors. Strauss (1972) has pointed out that immunization, if it is going to occur at all, will have shown itself by the time the patient has received 100 days or so of replacement therapy. There is no direct relation between amount or type of replacement therapy. Most patients are not destined to develop inhibitors, and justified infusions should not be withheld for fear of inducing this complication.

A recent survey of all Haemophilia Centres in the UK has shown the incidence of antibodies to be 6·15 per cent among haemophilia of all grades and 2·36 per cent among all patients with Christmas disease. In the age group up to 10 years 13 out of 318 with haemophilia (4·1 per cent) and 1 out of 34 with Christmas disease had antibodies. Even in the age group below 5 years they were present in 3 out of 91 haemophilic children.

Once an inhibitor has appeared it is important to restrict the use of replacement therapy to the absolute minimum, reserving it for haematomas threatening to compress nerves or blood vessels, for large haemarthroses and, of course, for unavoidable surgery. When red cell transfusions are needed the packed cells can be washed free of plasma. There is a tendency for the antibodies to diminish over a period of years, but they rapidly reappear within a week of giving further Factor VIII.

If it is essential to give replacement therapy massive doses may be needed using human concentrates, or even animal concentrates in dire emergency. The management of such patients has recently been described by Rizza and Biggs (1973), using a newly developed quantitative *in vitro* measurement of the antibody level, based upon the earlier methods of Biggs and Bidwell (1959). Patients with less than 5 units/ml of antibody by this test show some response to treatment with Factor VIII in terms of postinfusion rise, accompanied by a good clinical response. Unfortunately the activity of the antibody tends to rise rapidly over a few days making continued treatment difficult. It is in those failing to respond that use of bovine or porcine Factor VIII becomes justifiable (Rizza and Matthews, 1972), since they are less susceptible than human Factor VIII to these antibodies. Recently the use of activated prothrombin complex concentrate has been described in such patients with good clinical response and without serious side effects (Kurczynski and Penner, 1974). At present their use is *sub judice*.

Other methods that have been suggested are attempts to suppress the antibodies by a combination of Factor VIII and cyclophosphamide (Green, 1971). Good results have been obtained in two children given 300 mg/m^2 of cyclophosphamide IV followed by concentrates and oral cyclophosphamide 3 mg/kg for 2–3 days (Lusher and Evans, 1971). The expected rise in antibody level after Factor VIII infusion was suppressed. Other heroic measures include exchange transfusion or plasmapheresis to reduce the antibody level (Abildgaard, 1969). It is clear that patients with antibodies should only be treated in experienced centres with more than usual facilities. The problems of management of such a patient are illustrated in Case 16.

Case 16. A boy of 5 (No. 186744) known to be a haemophiliac with a circulating inhibitor was admitted with a haematoma extending from the thigh to the ankle following a kick from another child. His weight was 18·8 kg. A dose of 6 bags of cryoprecipitate was given (which would normally raise the Factor VIII level to approx. 40 per cent). Pre- and postinfusion assays showed zero levels. Human Factor VIII concentrate (Hemofil) was therefore obtained and 6 vials (230 units each) were given (equivalent to 18–24 bags of Cryo). This caused a rise from zero to 15 per cent Factor VIII in the patient followed by disappearance of pain, diminution in the circumference of the thigh and return of full movement within 24 hours. One further dose of 6 vials of Factor VIII concentrate was given 24 hr after the first, giving a rise from zero to 13 per cent. There were no adverse side effects. No further replacement therapy was necessary, and was deliberately avoided so as not to stimulate a rise in inhibitor titre unnecessarily.

From the degree of rise in Factor VIII level, and assuming a plasma volume of 45 ml/kg, it was calculated that the level of inhibitor was approximately 1½ units/ml of the patient's plasma.

Other hereditary coagulation disorders

Far less common than haemophilia or Christmas disease they correspond in severity roughly to mild haemophilia, usually presenting as prolonged bleeding after dental extraction, trauma or surgery. Some may also present as bleeding from the umbilical stump in the neonatal period. Inheritance is autosomal recessive in most, but some show partial expression in the heterozygotes. All but deficiencies of Factor VII and Factor XIII (fibrin stabilizing factor) show up as defects of the intrinsic coagulation pathway in tests such as the kaolin clotting time of Margolis or the kaolin activated partial thromboplastin time (Figs. 18.4, 5 and 6). All are corrected *in vivo* by fresh-frozen plasma infusions, some also by stored plasma or whole blood.

DEFECTS OF THE CONTACT PHASE OF COAGULATION (FACTORS XI AND XII)

Deficiency of Factor XI ('plasma thromboplastin antecedent', PTA) was first described by Rosenthal, Dreskin and Rosenthal (1955) in a family with a mild haemorrhagic tendency manifest chiefly as excessive bleeding after dental extraction and surgery. It occurs in both sexes, inheritance being autosomal recessive with partial expression in heterozygotes. Most cases have been of Jewish origin.

Since it is the early 'contact activation' stage of coagulation which is impaired, those coagulation tests which employ preliminary kaolin activation (e.g. kaolin clotting time and kaolin activated PTT) are especially well suited to detecting both Factor XI or XII deficiency. The normal activation product is not formed. Specific coagulation tests for detecting Factor XI and XII deficiencies and distinguishing between the two have been developed by Nossel (1964). Details of the methods are also given by Hardisty and Ingram (1965).

Infusion of fresh or stored plasma (15 ml/kg) gives satisfactory correction with a half-life of 40–84 hours (Rosenthal and Sloan, 1965). Bennett and Dormandy (1966) also described an elderly male with 4 per cent Factor XI who was well controlled by the use of the residual plasma from which cryoprecipitate had been prepared (so-called exhausted plasma). Since the effect of infusions was cumulative daily infusions of only 10 ml/kg maintained the level between 30 and 50 per cent permitting a nephrectomy to be performed without serious haemorrhage. For treatment of spontaneous bleeding a level of 20 per cent is satisfactory, and a single infusion may be all that is necessary.

Factor XII deficiency hardly ever gives rise to a bleeding tendency, even after a haemostatic challenge such as tonsillectomy (Abildgaard et al., 1963). Originally described by Ratnoff and Colopy in 1955, this first case was a Mr Hageman, who later had a coronary thrombosis. It is inherited as an autosomal recessive character. The striking feature is prolongation of the whole blood clotting time. The abnormality is more likely to be picked up fortuitously as the result of preoperative coagulation tests than because of investigation of a bleeding tendency. Providing the precise diagnosis can be established no particular therapy is needed during surgery.

DEFICIENCIES OF FACTORS IN THE PROTHROMBIN COMPLEX (FACTORS II, V, VII AND X)

True prothrombin (Factor II) deficiency is excessively rare. Haemorrhagic symptoms can be mild (Borchgrevink et al., 1959) or severe (Bruning and Loeliger, 1971). A two-stage prothrombin assay is necessary to distinguish it from the commoner Factor VII or X deficiencies. When Factor II levels of around 10 per cent are present as an isolated deficiency, tests such as Quick's prothrombin time may be nearly normal. Treatment of a severe case with a Factor II containing concentrate showed a half-life *in vivo* of 4 days (Bruning and Loeliger, 1971).

Factor VII (proconvertin) deficiency results in a relatively severe haemorrhagic state in homozygotes, with milder symptoms in heterozygotes, inheritance being autosomal. A recent case report by Falter and Kaufmann (1971) described a boy of $6\frac{1}{2}$ years whose only symptom was epistaxis. The Quick's prothrombin time was 38 seconds in the patient; 17 and 18 seconds in the parents (normal 12–14 seconds). Assay of Factor VII showed 3 per cent in the patient; 44 and 45 per cent in the parents (normal 75 to 100 per cent). The PTT was normal in all, as expected, since Factor VII does not lie on the intrinsic pathway (Fig. 18.6). The whole blood clotting time is also normal for the same reason.

Other cases have presented as a haemorrhagic state in the neonatal period (Rabiner et al., 1960) at which time it is difficult to distinguish from haemorrhagic disease of the newborn, which also involves Factor VII deficiency. Surgical management in this deficiency has been reviewed by Strauss (1965). Levels of 10 per cent or more are necessary for haemostasis. This can be obtained with fresh or even stored plasma, since Factor VII is stable, unlike Factors V or VIII. Frequent infusions, however, may be necessary since the

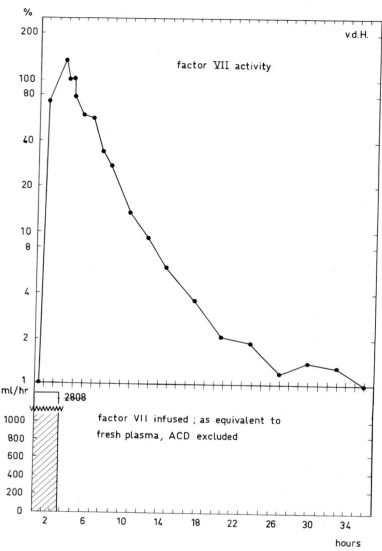

Fig. 18.11 *In-vivo* survival of Factor VII concentrate (prothrombal) in a patient with severe Factor VII deficiency. (Reproduced from *British Journal of Haematology* (1971), **21**, 391, by permission of the authors Bruning and Loeliger).

half-life *in vivo* is approximately 3 hours (Fig. 18.11) whether after infusion of plasma (Hitzig and Zollinger, 1958; Hjort *et al.*, 1961) or of a concentrate (Bruning and Loeliger, 1971).

Factor X (Stuart-Prower) deficiency was originally confused with that of Factor VII, Hougie *et al.* (1957) defining the distinction. Unlike Factor VII, Factor X lies on the intrinsic pathway. When deficient the PTT is prolonged with a 'serum' defect in the TGT. Quick's prothrombin time is prolonged but corrected by normal serum. The haemorrhagic state is relatively severe in homozygotes, the inheritance being autosomal recessive. Fresh or stored plasma will correct haemostasis. Half-life of the transfused factor is 1–2 days (Biggs and Denson, 1963). Kroll *et al.* (1964) reported the strange association of carotid body tumours with Factor VII and X deficiency.

Factor V (proaccelerin) deficiency was originally termed 'parahaemophilia' (Redner *et al.*, 1953) with mild to moderate haemorrhagic symptoms mainly after surgery. Inheritance is autosomal recessive. Coagulation results are similar to those in Factor X deficiency but it is the patients' adsorbed plasma that gives an abnormal result in the TGT. Also the prolonged Quick's prothrombin time is corrected by normal adsorbed plasma. Factor V assay (Stefanini, 1950) will confirm the diagnosis, assuming consumptive coagulopathy and fibrinolysis can be excluded as acquired causes of low Factor V levels. Fresh frozen plasma must be used to correct the deficiency since Factor V is labile under normal storage conditions. Satisfactory haemostasis is obtained with levels of 25 per cent or above, and the half-life *in vivo* is 36 hours (Webster *et al.*, 1964).

A family with elevated levels of Factor V associated with a tendency to thrombosis has also been described (Gaston, 1966). The proband was a 6-year-old girl who underwent successful iliofemoral thrombectomy. Her Factor V level ranged between 156 and 200 per cent.

Combined deficiencies of Factor V and Factor VIII have been described in a number of families associated with haemorrhagic symptoms of varying severity. Haematomas and haemarthroses were present in two severely affected patients, a boy and a girl, reported by Gobbi *et al.* (1967). In this family the Factor VIII was very low (2 per cent and less than 1 per cent) and the Factor V only moderately so (25 and 27 per cent). Family studies disclosed that both classical haemophilia and pure Factor V deficiency were present in relatives. It was postulated that the two defects had been inherited independently. Various genetic hypotheses were invoked by these authors to explain the occurrence of haemophilia in the girl. This report contrasted with that of Jones, Rizza, Hardisty, Dormandy and Macpherson (1962) where the Factor VIII levels were 6 and 11 per cent, and Factor V 3 and 10 per cent with a milder haemorrhagic state without haemarthroses. These and other authors have considered that the double defect was an example of pleiotropism, both depending upon a single mutant gene presumably responsible for the synthesis of a common protein precursor to both Factors V and VIII. A recent study of a family of over 40 members showed that the two deficiencies segregated together (Smit Sibinga *et al.*, 1972). Previous reported cases and genetic hypothesis in the literature are reviewed and these authors suggest an autosomal recessive mode of inheritance with a marked degree of penetrance and varying expressivity in heterozygotes.

One case of congenital combined deficiency of prothrombin, Factors VIII, IX and X has also been reported by McMillan and Roberts (1966).

DEFECTS OF FIBRINOGEN AND FIBRIN STABILIZATION (FACTORS I AND XIII)

Totally incoagulable blood even on addition of thrombin is characteristic of the rare disorder congenital afibrinogenaemia (Frick and McQuarrie, 1954; Werder, 1963). It should be pointed out that coagulation screening using only two-stage tests such as the TPST will fail to disclose this deficiency since fibrinogen is added to the system in the normal plasma used as 'substrate'. If it is not to be missed the thrombin time or fibrinogen titre must be performed on the patient's plasma, or PTT or clotting time determined, since any of these would be grossly abnormal. Fibrinogen survival is normal (Fig. 18.12) with a half-life of approximately 4 days (Tytgat *et al.*, 1972).

Clinically the disorder may present in the neonatal period as bleeding fom the umbilical stump. In later life the haemorrhagic state is relatively mild. Patients suffer more from bleeding following trivial cuts or minor surgery than they do from major surgery since the coagulation defect is promptly corrected by blood transfusion by virtue of its contained and stable fibrinogen. Haemarthroses seldom occur and menorrhagia is not a problem in later life. Inheritance is autosomal recessive, but heterozygotes may have subnormal fibrinogen concentrations. Since there is an absolute deficiency of fibrinogen synthesis

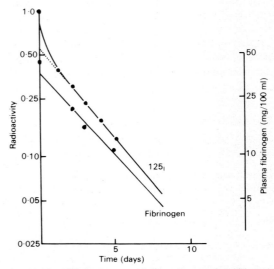

Fig. 18.12 Fibrinogen metabolism in a patient (7 year-old male) with congenital afibrinogenaemia. The labelled fibrinogen was injected after administration of blood and plasma. (Reproduced from *British Journal of Haematology* (1972), **22**, 714, by permission of the authors Tytgat *et al.*).

antifibrinogen antibodies may develop in some patients following replacement therapy, reducing the survival of infused fibrinogen.

A similar type of defect with prolonged thrombin time and apparently low fibrinogen when determined by thrombin clottability can occur due to *dysfibrinogenaemia* (von Felten *et al.*, 1966; Blombäck *et al.*, 1968). Structurally abnormal fibrinogen is synthesized that is still detectable by immunological assay although not reacting normally to thrombin. There is a mild to moderate haemorrhagic state. Inheritance is autosomal dominant, unusual among the coagulation disorders. Such cases could easily be confused with hereditary afibrinogenaemia.

Factor XIII (fibrin stabilizing factor) is an enzyme present in normal plasma which catalyses the formation of gamma-glutamyl-epsilon-lysine bridges between fibrin units rendering a firmer, more closely knit cross-linked form of fibrin which becomes insoluble in 5 M urea or 1 per cent monochloacetic acid in the process (Lorand *et al.*, 1968). Pure fibrinogen clotted by pure thrombin gives a loose form of fibrin still soluble in these reagents (Laki and Lorand, 1948).

Duckert *et al.* (1960) described a 7-year-old boy with a deficiency of this factor who showed a delayed haemorrhage from the umbilical stump, occurring during the second week of life. This was followed by a persisting history of increased bleeding usually starting 2–3 days after injury. This was accompanied by delayed healing and excessive retracted scar tissue. These manifestations fit in well with the concept of structurally impaired fibrin formation. Subsequent case reports have emphasized the characteristic sign of umbilical haemorrhage at the time of separation of the cord, the delayed nature of the bleeding, from several hours to 4 days after trauma, and have also shown a high incidence of intracranial haemorrhage in these children (Hanna, 1970). Haemarthrosis is uncommon and does not cause crippling. Gastrointestinal bleeding can occur. Habitual abortions can occur due to Factor XIII deficiency, but can be corrected by regular prophylactic plasma transfusions (Fisher *et al.*, 1966). A recent study of 4 patients in 2 Pakistani families with this deficiency supports the probable autosomal recessive pattern of inheritance (Aziz and Siddiqui, 1972).

All usual coagulation tests of the intrinsic and extrinsic coagulation pathways give normal results in this deficiency. Only if the test in which 0.2 ml of the patient's plasma is recalcified and clotted at $37° C$ with 0.2 ml of $M/_{40}CaCl_2$ and then incubated with 3–5 ml of 5M urea is performed will it be detected. In Factor XIII deficiency the clots will dissolve in 1–2 hours, whereas normal clots remain undissolved after 24 to 48 hours' incubation at RT. Correction experiments show that addition of 0.6 to 1.2 per cent of normal plasma to the mixture are sufficient to render the clots insoluble (Aziz and Siddigui, 1972). Transfusion of all blood products will likewise correct the haemostatic defect. Amris and Hilden (1968) have described the advantages of using cryoprecipitate for this purpose. Two 14-year-old patients were treated with 2 to 4 units at 3 to 4 week intervals. It is suggested that this may be justifiable in children because of the danger of intracranial haemorrhage (Hanna, 1970).

The clinical disorders due to Factor XIII deficiency have been reviewed by Duckert and Beck (1968).

REFERENCES

Abell, J. M. & Bailey, R. W. (1960) Hemophilic pseudotumor. *Arch. Surg.*, **81**, 569.

Abildgaard, C. F., Cornet, J. A., Alcalde, V. & Schulman, I. (1963) Hageman factor deficiency in a child. *Pediatrics*, **32**, 280.

Abildgaard, C. F., Simone, J. V. & Schulman, I. (1965) Steroid treatment of hemophilic hematuria. *J. Pediat.*, **66**, 117.

Abildgaard, C. F. (1969) The management of bleeding in hemophilia. *Advances Pediat.*, **16**, 365.

Ali, A. M., Gandy, R. H., Britten, M. I. & Dormandy, K. M. (1967) Joint haemorrhage in haemophilia: Is full advantage taken of plasma therapy? *Brit. med. J.*, **iii**, 828.

Amris, C. J. & Hilden, M. (1968) Treatment of factor XIII deficiency with cryoprecipitate. *Thromb. Diath. Haem.*, **20**, 528.

Aziz, M. A. & Siddiqui, A. R. (1972) Congenital deficiency of fibrin-stabilizing factor (factor XIII): A report of four cases (two families) and family members. *Blood*, **40**, 11.

Baehner, R. L. & Strauss, H. S. (1966) Hemophilia in the first year of life. *New Eng. J. Med.*, **275**, 524.

Bennett, E. & Dormandy, K. (1966) Pool's cryoprecipitate and exhausted plasma in the treatment of von Willebrand's disease and factor XI deficiency. *Lancet*, **ii**, 731.

Bennett, E., Dormandy, K. A., Churchill, W. G., Coward, A. R., Smith, M. & Cleghorn, T. E. (1967) Cryoprecipitate and the plastic blood-bag system: Provision of adequate replacement therapy for routine treatment of haemophilia. *Brit. med. J.*, **ii**, 88.

COAGULATION DISORDERS. 1. HEREDITARY 331

Bennett, E. & Huehns, E. R. (1970) Immunological differentiation of three types of haemophilia and identification of some female carriers. *Lancet*, **ii**, 956.

Bennett, B. & Grove, G. E. B. (1973) Antigen/Biological-activity ratio for factor VIII. *Lancet*, **i**, 777.

Bennett, A. E., Ingram, G. I. C. & Inglish, P. J. (1973) Antifibrinolytic treatment in haemophilia: A controlled trial of prophylaxis with tranexamic acid. *Brit. Jl Haemat.*, **24**, 83.

Bennett, B. & Ratnoff, O. D. (1973) Detection of the carrier state for classical haemophilia. *New Eng. J. Med.*, **288**, 342.

Bennett, B. (1974) Annotation: Anti-haemophilic factor, normal or abnormal. *Brit. J. Haemat.*, **26**, 1.

Bigg, R. & Douglas, A. S. (1953) The thromboplastin generation test. *J. Clin. Path.*, **6**, 23.

Biggs, R. (1957) Assay of antihaemophilic globulin in treatment of haemophilic patients. *Lancet*, **ii**, 311.

Biggs, R. & Bidwell, E. (1959) A method for the study of antihaemophilic globulin inhibitors with reference to six cases. *Brit. J. Ha.mat.*, **5**, 379.

Biggs, R. P. & Denson, K. W. E. (1963) The fate of prothrombin and factors VIII, IX, and X transfused to patients deficient in these factors. *Brit. J. Haemat.*, **9**, 523.

Biggs, R. & Macfarlane, R. G. (1966) *Treatment of Haemophilia and Other Coagulation Disorders*. Oxford: Blackwell Scientific Publications.

Blombäck, M., Blombäck, B., Mammen, E. F. & Prasad, A. S. (1968) Fibrinogen Detroit—a molecular defect in the N-terminal disulphide knot of human fibrinogen. *Nature*, **218**, 134.

Bloom, A. L., Giddings, J. C. & Peake, I. R. (1973) Low-molecular-weight factor VIII. *Lancet*, **i**, 661.

Bond, T. P., Levin, W. C., Celander, D. R. & Guest, M. M. (1962) 'Mild haemophilia' affecting both males and females. *New Eng. J. Med.*, **266**, 220.

Borchgrevink, S. G., Egeberg, O., Pool, J. G., Skulason, T., Stormorken, H. & Waaler, B. (1959) A study of a case of congenital hypoprothrombinaemia. *Brit. J. Haemat.*, **5**, 294.

Bowie, E. J. W., Thompson, J. H., Didisheim, P. & Owen, C. A. (1967) Disappearance rates of coagulation factors: Transfusion studies in factor-deficient patients. *Transfusion*, **7**, 174.

Boyer, S. H., Siggers, D. C. & Krueger, L. J. (1973) Caveat to protein replacement therapy for genetic disease. Immunological implications of accurate molecular diagnosis. *Lancet*, **iii**, 654.

Britten, A. F. H. & Salzman, E. W. (1966) Surgery in congenital disorders of blood coagulation. *Surg. Gynec. and Obst.*, **123**, 1333.

Brown, D. L., Hardisty, R. M., Kosoy, M. H. & Bracken, C. (1967) Antihaemophilic globulin: Preparation by an improved cryoprecipitation method and clinical use. *Brit. med. J.*, **ii**, 79.

Bruning, P. F. & Loeliger, E. A. (1971) Prothrombal: A new concentrate of human prothrombin complex for clinical use. *Brit. J. Haemat.*, **21**, 377.

Buchholz, D. H. (1974) Blood transfusion: Merits of component therapy. II. The clinical use of plasma and plasma components. *J. Pediat.*, **84**, 165.

Cade, J. F., Hirsh, J. & Martin, M. (1969) Placental barrier to coagulation factors: Its relevance to the coagulation defect at birth and to haemorrhage in the newborn. *Brit. med. J.*, **ii**, 291.

Clark, K. G. A. (1973) Haemophilic women. *Lancet*, **i**, 1388.

Colman, R. W. (1973) Immunologic heterogeneity of hemophilia. *New Eng. J. Med.*, **288**, 369.

Corrigan, J. J. (1972) Oral bleeding in hemophilia: Treatment with epsilon aminocaproic acid and replacement therapy. *J. Pediat.*, **80**, 124.

Curran, J. P. & Jung-Shung Wang (1971) Fatal intracranial hemorrhage as the first sign of hemophilia B in an infant. *Amer. J. Dis. Child.*, **122**, 63.

Dallman, P. R. & Pool, J. G. (1968) Treatment of hemophilia with factor VIII concentrates. *New Eng. J. Med.*, **278**, 199.

Davie, E. W. & Ratnoff, O. D. (1964) Waterfall sequence for intrinsic blood clotting. *Science*, **145**, 1310.

Davie, E. W., Hougie, C. & Lunblad, R. L. (1969) Mechanisms of blood coagulation, Chap. 2. In *Recent Advances in Blood Coagulation*. Edited by L. Poller. London: Churchill.

Davies, S. H., Turner, J. W., Cumming, R. A., Gillingham, F. J., Girdwood, R. H. & Darg, A. (1966) Management of intracranial haemorrhage in haemophilia. *Brit. med. J.*, **iv**, 1627.

Denson, K. W. E. & Ingram, G. I. C. (1973) Antigen/Biological-activity ratio for factor VIII. *Lancet*, **i**, 157.

Deykin, D. (1970) The clinical challenge of disseminated intravascular coagulation. *New Eng. J. Med.*, **283**, 636.

Didisheim, P. & Lewis, J. H. (1958) Congenital disorders of the mechanism for coagulation of blood. *Pediat.*, **22**, 478.

Dike, G. W. R., Bidwell, E. & Rizza, C. R. (1972) The preparation and clinical use of a new concentrate containing factor IX, prothrombin and factor X and of a separate concentrate containing factor VII. *Brit. J. Haemat.*, **22**, 469.

Dormandy, K. M. & Hardisty, R. M. (1961) Coagulation tests on capillary blood. A screening procedure for use in small children. *J. Clin. Path.*, **14**, 543.

Dormandy, K. M. (1973) Pain in haemophilia. *Lancet*, **ii**, 931.

Duckert, F., Jung, E. & Shmerling, D. H. (1960) A hitherto undescribed congenital haemorrhagic diathesis probably due to fibrin stabilizing factor deficiency. *Throm. Diath. Haem.*, **5**, 179.

Duckert, F. & Beck, E. A. (1968) Clinical disorders due to the deficiency of factor XIII (Fibrin stabilizing factor, fibrinase). *Sem. Haemat.*, **5**, 83.

Duthie, R. B., Matthews, J. M., Rizza, C. R., Steel, W. M. & Woods, C. G. (1972) *The Management of Musculo-Skeletal Problems in the Haemophilias*. Oxford: Blackwell Scientific Publications.

Falter, McL. & Kaufmann, M. F. (1971) Congenital factor VII deficiency. *J. Pediat.*, **79**, 298.

Felten, A. von, Duckert, F. & Frick, P. G. (1966) Familial disturbance of fibrin monomer aggregation. *Brit. J. Haemat.,* **12**, 667.

Fisher, S., Rikover, M. & Naor, S. (1966) Factor 13 deficiency with severe hemorrhagic diathesis. *Blood,* **28**, 34.

Fletcher, A. P., Biederman, O., Moore, D., Alkjaersig, N. & Sherry, S. (1964) Abnormal plasminogen-plasmin system activity (fibrinolysis) in patients with hepatic cirrhosis: its cause and consequences. *J. clin. Invest.,* **43**, 681.

Forbes, C. D., Barr, R. D., Reid, G., Thomson, C., Prentice, C. R. M., McNicol, G. P. & Douglas, A. S. (1972) Tranexamic acid in control of haemorrhage after dental extraction in haemophilia and Christmas disease. *Brit. med. J.,* **ii**, 311.

Frick, P. G. & McQuarrie, I. (1954) Congenital afibrinogenemia. *Pediatrics,* **13**, 44.

Gaston, L. W. (1966) Studies on a family with an elevated plasma level of factor V (proaccelerin) and a tendency to thrombosis. *J. Pediat.,* **68**, 367.

Gilchrist, G. S., Liebermann, E., Ekert, H., Fine, R. N. & Grushkin, C. (1969) Heparin therapy in the haemolytic uraemic syndrome. *Lancet,* **1**, 1123.

Gilchrist, G. S., Ekert, H., Shawbrom, E. & Hammond, D. (1969) Evaluation of a new concentrate for the treatment of factor IX deficiency. *New Eng. J. Med.,* **280**, 291.

Gobbi, F., Ascari, E. & Barbieri, U. (1967) Congenital combined deficiency of factor VIII (antihaemophilic globulin) and factor V (proaccelerin) in two siblings. Clinical study and genetic speculations. *Thromb. Diathesis Haem.,* **17**, 194.

Gordon, A. M., McNicol, G. P., Dubber, A. H. C., McDonald, G. A. & Douglas, A. S. (1965) Clinical trial of epsilon-aminocaproic acid in severe haemophilia. *Brit. med. J.,* **ii**, 1632.

Green, D. (1971) Suppression of an antibody to factor VIII by a combination of factor VIII and cyclophosphamide. *Blood,* **37**, 381.

Hanna, M. (1970) Congenital deficiency of factor XIII: Report of a family from Newfoundland with associated mild deficiency of factor XII. *Pediatrics,* **46**, 611.

Hardisty, R. M. (1957) Christmas disease in a woman. *Brit. med. J.,* **i**, 1039.

Hardisty, R. M. & Ingram, G. I. C. (1965) *Bleeding Disorders. Investigation and Management.* Oxford: Blackwell Scientific Publications.

Hartmann, J. R. & Diamond, L. K. (1957) Haemphilia and related haemorrhagic disorders. *Practitioner,* **178**, 179.

Hartman, J. R. (1965) Letter to the Editor. *J. Pediat.,* **66**, 1107.

Harvey, G. P. (1973) Little relief for pain of haemophilia. *Lancet,* **ii**, 776.

Hirschman, R. J., Hscoitz, S. B. & Shulman, N. R. (1970) Prophylactic treatment of factor VIII deficiency. *Blood,* **35**, 189.

Hitzig, W. H. & Zollinger, W. (1958) Kongenitaler factor VII mangel: Familienuntersuchung und physiologische Studien über den Factor VII. *Helv. Paed. Acta,* **13**, 189.

Hjort, P. F., Egeberg, O. & Mikkelsen, S. (1961) Turnover of prothrombin, factor VII and factor IX in a patient with hemophilia A. *Scandinav. J. Clin. Lab. Invest.,* **13**, 668.

Hoag, M. S., Johnson, F. F., Robinson, J. A. & Aggeler, P. M. (1969) Treatment of hemophilia B with a new clotting factor concentrate. *New Eng. J. Med.,* **280**, 581.

Honig, G. R., Forman, E. N., Johnston, C. A., Seeler, R. A., Abildgaard, C. F. & Schulman, I. (1969) Administration of single doses of AHF (factor VIII) concentrates in the treatment of hemophilic hemarthroses. *Pediatrics,* **43**, 26.

Hougie, C., Barrow, E. M. & Graham, J. B. (1957) Stuart clotting defect. I. Segregation of an hereditary hemorrhagic state from the heterogeneous group heretofore called stable factor'' (SPCA, Proconvertin, Factor VII) deficiency. *J. Clin. Invest.,* **36**, 485.

Hougie, C. & Sargeant, R. (1973) Antigen/Biological-activity ratio for factor VIII. *Lancet,* **i**, 616.

Ikkala, E. (1960) Haemophilia. A study of its laboratory, clinical, genetic and social aspects based on known haemophiliacs in Finland. *Scand. J. Clin. Lab. Invest.,* **12**, Suppl. 45.

Israëls, M. C. G., Lempert, H. & Gilbertson, E. (1951) Haemophilia in the female. *Lancet,* **i**, 1375.

Johnson, A. J., Karpatkin, M. H. & Newman, J. (1971) Clinical investigation of intermediate and high purity antihaemophilic factor (factor VIII) concentrates. *Brit. J. Haemat.,* **21**, 21.

Jones, J. H., Rizza, C. R., Hardisty, R. M., Dormandy, K. M. & MacPherson, J. C. (1962) Combined deficiency of factor V and factor VIII (antihaemophilic globulin). A report of three cases. *Brit. J. Haemat.,* **8**, 120.

Josso, F., Prou-Wartelle, O., Alagille, D. & Soulier, J. P. /1964) Le déficit congénital en facteur stabilisant de la fibrine (facteur XIII). *Nouv. Rev. franç. Hemat.,* **4**, 267.

Kasper, C. K., Dietrich, S. L. & Rapaport, S. I. (1970) Hemophilia prophylaxis with AHF concentrate. *Arch. Intern. Med.,* **125**, 1004.

Kernoff, P. B. A. & Rizza, C. R. (1973) Antigen/Biological-activity ratio for factor VIII. *Lancet,* **1**, 777.

Kisker, C. T. & Burke, C. (1970) Double-blind studies on the use of steroids in the treatment of acute haemarthrosis in patients with hemophilia. *New Eng. J. Med.,* **282**, 639.

Kowalski, E. (1968) Fibrinogen derivatives and their biologic activities. *Sem. Hemat.,* **5**, 45.

Kozinn, P. J., Ritz, N. & Horowitz, A. W. (1963) Scalp hemorrhage as an emergency in the newborn. *J.A.M.A.,* **194**, 567.

Kroll, A. J., Alexander, B., Cochios, F. & Pechet, L. (1964) Hereditary deficiencies of clotting factors VII and X associated with carotid-body tumours. *New Eng. J. Med.,* **270**, 6.

Kurczynski, E. M. & Penner, J. A. (1974) Activated prothrombin concentrate for patients with factor VIII inhibitors. *New Eng. J. Med.,* **291**, 164.

Laki, K. & Lorand, L. (1948) On the solubility of fibrin clots. *Science,* **108**, 280.

Lancet (1973A) Leading Article: Treatment of haemophilia. *Lancet*, **ii**, 648.

Lancet (1973B) Pain in haemophilia. *Lancet*, **ii**, 757.

Lancet (1973C) Editorial: Haemophilia in Women. *Lancet*, **ii**, 1305.

Larrieu, M. J., Rigollot, C. & Marder, V. J. (1972) Comparative effects of fibrinogen degradation fragments D and E on coagulation. *Brit. J. Haemat.*, **22**, 719.

Lazerson, J. (1973) Hemophilia home transfusion program: Effect of cryoprecipitate utilization. *J. Pediat.*, **82**, 857.

Levine, P. H. (1974) Efficacy of self-therapy in hemophilia: A study of 72 patients with Hemophilia A and B. *New Eng. J. Med.*, **291**, 1381.

Lorand, L., Rule, N. G., Ong, H. H., Furlanetoo, R., Jacobsen, A., Downey, H., Oner, N. & Bruner-Lorand, J. (1968) Amine specificity in transpeptidation inhibition of fibrin cross-linking. *Biochem.*, **7**, 1214.

Lusher, J. M. & Evans, R. K. (1971) Effective suppression of factor 8 antibody with cyclophosphamide. *Blood*, **38**, 818.

McMillan, C. W. & Roberts, H. R. (1966) Congenital combined deficiency of coagulation factors II, VII, IX, and X: Report of a case. *New Eng. J. Med.*, **274**, 1313.

Macfarlane, R. G. (1964) An enzyme cascade in the blood clotting mechanism, and its function as a biochemical amplifier. *Nature*, **202**, 495.

Macfarlane, R. G. (1968) How does blood clot? *Hospital Medicine*, **4**, 29.

Macpherson, J. C. & Hardisty, R. M. (1961) A modified thromboplastin screening test. *Thromb. Diath. Haem.*, **6**, 492.

Margolis, J. (1961) Some experiences with a simplified micromethod for coagulation studies. *Brit. J. Haemat.*, **7**, 21.

Mason, D. Y. & Ingram, G. I. C. (1971) Management of hereditary coagulation disorders. *Sem. Haemat.*, **8**, 158.

Mazza, J. J., Bowie, E. J. W., Hagedorn, A. B., Didisheim, P., Taswell, H. F., Peterson, L. F. A. & Owen, C. A. (1970) Anti-hemophilic factor VIII in hemophilia. *J.A.M.A.*, **211**, 1818.

Mersky, C., Johnson, A. J., Pert, J. H. & Wohl, H. (1964) Pathogenesis of fibrinolysis in defibrination syndrome: Effect of heparin administration. *Blood*, **24**, 701.

Mersky, C., Kleiner, G. J. & Johnson, A. J. (1966) Quantitative estimation of split products of fibrinogen in human serum, relation to diagnosis and treatment. *Blood*, **28**, 1.

Miller, J. (1973) Haemophilia: A challenge to social work. *Social Work Today*, **4**, 501.

Nilsson, I. M., Sjoerdsma, A. & Waldenström, J. (1960) Antifibrinolytic activity and metabolism of E-aminocaproic acid in man. *Lancet*, **1**, 1322.

Nossel, H. L. (1964) *The Contact Phase of Blood Coagulation*. Oxford: Blackwell Scientific Publications.

Owren, P. A. & Aas, K. (1951) The control of dicoumarol therapy and the quantitative determination of prothrombin and proconvertin. *Scand. J. Clin. Lab. Invest.*, **3**, 201.

Owren, P. A. (1959) Thrombotest, a new method for controlling anticoagulant therapy. *Lancet*, **ii**, 754.

Patek, A. J. & Stetson, R. J. (1936) Hemophilia. I. The abnormal coagulation of blood and its relation to blood platelets. *J. Clin. Invest.*, **15**, 531.

Pool, J. G. & Shannon, A. E. (1965) Production of high-potency concentrates of antihemophilic globulin in a closed-bag system. *New Eng. J. Med.*, **273**, 1443.

Prentice, C. R. M., Breckenridge, R. T., Forman, W. B. & Ratnoff, O. D. (1967) Treatment of haemophilia (factor-VIII deficiency) with human antihaemophilic factor prepared by the cryoprecipitate process. *Lancet*, **i**, 457.

Quesne, B. le, Britten, M., Maragaki, C. & Dormandy, K. (1974) Home treatment for patients with haemophilia. *Lancet*, **ii**, 507.

Rabiner, S. F., Winick, M. & Smith, C. H. (1960) Congenital deficiency of factor VII associated with hemorrhagic disease of the newborn. Report of a case. *Pediatrics*, **25**, 101.

Rabiner, S. F. & Telfer, M. C. (1970) Home transfusion for patients with haemophilia A. *New Eng. J. Med.*, **283**, 1011.

Rainsford, S. G. & Hall, A. (1973) A three-year study of adolescent boys suffering from haemophilia and allied disorders. *Brit. J. Haemat.*, **24**, 539.

Rapaport, S. I., Ames, S. B., Mikkelsen, S. & Goodman, J. R. (1960) Plasma clotting factors in hepatocellular disease. *New Eng. J. Med.*, **263**, 278.

Rapaport, S. I., Patch, M. J. & Moore, F. J. (1960) Antihemophilic globulin levels in carriers of hemophilia A. *J. Clin Invest.*, **39**, 1619.

Ratnoff, O. D. & Colopy, J. E. (1955) A familial hemorrhagic trait associated with a deficiency of a clot-promoting fraction of plasma. *J. Clin. Invest.*, **34**, 602.

Redner, B., Scalettar, H. & Weiner, M. (1953) Parahaemophilia (Owren's disease). *Pediatrics*, **12**, 5.

Rizza, C. R. & Biggs, R. (1971) Haemophilia today. *Brit. J. Hosp. Med.*, **6**, 343.

Rizza, C. R. & Matthews, J. M. (1972) Management of the haemophilic child. *Arch. Dis. Childh.*, **47**, 451.

Rizza, C. R. & Biggs, R. (1973) The treatment of patients who have factor-VIII antibodies. *Brit. J. Haemat.*, **24**, 65.

Robbins, K. C. (1944) A study on the conversion of fibrinogen to fibrin. *Amer. J. Physiol.*, **152**, 581.

Rodman, N. F., Barrow, E. M. & Graham, J. B. (1958) Diagnosis and control of the haemophiloid states with the partial thromboplastin time (PTT) test. *Amer. J. clin. Path.*, **29**, 525.

Rosenthal, R. L., Dreskin, O. H. & Rosenthal, N. (1955) Plasma thromboplastin antecedent (PTA) deficiency: Clinical, coagulation, therapeutic and hereditary aspects of a new hemophilia-like disease. *Blood*, **10**, 120.

Rosenthal, R. L. & Sloan, E. (1965) PTA factor (XI) levels and coagulation studies after plasma infusions in PTA deficient patients. *J. Lab. Clin. Med.*, **66**, 709.

Sharp, A. A., Howie, B., Biggs, R. & Methven, D. T. (1958) Defibrination syndrome in pregnancy. Value of various diagnostic tests. *Lancet*, **ii**, 1309.

Sharp, A. A. & Eggleton, M. J. (1963) Haematology and the extracorporeal circulation. *J. clin. Path.*, **16**, 551.

Simpson, N. E. & Biggs, R. (1962) The inheritance of Christmas factor. *Brit. J. Haemat.*, **8**, 191.

Sjølin, K.-E. (1960) *Haemophilic Disease in Denmark. A Classification of the Clotting Defects in 78 Haemophilic Families.* Oxford: Blackwell Scientific Publications.

Smit Sibinga, C. Th., Gökemeyer, J. D. M., Kate, L. P. ten & Bos-van Zwol, F. (1972) Combined deficiency of factor V and factor VIII: Report of a family and genetic analysis. *Brit. J. Haemat.*, **23**, 467.

Stark, S. N., White, J. G. & Langer, L. (1965) Epsilon-aminocaproic acid therapy as a cause of intrarenal obstruction in haematuria of haemophilics. *Scandinav. J. Haemat.*, **2**, 99.

Steinle, C. J. & Kisker, C. T. (1970) Pediatric dentistry for the child with haemophilia. *New Eng. J. Med.*, **283**, 1325.

Stephanini, M. (1950) New one-stage procedures for the quantitative determination of prothrombin and labile factor. *Amer. J. clin. Path.*, **20**, 233.

Stites, D. P., Hershgold, E. J., Perlman, J. D. & Fudenberg, H. H. (1971) Factor VIII detection by hemagglutination inhibition: Hemophilia A and von Willebrand's disease. *Science*, **171**, 196.

Stormorken, H. & Owren, P. A. (1971) Physiopathology of hemostasis. *Sem. Hemat.*, **8**, 3.

Strauss, H. (1965) Clinical pathological conference. *J. Pediat.*, **66**, 443.

Strauss, H. S. (1965) Surgery in patients with congenital factor VII deficiency (congenital hypoproconvertinemia). Experience with one case and review of the literature. *Blood*, **25**, 325.

Strauss, H. S. (1972) Diagnosis and treatment of inherited bleeding disorders. *Ped. Clin. N. Amer.*, **19**, 1009.

Stuart, J., Davies, S. H., Cumming, R. A., Girdwood, R. H. & Darg, A. (1966) Haemorrhagic episodes in haemophilia: A 5-year prospective study. *Brit. med. J.*, **iv**, 1624.

Tavenner, R. W. H. (1968) Epsilon-aminocaproic acid in the treatment of haemophilia and Christmas disease with special reference to the extraction of teeth. *British Dental Journal*, **124**, 19.

Tavenner, R. W. H. (1972) Use of tranexamic acid in control of haemorrhage after extraction of teeth in haemophilia and Christmas disease. *Brit. med. J.*, **ii**, 314.

Tytgat, G. N., Collen, D. & Vermylen, J. (1972) Metabolism and distribution of fibrinogen. II. Fibrinogen turnover in polycythaemia, thrombocytosis, haemophilia A, congenital afibrinogenaemia and during streptokinase therapy. *Brit. J. Haemat.*, **22**, 701.

Walsh, P. N., Rizza, C. R., Matthews, J. M., Eipe, J., Kernoff, P. B. A., Coles, M. D., Bloom, A. L., Kaufman, B. M., Beck, P., Hanan, C. M. & Bigg, R. (1971) Epsilon-aminocaproic acid therapy for dental extractions in haemophilia and Christmas disease: A double blind controlled trial. *Brit. J. Haemat.*, **20**, 463.

Wanken, J. J., Eyring, E. J. & Kontras, S. B. (1969) Should haemophilic hemarthroses be aspirated? *Lancet*, **ii**, 1253.

Webster, W. P., Roberts, H. R. & Penick, G. D. (1964) Hemostasis in factor V deficiency. *Am. J. Med. Sci.*, **248**, 194.

Webster, W. P., Roberts, H. R. & Penick, G. D. (1968) Dental care of patients with hereditary disorders of blood coagulation. *Mod. Treat.*, **5**, 93.

Werder, E. (1963) Kongenitale Afibrinogenämie. *Helv. Paediat. Acta*, **18**, 208.

Zimmerman, T. S., Ratnoff, O. D. & Powell, A. E. (1971A) Immunologic differentiation of classic hemophilia (factor VIII deficiency) and von Willebrand's disease. *J. Clin. Invest.*, **50**, 244.

Zimmerman, T. S., Ratnoff, O. D. & Littell, A. S. (1971B) Detection of carriers of classic hemophilia using an immunologic assay for antihemophilic factor (factor VIII). *J. Clin. Invest.*, **50**, 255.

19. Coagulation Disorders. II. Acquired

Impaired hepatic synthesis, Vitamin K, Coagulation status in the newborn, Haemorrhagic disease of the newborn, Vitamin K deficiency beyond the neonatal period, Hepatocellular disease | Disseminated intravascular coagulation (DIC), *Fibrin degradation products (FDPs), Diagnosis of DIC, General considerations, Specific therapy for DIC. DIC in the neonatal period, Causes of intravascular coagulation beyond the newborn period* | Acquired inhibitors of coagulation.

In paediatric practice these are of two main types: (a) Impaired hepatic synthesis of vitamin K dependent Factors II, VII, IX and X, (b) Consumption of Factors I (fibrinogen), II, V, VIII and platelets due to intravascular clotting, often with secondary fibrinolysis.

Other types of abnormality such as primary fibrinolysis or the appearance of specific inhibitors of coagulation (McMillan *et al.*, 1972) are of great rarity in this age group.

IMPAIRED HEPATIC SYNTHESIS

Disorders in this category include haemorrhagic disease of the newborn, malabsorption states and liver disease.

Vitamin K

Both normal hepatocellular function and an adequate hepatic supply of vitamin K are necessary for the synthesis of Factors II (prothrombin), VII, IX, and X, conveniently referred to as the 'prothrombin complex'. At the biochemical level vitamin K catalyses oxidative phosphorylation and electron transport (Martius, 1967). Naturally occurring K vitamins are fat soluble. K_1 is present in green leafy vegetables and has a phytyl side chain (2-Methyl-3-phytyl-1,4-naphthoquinone). K_2 is derived from intestinal bacteria and has a similarly fat soluble difarnesyl substitution at the 3 position. It is questionable how much of this intestinally synthesized vitamin is absorbed from the colon in man. The water soluble analogues of vitamin K have the same 2-Methyl-1, 4-naphthoquinone nucleus but lack the hydrophobic side chains at the 3 position. Unlike the natural vitamin they may produce haemolysis in the newborn if given to the infant or its mother in large doses.

Pharmaceutical preparations of the naturally occurring vitamin K_1 include Konakion and Aqua Mephyton (colloidal suspensions that can be given orally, IM, SC, or IV), Phytonadione and Mephyton (oily preparations that can be given orally or IV). Water soluble analogues include Synkavite, Hykinone, Menadione and its sodium disulphite derivatives. Further details of these compounds are given in the Report of the Committee on Nutrition of the American Academy of Pediatrics (1961).

Table 19.1 Coagulation test in term neonates

Test	Mean	Standard deviation	No. of neonates	Mean adult value
P.T. (seconds)	17·5	3·2	66	15
per cent	78	—	66	100
K.P.T.T. (seconds)	71	21	66	50
Factor II (per cent)	60	38	12	100
Factor V (per cent)	92	41	66	100
Factors VII and X (per cent)	56	35	66	100
Factor VIII (per cent)	70	56	62	100
Factor X (per cent)	55	42	63	100
Fibrinogen (mg/100 ml)	193	102	64	290

Reproduced by permission of the author and the editor from Cade (1969), Brit. med. J., **ii,** *282.*

Coagulation status in the newborn

The normal full term infant is born with levels of Factors II, VII, IX and X that are low by adult standards (Hathaway, 1970A) (Table 19.1). In a series of 250 healthy term infants in Glasgow a quarter had thrombotest levels of 10 per cent or less, and in half these it was 5 per cent or less. The coagulation factors fall even lower over the first few days of life reaching their nadir on about the third day. It is thought that this postnatal fall is due to the low body stores of vitamin K at birth (*B.M.J.*, 1971). Although as little as 25 micrograms of vitamin K can prevent this fall in the prothrombin complex (Aballi and de Lamerens, 1962A) the infant's intake may be less than this if breast fed.

Table 19.2   Coagulation tests in premature neonates according to gestational age

Weeks	35 and 36	33 and 34	29–32	< 29
P.T. (seconds)	16·3	17·9	21·8	35·4★
Per cent	88	75	40	14
S.D.	2·3	4·2	12·8	21·6
K.P.T.T. (seconds)	73	100	104★	147★
S.D.	19	50	41	42
Factor II (per cent)	79	46	53	47
S.D.	37	10	45	30
Factor V (per cent)	51	49	58	65
S.D.	20	30	39	48
Factors VII and X (per cent)	45	37	36	27
S.D.	26	34	29	18
Factor VIII (per cent)	67	21	46	57
S.D.	97	39	41	61
Factor X (per cent)	35	12	45	46
S.D.	26	13	34	31
Fibrinogen (mg/100 ml)	185	179	267	224
S.D.	72	83	146	187

S.D. = Standard deviation.
★Indicates significant difference (P < 0·05) in P.T. and K.P.T.T. compared with term neonates.
Reproduced by permission of the author and the editor from Cade (1969), Brit. med. J., **ii,** *282.*

Table 19.3   Coagulation tests in premature neonates according to birth weight

Birth weight (g.)	2,001–2,500	1,501–2,000	1,001–1,500	< 1,000
P.T. (seconds)	16·6	17·3	26·6★	37·0
Per cent	86	79	21	13
S.D.	2·7	3·2	17·3	23·5
K.P.T.T. (seconds)	77	113	117★	132★
S.D.	17	50	46	41
Factor II (per cent)	99	70	47	13
S.D.	49	—	32	12
Factor V (per cent)	66	67	64	26
S.D.	38	22	41	17
Factors VII and X (per cent)	48	37	42	10
S.D.	28	36	26	2
Factor VIII (per cent)	21	44	50	45
S.D.	26	43	57	42
Factor X (per cent)	22	29	39	46
S.D.	19	30	33	39
Fibrinogen (mg/100 ml)	202	233	215	294
S.D.	34	133	109	226

S.D. = Standard deviation.
★Indicates significant difference (P < 0·05) in P.T. and K.P.T.T. compared with term neonates.
Reproduced by permission of the author and the editor from Cade (1969), Brit. med. J., **ii,** *282.*

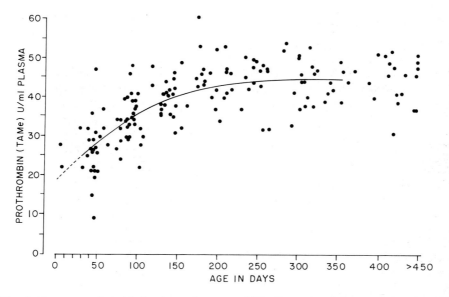

Fig. 19.1 The rise in true prothrombin level over first year of life. (Reproduced from *American Journal of Diseases Children* (1964), **107**, 614, from a paper by Glueck *et al.* by permission of the authors).

The vitamin K content of cow's milk is about 6 micrograms per 100 ml and that of breast milk 1·5 micrograms per 100 ml (Dam *et al.*, 1942). It is the combination of low initial stores and subsequent poor intake of vitamin K that occasionally produces an exaggeration of the coagulation defect, causing primary haemorrhagic disease of the newborn (Aballi and de Lamerens, 1962B).

In premature infants of low birth weight both the vitamin K stores and the level of coagulation factors are even lower than in term infants (Tables 19.2 and 3). The response to vitamin K is slow and inconstant (Aballi *et al.*, 1957; van Creveld *et al.*, 1954) suggesting that the immature liver has reduced synthetic capability. This is supported by experimental work with liver slices from immature rats (Pool and Robinson, 1959). In clinical terms this puts the low birth weight infant with low prothrombin complex levels in a slightly different class from the breast fed, otherwise healthy, full term infant with haemorrhagic disease.

Platelet count and most other readily measured coagulation factors are normal even in the premature infant. Minor abnormalities in Factors V and VIII have, however, been reported in premature infants. Cade *et al.* (1969) found a mean Factor V level of 67 per cent; McMillan and Elston (1968) a mean Factor VIII of 77 per cent, with a range of 31 to 123 per cent in prematures. The prolonged thrombin time found in the newborn in spite of normal fibrinogen levels (Roberts *et al.*, 1966) is attributed to a qualitative abnormality of 'foetal fibrinogen' (Witt *et al.*, 1969). Hathaway (1970A) has also pointed out that the rather low levels of Factors IX, XI and XII result in a modest prolongation of the PTT to 71 seconds in term infants, and to 90 seconds in premature infants (normal 37–50 seconds).

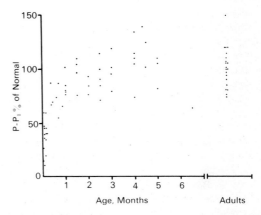

Fig. 19.2 Prothrombin—proconvertin (P and P) values during the first year of life. (Uncorrected for haematocrit). (Reproduced from *Acta Paediatrica Scandinavia* (1971), **60**, 269, from a paper by Norén *et al.* by permission of the authors).

Over the first year of life there is a gradual rise in both true prothrombin and the 'P and P' percentage to normal adult values (Glueck *et al.*, 1964; Noren *et al.*, 1971) (Figs. 19.1 and 2). Factor IX is also normal by 3 months.

Haemorrhagic disease of the newborn

This term was originally used by Townsend as long ago as 1894 to distinguish those haemorrhagic states confined to the neonatal period from the life-long bleeding states such as haemophilia. Brinkhouse and colleagues first related this disorder to hypoprothrombinaemia in 1937, and Waddell *et al.* to vitamin K deficiency (1939). Aballi *et al.* (1959) described 26 infants with gastrointestinal haemorrhage, epistaxis, cephalhaematoma or umbilical haemorrhage in the first 3 days of life. They suggested that it was a low Factor IX or X which distinguished those who bled from those who did not.

Nowadays it is profitable to **distinguish** *primary* haemorrhagic disease of the **newborn**, due to vitamin K deficiency, from **the** *secondary* form occurring in sick or premature **infants** and not due to simple vitamin K deficiency (Aballi and de Lamerens, 1962A, B).

The overall incidence of haemorrhagic disease is in the order of 1 in 200 to 1 in 400 births (Smith 1960) but a strong association with poor socioeconomic conditions has been noted, with a high incidence in areas such as Cuba (Aballi *et al.*, 1959) and the southern states of America. This may be due to the more common use of breast feeding in these areas, but maternal nutritional status could also play a part.

Aballi and de Lamerens (1962B), working in Memphis, Tennessee, encountered 21 infants with the primary form of haemorrhagic disease. Nineteen were full term, none had been given vitamin K and none had clinical evidence of infection or hypoxia. Haemorrhagic symptoms developed between the 2nd and 4th day of life. These consisted of gastrointestinal haemorrhage in 6, bleeding from the nose in 7 and subgaleal haemorrhage in 4. Only 1 infant died. Quick's prothrombin time was prolonged in all, with deficiencies of Factors II, VII, IX and X in many. Factor V was normal. There was a rapid response in the coagulation defect after giving 1 to 10 mg of vitamin K_1 or after whole blood transfusion. They concluded that these cases represented an exaggeration of the vitamin K deficiency normally seen in the neonatal period.

Contrasted with this group the same authors described 25 infants with haemorrhage of whom 21 were premature, with clinical evidence of hypoxia or infection in most. All had received vitamin K. The site of bleeding differed with 14 having pulmonary haemorrhage and 12 CNS haemorrhage of which 10 were intraventricular.

All but one of the infants died. Coagulation defects were more variable than in the primary group. Quick's prothrombin time was only moderately prolonged, Factor VII and V were usually low. Platelets were reduced in number or sometimes in function with a prolonged bleeding time in most infants. There was a poor response to vitamin K. They classified this group as having the secondary form of haemorrhagic disease which they regarded as due to 'an intensification of the peculiarities associated with immaturity'. Nowadays we would probably recognize these infants as having the stigmata of intravascular coagulation.

In addition they described 4 infants as having the features of both groups, consistent with the concept that premature infants are also prone to vitamin K deficiency and may respond suboptimally to the vitamin. Gray *et al.* (1968) similarly found low thrombotest results in low birth weight, hypoglycaemic infants with previous intrapartum hypoxia and liability to intracranial haemorrhage (intraventricular or subarachnoid). Poor response to IM vitamin K was also noted.

Sutherland, Glueck and Gleser (1967), in Cincinnati, studied 3,338 full term infants for clinical evidence of haemorrhage. They were randomized to receive placebo, 100 micrograms of vitamin K or 5 mg of vitamin K. Some were breast fed, others were on a cow's milk formula. Mild bleeding was seen in 5 per cent or more in all 3 groups, but severe bleeding occurred in 8 out of the 1,143 (0·7 per cent) in the placebo group and in none out of the 1,137 given 100 micrograms or the 1,063 given 5 mg of vitamin K. All but one of the infants with serious bleeding had been breast fed. In 4 the bleeding occurred after circumcision. The authors concluded that 'the breast fed infant who does not receive vitamin K has a 5 per cent increased risk of bleeding, increased to 10 per cent if subjected to a lacerating injury such as circumcision'. 100 micrograms was as effective as 5 mg. Also 'breast feeding is a prerequisite of vitamin K deficient haemorrhagic disease'. The reason for this is the much lower content of the vitamin in breast milk compared to cow's milk mentioned above (Dam *et al.*, 1942). Sutherland and coworkers also recognized a second type of neonatal bleeding characterized by a normal coagulation mechanism, independent of vitamin K administration and frequent among breast fed infants. This group may correspond to the 'secondary' haemorrhagic disease of Aballi and de Laverens.

The role of dietary intake during the first days of life in the genesis of this disorder has recently been confirmed by Keenan *et al.* (1971). In healthy full term infants without bleeding the Quick's prothrombin time remained prolonged after 24 hours on sterile water or breast milk whereas it was shortened 24 hours after feeding with cow's milk or injection of vitamin K. With respect to the earlier theory that neonatal hypoprothrombinaemia was caused by lack of vitamin K synthesis by intestinal flora in the sterile gut of the newborn Keenan and colleagues comment that 'whatever the exact role of the enteric flora in the production of vitamin K by the human host the very rapid response of prothrombin activity within a few hours of the first feeding of sterilized cow's milk, probably before the milk could have much effect upon the enteric flora, supports the hypothesis that the dietary supply of vitamin K is of pre-eminent importance, at least in the first few days of extrauterine life'. They recommend the parenteral administration of 100 micrograms of vitamin K_1 to every newborn infant shortly after birth. This dose of the natural K_1 does not carry the risk of haemolysis seen with larger doses of the synthetic analogues yet will eliminate primary haemorrhagic disease. In this way it will also aid in the recognition of other causes of bleeding at this age, such as thrombocytopenia, intravascular coagulation or an inherited haemorrhagic state. This recommendation is also closely in line with that of the Committee on Nutrition of the American Academy of Pediatrics: 'A single parenteral dose of 0·5 to 1 mg or oral dose of 1·0 to 2·0 mg (of vitamin K_1) is probably adequate for prophylaxis'. Administration to the baby is recommended as being more certain of effect than administration to the mother. Oski and Naiman (1972) point out that deaths due to vitamin K deficiency in the newborn still occur and should be prevented by adoption of the Committee's recommendations. It would seem that this is more particularly true when the infant is being breast fed, which applies to a minority these days. The lack of agreement on the advisability of giving vitamin K prophylaxis (Craig, 1961; McElfresh, 1961) has partly arisen from failure to distinguish between the two types of haemorrhagic disease (*B.M.J.*, 1971) and also from the early experience of inducing haemolysis and jaundice by the use of doses of 10 mg or more of the water-soluble vitamin K analogues in premature infants (Allison, 1955; Sutherland, 1963).

INTRAPARTUM AND PERINATAL BLEEDING

Ahuja *et al.* (1969) made the point that the haemostatic challenge of vacuum extraction during delivery could result in massive subaponeurotic haemorrhage if the vitamin K dependent coagulation factors were low, viz. when the thrombotest was 10 per cent or less. Levels of 10 per cent or less are found in approximately one quarter of otherwise healthy newborn infants. A similar intrapartum haemostatic challenge exists with foetal blood sampling, and Hull (1972) has emphasized that when undue bleeding occurs after this procedure one should look to the coagulation status of the infant rather than to local factors such as the depth of the stab, which is probably irrelevant. In the absence of asphyxia the coagulation defect in such infants is more likely to be deficiency of the vitamin K dependent factors than DIC, especially in black infants in whom this 'early' form of haemorrhagic disease seems to be unduly common. Hull and Wilson (1972) reported one such black infant who bled excessively at birth from a scalp stab despite prolonged pressure over the area. After 3 hours the wound was sutured but by 18 hours a huge subaponeurotic haematoma had formed. At this time the haemoglobin had fallen to 8·7 g/100 ml and coagulation tests suggested severe primary haemorrhagic disease, with a Quick's prothrombin time of 110 seconds. The haemorrhage and the coagulation defect responded to vitamin K and blood transfusion. Hull (1972) points out that local pressure and not sutures should be used in such cases and that the early infusion of fresh frozen plasma, 10 ml/kg, might be used as advocated by Ahuja *et al.* (1969) on the basis that vitamin K alone acted too slowly to prevent serious and life-threatening haemorrhage.

MATERNAL DRUG INGESTION

Other causes of neonatal hypoprothrombinaemia include that secondary to maternal ingestion of oral anticoagulants, which can cause death *in utero* (Gordon and Dean, 1955). Fillmore and McDavitt (1970) reported 4 stillbirths among 36 mothers on oral anticoagulants. The maternal Quick's prothrombin time was in excess of 3 times normal in these 4 instances. They suggest that the outcome can be satisfactory if the maternal level is well controlled and there is no abnormal obstetric history and a normal delivery. Breast feeding when the mother is taking oral anticoagulants can also cause a haemorrhagic state in the baby. Eckstein and Jack (1970) recorded scrotal haematoma and retroperitoneal bleeding following a hernia operation at 4 weeks in one such baby.

Maternal ingestion of anticonvulsants can also cause bleeding in the infant. Mountain *et al.* (1970) reported 16 such neonates with severe deficiency of the prothrombin complex in 7 and with bleeding in 2. Evans *et al.* (1970) reported 5 further infants with bleeding and low vitamin K dependent clotting factors. Their mothers had taken 2 or more of the following drugs: phenytoin, primidone or phenobarbitone. In 2 instances the mothers had more than one affected baby.

DIAGNOSIS

Diagnosis of primary haemorrhagic disease of the newborn is facilitated by recognizing the relationship with breast feeding, the time of onset between 2 and 4 days of life in otherwise healthy infants and the typical sites of bleeding: gastrointestinal (melaena or haematemesis), nose, scalp, umbilicus skin puncture or circumcision site. When the only evidence of bleeding is fresh blood from the mouth or passed per rectum this must be distinguished from ingested maternal blood swallowed at delivery or later from a cracked nipple, by the following test for foetal haemoglobin:

The bloody stool is mixed with water to produce a pink solution containing haemoglobin. After centrifugation 5 ml of the supernatant fluid is mixed with 1 ml of 1 per cent sodium hydroxide solution. A brownish yellow colour indicates Hb A. With Hb F, indicating the infant's blood, the solution remains pink (Keay and Uttley, 1973).

If a haemorrhagic state is present the simplest way of determining whether or not there is a serious depletion of the vitamin K dependent coagulation factors is to perform a thrombotest estimation. This test was developed to measure the overall activity of the four Factors II, VII, IX and X for purposes of control of oral anticoagulant therapy in adults (Owren, 1959) and is ideally suited to measuring the same four factors in the newborn. A further very practical advantage is that the test can be performed on capillary blood, obtained from a heel stab. The test is performed at the cot side using a portable water bath, and result in percentage of normal activity is read off a graph within a matter of minutes of performing the heel stab. The 'P and P' test of Owren and Aas (1951) is an alternative to the thrombotest, measuring the combined activity of Factors II and VII, and also performed on capillary blood (Stuart et al., 1973). Both tests, however, need to be corrected for the high PCV (haematocrit) found in newborn babies (a correction graph is supplied with thrombotest reagent).

Additional tests that should always be performed when investigating a haemorrhagic state in an infant include a platelet count, haemoglobin estimation and blood film, all these tests of course also being performed on capillary blood. A normal platelet count is expected in primary haemorrhagic disease, even in premature babies. If below $100,000/mm^3$ and falling then intravascular coagulation and/or infection would be considered, as in the secondary type of haemorrhagic disease. More detailed coagulation investigations including measurement of FDPs, fibrinogen and, ideally, Factor V would be desirable. A haemoglobin estimation would clearly be helpful as a baseline to help in assessing the severity of occult blood loss and the possible need for transfusion, although it can take some hours to fall after blood loss. The blood film might show toxic granulations or neutropenia in septicaemia and excessive numbers of fragmented burr cells in disseminated intravascular coagulation. In primary haemorrhagic disease it would show only an increase in normoblasts and polychromasia as a response to acute blood loss. The remote possibility of an inherited coagulation defect such as haemophilia is more likely to be suspected from the family history than as a result of initial coagulation tests on the infant. All screening tests of the intrinsic pathway such as the PTT, TPST or kaolin clotting time give abnormal results in the first few weeks of life due to the low levels of Factors IX and X. Only by a specific assay for Factor VIII would an early diagnosis of haemophilia be possible. In this context it should be remembered that afibrinogenaemia and Factor XIII deficiency may also present as excessive bleeding from the cord, and could be diagnosed by specific assays.

TREATMENT

Treatment is by the parenteral administration of vitamin K_1 in a dose of 1–2 mg. This should preferably be given intravenously so as to avoid haematoma formation, especially if there are possible alternative diagnoses such as DIC or haemophilia not fully excluded at the time (Oski and Naiman, 1972). A rapid response to vitamin K with rise in thrombotest to haemostatic levels in 4 to 8 hours and cessation of bleeding is valuable confirmatory evidence of the original diagnosis. A failure to respond would suggest suppression of hepatocellular function, due to immaturity, sepsis or hypoxia, or that an alternative diagnosis should be considered, in particular, secondary haemorrhagic disease.

Transfusion of whole blood will be needed in infants where substantial blood loss has occurred. The plasma component is of value in addition to the red cells, as replacement therapy of the deficient factors. As Factors VII, IX and X are stable normally stored blood of a few days' age is still effective.

If there is a life-threatening haemorrhage such as the subaponeurotic scalp haematomas that can follow vacuum ('ventouse') extraction in infants with low prothrombin complex levels then rapid infusion of fresh frozen plasma, 10 ml/kg body weight, is recommended as well as vitamin K_1 (Ahuja et al., 1969). This will elevate the factors to a haemostatic level more rapidly than vitamin K alone. Without vitamin K, however, the effect of plasma would be short lived due to the short half-life of Factor VII (Fig. 18.11).

The 'P and P' test (measuring both Factors II and VII) is equally satisfactory for purposes of diagnosis and determining response to therapy, possessing much the same advantages in this respect as the thrombotest. Quick's prothrombin time may also be used but suffers from the defect that it is partly measuring two factors (V and fibrinogen) irrelevant to vitamin K deficiency, while not in any way affected by the Factor IX level which may be an important determinant of the severity of bleeding in this syndrome. All three of these tests would show a grossly abnormal result in primary haemorrhagic disease of the newborn e.g.

Thrombotest	at least < 10 per cent
P and P test	at least < 10 per cent
Quick's prothrombin time	at least > 60 seconds

A baby (b.wt. 3·58 kg) with haemorrhagic disease of the newborn (QMH PD No. 11252) presented with spontaneous bleeding from the gums at the age of 24 hr. The thrombotest was 5 per cent at 9.30 a.m. of its second day of life, 16 per cent at mid-day ($1\frac{1}{2}$ hr after 5 mg vit. K_1 plus 360 ml FFP), 21 per cent 4 hours later and 45 per cent the next morning. The platelet count remained normal throughout.

Vitamin K deficiency beyond the neonatal period

Following the neonatal depression of vitamin K dependent factors, with the nadir in the middle of the first week of life, there is a rise towards normal in the second week but adult levels may not be reached for weeks or even months (Aballi and de Lamerens, 1962A; Hartmann et al., 1956; McElfresh, 1961). The low levels of Factor IX that can be found in normal infants up to 3 months of age can cause difficulties in the early diagnosis of Christmas disease.

Nammacher et al. (1970) reported 4 full term infants aged 5 to 8 weeks with a haemorrhagic syndrome and coagulation changes similar to haemorrhagic disease of the newborn. Quick's prothrombin times were 53, 60, 73 and 119 seconds before vitamin K administration but normal after vitamin K. Factor II, IX and X levels in the 1 to 7 per cent range were recorded, but V was normal in the two cases tested. Platelet count was normal in all. Three of the four were breast fed. Haemorrhagic manifestations included purpura and suggestive evidence of intracranial haemorrhage in two. Decreased vitamin K intake or malabsorption and changes in intestinal flora secondary to antibiotic therapy were proposed as causes of this syndrome. Goldman and Deposito (1966) also reported 5 cases with similar coagulation changes and haemorrhage occurring between the ages of 10 days to 7 weeks. Similar cases have been described in association with antibiotic therapy (Lelong et al., 1964) or as a seasonal syndrome in Iraq associated with fever, vomiting, diarrhoea, anorexia and anaemia, but without antibiotic therapy (Taj-Eldin et al., 1967).

Diarrhoea alone (Matoth, 1950; Rapaport and Dodd, 1946) or associated with kwashiorkor (Merskey and Hansen, 1957) can produce a similar coagulation defect in infants and young children. This could well be due to disturbance of intestinal flora since it has been shown that at least water soluble vitamin K analogues can be absorbed from the colon in infants (Aballi et al., 1966). When poor intestinal synthesis is accompanied by poor dietary intake the resultant deficiency might be severe enough to produce a haemorrhagic state.

In older children the commonest cause of vitamin K deficiency is malabsorption due to coeliac disease, fibrocystic disease, chronic diarrhoea, biliary atresia or obstruction of the gastrointestinal tract (McMillan et al., 1972). Although the factors of the prothrombin complex may be lowered in these diseases they seldom give rise to spontaneous haemorrhage. If intestinal biopsy or liver puncture is being performed it would be wise to exclude such a deficiency by performing the thrombotest beforehand. Correction by parenteral vitamin K would be expected. Indeed the rapid correction of prothrombin complex by parenteral but not by oral vitamin K has been used as a means of distinguishing between obstructive jaundice and hepatocellular disease (Owren, 1949). In hepatocellular disease there is only a slow and partial response to vitamin K by either route.

Asparaginase administration, in the treatment of leukaemia, has been associated with multiple coagulation deficiencies, including low fibrinogen, V, VII, X, IX and plasminogen with elevated FDPs. The changes were attributed to defective synthesis plus limited DIC (Gralnick and Henderson, 1971). Two out of 13 patients developed haemorrhage or thrombosis.

Finally the possibility of accidental or deliberate ingestion of anticoagulant tablets belonging to a grandparent or parent should not be forgotten (Agle et al., 1970). Other drugs that antagonize vitamin K such as aspirin, tetracycline and sulphonamides are unlikely to depress the coagulation factors sufficiently to produce overt haemorrhage.

Hepatocellular disease

Not only the vitamin K dependent factors but also Factor V, fibrinogen, plasminogen and perhaps Factor VIII are all synthesized in the liver. This organ also probably clears circulating fibrinolytic

of acute haemorrhagic disorder due to hepatocellular disease is Reye's syndrome. This consists of acute encephalopathy and fatty degeneration of the liver of unknown aetiology. Although DIC was suspected a recent investigation by Schwartz (1971) showed low levels of Factors I (fibrinogen), II (prothrombin), V, VII, IX and X with normal FDPs, platelet count and Factor VIII. This pattern strongly suggested simple failure of synthesis of hepatic factors, without evidence of DIC. Rather similar results have recently been found at the Royal Hospital for Sick Children in Glasgow in two infants dying of acute hepatic failure; one with Reye's syndrome, the other with acute hepatitis (Table 19.4). Exchange transfusion with normal

Table 19.4   Coagulation data in Reye's syndrome and acute hepatic failure in young children

$1\frac{3}{4}$-year-old girl with Reye's syndrome			
Thrombotest	5 p.m.	33 per cent	
	10 a.m.	25 per cent	
	12 mid-day	11 per cent	
Platelets	220,000/mm³		
FDPs	50 μg/ml		
		Initial	Following plasma exchange
1-year-old boy with acute hepatic failure of unknown cause			
Thrombotest		7 per cent	31 per cent
Quick's prothrombin time (N = 14″)		>120″	19″
Two-stage prothrombin		0 per cent	74 per cent
Factor IX assay		13 per cent	42 per cent
Factor V assay		5·5 per cent	60 per cent
Fibrinogen		90 mg/100 ml	142 mg/100 ml
Plasminogen		0·66 cu/ml	3·2 cu/ml
FDPs		20 μg/ml	5 μg/ml

activator (von Kaulla, 1964; Fletcher et al., 1964) and coagulant substances (Deykin, 1966).

The Quick's prothrombin time and the TAMe esterase prothrombin assay have been shown to be excellent liver function tests for the detection and grading of severity of hepatic parenchymal damage in children (Glueck et al., 1970). It has been our impression that the same can be said for the thrombotest. When Factor V falls in addition to Factors II, VII, IX and X this is indicative of more severe, decompensated liver failure (Owren, 1949; Rapaport et al., 1960). Low fibrinogen has a similar significance. Dysfibrinogenaemia has been found in a patient with primary hepatoma (von Felten et al., 1969).

Although abnormal coagulation tests could be found in 85 per cent of patients with parenchymal liver disease in one series only 15 per cent had abnormal bleeding (Deutsch, 1965). In the paediatric context one of the most dramatic examples

plasma or infusion of prothrombin concentrates containing Factors II, VII, IX and X (Dike et al., 1972; Bruning and Loeliger, 1971; Tullis et al., 1965) are worthy of trial in such cases if control of haemorrhage is a major clinical problem. Both measures were employed in our second case with temporary benefit. A commercially available concentrate containing these factors is Konyne (Cutter).

Chronic hepatocellular disease such as cirrhosis is only rarely encountered in childhood. In a personally studied case due to Wilson's disease a complex disorder existed with (a) deficiency of the vitamin K dependent factors, (b) increased circulating activator, (c) moderate thrombocytopenia due to hypersplenism. In addition to replacement therapy for the prothrombin complex deficiency antifibrinolytic therapy with tranexamic acid was needed to achieve haemostasis firstly following dental extraction and later during abdominal surgery. Antifibrinolytic therapy with EACA in the management of cirrhotic bleeding was first described by Grossi et al. (1961, 1964).

Gilbert's syndrome (constitutional hepatic dysfunction) has been reported with low Factor VII (19 per cent), but normal prothrombin, IX and X. (Seligsohn et al., 1970). Similar changes were present in the Dubin-Johnson syndrome.

A more common situation in paediatric practice is the management of splenectomy and lienorenal anastomosis in children with portal hypertension and a variable degree of hepatic dysfunction. In addition to a trial of parenteral vitamin K for a few days beforehand, replacement therapy for any deficiency of coagulation factors is given immediately before operation and repeated as necessary in the postoperative period. A platelet concentrate is also infused immediately after the splenic pedicle has been clamped. No undue operative or postoperative bleeding has been encountered in such cases with this schedule.

Questionably related to concomitant liver damage is the Factor IX deficiency (5–28 per cent) with other factors normal reported in the nephrotic syndrome by Handley and Lawrence (1967). Factor IX was not detected in the urine of these patients. Paradoxically a high level of Factor VIII has been found in bad prognosis cases of glomerulonephritis (Ekberg and Nilsson, 1975). The origin of this Factor VIII may be vascular (Hoyer et al., 1974).

DISSEMINATED INTRAVASCULAR COAGULATION (DIC)

When blood clots *in vitro* the platelets, fibrinogen, Factors II (prothrombin), V and VIII are consumed, whereas Factors VII, IX, X, XI and XII are still present in the serum. Analogous changes in the circulating blood have been termed 'consumptive coagulopathy' (Rodriguez-Erdmann, 1965) and have widely been interpreted as indicating disseminated intravascular coagulation, with intravascular deposition of insoluble fibrin in the small blood vessels. It has also been assumed that the appearance of fibrin degradation products in the serum of such cases represented a fibrinolytic response by the body leading to dissolution of the deposited intravascular fibrin. Although it is convenient to retain the term DIC in our present state of knowledge it is becoming increasingly apparent that similar changes in the circulating clotting factors can occur with *localized* intravascular coagulation such as in giant haemangiomas, renal vein thrombosis or arterial aneurysms. 'DIC' may therefore not necessarily be disseminated. It is a reasonable proposition that the demonstration of rapidly falling platelet count, fibrinogen, Factor V and Factor VIII levels, and elevated FDPs, indicate *intravascular coagulation* (Merskey et al., 1964, 1967) but that whether this is *localized* or *disseminated* can only be judged by consideration of clinical or other evidence of multiple organ or tissue involvement.

In fact the fundamental coagulation processes involved in DIC are probably more complicated than implied above, and the following account is taken from the reviews of Deykin (1970) and the *Lancet* (1972) on the subject. *Simultaneous* activation of both the coagulant pathway *and* the fibrinolytic pathway can occur as a result of vascular damage by endotoxin, both being mediated through Factor XII (Ogston et al., 1969). This will result in the *simultaneous* production of both thrombin and plasmin, each of which attacks fibrinogen but with different products (Fig. 19.3).

The simultaneous production of fibrin monomer and the products of plasmin digestion of fibrinogen

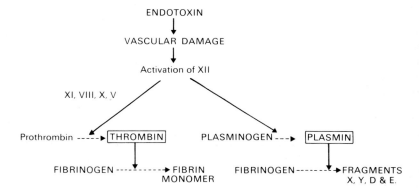

Fig. 19.3 Simultaneous activation of the coagulant and fibrinolytic pathway.

or fibrin (X, Y, D and E fragments) creates a complex situation where a number of possible alternative reactions exist for fibrin monomer in addition to the normal polymerization to form insoluble fibrin (Table 19.5).

The anticoagulant properties of the 'early' fragments X, and particularly Y, are thought to be due to their formation of complexes with fibrin monomer that are unclottable by thrombin (Marder

with latex particles coated with antifibrin antibody, and macroscopic agglutination recorded (Thrombo-Wellcotest; Wellcome Reagents, Ltd.), and the formal assay using tanned sheep red cells coated with fibrinogen (Merskey *et al.*, 1966). The reagents for this assay can also now be obtained commercially ('FDP Kit', Wellcome Reagents, Ltd). Similar results are found by the two methods (Thomas *et al.*, 1970).

Table 19.5 Possible reactions of fibrin monomer, normal and pathological

Fibrin monomer + Fibrin monomer	——→	Insoluble fibrin (normal product)
Fibrin monomer + Fragments X or Y	——→	Unclottable complexes ('FDPs', also antithrombin)
Fibrin monomer + Fragments D or E	——→	Defective fibrin (haemostatically defective)
Fibrin monomer + Fibrinogen	——→	Soluble complexes (clottable by thrombin)

*After Deykin (1970), by permission from New England J. Medicine, **283**, 636 (1970).*

and Shulman, 1969). They may also neutralize thrombin by adsorption and impair platelet function. Of the 'later' fragments D inhibits fibrin monomer polymerization while E appears to be a competitive inhibitor of the clotting action of thrombin on fibrinogen (Larrieu *et al.*, 1972). The effect of 'balanced' DIC with simultaneous production of thrombin and plasmin may be that *fibrinogen and other coagulation factors are consumed but no insoluble fibrin is necessarily formed.* This may explain the negative histological findings in some instances. It is envisaged that there is a variable balance between coagulation and fibrinolysis so that one or other may be predominant in different pathological situations. Fragments D or E will be incorporated into any fibrin that is laid down in their presence resulting in its abnormal ultrastructure and defective haemostatic function (Bang *et al.*, 1962).

Fibrin degradation products (FDPs)

Normal serum, treated with adequate thrombin, contains only traces $(1–2 \mu g/ml)$ of immunologically detectable material reacting with antifibrin antisera providing that *in vitro* fibrinolysis is prevented by collection into EACA or trasylol (Mersky *et al.*, 1966; Thomas *et al.*, 1970). A considerable correspondence has emphasized the importance of these precautions, especially when examining cord blood (Hathaway, 1970B; Ekert, 1970; Chessels and Pitney, 1970; Ekelund *et al.*, 1970; Karpatkin, 1970).

The most widely used assays are the rapid screening test where dilutions of serum are mixed

Typical figures are given in Table 19.6 from Sack and Buraschi (1971). Grossly elevated values (over $100 \mu g/ml$) are usual in consumptive coagulopathy (DIC) but moderate elevations occur in a number of other conditions including local thrombosis. In the paediatric context this includes renal vein thrombosis in infancy (Murphy and Willoughby, 1975). Elevated FDPs have also sometimes been found in normal newborn infants, or mildly ill infants without other evidence of DIC (Bonifaci *et al.*, 1968). Hathaway *et al.* (1969) confirmed this point finding $10–50 \mu g/ml$ in most of their infants with mild illness and no other evidence of DIC. Elevated FDPs are therefore suggestive but not diagnostic of DIC unless accompanied by other evidence such as a falling platelet count, fibrinogen or other consumable coagulation factors. This applies particularly to the newborn.

FDPs were originally thought to result from lysis of intravascularly deposited fibrin. It is clear, however, from the concept of simultaneous activation of coagulant and fibrinolytic pathways (Deykin, 1970) that they can represent fibrin monomer combined with fragments X or Y to form soluble unclottable complexes. Other smaller fragments such as D and E may similarly assay as FDPs (*Lancet*, 1972). None of the routine techniques distinguish between fibrinogen and fibrin degradation products although there is some hope that a specific assay for D-dimer may be indicative of lysis of fibrin that has been cross-linked by Factor XIII (Gaffney, 1972).

The specific assay for circulating fibrin monomer ('fibrin') in the plasma recently developed by

Table 19.6 Assay of FDP by the improved TRCHII

Group	No. of cases	TRCHII Assay*
Normal subjects	35	1·40 ± 0·20
Consumption coagulopathy	35	148·74 ± 48·94
Laennec's cirrhosis	29	82–41 ± 26·45
Cancer	39	70·70 ± 14·88
Recent myocardial infarction	23	27·26 ± 10·56
Peripheral vascular occlusions	10	42·90 ± 31·80
Pulmonary embolism	8	140·04 ± 80·27
CVA of thrombotic aetiology	13	88·24 ± 30·24†
CVA of haemorrhagic or embolic origin	10	18·58 ± 6·27†

*Mean ±SEM—results expressed in μg/ml.
†Significant (P < 0·05) by Cochran & Cox method for comparing means with unequal variances.
Reprinted, by permission, from The New England Journal of Medicine (1971), **284**, *1441.*

Kisker and Rush (1971) should in the future provide a far more certain index of intravascular coagulation than the conventional FDP level, and could also be useful for monitoring the progress of DIC and its response to therapy. Cryofibrinogen estimation and ethanol gelation tests are similarly thought to depend upon circulating fibrin monomer and to indicate intravascular fibrin formation (Breen and Tullis, 1969). Conventional FDP measurement are inevitably restricted to serum and may underestimate the circulating fibrin complexes (*Lancet*, 1972).

Diagnosis of DIC

Clinical features suggesting DIC include shock and generalized bleeding particularly from skin puncture sites. Accompanying the haemorrhage there may be thrombotic or ischaemic lesions affecting such tissues as the skin, kidney and brain resulting in a complex clinical picture. In many cases a known precipitating factor such as gram negative septicaemia may be present.

Serial haematological measurements are more informative than single determinations in making this diagnosis since it is the rapid and progressive fall of consumable coagulation components that is sought, and previous levels for instance of platelets or fibrinogen are not necessarily known (Deykin, 1970).

The characteristic features of consumptive coagulopathy are as follows:
1. Falling platelet count
2. Falling fibrinogen level and prolonged thrombin time
3. Elevated FDPs
4. Falling Factor V and sometimes Factor VIII
5. Low plasminogen.

Low Factor II also occurs in DIC but is not a specific finding since, being a vitamin K dependent factor it could be due to impaired hepatic synthesis.

Conversely fibrinogen and V can be low in severe hepatic failure. A falling Hb and fragmented 'burr' red cells may appear when partial occlusion of microvasculature by intravascular fibrin occurs (Baker *et al.*, 1968). Red cell fragmentation is not necessarily an *early* sign of DIC. Fragmented RBCs may not appear until 48 hours after the platelets and coagulation factors have fallen (Willoughby *et al.*, 1972A), presumably only *following* the deposition of intravascular fibrin.

Laboratory evidence of *consumptive coagulopathy* is indicative of the clinical state of intravascular coagulation, usually disseminated (i.e. DIC), but sometimes local (e.g. giant haemangioma or bilateral renal vein thrombosis). Although final confirmation of consumptive coagulopathy must rest upon specific assays of fibrinogen, Factors V and VIII, especially in the newborn (Hathaway *et al.*, 1969) an appropriately selected set of screening tests which can be performed rapidly on a capillary sample of blood can give practical guidance in the early recognition of DIC. At the Royal Hospital for Sick Children in Glasgow the following initial tests are performed:

1. Platelet count (Normal: 150,000–400,000/mm^3)
2. Thrombin time (Normal: 13 to 21 seconds)
3. Fibrinogen titre (Normal: 1/160)
4. TPST (Normal: min. substrate CT < 9 sec)
5. FDPs (Normal: up to 10 μg/ml)
6. Thrombotest (Normal: 50 to > 100 per cent).

These tests are performed upon 0·2 ml of capillary blood collected from a warmed finger or heel directly into 1·8 ml saline containing 0·1 per cent citrate as described by Dormandy and Hardisty (1961). PCV and Hb are also determined and a blood film made. After centrifugation of the citrated plasma (dilution approx. 1/20, depending upon the PCV) 0·2 ml is used for the TPST and 0·5 ml for preparing a series of dilutions for the

For research purposes it is ideal to measure the survival and turnover of platelets and fibrinogen (Brodsky et al., 1972; Harker and Slichter, 1972). This allows clear distinction between thrombocytopenia due to intravascular coagulation from that due to selective platelet sequestration (Fig. 19.4).

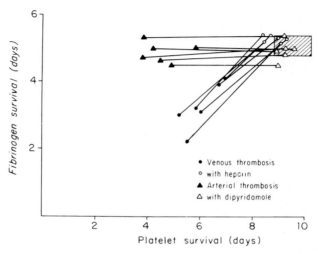

Fig. 19.4 Platelet and fibrinogen consumption *in vivo*. The effects of heparin and dipyridamole. In venous thrombosis, platelet and fibrinogen survival are shortened proportionately and corrected by heparin. In arterial thrombosis, it is only platelet survival that is shortened, reversed by dipyiridamole. The converse therapeutic corrections do not hold. (Reproduced from the *New England Journal of Medicine* (1972), **287**, 999, by permission of the authors Harker and Slichter).

fibrinogen titre. 0·1 ml of thrombin (50 units/ml) is added to each 0·5 ml of plasma dilution, and the thrombin time determined on the first tube. A normal control is tested in parallel.

The TPST may sometimes be spuriously short due to the presence of activated intermediate products such as Factor X if there has been a slow or imperfect collection of the capillary blood sample. The application of this technique to the investigation of coagulation defects in newborns is described by Stuart et al. (1973).

The thrombotest is of value since it is usually normal in DIC, Factor II being the only 'consumable' factor measured by this test. If the TPST is grossly abnormal when the thrombotest is close to normal there is a strong probability that Factor V or VIII are low, in the case of acquired coagulation disorders.

Where possible, it is desirable to collect venous blood (9 parts of blood + 1 part of 3·8 per cent Na citrate in a siliconized tube in melting ice) for separation of plasma aliquots (stored at −30° C) for subsequent confirmatory assay of fibrinogen, V and VIII.

General considerations

DIC is always secondary to an underlying disease process. Therapy of the primary condition is therefore of first importance, including administration of antibiotics, correction of acidosis, electrolyte imbalance and shock (Karpatkin, 1971). Before deciding upon therapy designed to intervene upon the process of DIC, usually heparin, one must consider: (a) Is the DIC endangering the patient by virtue of either progressive thrombosis or uncontrollable haemorrhage? (b) Is the DIC continuing or has it already ceased? (c) Has the patient a recoverable disease if protected from the consequences of DIC? These questions are not always easy to answer, but require consideration in each individual case. The decision to give heparin is made more difficult if there is a recent surgical or other wound that could give rise to serious haemorrhage.

Specific therapy for DIC

The primary object is to interrupt the generation of thrombin. It is generally agreed that heparin is the most active drug for this purpose and is the first choice in the treatment of DIC (Mersky et al., 1964; Abildgaard, 1969; Deykin, 1970; Karpatkin, 1971; McMillan et al., 1972). Oral anticoagulants such as warfarin are ineffective. Mosesson, Colman and Sherry (1968) showed in a case of chronic DIC that changing from heparin to warfarin was followed by a fall in fibrinogen and platelet count, and that these were brought back to normal by giving heparin. Antifibrinolytic drugs are contraindicated since these could upset the balance between coagulation and fibrinolysis leading to widespread intravascular deposition of fibrin (Deykin, 1970). Indeed, there is currently greater interest in the possible use of fibrinolytic agents such as urokinase or streptokinase when there is thought to be actual fibrin deposition (Monnens, 1973).

Replacement therapy of the depleted fibrinogen, Factor V, VIII or platelets is seldom necessary since the rate of synthesis or formation is usually adequate, the platelet count being capable of rising 30,000/mm^3 per day when consumption is halted. In any event it should not be given until after adequate heparinization. For instance, Winkelstein et al. (1969) have pointed out that Dextran is safer than plasma in the treatment of shock in meningococcal septicaemia when DIC is suspected.

Corticosteroid therapy has been thought to be inadvisable in the presence of DIC since Thomas and Good (1952) found enhancement of the Shwartzman reaction by cortisone in rabbits. Later workers, however, have failed to confirm this effect (Corrigan et al., 1967). Corticosteroids (e.g. IV hydrocortisone) should probably therefore not be withheld when the underlying condition or concomitant shock would benefit, particularly if the intravascular clotting is blocked by prior or simultaneous administration of heparin (Abildgaard, 1969; Karpatkin, 1971).

Exchange transfusion with citrated whole blood has been successfully employed in the treatment of infants with presumed DIC by Gross and Melhorn (1971). The idea of 'washing out' the circulating products of coagulation and fibrinolysis is certainly commendable. Others have used fresh heparinized blood in this way.

HEPARIN THERAPY

Heparin has been well established for many years as a potent antagonist to thrombin, this effect requiring the presence of plasma heparin cofactor or antithrombin III. More recently it has been recognized that even at low plasma levels heparin has an additional anticoagulant effect brought about by stimulating the inhibition of activated Factor X (Xa) by the natural plasma Factor Xa inhibitor (Biggs et al., 1970). The two heparin cofactors antithrombin III and Factor Xa inhibitor may be identical (Yin et al., 1971). Inhibition at this point lies at the junction of the intrinsic and extrinsic arms of the coagulation system (Fig. 18.4). Heparin may therefore inhibit the *formation* of thrombin as well as blocking its reaction with fibrin. This could be relevant to its use in DIC since thrombin, once formed has multiple activities including aggregation of platelets and activation of Factor XIII (fibrin stabilizing factor) as well as being 'autocatalytic' by virtue of its stimulation of earlier steps of the coagulation cascade.

It has been claimed that heparin, injected *in vivo*, reduces platelet adhesiveness (Negus et al., 1971) and response to collagen (Rowsell et al., 1967) but this has not been confirmed by others. The question of whether heparin exerts a direct effect upon the platelet membrane and function is currently *sub judice* and the subject of much debate (O'Brien et al., 1972A; Eika, 1972; O'Brien et al., 1972B; de Gaetano and Vermylen, 1972). The most provocative claim is that heparin plus Factor Xa inhibitor form a potent anti-platelet inhibitor (Yin et al., 1973A).

There is no firm evidence that heparin enhances fibrinolysis *per se* but Kakkar et al. (1972) have pointed out that fibrin laid down at a time of thrombin inhibition may be less tightly cross-linked since thrombin is necessary for Factor XIII activity. Such clots will be more susceptible to normal fibrinolysis.

The dose of heparin required to produce a given degree of anticoagulation will depend upon a number of factors which are liable to vary during an episode of intravascular coagulation. These include levels of heparin cofactors (antithrombin II or III) (Abildgaard, 1968) and Factor Xa inhibitor (Yin et al., 1971), platelet factor 4 (heparin neutralizing activity) (Gérard et al., 1973), rate of renal excretion (Karpatkin, 1971) and most probably the rate of thrombin formation and Factor X activation.

CONTROL AND DOSAGE OF HEPARIN

The whole blood clotting time or the thrombin time have conventionally been used to monitor the level of anticoagulation during heparin therapy (Margolius et al., 1961). When performed on fresh platelet-free plasma great sensitivity is attainable (Eika et al., 1972). In recent years the Kaolin-activated PTT (Fig. 19.5) of Proctor and

Rapaport (1961) has gained widespread favour for the purpose of controlling heparin therapy in the treatment or prophylaxis of thrombosis (Estes, 1970; Stuart and Michel, 1971; Deykin, 1972;

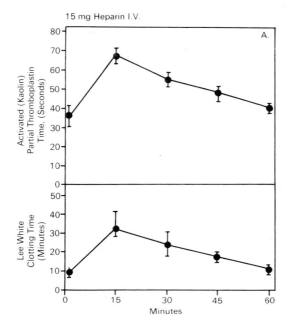

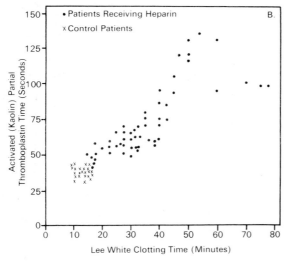

Fig. 19.5 Relationship between activated partial thromboplastin time and Lee and White clotting time for heparin control. A, Mean and range of activated PTT and L-W coagulation time obtained serially during heparin tolerance tests in four patients. B, Overall comparison of activated PTT and L-W coagulation time in 78 patients (23 normal and 55 receiving heparin). (Reproduced from the *Journal of the American Medical Association* (1967), **201**, 157, by permission of the authors Spector and Corn).

Lancet, 1972). First proposed for this purpose by Spector and Corn (1967) because of greater precision and reproducibility a prospective study by Basu *et al.* (1972) showed that their patients who developed a recurrent thrombosis had been allowed to fall below the suggested therapeutic range of $1\frac{1}{2}$ to $2\frac{1}{2}$ the normal APTT (normal 39–41 seconds, therapeutic range 60–100 seconds). Keeping within this therapeutic range did not unfortunately prevent a number of haemorrhagic incidents. A disadvantage in the use of APPT or thrombin time for control of heparin in DIC is that both are liable to give abnormal pretherapy 'base-line' results due to the underlying coagulation disorder. A practical difficulty in young children is that both tests require venous blood.

Great sensitivity, with detection of 0·01 units/ml of heparin or less, has been achieved with a recently described assay based upon the specific enhancement of Factor Xa inhibition described above (Yin *et al.*, 1973B). This would appear ideal for monitoring treatment of DIC but is probably too complex for widespread availability. It is apparently capable of showing the effects of small doses of heparin undetected by the APTT (Kakkar *et al.*, 1972) (Fig. 19.6).

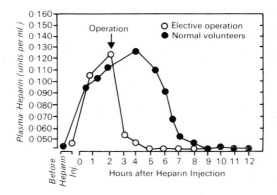

Fig. 19.6 Typical circulating plasma-heparin levels, by specific assay, after administration of 5000 units of heparin (s.c.) to healthy volunteers and patients having major elective operations. (Reproduced from *Lancet* (1972), **2**, 101, from a paper by Kakkar *et al.* by permission of the authors).

Unless this sophisticated assay is available the whole blood clotting time, and in particular the capillary method, is probably adequate to prevent serious over-heparinization. The particular advantage in children is that separate repeated venepunctures are unnecessary. The test is performed from a finger or heel stab as often as clinically indicated and the answer is obtained at the bedside using a portable water bath. The normal clotting time by this method is $2\frac{3}{4} \pm \frac{1}{4}$ minute and has not been found to be increased in the presence of untreated DIC. On heparin doses of 25 to 35 units/kg/hour capillary clotting times of 4 to 7 minutes are attained. Heparinization producing clotting times of this order have accompanied apparent reversal of DIC without overt haemorrhage (Willoughby *et al.*, 1972A and 1972B). Ekert and Seshadri (1973) found that an average initial dose of approximately 30 units/kg/hr prolonged the PTT to $1\frac{1}{2}$–$2\frac{1}{2}$ times normal in children with HUS. In patients with overt DIC a similar initial dose was needed to shorten the PTT. This could then be maintained in the normal range by 25 units/kg/hr.

The optimum dose of heparin or degree of anticoagulation for the treatment of DIC is not certainly known. In practice it is partly determined by the clinical and haematological response, especially looking for a rising platelet count, and terminating the heparin when both clinical and coagulation findings suggest that DIC has ceased.

A widely quoted dosage schedule for children is 100 units/kg given by IV 'bolus' every 4 hours. This was the dose originally shown by Abildgaard *et al.* in 1967 to be effective in a case of meningo-coccal septicaemia with DIC. Excretion of intra-venously administered heparin is usually complete by 4–6 hours, providing renal function is normal (Karpatkin, 1971). It would seem more logical to aim at a constant level of anticoagulation by continuous infusion, e.g. at 25 units/kg/hour, thereby avoiding the 'peaks of dangerously high heparin levels and the 'troughs' of inadequate or non-existent heparinization'. This will also allow control of the degree of heparinization in a way that is impossible with intermittent therapy. Although continuous infusion is widely recommended in both DIC (McMillan *et al.*, 1972) and venous thrombosis (Basu *et al.*, 1972; Gieske, 1972) no controlled trial had actually been undertaken to compare it with intermittent IV doses. Now Salzman *et al.* (1975) have reported one such trial, just completed, which showed that major bleeding was seven times more frequent with intermittent than with continuous infusion, yet was no more effective for prevention of thromboembolism. The intramuscular route, whether for heparin or other drugs, is contraindicated since these patients usually have both thrombocytopenia and a systemic coagulation defect.

The degree of anticoagulation that should be aimed at is somewhat uncertain. An increase in the whole blood (Lee and White) clotting time to between 2 and 3 times the normal of 8–10 minutes is recommended by some authors, Karpatkin (1971) favouring the higher value of 30 min, in order to arrest the coagulopathy with certainty. It has been my experience, however, that reversal of the changes of DIC can occur with more modest prolongation of the capillary clotting time from the pretherapy level of $2\frac{3}{4}$ minutes up to the 4 minutes or so that is commonly attained at a dose of 25 units/kg/hr. Good results with clinical and haematological evidence of resolution of DIC have also been obtained by Gérard *et al.* (1973) in children with meningococcal purpura given even lower doses of heparin. In order to relate the dose to the antiheparin activity of the circulating platelets they used the formula:

$$\text{Daily dose in units/kg} = \frac{\text{Platelet count per mm}^3}{500}$$

e.g. if platelet count 60,000 dose equals 120 units kg/day or 5 units/kg/hr.

This dose would produce a negligible or un-detectable change in monitoring tests such as the whole blood clotting time or APTT, being of the same daily magnitude as the micro-doses of heparin currently proving effective in the prevention of postoperative thrombosis and pulmonary embolism (Kakkar *et al.*, 1972; Lahnborg *et al.*, 1974). The dose of 5,000 units SC b.d. given to adults in these trials corresponds to an average dose of approxi-mately 6 units/kg/hr. One cannot extrapolate from the prevention of deep vein thrombosis and embolism to the correction of DIC, but the value of smaller and safer doses of heparin warrants further exploration.

Recommended heparin therapy for DIC in the present state of knowledge is:

100 units/kg IV stat. followed by

25 units/kg/hr by continuous IV infusion

adjusting the dose at 12 or 24 hr intervals so as to keep the capillary clotting time 1 to 2 minutes longer than pretreatment result (i.e. 4 to 5 minutes compared with about 3 minutes pretreatment).

The heparin is dissolved in $\frac{1}{2}$ strength saline or similar electrolyte solution and the volume infused per hour determined from considerations of the required fluid intake.

DIC in the neonatal period

Aballi and de Lamerens (1962A and B) first used the term 'secondary haemorrhagic disease of the newborn' to describe the haemorrhagic state that occurs in 'sick' premature infants often with evidence of hypoxia at birth, respiratory distress, acidosis, infection or hypothermia. Coagulation investigations showed low factor V and platelets in addition to the usual depletion of vitamin K dependent factors. The response to vitamin K was poor and there is little doubt that many of these infants would have shown evidence of DIC by current techniques. Of 25 such infants 14 had pulmonary haemorrhage and 12 CNS bleeding including 10 intraventricular. All had received vitamin K and all but one died. This contrasts with primary haemorrhagic disease which typically occurs in otherwise healthy term infants not given vitamin K.

More recently, Boyd (1967) found histological evidence of intravascular fibrin deposition in infants dying within 48 hours, and Hathaway et al. (1969) reported coagulation data suggestive of DIC in 11 of 19 sick newborn infants. Of the affected infants 1 had disseminated herpes simplex, 1 cytomegalovirus infection, 1 rubella syndrome and the remainder had severe respiratory distress syndrome (RDS, hyaline membrane disease) or were born to mothers with toxaemia of pregnancy or abruptio placentae. Most were of low birth weight. In 5 of the 7 fatal cases microthrombi were found. Chessells and Wigglesworth (1970) reported clinical, laboratory and autopsy findings in 5 newborn infants who died with a haemorrhagic state developing within 24 hours of birth. Four were premature, 3 had birth asphyxia, 3 became hypothermic and 2 had Rhesus disease. Low platelet counts (32,000 to 131,000/mm³), low fibrinogen (112 to 163 mg/100 ml), low Factor V (5 and 28 per cent) and prolonged thrombin times together with variable levels of FDPs and Factor VIII were found among these infants, suggestive of DIC. The thrombotest was also low, but this test largely reflects the vitamin K dependent factors commonly diminished in the newborn. Autopsy showed thick subarachnoid clot in all, with intravascular fibrin deposition in 4 of the 5 infants. A possible role of DIC in the genesis of intraventricular haemorrhage, seen in premature infants is suggested by the finding of Towbin (1968) that this is frequently secondary to subependymal venous infarcts.

From these and other reports it is clear that multiple factors are concerned in the genesis of this syndrome, including the following:

Prematurity. Gestational age alone does not account for the haemorrhagic state. Corrigan and Sell (1971) compared the coagulation changes in 93 sick newborns with 106 age-matched controls. Consumption of Factors II, V, VIII and fibrinogen with or without thrombocytopenia occurred only in the sick infants although the lower the gestational age the lower the vitamin K dependent factors and Factor XIII with a similar trend in Factor VIII. A recent account of the development of haemostasis and coagulation in relation to gestation is that of Bleyer et al. (1971).

Asphyxia and acidosis. Skyberg and Jacobsen (1969) have described a newborn with severe birth asphyxia developing coagulation evidence of DIC and successfully treated by exchange transfusion with fresh heparinized blood, and in Case 2 of Berglund (1970) intrauterine anoxia was the probable cause of similar coagulation changes. Coagulation studies on 9 severely asphyxiated newborns by Chessells and Wigglesworth (1971A) showed low fibrinogen, elevated FDPs and low or rising platelet count. Two of these 3 died and showed fibrin emboli in the liver and adrenals. Table 19.7 shows coagulation findings in two infants personally observed who suffered severe pure asphyxia during birth. Hardaway et al. (1964) suggested that acidosis, which accompanies hypoxia, accelerates coagulation. Gaynor et al. (1968) suggested that anoxic damage to small blood vessels predisposed to fibrin deposition.

Hypothermia. Among the 9 infants with asphyxia studied by Chessells and Wigglesworth only 4, including the 3 with evidence of DIC, had experienced a fall in body temperature to 34° C. Having previously noted an association of hypothermia with 'secondary haemorrhagic disease' these authors have suggested (1971A) that acidosis and hypothermia may have a synergistic action in causing DIC.

Infection. As in other age groups septicaemia, especially with gram negative organisms, is a potent cause of DIC (Corrigan et al., 1968). An example of *Coliform* septicaemia causing generalized purpura with both haematological and pathological evidence of DIC is shown in Fig. 19.7. Whaun et al (1971) found gram negative sepsis to be the commonest cause of DIC in the newborn.

Viraemic infections, including disseminated herpes simplex (Miller et al., 1970), cytomegalovirus and rubella syndrome (Hathaway et al., 1969), have also produced DIC in the newborn.

Severe Rhesus disease. Haemorrhagic manifestations occurred after exchange transfusion in 4 out of 502 Rhesus affected infants in a survey by Panagopoulos et al. (1969), and this was usually related to transient thrombocytopenia. Any deficiency of vitamin K dependent coagulation factors at birth will temporarily be corrected by the exchange transfusion. It is probably only the most severely affected infants that are at risk of bleeding

COAGULATION DISORDERS. 2. ACQUIRED   351

Table 19.7 Examples of consumptive coagulopathy in the neonatal period

1. Severe birth asphyxia due to prolapsed cord
   Bleeding into eye and subdural haemorrhage. Survived mentally retarded. At 24 hr and following 50 ml FFP because of low thrombotest (7 per cent) at birth:

Platelets	62,000/mm³
Thrombotest	< 5 per cent
Fibrinogen	70 mg/100 ml
Plasminogen	< 1·0 cu/ml
Factor V	2 per cent of normal
Factor VIII	135 per cent of normal
FDPs	80 µg/ml

2. Severe birth asphyxia due to precipitate labour with simultaneous delivery of baby and placenta
   Baby died.   No P.M.   At 12 hr:

Platelets	88,000/mm³
Thrombotest	13·5 per cent
Fibrinogen	70 mg/100 ml
Plasminogen	0·3 cu/ml
Factor V	4 per cent of normal
Factor VIII	100 per cent of normal
FDPs	160 µg/ml

3. Hypothermia in a 34-week premature infant with oesophageal atresia. 33° C recorded at age of 13½ hr
   At age of 1½ days:

Platelets	17,000/mm³
Thrombotest	17 per cent
Fibrinogen	96 mg/100 ml
Plasminogen	1·1 cu/ml
Factor V	10 per cent of normal
Factor VIII	26 per cent of normal
FDPs	20 µg/ml

(Diamond et al., 1952). Nevertheless, Chessells and Wigglesworth (1971B) point out that haemorrhage still constitutes a major finding among fatal cases. This was most commonly intracranial, but was often accompanied by bleeding into the lungs or oozing from umbilicus and injection sites. In 4 cases with cord blood Hb levels of 3–5 g/100 ml there was laboratory evidence (thrombocytopenia, low fibrinogen levels, abnormal TPST and elevated FDPs) suggestive of DIC, and in 9 out of 17 fatal cases intravascular fibrin was found at autopsy. It is clear most were excessively severe cases and that problems associated with prematurity and very low K dependent factors played a part in others. Hathaway (1970A) reported detailed coagulation results on two hydropic Rhesus affected babies. Platelet counts of 37,800 and 45,000/mm³ were accompanied by Factor V levels of 24 and 33 per cent, fibrinogen of 231 and 159 mg/100 ml and FDPs of 20 and 15 µg/ml. Because the Factor VIII levels were normal (120 and 80 per cent) he favoured impaired hepatic synthesis and increased fibrinolysis rather than DIC in these infants. Equally one could argue that Factor VIII is less sensitive to depletion in DIC compared to Factor V and fibrinogen. Low platelet counts in severe Rhesus disease may perhaps have an immunological basis before exchange transfusion, while they are to be expected following exchange because of the paucity of platelets in the transfused blood.

RESPIRATORY DISTRESS SYNDROME (RDS, HYALINE MEMBRANE DISEASE)

Because the pulmonary hyaline membrane consists of fibrin there have been extensive studies of the fibrinolytic system (Ambrus et al., 1963; Ambrus et al., 1965; von Kualla et al., 1965) and of fibrinogen turnover rate (Karitzky et al., 1971) in premature infants with or without RDS, and in normal infants (Beller et al., 1966) and foetuses (Ekelund et al., 1970). A shortened half-life of circulating ^{125}I fibrinogen occurs in premature infants, particularly those with RDS, with accumulation of radioactivity over the lungs during the first day of life (Karitzky et al., 1971). Plasma plasminogen levels are low in all newborns, as compared to adults (Phillips and Skrodelis, 1958); lower in healthy prematures and lowest in prematures with RDS (Ambrus et al., 1963). The premature infant therefore has a lower fibrinolytic potential should the physiological need arise, and is less able to achieve lysis of fibrin whether deposited in the alveoli or intravascularly. Encouraging results have been obtained by the infusion of plasminogen (7·5 RPMI units) in the prevention of RDS (Ambrus *et al.*, 1974). In a placebo group 5 out of 51 infants (b.wt. 1–2·5 kg) died with hyaline membrane disease, compared to 0 out of 49 given plasminogen. There was also a lower incidence of clinical RDS.

The hypothesis that DIC was the underlying cause of RDS was proposed by Stark *et al.* in 1968. They described one such infant, delivered by Caesarean section for abruptio placentae, with low fibrinogen, prothrombin and Factor V levels who appeared to benefit from heparin therapy. RDS was also present in many of the infants with laboratory or pathological evidence of *intravascular* fibrin deposition reported by Hathaway *et al.* (1969). Detailed investigations by Markarian and colleagues (1971A) showed that a state of hypercoagulability, as shown by thromboelastograph tracings, was common in RDS and was associated with decreased fibrinolytic activity and lowered median levels of Factors V and VIII, particularly in those infants who died with haemorrhage. Massive thrombosis following umbilical artery catheterization has also been described in RDS (Du *et al.*, 1970), perhaps related to this hypercoagulable state. A controlled trial of the prophylactic use of heparin in low birth weight infants (Markarian *et al.*, 1971B) showed no influence on the incidence of hyaline membranes at autopsy, but there was a reduction in mortality and of severe CNS haemorrhage in the treated group (excluding moribund infants and those under 1 kg). The relevance of DIC to RDS may perhaps best be summarized by the finding in the recent prospective study of Margolis *et al.* (1973). Only two out of 11 infants showed definite evidence of DIC, with low platelets *or* fibrinogen, and low Factors V and VIII. Both these infants were born after abruptio placentae. Three others died and their autopsies failed to show disseminated fibrin emboli although all three had extensive atelectasis and hyaline membranes, and 2 had intracranial haemorrhages. This haemorrhagic complication can therefore occur without DIC.

The conclusion appears to be that DIC is not a consistent finding in RDS, although it is a frequent consequence of one of the main precipitating causes of RDS, viz. neonatal asphyxia in premature infants, a particular cause of which is abruptio placentae. Heparin therapy may be of value in this

minority of infants who develop DIC, but not in the majority either for prophylaxis or therapy. It is also unlikely that heparin therapy would prevent intracranial haemorrhage in RDS. For a general discussion of the different types of neonatal intracranial haemorrhage, and some of the non-haematological factors in their pathogenesis, the reader is referred to a recent Editorial by Volpe (1974).

MATERNAL AND INTRAUTERINE CAUSES OF NEONATAL DIC

The association of DIC or 'defibrination syndrome' in the infant born after maternal abruptio placentae was specifically documented by Edson *et al.* (1968). Other examples are included in the reports of Hathaway *et al.* (1969), and Margolis *et al.* (1973). The common factor is probably foetal asphyxia. Toxaemia of pregnancy has similarly been associated with the coagulation changes of DIC, the infant showing temporary improvement after exchange transfusion with heparinized blood (Leissring and Vorlicky, 1968). Prenatal infection has already been mentioned. Maternal diabetes (Hathaway, 1970C), dead twin foetus syndrome (Moore *et al.*, 1969) and perhaps liberation of thromboplastin from placental infarction in a postmature infant (Markarian *et al.*, 1971C) have been associated with the changes of DIC, the last case showing a response in coagulation changes and survival after heparin (50 units/kg every 3 hours for $2\frac{1}{2}$ days, then 50 units/kg every 6 hours for a further 2 days). The authors state that 'within an hour after the heparin was started, the oozing of the blood from the cord ceased'.

In conclusion, DIC in the newborn is commonly precipitated by anoxia or infection, particularly in the premature infant. These factors occur in a wide range of clinical circumstances, including RDS, placental abruption and severe Rhesus disease. Associated features may be acidosis and hypothermia. When haemorrhagic symptoms are prominent this syndrome is conveniently termed secondary haemorrhagic disease of the newborn in contrast to the primary form due to vitamin K deficiency in full term infants.

Causes of intravascular coagulation beyond the newborn period

RENAL VEIN THROMBOSIS AND HYPERTONIC DEHYDRATION

This condition arises in young infants usually in the first 4 weeks of life. The precipitating factor seems most commonly to be hypertonic (hyperosmolar or hypernatraemic) dehydration, usually due to intestinal or other infection. Another association is with cyanotic heart disease and angiocardiography. Presenting features are oliguria, haematuria and palpable renal swelling, usually bilateral. In a recent review of 113 cases the mortality was 66 per cent (Arneil *et al.*, 1973). It is well recognized that bilateral renal vein thrombosis is a cause of thrombocytopenia in infancy but only more recently has the association with consumptive coagulopathy (Renfield and Kraybill, 1973), MAHA and raised FDPs (Arneil *et al.*, 1973) been reported. Haematological data in 7 infants we have seen with renal vein thrombosis are shown in Table 19.8.

Although the coagulation changes are the same as in DIC it is clear that in many of these infants it is *local* rather than *disseminated* intravascular coagulation.

GIANT HAEMANGIOMA (KASABACH-MERRITT SYNDROME)

This is another form of localized intravascular consumption of platelets and coagulation factors that can occur in the neonatal period, or in later life. The clinical diagnosis is immediately apparent unless the haemangioma is confined to an internal viscera such as the spleen or liver.

The syndrome was originally described by Kasabach and Merritt (1940) in a 2-month-old

Table 19.8   Haematological data on 7 infants with renal vein thrombosis

	Throm-bosis	Age weeks	Platelets mm^3	Fibrino-gen mg/100 ml	FDPs μg/ml	Factor V per cent	Factor VIII per cent	Plasmino-gen cu/ml	Hb g/100 ml	Burr cells
F.F.	Bilateral	7	4,000	30	300	3	20	0·5	20·8 → 9·4	+
D.B.	Bilateral	28	10,000	42	160	15	250	1·6	10·8 → 5·4	+
C.C.	Right	1½	24,000	(128)★	160	(130	110	1·4)★	23·6 →19·6	—
M.D.	Bilateral	29	46,000	124	40	240	90	3·0	13·0 →10·8	+
H.McN.	Right	2	83,000	100	20	35	62	2·0	16·2 → 9·8	+
L.C.	Bilateral	1½	60,000	142	40	190	100	1·3	16·8 →14·2	—
J.W.	Right	2	195,000	230	20	48	170	1·3	19·0 →13·0	—
	Normal values		>150,000	>200	<20	50–200	50–200	>2·0	10–15	—

★Assayed only after heparin therapy. Screening tests suggested more marked coagulation defect prior to heparin. From Murphy and Willoughby (1976).

Heparin, rather than nephrectomy, is now recommended initial therapy (Touloukian, 1969), especially in the presence of thrombocytopenia or consumption of coagulation factors (Arneil *et al.*, 1973; Renfield and Kraybill, 1973). We have seen a striking improvement in survival rate since adopting the policy of giving heparin 100 units/ kg stat., followed by a continuous infusion of 25 units/kg/hour and adjusting the dose daily so as to maintain an increase in the capillary clotting time from 2½–2¾ minutes to 4–5 minutes. This is started as soon as the diagnosis is made and is continued until the platelets are rising and renal function improving.

Similar coagulation changes and MAHA are found in a proportion of infants with hypertonic dehydration without overt renal vein thrombosis (Murphy and Willoughby, 1976). We interpret this as indicating that these two clinical conditions are part of a continuous spectrum that may or may not progress to actual thrombosis. On this basis it is our policy to give a continuous heparin infusion in such infants showing thrombocytopenia, elevated FDPs and consumption of coagulation factors.

infant with extensive haemangioma of the thigh with thrombocytopenia and a haemorrhagic diathesis. More recent investigations have shown associated depletion of fibrinogen, Factor V and VIII with reversal after heparin therapy (Blix and Aas, 1961; Hillman and Phillips, 1967; Verstraete *et al.*, 1965). Platelets labelled with ^{51}Cr have been shown to be sequestrated in the haemangioma (Brizel and Raccuglia, 1965) and ^{131}I-fibrinogen to have a reduced half-life with retention in the tumour (Thatcher *et al.*, 1968). Elevated FDPs were also found. All the coagulation abnormalities return to normal after heparin (Wochner *et al.*, 1967), surgical removal or irradiation of the haemangioma (Thatcher *et al.*, 1968). Burr cells are present in some cases (Brizel and Raccuglia, 1965). Decrease in size of the tumour, probably due to thrombosis, followed the use of the fibrinolytic inhibitor EACA in one patient (Henriksson *et al.*, 1971). This therapy was only justified by the fact that the intravascular coagulation and reactive fibrinolysis were local rather than disseminated. The successful use of prednisone, which may act primarily on the vasculature, has been reported

354 PAEDIATRIC HAEMATOLOGY

by Frost and Esterly (1968); and the successful use of local irradiation by Duncan and Halnan (1964).

I have encountered one such patient who only showed thrombocytopenia, MAHA and elevated FDPs when her haemangioama was infected, and not at other times. I have seen a convincing response to prednisolone in another case.

CONGENITAL HEART DISEASE (CHD)

Cyanotic congenital heart disease with secondary polycythaemia predisposes both to thrombosis and also to a haemorrhagic state after corrective surgery (Kontras et al., 1966; Naiman, 1970). Since thrombocytopenia is common in such children it is an attractive hypothesis to attribute these manifestations to DIC. This received support from the report of Dennis et al. (1967) in which the pattern of consumptive coagulopathy was found in 5 children with cyanotic congenital heart disease and a haemorrhagic diathesis. Heparin appeared beneficial, raising the Factor V from 1 to 80 per cent and the Factor VIII from 10 to 70 per cent in a case of transposition of the great vessels. Similar but less spectacular changes occurred in the other cases. The platelet count rose in all and FDPs disappeared in the 3 who were tested. Nevertheless, the results of this study must partly be discounted on a point of technique. These workers used the standard ratio of 1 part of 3·8 per cent citrate to 9 parts of blood without regard to the fact that the high haematocrit would then result in an excess of citrate, which grossly distorts the results of one-stage coagulation tests such as the Quick's prothrombin time, PTT or certain assays (Naiman, 1970). Subsequent workers have adjusted the volume of added citrate by using the following or a similar formula:

Volume of blood added to

0·25 ml of 3·8 per cent trisodium citrate

$$= 2 \cdot 25 \text{ ml} \times \frac{100 - \text{Normal PCV}}{100 - \text{Patient's PCV}}$$

(Ihenacho et al., 1973),

the 'normal' PCV in infants beyond the first month of age being taken as 38 per cent.

Subsequent investigations using the above precautions have produced conflicting results. Komp and Sparrow (1970) found moderately decreased levels of platelets, Factor V, Factor VIII and fibrinogen, and the presence of cryofibrinogen and FDPs in cyanotic congenital heart disease where the PCV was over 50 per cent, but not when it was below this level. These results, however, showed only a statistical trend within the group, with many of the individual values still in the normal range. From their data it cannot be seen that any single patient showed the full pattern of consumptive coagulopathy. Much the same can be said of the more recent study by Ihenacho et al. (1973) from Birmingham. The mean platelet count was 201,400/mm³ and Factor V 85 per cent in 55 children with cyanotic CHD. Both these reports showed that the thrombocytopenia and coagulation abnormalities occurred in cyanotic rather than acyanotic CHD. Both groups of workers interpreted their results to indicate low-grade chronic intravascular coagulation or consumption of platelets and coagulation factors in at least some of the cyanotic and polycythaemic patients. Ihenacho et al. (1973) found a rise in factor levels following venesection in 2 patients and heparinization in 4 out of 5 patients (25–40 units/kg/hr by continuous IV infusion). They suggest that in cyanotic CHD the pulmonary microvasculature may possibly be the major area of localized intravascular coagulation, and that other factors such as liver cell hypoxia and the marrow reserve will determine the day-to-day balance between production and consumption as reflected by plasma levels and platelet count. This point is probably relevant to DIC in other clinical situations.

By contrast a number of other investigations have failed to show evidence of DIC in cyanotic CHD (Johnson et al., 1968; Ekert and Gilchrist, 1968; Iolster, 1970: Ekert et al., 1970; Maurer et al., 1972). Johnson, Abildgaard and Schulman (1968) investigated 10 children with cyanotic CHD and thrombocytopenia (30,000 to 135,000/ mm³). The *lowest* Factor V was 93 per cent, Factor VIII 93 per cent, and fibrinogen 200 mg/ 100 ml. Only one had questionably positive FDPs. Ekert, Gilchrist, Stanton and Hammond (1970) likewise found that the pattern of haemostatic abnormalities in 28 children with cyanotic CHD did not indicate 'decompensated' intravascular coagulation. Heparin did not correct the haemostatic defect in one patient and the half-time of I¹²⁵-fibrinogen was normal in another. Iolster (1970) found low prothrombin, Factor VII and fibrinogen pointing more to anoxic liver dysfunction than to DIC.

All reports show a high incidence of thrombocytopenia in cyanotic, but not acyanotic, CHD. Ekert and Gilchrist (1968) question whether the low platelet counts necessarily reflect a true reduction in the circulating platelet pool and suggest that margination of platelets in the small blood vessels may occur in the presence of a high haematocrit. They also found no correlation between the presence of a prolonged bleeding time and a low platelet count proposing that a platelet functional defect may exist. This has recently been found to be the case by Maurer *et al.* (1972). They showed that approximately 11 per cent of 65 children with CHD had mild bleeding symptoms and 9 per cent had prolonged bleeding times in spite of normal platelet counts. Fourteen of 37 (38 per cent) with cyanotic CHD and 4 of 28 with acyanotic CHD showed impaired platelet aggregation by ADP, noradrenalin and collagen. This abnormality was present in all the patients with a prolonged bleeding time and in all those with a bleeding tendency. In the cyanotic patients this impairment was correlated with the severity of hypoxia. Their data did not support DIC as a frequent occurrence in cyanotic CHD and my own observations would support this conclusion.

Postoperative haemorrhage after cardiac surgery. Clinically the most important question is the relation of these abnormalities to the serious postoperative bleeding that often occurs following corrective surgery in these children. Ekert and Gilchrist (1968) pointed out that since it was postoperative rather than preoperative bleeding that occurred it was doubtful whether their preoperative abnormal laboratory data had much relation to their haemostatic status. Likewise O'Neill and Hutton (1966) and Maurer *et al.* (1972) found that, strangely, none of their patients with a prolonged bleeding time or impaired platelet aggregation appeared to bleed excessively during palliative or corrective surgery.

Management of the haemostatic defects in these patients undergoing surgery has been discussed by Naiman (1970), Ekert *et al.* (1970) and Inglis *et al.* (1975). Inglis and coworkers made a serial study of cyanotic and acyanotic patients postoperatively. Cyanotic patients who subsequently died showed lower platelet counts, Factor V, and fibrinogen with higher FDPs in the first 24 hr postoperatively compared to similar estimations in cyanotic patients who subsequently survived. Seven of the 12 cyanotic patients who died showed a combination of low skin temperature, low urine output, excessive bleeding, low coagulation factor levels and elevated FDPs suggesting DIC. There was no evidence of increased fibrinolysis. The factor levels in the patients who died either remained low or fell further until death, in contrast to the rebound towards normal that occurred in those who survived. These authors attributed the coagulation defect to the hypoxia of poor tissue perfusion caused by low cardiac output. Whether the DIC aggravates this process is unknown. It is uncertain whether infusion of coagulation factors will be beneficial. Likewise post-operative heparinization will carry risks of local bleeding.

Practical guidelines that emerged from this study were that 'any patient who shows poor tissue perfusion with persistently low skin temperature 4 to 20 hours postoperatively, with or without excess haemorrhage, is likely to develop DIC'. In contrast if a patient bleeds excessively within the first 4 postoperative hours then a more likely cause is heparin rebound, a specific bleeding site, or thrombocytopenia.

Attempts at preoperative correction of the coagulation status by the relatively physiological method of reducing red cell mass by erythropheresis (exchanging some of the red cells with plasma) have been proposed (von Kaulla *et al.*, 1967). Improvement in platelet count and coagulation factor level after venesection has been documented in 2 such children by Ihenacho *et al.* (1973). In the present state of knowledge these approaches are thought to be more justified than heparin therapy (Naiman, 1970).

OTHER VASCULAR DISORDERS

Related to cardiac disease is the shortened platelet survival in patients with prosthetic heart valves (Harker and Slichter, 1970; 1972; Weily *et al.*, 1974) or rheumatic heart disease (Steele *et al.*, 1974). Selective consumption of platelets rather than fibrinogen has been shown to occur with prosthetic heart valves, this being corrected by dipyridamole. Aspirin alone has little effect although it potentiates that of dipyridamole. In patients with rheumatic heart disease platelet survival is normal with aortic stenosis, in which thromboembolism is rare, but shortened in mitral stenosis in which thromboembolism is common. In anoxic newborns platelet thromboses or vegetations upon the atrioventricular valves have recently been described which are quite distinct from DIC, being thought to originate from platelet adhesion to vascular endothelium damaged by anoxia (Favara *et al.*, 1974).

Other vascular derangements can produce similar effects. A shortened platelet lifespan has been found in 5 out of 12 children with ventriculojugular shunts for hydrocephalus (Stuart *et al.*, 1972). The presence of a silastic catheter in the circulation results in platelet aggregation which is the forerunner of thrombus formation. Aspirin, 10 mg/kg per day and dipyridamole 1·5 mg/kg per day caused the platelet survival to return to normal. FDPs were seldom elevated in these patients. In homocystinaemia a three-fold isolated shortening of platelet survival has been demonstrated, which is attributed to a primary damage to arterial vascular endothelium by the circulating homocystine (Harker *et al.*, 1974). Presumably this is related to the tendency to arterial thrombosis. Platelet survival was improved by dipyridamole.

A good recent review by Maurer (1972) of the haematological effects of cardiac disease discusses not only the disturbances of haemostasis but also the red cell fragmentation and haemolytic anaemia due to cardiac prostheses.

THE HAEMOLYTIC URAEMIC SYNDROME (HUS)

This is predominantly a paediatric disease, originally described by Gasser *et al.* (1955), and characterized by acute renal failure, a micro-angiopathic haemolytic anaemia with numerous burr cells on the blood film and thrombocytopenia.

The manifestations of the prodromal and acute phases of HUS have been listed by Hammond and Lieberman (1970) (Table 19.9).

Prognostically it has been found by a multi-variate analysis of admission data from 31 children that features associated with death from progressive renal failure were the presence of anuria, hepatomegaly and purpura, and the absence of preceding gastrointestinal symptoms (Stuart *et al.*, 1974).

Pathological findings essentially show fibrin thrombi in the capillaries and pre-capillary arterioles of the glomeruli (Craig and Gitlin, 1957). In addition the endothelial cells are swollen and, in the glomeruli, separated from the basement membrane by an accumulation of material reacting with antifibrin fluorescent antibody (Gervais *et al.*, 1971). Platelet accumulation in the glomeruli has

Table 19.9   Clinical manifestations of HUS

Prodrome	
Diarrhoea, vomiting, mild fever, upper respiratory tract infection	
Acute phase	
Anaemia:	pallor, weakness
Bleeding:	urine, stool, vomitus, skin
Renal failure:	oliguria, proteinuria, azotaemia, hyperkalaemia
Cardiovascular:	heart failure, hypertension, hepatomegaly
CNS symptoms:	irritability, stupor, seizures

Reproduced, by permission, from Hammond and Lieberman (1970), Arch. Int. Med., 126, 816.

Age incidence. In the large series of 162 cases reported from Argentina the mean age at onset was 12.4 months with a range of 2 months to 5 years (Gianantonio *et al.*, 1966). Two thirds presented before the age of 12 months, with the youngest at one month in the series of 114 cases reported by Piel and Phibbs (1966). A collection of 278 cases from the literature showed a skew age distribution extending throughout childhood with the highest incidence in infants less than a year, the peak being at about 7 months (Brain, 1969).

Clinical features. A prodromal febrile illness is usual 3 to 14 days before the onset of the main syndrome. In infants this is usually gastrointestinal; in older children it is more often upper respiratory. Although these infections have on occasions been proved to be viral a number of different viruses have been incriminated (Gianantonio *et al.*, 1964) including the Coxsackie group (Glasgow and Balduzzi, 1965; Ray *et al.*, 1970). Small epidemics have also been recorded (McLean *et al.*, 1966; Ray *et al.*, 1970; Ruthven and Fyfe, 1968). HUS has also followed inoculations with triple vaccine (diphtheria, tetanus and pertussis), polio, measles and smallpox vaccination (Brain, 1969).

been demonstrated by electron microscopy (Courtecuisse *et al.*, 1967). Although intravascular coagulation is typically localized to the kidney in HUS other tissues are involved in a proportion of cases (Piel and Phibbs, 1966; Lieberman *et al.*, 1966).

The mechanism of pathogenesis of HUS is unknown but Brain (1969) supports the hypothesis that an abnormal immunological response to infection results in the persistence of circulating soluble immune complexes. Such complexes, due to incomplete antibody production, have been shown by Lee (1963) to produce intravascular coagulation and glomerular thrombosis when injected into rabbits. Consistent with this hypothesis is the finding that administration of the interferon-inducing agent polycarboxylate in chronic measles encephalitis produces a viral-like illness, followed by a fall in Factor V and fibrinogen and later thrombocytopenia, burr cell formation, haemolysis, oliguria and rising blood urea (Leavitt *et al.*, 1971). An alternative pathogenesis in HUS would be primary endothelial damage to the renal microvasculature by an unknown agent or toxin.

Haematological findings. The characteristic blood

film appearances with numerous burr cells, triangular cells and some spherocytes, associated with increased osmotic fragility, polychromasia, negative Heinz body test and negative direct Coombs test were well described in 7 children with fatal HUS by Lock and Dormandy (1961). The haemoglobin level is usually between 4 and 10 g/100 ml, the bilirubin elevated and the platelet count well below 100,000/mm³ except in the mildest cases. The peripheral blood findings are, in short, those of MAHA by current terminology, but by definition in HUS there is also a grossly raised blood urea. Recent reports show that serum FDPs are virtually always raised.

Coagulation investigations. The association of burr cells and thrombocytopenia strongly suggests the intravascular deposition of fibrin in small vessels (Baker *et al.*, 1968) and this is, in fact,

another severe case, but normal factor levels in the two mildest cases. FDPs were elevated in all 4 (16—160 μg/ml).

More precise data has been provided by *in vivo* kinetic studies of labelled platelets, fibrinogen and plasminogen (Harker and Slichter, 1972; George *et al.*, 1974), designed to delineate the relative contribution of platelet consumption, intravascular coagulation and fibrinolysis respectively. By these methods selective platelet consumption with normal fibrinogen survival was found in 4 patients with HUS, this being the same pattern as in patients with prosthetic heart valves, AV silastic catheters, vasculitis, TTP or arterial thrombosis. Platelet survival was improved by dipyridamole but not by heparin in this group (although the HUS patients were only tested with heparin) (Harker and Slichter, 1972). Table 19.10 gives

Table 19.10 *In vivo* survival* of platelets, fibrinogen and plasminogen in the haemolytic uraemic syndrome

	No.	Platelet	Fibrinogen	Plasminogen
Normal	16	8·4 $\pm$ 0·8	5·1 $\pm$ 0·2	2·3 $\pm$ 0·2
HUS	7	2·0 $\pm$ 0·5†	3·5 $\pm$ 1·4†	1·7

*Days (mean $\pm$ ISD).
†Significant to P < 0·001 (Student's t-test, as compared to normal.)
All 7 HUS patients had shortened platelet survival.
From George *et al.* (1974).
Reproduced, by permission, from The New England Journal of Medicine (1974), **291,** *1111.*

found in the kidney histologically. Lanzkowsky and McCrory (1967) questioned whether DIC played a role in HUS, stimulating a number of investigations to determine this point.

Sanchez Avalos *et al.* (1970) found elevated Factors V, VIII, IX and XI accompanied by thrombocytopenia in 26 children, suggesting a hypercoagulable state. But in 3 patients with a severe or fatal course they found concomitant falls in fibrinogen, platelets, Factor V and Factor VIII with the appearance of FDPs in the serum at the height of the consumptive process. Katz *et al.* (1971) similarly found elevated V and VIII in 3 out of 10 relatively mild cases of HUS. FDPs were elevated but none showed consumption of coagulation factors. Willoughby *et al.* (1972B) found typical changes of consumptive coagulopathy early in one severe case (fibrinogen 61 mg/100 ml, Factor V, 17 per cent, FDPs 160 μg/100 ml, platelets 40,000/mm³), sequential coagulation factor changes suggestive of a response to heparin in

more recent data on a total of 7 patients with HUS reported by the same group of workers (George *et al.*, 1974). This in fact shows a four-fold shortening of platelet survival compared to normal (P < 0·001) and a more modest shortening in fibrinogen survival, also significant (P < 0·001). In a number of other renal disorders including membranoproliferative glomerulonephritis, glomerulosclerosis, diabetic nephropathy and other glomerular diseases a pattern indicative of isolated platelet consumption was found in a proportion of the patients. These authors conclude therefore that platelet consumption is a secondary consequence of primary intrarenal endothelial damage in these disorders. They point out that the role of this platelet consumption in perpetuating renal damage is uncertain and that controlled trials with anti-platelet agents are needed. In two patients with HUS the administration of dipyridamole improved the platelet survival from 1·9 to 3·4 days and from 2·4 to 6·2 days. Heparin produced no change in platelet survival in these same patients.

Katz *et al.* (1973) have found normal *in vivo* platelet survival in 4 infants within 3 to 6 days from the onset of prodromal symptoms, suggesting that consumption is no longer occurring by the time that the diagnosis is made. But these were mild cases as judged by their blood urea levels and these findings do not apply to all cases (Table 19.10).

Treatment. It is clear that management of the acute renal failure and electrolyte disturbances with subsequent provision of adequate protein and calorie intake is of prime importance. Together with the introduction of early peritoneal dialysis this has resulted in reduction of the mortality in the acute stage to 6·25 per cent in expert hands (Gianantonio *et al.*, 1973).

Heparin therapy was advocated by Gilchrist *et al.* (1969) with the aim of halting further renal damage and continued deposition of fibrin and platelets. Apparent reversal of thrombocytopenia (Kibel and Barnard, 1964; Kunzer and Aalam, 1964; Desmit and Hart, 1966; Hitzig *et al.*, 1968; Sharpstone *et al.*, 1968; Moncrieff and Glasgow, 1970), fall in FDPs (Uttley, 1970) and rise in fibrinogen (Desmit and Hart, 1966), Factor V and Factor VIII (Willoughby *et al.*, 1972B) during heparin therapy give some support to this proposition. But spontaneous correction has also been seen (Monnens and Schretlen, 1967; Sanchez Avalos *et al,*. 1970) leaving the contribution of heparin uncertain. It is clear that it would need to be given in as early a stage in the evolution of the syndrome as possible. It is also important that its use does not compromise the institution of peritoneal dialysis when needed. However, with a dose of 25–35 units heparin/kg hr, resulting in prolongation of the capillary clotting time to 4–7½ min (normal $2\frac{3}{3}\pm\frac{1}{4}$ min) we have been able to proceed with peritoneal dialysis without complication (Cases 2, 3 and 4, Willoughby *et al.*, 1972).

A beneficial effect of heparin upon survival has, however, been questioned (Kaplan *et al.*, 1971) and remains unproven in the absence of controlled trials. Comparison of results from different centres can be misleading because of geographical differences in the severity of the syndrome (Tune *et al.*, 1973). Other approaches that are being investigated include the use of drugs directed at suppressing tissue damage or platelet aggregation (Clarkson *et al.*, 1970) or fibrinolytic agents with the object of removing intravascular fibrin already deposited. Corticosteroids have been followed by rapid and alarming deterioration (Mandal and McNulty, 1971). The use of streptokinase followed by heparin was pioneered in HUS by Monnens and Schretler (1968). Subsequently Rosen *et al.* (1970) used simultaneous urokinase (100,000 units/24 hr) and heparin (20,000 units/24 hr) in an anuric 9-year-old boy with rapid diuresis and ultimate success. Lately direct infusion into renal arteries has been used. Bergstein *et al.* (1972) reported 3 severe cases who recovered after initial treatment with streptokinase followed by heparin. The dose of streptokinase was calculated as the number of units necessary to lyse the clot from 1 ml of the patient's plasma, multiplied by the estimated plasma volume. This dose was then continued hourly by constant infusion. Courses of 5 days, 56 hours and 102 hours were given to the different children, followed by heparin 100 units/kg/4-hourly. Fibrinolysis was shown to be occurring in the glomeruli in tissue obtained by renal biopsy. The authors postulated that defective fibrinolytic capability of the kidney was the key factor determining whether recovery occurred in HUS, and that this therapy could restore this capacity. Winterborn *et al.* (1972) reported a similarly treated child in which the absence of intravascular fibrin was demonstrated by renal biopsy at 28 days from the onset. Results of this therapy in 36 children with HUS have recently been reported by Monnens (1973). All but 2 survived of a group of 15 presenting with anuria (< 10 ml/24 hr). It does appear, however, that more severe bleeding is to be expected with fibrinolytic therapy than heparin. Monnens aims to maintain the thrombin time at 2–4 times the normal value during the period of 72 hours on streptokinase. A practical point is that it is better to compare these serial thrombin times with that of pooled normal plasma rather than the patient's pre-treatment plasma, since this may show a prolonged thrombin time, presumably due to FDPs (Stuart *et al.*, 1974).

Emphasis has now shifted from improvement of the short term survival, which is now 80–90 per cent, to efforts to improve the long term results by preventing ischaemic glomerular scarring. It is possible that this is determined by the extent of fibrin deposition and that heparin and/or fibrinolytic agents may modify this (Gianantonio *et al.*, 1973; Monnens, 1973). Powell and Ekert (1974) made a retrospective analysis of the results of trertment of HUS over a 10-year period. This suggested that heparin reduced the mortality rate in the acute phase. Heparin alone did not prevent the late occurrence of chronic renal disease, but

COAGULATION DISORDERS. 2. ACQUIRED 359

Table 19.11 Comparison of treatment regimes in HUS

Treatment	Total no. of cases	Deaths during acute illness	Chronic renal disease follow-up	Normal at follow-up
Symptomatic only	22	9	5	8
Heparin for less than 7 days	6	3	2	1
Heparin for 7 or more days	8	2	2	4
Streptokinase, heparin, aspirin and dipyridamole	8	2	0	6

(Aspirin 10–20 mg/kg on alternate days, dipyridamole 5 mg/kg per day)
All four treatment groups received dialysis and blood transfusions as necessary. There was no marked difference in treatment other than as indicated.
Data reproduced, with permission, from Powell and Ekert (1974), J. Pediat., **84**, *347.*

may have done so when combined with streptokinase and antiplatelet agents (Table 19.11).

As mentioned above, a controlled trial of dipyridamole, aspirin or other antiplatelet agent is needed (George *et al.*, 1974).

THROMBOTIC THROMBOCYTOPENIC PURPURA (TTP)

Typically a condition of adults this disorder has many features in common with childhood HUS including, in particular, the combination of rapidly developing MAHA and renal involvement. Unlike the typical case of HUS, TTP shows thrombotic lesions of many tissues including especially the brain, giving rise to a fluctuating neurological picture (Amorosi and Ultman, 1966). Nevertheless it is still an open question whether HUS and TTP are different ends of the same spectrum.

A few reports of TTP in childhood can be found (McWhinney *et al.*, 1962). Berberich *et al* (1974) also described 3 children aged 6, 14 and 15 years who survived an acute illness closely resembling TTP. Their platelet counts were 8,900 to 12,000/ mm^3. Coagulation monitoring and kinetic measurements of platelet and fibrinogen survival gave no evidence of any beneficial effect from heparin, aspirin or dipyridamole. Significant increases in antibody titre to Coxsackie B virus developed in 2 of the 3 children. These negative findings were at variance with the responses to heparin (Bernstock and Hirson, 1960) and dipyridamole plus aspirin (Giromini *et al.*, 1972) previously thought to occur in adult TTP. Amir and Krauss (1973) have reported response to dipyridamole (100 mg 6-hourly) plus aspirin (900 mg 6-hourly) in a 17-year-old boy previously unresponsive to heparin.

Recent detailed coagulation investigations in 12 adults with this disease showed no coagulation abnormalities in 6, minimal abnormalities in 3 and major changes compatible with DIC in only 3. From

temporal relationships it was suggested that the DIC, when present, resulted from the haemolysis rather than being causal to this or the disease (Jaffe *et al.*, 1973). The study of Neame *et al.* (1973) showed that the multiple vascular occlusions are primarily due to densely packed platelet aggregates with fibrin playing a secondary and variable part in the process. 'Disseminated intravascular platelet aggregation' is the term used by these authors, and could possibly be relevant to certain other syndromes previously attributed to DIC, including perhaps HUS.

SEPTICAEMIA–BACTERIAL, VIRAL, FUNGAL, RICKETTSIAL, PROTOZOAL

Corrigan *et al.* (1968) made detailed coagulation investigations in 36 children with various types of septicaemia. They found that the pattern of coagulation changes characteristic of DIC were present in the group of 11 patients with hypotension and shock but not in the 25 normotensive patients. The most reliable laboratory indices for this purpose were thrombocytopenia, reduced Factor V and elevated serum FDPs. The organisms associated with shock and DIC were: *Meningococcus, Haemophilus influenzae, Aerobacter, Herellea* and *beta haemolytic streptococci*. Clinical features in this group included anuria or oliguria, gastrointestinal bleeding and, in the case of meningococci, necrotic skin lesions. Five of the 11 died. The group without shock or DIC included cases with 3 of the same organisms, viz. *Meningococci, Haemophilus influenzae* and *Aerobacter*, as well as *Staphylococcus aureus, pneumococci*, typhoid and Rocky Mountain spotted fever. Two out of 25 died. It was therefore the state of shock, not the organism, that correlated with coagulation changes of DIC and poor prognosis. Intravascular coagulation due to *Pseudomonas* septicaemia has also been reported and an analogy with the Shwartzman reaction suggested (Rapaport *et al.*, 1964). An example of intravascular coagulation due to coliform septicaemia in a neonate is shown in Fig. 19.7.

A subsequent investigation by Corrigan and Jordan (1970) in 25 children with septic shock showed evidence of DIC in all but one. In addition to standard therapy 24 were given heparin, yet 14 (58 per cent) still died in shock. Laboratory evidence of improvement in the coagulation defects occurred in all who survived but in only 3 of the 14 who died. They concluded that heparin or reversal of the coagulation defect did not improve survival. It was not clear whether DIC produced shock or the reverse. They suggested that improving hypotension might have a major role in correcting the DIC. Acting on this assumption the same authors (Corrigan et al., 1974) treated 3 subsequent children with septic shock (2 meningococcal, 1 probable gram negative) without heparin but with IV antibiotics, dextran (10 ml/kg Dextran 75) and fresh frozen plasma (10 ml/kg). The blood pressure rapidly responded in the 3 children. Sequential coagulation data showed that concomitantly with the correction of the shock there was reversal of consumptive coagulopathy. They concluded that the state of shock was the cause of the DIC. Kisker and Rush (1973) also found that abolition of DIC in meningococcaemia did not ensure survival.

Other workers, however, have felt that demonstrable intravascular deposition of fibrin was an important cause of death in meningococcal septicaemia and that attempts at reversal with heparin should be made. Abildgaard et al. (1967) reported an early success with heparin. Winkelstein et al. (1969) found that 26 such patients had platelet counts of 90,000/mm^3 or more and survived; but 3 had platelet counts below this level and died. Three other patients with thrombocytopenia and coagulation defects were treated with heparin and survived. They favoured Dextran 70 rather than plasma for treatment of the shock since the anticoagulant effect of this product could be valuable in DIC while avoiding the hazards of adding more consumable coagulation factors. Retrospective histology on the previous 12 patients who had died of this infection showed fibrin microthrombi in all. Similar findings were reported by Denmark and Knight (1971) with 3 out of 10 children showing DIC but all surviving, 2 having heparin. Gérard et al. (1973) reported survival in 19 patients with the adverse features of shock, absence of meningitis and a normal white cell count, 17 of whom had thrombocytopenia and coagulation defects, treated with heparin 50 units/kg stat. followed by a small maintenance dose (daily units/kg = platelet count/500).

In a recent review of heparin therapy in acute meningococcaemia Hathaway (1973) suggests:
1. Antibiotic therapy
2. Treatment of shock with fluids, blood plasma, plasma expanders (especially Dextran), and vasoactive agents such as isoproterenol

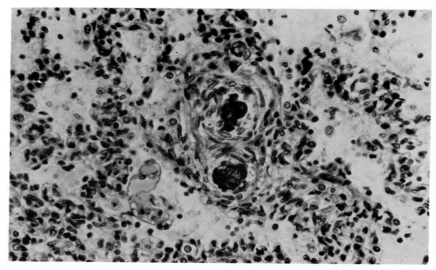

Fig. 19.7 Fibrin occlusion of pulmonary arterioles in a newborn with E. coli septicaemia. Haematological data Fibrinogen, 33 mg/100 ml; thrombin time, 35 sec.; Factor V, 6 per cent; Factor VIII, 45 per cent; plasminogen, 0·9 cu/ml; platelets, 90,000/mm^3 (a.m.), 12,000/mm^3 (p.m.); haemoglobin, 16·3 g/100 ml (a.m.), 12·2 g/100 ml (p.m.); film, red-cell fragmentation; no fibrinolysis on fibrin plates. (× 100).

3. Treatment of DIC if present (heparin and blood component replacement as needed)
4. Large doses of adrenosteroids if indicated.

I support this view having been impressed by the rapid clinical and coagulation response of a severely ill infant with this infection showing progressive necrotic cutaneous purpura and evidence of DIC before heparinization (Fig. 19.8 and Table 19.12) (Willoughby *et al.*, 1972A).

al., 1971), disseminated herpes simplex in the neonate (Miller *et al.*, 1970), Rocky Mountain spotted fever (Haynes *et al.*, 1970) and malignant tertian malaria (Borochovitz *et al.*, 1970). DIC of two grades of severity has been found in children with kwashiorkor and bleeding or purpura (Hassanein and Tankovsky, 1975). These children all had diarrhoea and most were dehydrated. Infection was probable in the majority. Their ages were 9 months

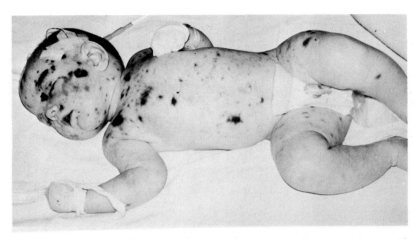

Fig. 19.8 Meningococcal septicaemia with progressive necrotic purpura and consumptive coagulopathy.

Table 19.12 Coagulation data from two children with meningococcal septicaemia with consumptive coagulopathy

	Case 1*	Case 2
	Aged 4 months	Aged 5 years
Platelets	35,000	54,000/mm³
Fibrinogen	227	56 mg/100 ml
Factor V	2 per cent	2 per cent
Factor VIII	23 per cent	6 per cent
Plasminogen	0·44	1·0 cu/ml
FDPs	160	160 μg/ml

*Clinical picture Fig. 19.8.

Since this case it is our policy to screen all seriously ill children with meningicoccaemia by performing daily or twice-daily platelet counts. Those whose platelet counts remain above 90,000–100,000/mm³ have uniformly recovered on conventional treatment, but three fatalities have occurred when the platelet count fell rapidly, closely parallel to Winkelstein's experience.

Other infections that may occur in childhood and which have been accompanied by DIC include miliary tuberculosis (Goldfine *et al.*, 1969), *Candida albicans* septicaemia (Philippidis *et*

to 3 years. The occurrence of DIC in virus diseases has been reviewed by McKay and Margaretten (1967), and the association of bleeding with infection, with or without DIC, has been discussed by Kisker and Mauer (1972). At a given level of platelet count the liability to spontaneous bleeding seems to be increased by the presence of bacterial infection. This point is of particular relevance in the management of acute leukaemia. The thrombocytopenic patient whose bleeding fails to respond to a platelet transfusion is likely to be infected.

PURPURA FULMINANS

This disorder is characterized by the sudden onset of rapidly spreading intracutaneous haemorrhage with bullae and subcutaneous necrosis (purpura gangrenosa) in patients recovering from a streptococcal infection or an exanthem, particularly varicella. Irreversible shock may supervene a few days from onset. In those who survive many require amputation of one or more legs or fingers for gangrene. Others require skin grafting.

Widespread cutaneous thrombosis occurs and an anology with the Shwartzman phenomenon has been proposed (Glass, 1962). Because of the unremitting and progressive course of the disease many desperate therapeutic measures have been tried. Supportive measures and steroids have often been used, the latter on the presumption that there is an underlying immunological cause. Dextran was used successfully by Paterson et al. (1965).

Thrombocytopenia and consumption of coagulation factors have been demonstrated in a number of individual cases (Hjort et al., 1964; Trueb et al., 1964; Paterson et al., 1963; Allen, 1966; Antley and McMillan, 1967) as expected from the pathology. In some instances the blood has been completely incoagulable and the fibrinogen zero (Hattersley, 1970).

Heparin therapy at a dose of 50–100 units/kg stat. followed by 100 units/kg 4-hourly was followed by a striking rise in depleted factors in the reports of Allen (1966) and Antley and McMillan (1967):

	Platelets 10^3/mm^3		Fibrinogen mg/100 ml		Prothrombin percentage		V percentage		VII percentage	
	Pre	Post	Pre	Post	Pre	Post	Pre	Post	Pre	Post
Allen (1966)	114	→180	15	→420	0	→100				
Antley (1967)	31	→500	<5	→174	<1	→200	10	→132	16	→143

Hattersley (1970) discusses the problems of monitoring the degree of heparinization since the PTT, thrombin time and clotting time are grossly prolonged by the disease itself. They relied mainly upon the fibrinogen level to monitor the correction of the consumptive process. When the fibrinogen rose the skin lesions improved. It is clear from these and other reports of the successful use of heparin in this disorder (Little, 1959; Hjort et al., 1964; Trueb et al., 1964) that early institution and a protracted course over several weeks is sometimes necessary with careful monitoring when it is finally stopped. Recurrence of clinical relapse has been seen on stopping heparin, with resolution on restarting it, thereby attesting to its efficacy.

This disease appears to be one of the clearest indications for the use of heparin in paediatric practice. Complete and permanent recovery has been recorded after heparin and Hattersley (1970) makes the point that the patient's 'life and limb' depend upon prompt diagnosis and treatment.

MISCELLANEOUS CAUSES OF DIC: *Acute liver failure, disseminated malignancy, acute intravascular haemolysis*

Flute and coworkers (Rake et al., 1971) found evidence of intravascular coagulation in four consecutive patients, 3 with fulminant hepatic failure and 1 with a severe relapse of serum hepatitis. They were treated with heparin plus fresh frozen plasma. Rapid correction of the coagulation disturbance was achieved and all 4 made a complete recovery. These patients showed a different haematological pattern from that usually seen in liver failure in that there was thrombocytopenia and a failure to correct the prothrombin time by giving blood or plasma transfusions. Also there was an increased disappearance rate of ^{125}I-labelled fibrinogen which was partly corrected by heparin. Heparin treatment has also been used in patients with a haemorrhagic state due to chronic liver disease, viz. extrahepatic portal hypertension and hepatic cirrhosis (Zetterquist and von Francken, 1963). Coagulation investigations had shown very high apparent levels of Factor VIII suggesting a hypercoagulable state. There was a good clinical response to heparin. A recent annotation on 'intravascular coagulation and the liver' is that by Bloom (1975).

Examples of malignant disease relevant to paediatric practice which can cause DIC include metastatic neuroblastoma (McMillan et al., 1968) and promyelocytic leukaemia (Verstrate et al., 1965). In the case of generalized malignancy such as neuroblastoma it is questionable whether attempts should be made to correct the DIC. In promyelocytic leukaemia at the time of presentation the situation may be different since the possibility of worthwhile remission exists. Originally the coagulation disturbance in this form of leukaemia was thought to be primary fibrinolysis, but more recently it has been recognized that the fibrinolysis is secondary to DIC. In a recent child with this form of leukaemia in Edinburgh heparin was given during the remission induction chemotherapy. As remission occurred the coagulation disorder and bleeding tendency resolved (Dr. Elizabeth Innes—personal communication). Another cause of a similar coagulation disturbance in leukaemia is gram negative septicaemia. The patients appear to have thrombocytopenic bleeding but unlike the usual situation, this fails to respond to adequate platelet transfusion. Strangely enough the full Shwartzman type reaction triggered by gram negative sepsis in such patients is contingent upon the presence of adequate circulating polymorphs and may be prevented by the severe neutropenia that is often present (Komp and Donaldson, 1970).

A major incompatibility in blood transfusion, resulting in acute intravascular haemolysis, is a cause of DIC (Krevans *et al.*, 1957) which it is hoped should not occur. Massive foeto-maternal haemorrhage from an A baby into an O mother can produce the same complication, resulting in otherwise inexplicable maternal 'defibrination' at the time of delivery. Since the foetal cells in the mother's circulation are rapidly destroyed they may not be found on a Kleihauer film of the mother's blood. Materno-foetal transfusion is less likely to harm the foetus, even when an 'A' mother bleeds into an 'O' baby, since Anti-A is seldom developed in a baby's serum at the time of birth. The possibility, however, exists. McKay (1965) has also suggested that intravascular clotting may play a role in some of the manifestations of sickle cell crises and acute haemolytic episodes in favism and PNH. It is an undoubted fact that a fall in platelet count parallels the drop in haemoglobin during infections in sickle cell anaemia. Massive haemolysis following fava bean ingestion or inhalation has been followed by a 'hypercoagulable state' with elevated fibrinogen and Factors V, and especially VIII. FDPs were not elevated (Mannucci *et al.*, 1969).

Additional causes of DIC that are given in the review by Hathaway (1970C), but have not been described above, include thermal and electrical burns, trauma, renal and hepatic transplants, fat embolism, hyperthermia, snake bite, acute anaphylaxis as well as a number of additional infections and other examples of disseminated malignancy. Elevated FDPs have been reported in certain 'collagen diseases' (Hedner and Nilsson, 1971).

ACQUIRED INHIBITORS OF COAGULATION

Specific inhibitors to individual Factors I (fibrinogen), II, V, VII, IX, XI and XIII have been described, but by far the commonest is that to Factor VIII developing in patients with classical haemophilia and described in Chap. 18. Inhibitors to the interaction of coagulation factors are also known to occur in DLE (Biggs and Denson, 1964) but the fully developed form of this disease is rare in childhood.

Recently, McMillan *et al.* (1972) have described two children aged 4 and 5, with acquired specific inhibitors to Factors II (prothrombin) and VIII. They were previously well but suddenly developed bruising and, in one case, vaginal bleeding. The haemorrhagic manifestations and coagulation defects (prolonged PTT and low specific assay results) subsided spontaneously and completely. No underlying disease was found, and DLE was specifically excluded.

REFERENCES

Aballi, A. J., López-Banús, V., Lamerens, S. de & Rozengvaig, S. (1957) Coagulation studies in the newborn period. I. Alterations of thromboplastin generation and effects of vitamin K on full-term and premature infants. *Am. J. Dis. Child.*, **94**, 594.

Aballi, A. J., López-Banús, V., Lamarens, S. de & Rosengvaig, S. (1959) Coagulation studies in the newborn period. III. Hemorrhagic disease of the newborn. *Am. J. Dis. Child.*, **97**, 524.

Aballi, A. J. & Lamerens, S. de (1962A) Coagulation changes in neonatal period and early infancy. *Ped. Clin. N. Am.*, **9**, 785.

Aballi, A. J. & Lamerens, S. de (1962B) Hemorrhagic disease of the newborn: Two forms with different hemostatic defects. *Am. J. Dis. Child.*, **104**, 475.

Aballi, A. J., Howard, C. E. & Triplett, R. F. (1966) Absorption of vitamin K from the colon in the newborn infant. *J. Pediat.*, **68**, 305.

Abildgaard, C. F., Corrigan, J. J., Seeler, R. A., Simone, J. V. & Schulman, I. (1967) Meningococcemia associated with intravascular coagulation. *Pediatrics*, **40**, 78.

Abildgaard, U. (1968) Highly purified antithrombin III with heparin cofactor activity prepared by disc electrophoresis. *Scand. J. Clin. Lab. Invest.*, **21**, 89.

Abildgaard, C. F. (1969) Recognition and treatment of intravascular coagulation. *J. Pediat.*, **74**, 163.

Agle, D. P., Ratnoff, O. D. & Spring, G. K. (1970) The anticoagulant malingerer. *Ann. Intern. Med.*, **73**, 67.

Ahuja, G. L., Willoughby, M. L. N., Kerr, M. M. & Hutchison, J. H. (1969) Massive subaponeurotic haemorrhage in infants born by vacuum extraction. *Brit. med. J.*, **iii**, 743.

Allen, D. M. (1966) Heparin therapy of purpura fulminans. *Pediat.*, **38**, 211.

Allison, A. C. (1955) Danger of vitamin K to newborn. *Lancet*, **i**, 669.

Ambrus, C. M., Weintraub, D. H., Dunphy, D., Dowd, J. E., Pickren, J. W., Niswander, K. R. & Ambrus, J. L. (1963) Studies on hyaline membrane disease: I. The fibrinolysin system in pathogenesis and therapy. *Pediatrics*, **32**, 10.

Ambrus, C. M., Weintraub, D. H., Niswander, K. R. & Ambrus, J. L. (1965) Studies on hyaline membrane disease: II. The ontogeny of the fibrinolysin system. *Pediatrics*, **35**, 91.

Ambrus, C. M., Weintraub, D. H., Choi, T. S., Eisenberg, B. *et al.* (1974) Plasminogen in the prevention of hyaline membrane disease. *Am. J. Dis. Child.*, **127**, 189.

American Academy of Pediatrics (1961) Report of the Committee on Nutrition. *Pediatrics*, **28**, 501.

Amir, J. & Krauss, S. (1973) Treatment of thrombotic thrombycytopenic purpura with anti-platelet drugs. *Blood*, **42**, 27.

Amorosi, E. L. & Ultmann, J. E. (1966) Thrombotic thrombocytopenic purpura: Report of 16 cases and review of the literature. *Medicine*, **45**, 139.

Antley, R. M. & McMillan, C. W. (1967) Sequential coagulation studies in purpura fulminans. *New Eng. J. Med.*, **276**, 287.

Arneil, G. C., MacDonald, A. M., Murphy, A. V. & Sweet, E. M. (1973) Renal venous thrombosis. *Clinical Nephrology*, **1**, 119.

Baker, L. R. I., Rubenberg, M. L., Dacie, J. V. & Brain, M. C. (1968) Fibrinogen catabolism in microangiopathic haemolytic anaemia. *Brit. J. Haemat.*, **14**, 617.

Bang, N. U., Fletcher, A. P., Alkjaersig, N. & Sherry, S. (1962) Pathogenesis of the coagulation defect developing during pathological plasma proteolytic ('fibrinolytic') states. III. Demonstration of abnormal clot structure by electron microscopy. *J. Clin. Invest.*, **41**, 935.

Basu, D., Gallus, A., Hirsh, J. & Cade, J. (1972) A prospective study of the value of monitoring heparin treatment with activated partial thromboplastin time. *New Eng. J. Med.*, **287**, 324.

Beller, F. K., Douglas, G. W. & Epstein, M. D. (1966) The fibrinolytic enzyme system in the newborn. *Am. J. Obst. Gynec.*, **96**, 977.

Berberich, F. R., Cuene, S. A., Chard, R. L. & Hartman, J. R. (1974) Thrombotic thrombocytopenic purpura. Three cases with platelet and fibrinogen survival studies. *Pediatrics*, **84**, 503.

Berglund, G. (1970) Three cases of disseminated intravascular coagulation. *Acta Paediat. Scand.*, **59**, 664.

Bergstein, J. M., Edson, J. R. & Michael, A. F. (1972) Fibrinolytic treatment of the haemolytic-uraemic syndrome. *Lancet*, **i**, 448.

Bernstock, L. & Hirson, C. (1960) Thrombotic thrombocytopenic purpura. Remission on treatment with heparin. *Lancet*, **i**, 28.

Biggs, R. P. & Denson, K. W. E. (1964) The mode of action of a coagulation inhibitor in the blood of two patients with disseminated lupus erythematosus (DLE). *Brit. J. Haemat.*, **10**, 198.

Biggs, R., Denson, K. W. E., Akman, N., Borrett, R. & Hadden, M. (1970) Antithrombin III, antifactor Xa and heparin. *Brit. J. Haemat.*, **19**, 283.

Bleyer, W. A., Hakami, N. & Shepard, T. H. (1971) The development of hemostasis in the human fetus and newborn infant. *J. Pediat.*, **79**, 838.

Blix, S. & Aas, K. (1961) Giant haemangioma, thrombocytopenia, fibrinogenopenia, and fibrinolytic activity. *Acta Med. Scand.*, **169**, 63.

Bloom, A. L. (1975) Intravascular coagulation and the liver. *Brit. J. Haemat.*, **30**, 1.

Bonifaci, E., Baggio, P. & Gravina, E. (1968) Demonstration of split products of fibrinogen in the blood of normal infants. *Biol. Neonat.*, **12**, 29.

Borochovitz, D., Crosley, A. L. & Metz, J. (1970) Disseminated intravascular coagulation with fatal haemorrhage in cerebral malaria. *Brit. med. J.*, **ii**, 710.

Boyd, J. F. (1967) Disseminated fibrin thromboembolism among neonates dying within 48 hours of birth. *Arch. Dis. Childh.*, **42**, 401.

Brain, M. C. (1969) The haemolytic-uraemic syndrome. *Seminars in Haematology*, **6**, 162.

Breen, F. A. & Tullis, J. L. (1969) Ethanol gelation test improved. *Ann. Intern Med.*, **71**, 433.

Brinkhouse, K. M., Smith, H. P. & Warner, E. O. (1937) Plasma prothrombin level in normal infancy and hemorrhagic disease of the newborn. *Amer. J. Med. Sci.*, **193**, 475.

British Medical Journal (1971) Editorial: Haemorrhage in the newborn. *Brit. med. J.*, **iv**, 1.

Brizel, H. E. & Raccuglia, G. (1965) Giant hemangioma with thrombocytopenia. Radioisotopic demonstration of platelet sequestration. *Blood*, **26**, 751.

Brodsky, I., Ross, E. M., Kahn, S. B. & Petrov, G. (1972) Platelet and fibrinogen kinetics with (^{75}Se) Selenomethionine in thrombocytopenic states. II. *Brit. J. Haemat.*, **22**, 589.

Bruning, P. F. & Loeliger, E. A. (1971) Prothrombal: A new concentrate of human prothrombin complex for clinical use. *Brit. J. Haemat.*, **21**, 377.

Cade, J. F., Hirsh, J. & Martin, M. (1969) Placental barrier to coagulation factors: Its relevance to the coagulation defect at birth and to haemorrhage in the newborn. *Brit. med. J.*, **ii**, 281.

Chessels, J. M. & Pitney, W. R. (1970) Fibrin split products in serum of newborn: Possible technical errors. *Pediatrics*, **45**, 155.

Chessels, J. M. & Wigglesworth, J. S. (1970) Secondary haemorrhagic disease of the newborn. *Arch. Dis. Childh.*, **45**, 539.

Chessels, J. M. & Wigglesworth, J. S. (1971A) Coagulation studies in severe birth asphyxia. *Arch. Dis. Childh.*, **46**, 253.

Chessels, J. M. & Wigglesworth, J. S. (1971B) Haemostatic failure in babies with rhesus isoimmunization. *Arch. Dis. Childh.*, **46**, 38.

Clarkson, A. R., Fuster, V. & Cash, J. D. (1970) Heparin and the haemolytic-uraemic syndrome. *Brit. med. J.*, **iii**, 463.

Corrigan, J. J., Abildgaard, C. F., Seeler, R. A. & Schulman, I. (1967) Quantitative aspects of blood coagulation in the generalized Shwartzman reaction. II. Effect of cortisone. *Pediat. Res.*, **1**, 99.

Corrigan, J. J., Ray, W. L. & May, N. (1968) Changes in the blood coagulation system associated with septicemia. *New Eng. J. Med.*, **279**, 851.

Corrigan, J. J. & Jordan, C. M. (1970) Heparin therapy in septicemia with disseminated intravascular coagulation. Effect on mortality and on correction of hemostatic defects. *New Eng. J. Med.*, **283**, 778.

Corrigan, J. J. & Sell, E. J. (1971) Changes in the 'consumption' coagulation factors in normal and sick newborns as related to gestational age. *Blood*, **38**, 814.

Corrigan, J. J., Jordan, C. M. & Bennett, B. B. (1974) Disseminated intravascular coagulation in septic shock. Report of three cases not treated with heparin. *Am. J. Dis. Child.*, **126**, 629.

Courtecuisse, V., Habib, R. & Monnier, C. (1967) Non-lethal hemolytic and uremic syndrome in children: An electron microscopic study of renal biopsies from six cases. *Exp. Molec. Path.*, **7**, 327.

Craig, J. M. & Gitlin, D. (1957) The nature of the hyaline thrombi in thrombotic thrombocytopenic purpura. *Amer. J. Path.*, **33**, 251.

Craig, W. S. (1961) On real and apparent external bleeding in the newborn. *Arch. Dis. Childh.*, **36**, 575.

Creveld, S. van, Paulssen, M. M. P., Ens, J. C., Meij, C. A. M., Versteeg, P. & Verstegh, E. T. B. (1954) Proconvertin content in blood of newborn full-term and premature infants. *Étude. Néo-natal.*, **3**, 53.

Dam, H., Glavind, J., Larsen, H. & Plum, P. (1942) Investigations into the cause of physiological hypoprothrombinemia in newborn children. IV. The vitamin K content of woman's milk and cow's milk. *Acta Med. Scand.*, **112**, 210.

Denmark, T. C. & Knight, E. L. (1971) Cardiovascular and coagulation complications of group C meningococcal disease. *Arch. Intern. Med.*, **127**, 238.

Dennis, L. H., Stewart, J. L. & Conrad, M. E. (1967) Heparin treatment of haemorrhagic diathesis in cyanotic congenital heart disease. *Lancet*, **1**, 1088.

Desmit, E. M. & Hart, H. A. (1966) Behandeling van het hemolytisch-uremisch syndroom. *Nederl. T. Geneesk.*, **110**, 355.

Deutsch, E. (1965) Blood coagulation changes in liver disease. *Prog. Liver Dis.*, **2**, 69.

Deykin, D. (1966) Role of liver in serum-induced hypercoagulability. *J. Clin. Invest.*, **45**, 256.

Deykin, D. (1970) The clinical challenge of disseminated intravascular coagulation. *New Eng. J. Med.*, **283**, 636.

Deykin, D. (1972) Editorial: Regulation of heparin therapy. *New Eng. J. Med.*, **287**, 355.

Diamond, L. K., Allen, F. H., Vann, D. D. & Powers, J. R. (1952) Round table discussion: Erythroblastosis fetalis. *Pediatrics*, **10**, 337.

Dike, G. W. R., Bidwell, E. & Rizza, C. R. (1972) The preparation and clinical use of a new concentrate containing factor IX, Prothrombin and factor X and of a separate concentrate containing factor VIII. *Brit. J. Haemat.*, **22**, 469.

Dormandy, K. M. & Hardisty, R. M. (1961) Coagulation tests on capillary blood. A screening procedure for use in small children. *J. Clin. Path.*, **14**, 543.

Du, J. N. H., Briggs, J. N. & Young, G. (1970) Disseminated intravascular coagulopathy in hyaline membrane disease: Massive thrombosis following umbilical artery catheterization. *Pediat.*, **45**, 287.

Duncan, W. & Halnan, K. E. (1964) Giant haemangioma with thrombocytopenia. *Clin. Radiology*, **15**, 224.

Eckstein, H. B. & Jack, B. (1970) Breast feeding and anticoagulant therapy. *Lancet*, **i**, 672.

Edson, J. R., Blaese, R. M. & Krivit, W. (1968) Defibrination syndrome in an infant born after abruptio placentae. *J. Pediat.*, **72**, 342.

Eika, C. (1972) Heparin-induced platelet release and refractory platelets. *Lancet*, **i**, 1344.

Eika, C., Godal, H. C. & Kierulf, P. (1972) Detection of small amounts of heparin by the thrombin clotting-time. *Lancet*, **ii**, 376.

Ekberg, M. & Nilsson, I. M. (1975) Factor VIII and glomerulonephritis. *Lancet*, **i**, 1111.

Ekelund, H., Hedner, U. & Nilsson, I. M. (1970) Fibrin split products in serum of newborn: Possible technical errors. *Pediatrics*, **45**, 156.

Ekelund, H., Hedner, U. & Åstedt, B. (1970) Fibrinolysis in human foetus. *Acta Paediat. Scand.*, **59**, 369.

Ekert, H. & Gilchrist, G. S. (1968) Coagulation studies in congenital heart disease. *Lancet*, **ii**, 280.

Ekert, H. (1970) Fibrin split products in serum of newborn: Possible technical errors. *Pediatrics*, **45**, 154.

Ekert, H., Gilchrist, G. S., Stanton, R. & Hammond, D. (1970) Hemostasis in cyanotic congenital heart disease. *J. Pediat.*, **76**, 221.

Ekert, H. & Seshadri, R. (1973) Heparin treatment in childhood and its effect on monitoring tests. *Aust. paediat. J.*, **9**, 269.

Estes, J. W. (1970) Kinetics of the anticoagulant effect of heparin. *J.A.M.A.*, **212**, 1492.

Evans, A. R., Forrester, R. M. & Discombe, C. (1970) Neonatal haemorrhage following maternal anticonvulsant therapy. *Lancet*, **i**, 517.

Favara, B. E., Franciosi, R. A. & Butterfield, L. J. (1974) Disseminated intravascular and cardiac thrombosis of the neonate. *Am. J. Dis. Child.*, **127**, 197.

Felten, A. von, Straub, W. & Frick, P. G. (1969) Dysfibrinogenemia in a patient with primary hepatoma. First observation of an acquired abnormality of fibrin monomer aggregation. *New Eng. J. Med.*, **280**, 405.

Fillmore, S. J. & McDevitt, E. (1970) Effects of coumarin compounds on the fetus. *Ann. Int. Med.*, **73**, 731.

Fletcher, A. P., Biederman, O., Moore, D., Alkjaersig, N. & Sherry, S. (1964) Abnormal plasminogen-plasmin system activity (fibrinolysis) in patients with hepatic cirrhosis: Its cause and consequences. *J. Clin. Invest.*, **43**, 681.

Frost, N. C. & Esterly, N. B. (1968) Successful treatment of juvenile hemangiomas with prednisone. *J. Pediat.*, **72**, 351.

Gaetano, G. de & Vermylen, J. (1972) Effect of heparin on platelets. *Lancet*, **ii**, 376.

Gaffney, P. J. (1972) F.D.P. *Lancet*, **ii**, 1422.

Gasser, C. von, Gautier, E., Steck, A., Siebermann, R. E. & Oechslin, R. (1955) Hämolytisch-urämische Syndrome. Bilaterale Nierenrindennekrosen bei akuten erworbenen hämolytischen Anämien. *Schweiz. Med. Wschr.*, **85**, 905.

Gaynor, E., Bouvier, C. A. & Spaet, T. H. (1968) Circulating endothelial cells in endotoxin-treated rabbits. *Clinical Research*, **16**, 535.

George, C. R. P., Slichter, S. J., Quadracci, L. J., Striker, G. E. & Harker, L. A. (1974) Kinetic evaluation of hemostasis in renal disease. *New Eng. J. Med.*, **291**, 1111.

Gérard, O., Moriau, M., Bachy, A., Malvaux, P. & DeMeyer, R. (1973) Meningococcal purpura: Report of 19 patients treated with heparin. *J. Pediat.*, **82**, 780.

Gervais, M., Richardson, J. B., Chiu, J. & Drummond, K. N. (1971) Immunofluorescent and histologic findings in the hemolytic uremic syndrome. *Pediat.*, **47**, 352.

Gianantonio, C., Vitacco, M., Meddilaharzu, F., Rutty, A. & Mendilaharzu, J. (1964) The hemolytic-uremic syndrome. *J. Pediat.*, **64**, 478.

Gianantonio, C. A., Vitacco, M. & Mendilaharzu, F. (1966) The hemolytic-uremic syndrome. *Proc. 3rd Int. Congr. Nephrol. Washington*, **3**, 24.

Gianantonio, C. A., Vitacco, M., Mendilaharzu, F., Gallo, G. E. & Sojo, E. T. (1973) The hemolytic-uremic syndrome. *Nephron*, **11**, 174.

Gieske, J. C. (1972) Heparin therapy. *New Eng. J. Med.*, **287**, 1102.

Gilchrist, G. S., Ekert, H., Shawbrom, E. & Hammond, D. (1969) Evaluation of a new concentrate for the treatment of factor IX deficiency. *New Eng. J. Med.*, **280**, 291.

Giromoni, M., Bouvier, C. A., Dami, R., Denizot, M. & Jeannet, M. (1972) Effect of dipyridamole and aspirin in thrombotic microangiopathy. *Brit. med. J.*, **i**, 545.

Glasgow, L. A. & Balduzzi, P. (1965) Isolation of coxsackie virus, group A, type 4 from a patient with hemolytic uremic syndrome. *New Eng. J. Med.*, **273**, 754.

Glass, R. D. (1962) Purpura gangrenosa: Report of a case, with discussion of the Shwartzman phenomenon. *Med. J. Australia*, **49**, 300.

Glueck, H. I., Sutherland, J. & Gleser, G. (1964) Prothrombin levels during the first year of life. *Am. J. Dis. Child.*, **107**, 612.

Glueck, H. I., Will, R. M., McAdams, A. J. & Gleser, G. (1970) Measurement of prothrombin. A neglected liver function test in infancy and childhood. *J. Pediat.*, **76**, 914.

Goldfine, I. D., Schachter, H., Barclay, W. R. & Kingdon, H. S. (1969) Consumption coagulopathy miliary tuberculosis. *Ann. Intern. Med.*, **71**, 775.

Goldman, H. I. & Deposito, F. (1966) Hypoprothrombinemic bleeding in young infants. *Am. J. Dis. Child.*, **111**, 430.

Gordon, R. R. & Dean, T. (1955) Foetal deaths from antenatal anticoagulant therapy. *Brit. med. J.*, **ii**, 719.

Gralnick, H. R. & Henderson, E. (1971) Hypofibrinogenemia and coagulation factor deficiencies with L-asparaginase treatment. *Cancer*, **27**, 1313.

Gray, O. P., Ackerman, A. & Fraser, A. J. (1968) Intracranial haemorrhage and clotting defects in low-birth-weight infants. *Lancet*, **i**, 545.

Gross, S. & Melhorn, D. K. (1971) Exchange transfusion with citrated whole blood for disseminated intravascular coagulation. *J. Pediat.*, **78**, 415.

Grossi, C. E., Moreno, A. H. & Rousselot, L. M. (1961) Studies on spontaneous fibrinolytic activity in patients with cirrhosis of the liver and its inhibition by epsilon amino caproic acid. *Ann. Surg.*, **153**, 383.

Grossi, C. E., Rousselot, L. M. & Panke, W. F. (1964) Control of fibrinolysis during portocaval shunts. *J. Am. Med. Ass.*, **187**, 1005.

Hammond, D. & Lieberman, E. (1970) The hemolytic uremic syndrome. Renal cortical thrombotic microangiopathy. *Arch. Intern. Med.*, **126**, 816.

Handley, D. A. & Lawrence, J. R. (1967) Factor-IX deficiency in the nephrotic syndrome. *Lancet*, **i**, 1079.

Hardaway, R. M., Elovitz, M. J., Brewster, W. R. & Houchin, D. N. (1964) Clotting time of heparinized blood. *Archives of Surgery*, **89**, 701.

Harker, L. A. & Slichter, S. J. (1970) Studies of platelet and fibrinogen kinetics in patients with prosthetic heart valves. *New Eng. J. Med.*, **283**, 1303.

Harker, L. A. & Slichter, S. J. (1972) Platelet and fibrinogen consumption in man. *New Eng. J. Med.*, **287**, 999.

Harker, L. A., Slichter, S. J., Scott, C. R. & Ross, R. (1974) Homocystinemia. Vascular injury and arterial thrombosis. *New Eng. J. Med.*, **291**, 537.

Hartmann, J. R., Howell, D. A. & Diamond, L. K. (1955) Disorders of blood coagulation during the first week of life. *Am. J. Dis. Child.*, **90**, 594.

Hassanein, E. A. & Tankovsky, I. (1974) Disseminated intravascular clotting in kwashiorkor. *Arch. Dis. Childh.*, **50**, 308.

Hathaway, W. E., Mull, M. M. & Pechet, C. S. (1969) Disseminated intravascular coagulation in the newborn. *Pediatrics*, **43**, 233.

Hathaway, W. E. (1970A) Coagulation problems in the newborn infant. *Pediat. Clin. N. Amer.*, **17**, 929.

Hathaway, W. E. (1970B) Fibrin split products in serum of newborn: Possible technical errors. *Pediatrics*, **45**, 154.

Hathaway, W. E. (1970C) Care of the critically ill child: The problem of disseminated intravascular coagulation. *Pediatrics*, **46**, 767.

Hathaway, W. E. (1973) Editorial: Heparin therapy in acute meningococcemia. *J. Pediat.*, **82**, 900.

Hattersley, P. G. (1970) Purpura fulminans: Complete recovery with intravenously administered heparin. *Amer. J. Dis. Child.*, **120**, 467.

Haynes, R. E., Sanders, D. Y. & Crablett, H. G. (1970) Rocky Mountain spotted fever in children. *J. Pediat.*, **76**, 685.

Hedner, U. & Nillson, I. M. (1971) Clinical experience with determination of fibrinogen degradation products. *Acta Med. Scand.*, **189**, 471.

Henriksson, P., Nilsson, I. M., Bergentz, S.-E., Ljungqvist, U. & Rosengren, B. (1971) Giant haemangioma with a disorder of coagulation. *Acta Paediat. Scand.*, **60**, 227.

Hillman, R. S. & Phillips, L. L. (1967) Clotting fibrinolysis in a cavernous hemangioma. *Amer. J. Dis. Child.*, **113**, 649.

Hitzig, W. H., Straub, P. W., Lo, S. S. & Frick, P. G. (1968) Clinical experience with anticoagulant therapy in the management of disseminated intravascular coagulation in children. *Proc. Roy. Soc. Med.*, **61**, 1138.

Hjort, P. F., Rapaport, S. I. & Jorgensen, L. (1964) Purpura fulminans. Report of a case successfully treated with heparin and hydrocortisone. Review of 50 cases from the literature. *Scandinav. J. Haemat.*, **1**, 169.

Hoyer, J. R., Michael, A. R. & Hoyer, L. W. (1974) Antihemophilic factor antigen: Localization in endothelial cells by immunofluorescent microscopy. *J. Clin. Invest.*, **52**, 2737.

Hull, M. G. R. (1972) Perinatal coagulopathies complicating fetal blood sampling. *Brit. med. J.*, **iv**, 319.

Hull, M. G. R. & Wilson, J. A. (1972) Massive scalp haemorrhage after fetal blood sampling due to haemorrhagic disease. *Brit. med. J.*, **iv**, 321.

Ihenacho, H. N. C., Breeze, G. R., Fletcher, D. J. & Stuart, J. (1973) Consumption coagulopathy in congenital heart disease. *Lancet*, **i**, 231.

Inglis, T. C. McN., Breeze, G. R., Stuart, J., Abrams, L. D., Roberts, K. D. & Singh, S. P. (1975) Excess intravascular coagulation complicating low cardiac output. *J. Clin. Path.*, **28**, 1.

Inness, Elizabeth. Personal communication.

Iolster, N. J. (1970) Blood coagulation in children with cyanotic congenital heart disease. *Acta Paediat. Scand.*, **59**, 551.

Jaffe, E. A., Nachman, R. L. & Merskey, C. (1973) Thrombotic thrombocytopenic purpura—coagulation parameters in twelve patients. *Blood*, **42**, 499.

Johnson, C. A., Abildgaard, C. F. & Schulman, I. (1968) Absence of coagulation abnormalities in children with cyanotic congenital heart disease. *Lancet*, **ii**, 660.

Kakker, V. V., Corrigan, T., Spindler, J., Fossard, D. P., Flute, P. T., Crellin, R. Q., Wessler, S. & Yin, E. T. (1972) Efficacy of low doses of heparin in prevention of deep-vein thrombosis after major surgery. *Lancet*, **ii**, 101.

Kaplan, B. S., Katz, J., Krawitz, S. & Lurie, A. (1971) An analysis of the results of therapy in 67 cases of the hemolytic uremic syndrome. *J. Pediat.*, **78**, 420.

Karitzky, D., Kleine, N., Pringsheim, W. & Kunzer, W. (1971) Fibrinogen turnover in the premature infant with and without idiopathic respiratory distress syndrome. *Acta Paediat. Scand.*, **60**, 465.

Karpatkin, M. (1970) Fibrin split products in serum of newborn: Possible technical errors. *Pediatrics*, **45**, 157.

Karpatkin, M. (1971) Diagnosis and management of disseminated intravascular coagulation. *Pediat. Clin. N. Amer.*, **18**, 23.

Kasabach, H. H. & Merritt, K. K. (1940) Capillary hemangioma with extensive purpura. *Am. J. Dis. Child.*, **59**, 1063.

Katz, J., Lurie, A., Kaplaw, B. S., Krawitz, S. & Metz, J. (1971) Coagulation findings in the hemolytic-uremic syndrome of infancy: Similarity to hyperacute renal allograft rejection. *J. Pediat.*, **78**, 426.

Katz, J., Krawitz, S., Sacks, P. V., Levin, S. E., Thomson, P., Levin, J. & Metz, J. (1973) Platelet, erythrocyte and fibrinogen kinetics in the hemolytic-uremic syndrome of infancy. *J. Pediat.*, **83**, 739.

Kaulla, K. N. von (1964) Liver in regulation of fibrinolytic activity. *Lancet*, **1**, 1046.

Kaulla, K. N. von, Kaulla, E. von & Butterfield, J. (1965) Fibrinolytic activity, thrombin inhibitor and kinetics of clot formation in premature infants with respiratory distress syndrome. *Acta Paediat. Scand.*, **54**, 587.

Kaulla, K. N. von, Paton, B. C., Rosenkrantz, J. G., Kaulla E. von, & Wasantapruek, S. (1967) Pre-operative correction of coagulation in tetralogy of Fallot. *Arch. Surg.*, **94**, 107.

Keay, A. J. & Uttley, W. S. (1973) Haemorrhagic disorders of the newborn. In *Textbook of Paediatrics*. Edited by Forfar, J. O. and Arneil, G. C. London: Churchill Livingstone.

Keenan, W. J., Jewett, T. & Glueck, H. I. (1971) Role of feeding and vitamin K in hypothrombinemia of the newborn. *Amer. J. Dis. Child.*, **121**, 271.

Kibel, M. A. & Barnard, P. J. (1964) Treatment of acute haemolytic-uraemic syndrome with heparin. *Lancet*, **2**, 259.

Kisker, C. T. & Rush, R. (1971) Detection of intravascular coagulation. *J. Clin. Invest.*, **50**, 2235.

Kisker, C. T. & Mauer, A. M. (1972) Bleeding and infection. *Am. J. Dis. Child.*, **124**, 483.

Kisker, C. T. & Rush, R. (1973) Circulating fibrin in meningococcemia. *J. Pediat.*, **82**, 787.

Komp, D. M. & Donaldson, M. H. (1970) Sepsis in leukemia and the Shwartzman reaction. *Amer. J. Dis. Child.*, **119**, 114.

Komp, D. M. & Sparrow, A. W. (1970) Polycythemia in cyanotic heart disease—a study of altered coagulation. *J. Pediat.*, **76**, 231.

Kontras, S. B., Sirak, H. D. & Newton, W. A. (1966) Hematologic abnormalities in children with congenital heart disease. *J.A.M.A.*, **195**, 611.

Krevans, J. R., Jackson, D. P., Cowley, C. L. & Hartman, R. C. (1957) The nature of the haemorrhagic disorder accompanying hemolytic transfusion reaction in man. *Blood*, **12**, 834.

Künzer, W. & Aalam, F. (1964) Treatment of the acute haemolytic uraemic syndrome with heparin. *Lancet*, **1**, 1106.

Lahnborg, G., Bergström, K., Friman, L. & Lagergren, H. (1974) Effect of low-dose heparin on incidence of post-operative pulmonary embolism detected by photoscanning. *Lancet*, **1**, 329.

Lancet (1972) Editorial: Control of heparin therapy. *Lancet*, **ii**, 524.

Lancet (1972) Editorial: FDP. *Lancet*, **ii**, 957.

Lanzkowsky, P. & McCrory, W. (1967) Disseminated intravascular coagulation as a possible factor in the patho-genesis of thrombotic microangiopathy (Hemolytic uremic syndrome). *J. Pediat.*, **70**, 460.

Larrieu, M. J., Rigollot, C. & Marder, V. J. (1972) Comparative effects of fibrinogen degradation fragments D and E on coagulation. *Brit. J. Haemat.*, **22**, 719.

Leavitt, T. J., Merigan, T. C. & Freeman, J. M. (1971) Hemolytic-uremic-like syndrome following polycarboxylate interferon induction—Treatment of Dawson's inclusion-body encephalitis. *Amer. J. Dis. Child.*, **121**, 43.

Lee, L. (1963) Antigen-antibody reaction in the pathogenesis of bilateral renal cortical necrosis. *J. Exp. Med.*, **117**, 365.

Leissring, J. & Vorlicky, L. (1968) Disseminated intravascular coagulation in a neonate. *Amer. J. Dis. Child.*, **115**, 100.

Lelong, M., Alagille, D. & Odievre, M. (1964) La forme neo-natale tardine de 1-avitaminase K aiguë idiopathique. *Nouv. Rev. Franç. Hemat.*, **4**, 173.

Lieberman, E., Heuser, E., Donnell, G. N., Landing, B. H. & Hammond, G. D. (1966) Hemolytic-uremic syndrome. Clinical and pathological considerations. *New Eng. J. Med.*, **275**, 227.

Little, J. E. (1959) Purpura fulminans treated successfully with anticoagulation. Post infective intravascular throm-bosis with gangrene. *J.A.M.A.*, **169**, 36.

Lock, S. P. & Dormandy, K. M. (1961) Red-cell fragmentation syndrome. A condition of multiple aetiology? *Lancet*, **1**, 1020.

McElfresh, A. E. (1961) Coagulation during the neonatal period. *Amer. J. Med. Sci.*, **242**, 771.

McKay, D. G. (1965) *Disseminated Intravascular Coagulation: An Intermediary Mechanism of Disease*. New York: Hoeber.

McKay, D. G. & Margaretten, W. (1967) Disseminated intravascular coagulation in virus diseases. *Arch. Intern. Med.*, **120**, 129.

McLean, M. M., Hilton-Jones, C. & Sutherland, D. A. (1966) Haemolytic-uraemic syndrome. *Arch. Dis. Childh.*, **41**, 76.

McMillan, C. W. & Elston, C. R. (1968) Plasma factor VIII activity in capillary and venous blood samples. *J. Lab. Clin. Med.*, **71**, 412.

McMillan, C. W., Gaudry, C. L. & Holemans, R. (1968) Coagulation defects and metastatic neuroblastoma. *J. Pediat.*, **72**, 347.

McMillan, C. W., Weiss, A. E. & Johnson, A. M. (1972) Acquired coagulation disorders in children. *Pediat. Clinics, N. Amer.*, **19**, 1029.

MacWhinney, J. B., Packer, J. T., Miller, G. & Greendyke, R. M. (1962) Thrombotic thrombocytopenic purpura in childhood. *Blood*, **19**, 181.

Mandal, B. K. & McNulty, M. (1971) Treatment of haemolytic-uraemic syndrome with phenformin and ethyl-oestrenol. *Lancet*, **11**, 1036. (Letter).

Mannucci, P. M., Lobina, G. F., Caocci, L. & Dioguardi, N. (1969) Effect on blood coagulation of massive intra-vascular haemolysis. *Blood*, **33**, 207.

Marder, V. J. & Shulman, N. R. (1969) High molecular weight derivatives of human fibrinogen produced by plas-min. II. Mechanism of their anticoagulant activity. *J. Biol. Chem.*, **244**, 2120.

Margolis, C. Z., Orzalesi, M. M. & Schwartz, A. D. (1973) Disseminated intravascular coagulation in the respiratory distress syndrome. *Am. J. Dis. Child.*, **125**, 324.

Margolius, A., Jackson, D. P. & Ratnoff, O. D. (1961) Circulating anticoagulants: A study of 40 cases and a review of the literature. *Medicine (Baltimore)*, **40**, 145.

Markarian, M., Githens, J. H., Rosenblüt, E., Fernandez, F., Jackson, J. J., Bannon, A. E., Lindley, A., Lubchenco, L. O. & Martorell, R. (1971A). Hypercoagulability in premature infants with special reference to the respira-tory distress syndrome and hemorrhage. I. Coagulation studies. *Biol. Neonate*, **17**, 84.

Markarian, M., Lubchenco, L. O., Rosenblüt, E., Fernandez, F., Lang, D., Jackson, J. J., Bannon, A. E., Lindley, A., Githens, J. H. & Martorell, R. (1971B) Hypercoagulability in premature infants with special reference to the respiratory distress syndrome and hemorrhage. II. The effect of heparin. *Biol. Neonate*, **17**, 98.

Markarian, M., Cohen, R. J. & Milbauer, B. (1971C). Disseminated intravascular coagulation in a neonate treated with heparin. *J. Pediatrics*, **78**, 74.

Martius, C. (1967) Chemistry and function of vitamin K. In *Blood Clotting Enzymology*. Edited by W. H. Seeger. New York: Academic Press.

Matoth, Y. (1950) Plasma prothrombin in infantile diarrhoea. *Am. J. Dis. Child.*, **80**, 944.

Maurer, H. M. (1972) Hematologic effects of cardiac disease. *Ped Clin. N. Amer.*, **19**, 1083.

Maurer, H. M., McCue, C. M., Caul, J. & Still, W. J. S. (1972) Impairment in platelet aggregation in congenital heart disease. *Blood*, **40**, 207.

Merskey, C. & Hansen, J. D. L. (1957) Blood coagulation defects in kwashiorkor and infantile gastroenteritis. *Brit. J. Haemat.*, **3**, 309.

Merskey, C., Johnson, A. J., Pert, J. H. & Wohl, H. (1964) Pathogenesis of fibrinolysis in defibrination syndrome: Effect of heparin administration. *Blood*, **24**, 701.

Merskey, C., Kleiner, G. J. & Johnson, A. J. (1966) Quantitative estimation of split products of fibrinogen in human serum, relation to diagnosis and treatment. *Blood*, **28**, 1.

Merskey, C., Johnson, A. J., Kleiner, G. J. & Wohl, H. (1967) The defibrination syndrome: Clinical features and laboratory diagnosis. *Brit. J. Haemat.*, **13**, 528.

Miller, D. R., Hanshaw, J. B., O'Leary, D. S. & Hnilicka, J. V. (1970) Fatal disseminated herpes simplex virus infection and hemorrhage in the neonate. Coagulation studies in a case and a review. *J. Pediat.*, **76**, 409.

Moncrieff, M. W. & Glasgow, E. F. (1970) Haemolytic-uraemic syndrome treated with heparin. *Brit. med. J.*, **iii**, 188.

Monnens, L. & Schretlen, E. (1967) Intravascular coagulation in an infant with the hemolytic-uremic syndrome. *Acta Paediat. Scandinav.*, **56**, 436.

Monnens, L. & Schretlen, E. (1968) Haemolytic-uraemic syndrome. *Lancet*, **2**, 735.

Monnens, L. A. H. (1973) Localized intravascular coagulation. *Postgrad. Medical Journal* (Aug. Supple. 73), 102.

Moore, C. M., McAdams, A. J. & Sutherland, J. (1969) Intrauterine disseminated intravascular coagulation: A syndrome of multiple pregnancy with a dead fetus. *J. Pediat.*, **74**, 523.

Mosesson, M. W., Colman, R. W. & Sherry, S. (1968) Chronic intravascular coagulation syndrome: Report of a case with special studies of an associated cryoprecipitate ('cryofibrinogen'). *New Eng. J. Med.*, **278**, 815.

Mountain, K. R., Hirsh, J. & Gallus, A. S. (1970) Neonatal coagulation defect due to anticonvulsant drug treatment in pregnancy. *Lancet*, **1**, 265.

Murphy, A. V. & Willoughby, M. L. N. (1976) (in press).

Naiman, J. L. (1970) Clotting and bleeding in cyanotic congenital heart disease. *J. Pediat.*, **76**, 333.

Nammacher, M. A., Willeman, M., Hartman, J. R. & Gaston, L. W. (1970) Vitamin K deficiency beyond the neonatal period. *J. Pediat.*, **76**, 549.

Neame, P. B., Lechago, J., Ling, E. T. & Koval, A. (1973) Thrombotic thrombocytopenic purpura: Report of a case with disseminated intravascular platelet-aggregation. *Blood*, **42**, 805.

Negus, D., Pintó, D. J. & Slack, W. W. (1971) Effect of small doses of heparin on platelet adhesiveness and lipoprotein-lipase activity before and after surgery. *Lancet*, **i**, 1202.

Noren, I., Carlsson, E., Kretzschmar, G. & Teger-Nilsson, A.-C. (1971) Prothrombin in newborns and during the first year of life. *Acta Paediat. Scand.*, **60**, 269.

O'Brien, J. R., Etherington, M., Jamieson, S. & Klaber, M. R. (1972A) Platelet function in venous thrombosis and low-dosage heparin. *Lancet*, **i**, 1302.

O'Brien, J. R., Etherington, M. & Jamieson, S. (1972B) Heparin-induced platelet release and refractory platelets. *Lancet*, **ii**, 233.

Ogston, D., Ogston, C. M., Ratnoff, O. D. & Forbes, C. D. (1969) Studies on a complex mechanism for the activation of plasminogen by kaolin and chloroform: The participation of Hageman factor and additional cofactors. *J. Clin. Invest.*, **48**, 1786.

O'Neill, B. J. & Hutton, R. A. (1966) Prolonged bleeding time in congenital heart disease. *J. Clin. Path.*, **19**, 99.

Oski, F. A. & Naiman, J. L. (1972) *Hematologic Problems in the Newborn*, p. 256. Philadelphia: Saunders.

Owren, P. A. (1949) The diagnostic and prognostic significance of plasma prothrombin and factor V levels in parenchymatous hepatitis and obstructive jaundice. *Scand. J. Clin. Lab. Invest.*, **1**, 131.

Owren, P. A. & Aas, K. (1951) The control of dicoumarol therapy and the quantitative determination of prothrombin and proconvertin. *Scand. J. Clin. Lab. Invest.*, **3**, 201.

Owren, P. A. (1959) Thrombotest, a new method for controlling anticoagulant therapy. *Lancet*, **ii**, 754.

Panagopoulos, G., Valoes, T. & Doxiadis, S. A. (1969) Morbidity and mortality related to exchange transfusion. *J. Pediat.*, **74**, 247.

Paterson, J. H., Pierce, R. B., Amerson, J. R. & Watkins, W. L. (1965) Dextran therapy of purpura fulminans. *New Eng. J. Med.*, **273**, 734.

Philippidis, P., Naiman, J. L., Sibinga, M. S. & Valdes-Dapnea, M. A. (1971) Disseminated intravascular coagulation in candida albicans septicaemia. *J. Pediat.*, **78**, 683.

Phillips, L. L. & Skrodelis, V. (1958) A comparison of the fibrinolytic enzyme system in maternal and umbilical cord blood. *Pediatrics*, **22**, 715.

Piel, C. F. & Phibbs, R. H. (1966) The hemolytic-uremic syndrome. *Pediat. Clin. N. Amer.*, **13**, 295.

Pool, J. G. & Robinson, J. (1959) *In vitro* synthesis of coagulation factors by rat liver slices. *Am. J. Physiol.*, **196**, 423.

Powell, H. R. & Ekert, H. (1974) Streptokinase and anti-thrombotic therapy in the hemolytic-uremic syndrome. *J. Pediat.*, **84**, 345.

Proctor, R. R. & Papaport, S. I. (1961) The partial thromboplastin time with kaolin. *Am. J. Clin. Path.*, **36**, 212.

Rake, M. O., Flute, P. T., Shilkin, K. B., Lewis, M. L., Winch, J. & Williams, R. (1971) Early and intensive therapy of intravascular coagulation in acute liver failure. *Lancet*, **ii**, 1215.

Rapaport, S. & Dodd, K. (1946) Hypoprothrombinemia in infants with diarrhoea. *Am. J. Dis. Child.*, **71**, 611.

Rapaport, S. I., Patch, M. J. & Moore, F. J. (1960) Antihemophilic globulin levels in carriers of hemophilia A. *J. Clin. Invest.*, **39**, 1619.

Rapaport, S. I., Tatter, D., Coeuv-Barron, N. & Hjort, P. F. (1964) Pseudomonas septicemia with intravascular clotting leading to the generalized Shwartzman reaction. *New Eng. J. Med.*, **271**, 80.

Ray, C., Tucker, V. L., Harris, D. J., Cuppage, F. E. & Chin, T. D. Y. (1970) Enterovirus associated with the hemolytic-uremic syndrome. *Pediatrics*, **46**, 378.

Renfield, M. L. & Kraybill, E. N. (1973) Consumptive coagulopathy with renal vein thrombosis. *J. Pediatrics*, **82**, 1054.

Roberts, J. T., Gray, O. P. & Bloom, A. L. (1966) An abnormality of the thrombinfibrinogen reaction in the newborn. *Acta Paediat. Scand.*, **55**, 148.

Rodriguez-Erdmann, F. (1965) Bleeding due to increased intravascular blood coagulation. Hemorrhagic syndromes caused by consumption of blood-clotting factors (consumption coagulopathies). *New Eng. J. Med.*, **273**, 1370.

Rosen, S. M., Robinson, P. J. A., Allison, C. J. & Standish, H. G. (1970) Microangiopathic haemolytic anaemia. *Brit. med. J.*, **iii**, 465.

Rowsell, H. C., Glynn, M. F. Mustard, J. F. & Murphy, E. A. (1967) Effect of heparin on platelet economy in dogs. *Am. J. Physiol.*, **213**, 915.

Ruthven, I. S. & Fyfe, W. M. (1968) The haemolytic uraemic syndrome—an epidemic disease? *Scot. Med. J.*, **13**, 162.

Sack, E. S. & Buraschi, J. (1971) Fibrin degradation products. *New Eng. J. Med.*, **284**, 1441.

Salzman, E. W., Deykin, D., Shapiro, R. M. & Rosenberg, R. (1975) Management of heparin therapy: Controlled prospective trial. *New Eng. J. Med.*, **292**, 1046.

Sanchez Avalos, J., Vitacco, M., Molinas, F., Penalver, J. & Gianantonio, C. (1970) Coagulation studies in the hemolytic-uremic syndrome. *J. Pediat.*, **76**, 538.

Schwartz, A. D. (1971) The coagulation defect in Reye's syndrome. *J. Pediat.*, **78**, 326.

Seligsohn, U., Shani, M. & Ramot, B. (1970) Gilbert syndrome and factor VII deficiency. *Lancet*, **i**, 1398.

Sharpstone, P., Evans, R. G., O'Shea, M., Alexander, L. & Lee, H. A. (1968) Haemolytic uraemic syndrome: Survival after prolonged oliguria. *Arch. Dis. Childh.*, **43**, 711.

Skyberg, D. & Jacobsen, C. D. (1969) Defibrination syndrome in a newborn, and its treatment with exchange transfusion. *Acta Paediat. Scand.*, **58**, 83.

Smith, C. H. (1960) *Blood Diseases of Infancy and Childhood*, p. 478. St Louis: Mosby.

Spector, I. & Corn, M. (1967) Control of heparin therapy with activated partial thromboplastin times. *J.A.M.A.*, **201**, 157.

Stark, C. R., Abramson, D. & Erkan, V. (1968) Intravascular coagulation and hyaline membrane disease of the newborn. *Lancet*, **i**, 1180.

Steele, P. P., Weily, H. S., Davies, H. & Genton, E. (1974) Platelet survival in patients with rheumatic heart disease. *New Eng. J. Med.*, **290**, 537.

Stuart, R. K. & Michael, A. (1971) Monitoring heparin therapy with activated partial thromboplastin time. *Canad. Med. Assn. J.*, **104**, 385.

Stuart, M., Stockman, J., Murphy, S., Schutt, L., Ames, M., Urmson, J. & Oski, F. (1972) Shortened platelet lifespan in patients with hydrocephalus and ventriculo jugular shunts: Results of preliminary attempts at correction. *J. Pediat.*, **80**, 21.

Stuart, J., Picken, A. M., Breeze, G. R. & Wood, B. S. B. (1973) Capillary-blood coagulation in the newborn. *Lancet*, **ii**, 1467.

Stuart, J., Winterborn, M. H., White, R. H. R. & Flinn, R. M. (1974) Thrombolytic therapy in haemolytic-uraemic syndrome. *Brit. med. J.*, **iii**, 217.

Sutherland, J. M. (1963) Observations on the relationships between drug therapy and neonatal jaundice. *Ann. N.Y. Acad. Sci.*, **111**, 461.

Sutherland, J. M., Glueck, H. I. & Gleser, H. (1967) Hemorrhagic disease of the newborn: Breast feeding as a necessary factor in the pathogenesis. *Am. J. Dis. Child.*, **113**, 524.

Taj-Eldin, S., Al-Nouri, L. & Fakri, O. (1967) Haemorrhagic diathesis in children associated with vitamin K deficiency. *J. Clin. Path.*, **20**, 252.

Thatcher, L., Clatanoff, D. & Stiehm, E. (1968) Splenic hemangioma with thrombocytopenia and afibrinogenemia. *J. Pediat.*, **73**, 345.

Thomas, L. & Good, R. A. (1952) The effect of cortisone on the Shwartzman reaction. The production of lesions resembling the dermal and generalized Shwartzman reaction by a single injection of bacterial toxin in cortisone treated rabbits. *J. Exper. Med.*, **95**, 409.

Thomas, D. P., Niewiarowski, S., Myers, A. R., Bloch, K. J. & Colman, R. W. (1970) A comparative study of four methods for detecting fibrinogen degradation products in patients with various diseases. *New Eng. J. Med.*, **283**, 663.

Touloukian, R. J. (1969) Idiopathic vena caval thrombosis with renal infarction in the newborn infant: Survival following nephrectomy. *Surgery*, **65**, 978.

Towbin, A. (1968) Cerebral intraventricular hemorrhage and subependymal matrix infarction in the fetus and premature infant. *Amer. J. Path.*, **52**, 121.

Townsend, C. W. (1894) The hemorrhagic disease of the newborn. *Arch. Pediat.*, **11**, 559.

Trueb, O., Willi, H., Siebenmann, R., Hitzig, W. H. & Frick, P. G. (1964) Purpura fulminans bei einem neugeborenen. Ein therapieversuch mit antikoagulantien. *Helv. Paediat. Acta*, **19**, 223.

Tullis, J. L., Melin, M. & Jurigian, P. (1965) Clinical use of human prothrombin complexes. *New Eng. J. Med.*, **273**, 667.

Tune, B. M., Levitt, T. J. & Gribble, T. J. (1973) The hemolytic-uremic syndrome in California. A review of 28 non-heparinised cases with long-term follow-up. *J. Pediat.*, **82**, 304.

Uttley, W. S. (1970) Serum levels of fibrin/fibrinogen degradation products in the haemolytic-uraemic syndrome. *Arch. Dis Childh.*, **45**, 587.

Verstraete, M., Vermylen, C., Vermylen, J. & Vandenbroucke, J. (1965) Excessive consumption of blood coagulation components as cause of hemorrhagic diathesis. *Am. J. Med.*, **38**, 899.

Volpe, J. (1974) Neonatal intracranial hemorrhage—iatrogenic etiology? *New Eng. J. Med.*, **291**, 43.

Waddell, N. W., Guerry, P. du, Bray, W. E. & Kelley, O. R. (1939) Possible effects of vitamin K on prothrombin and clotting time in newly-born infants. *Proc. Soc. Exp. Biol. Med.*, **40**, 432.

Weily, H. S., Steele, P. P., Davies, H., Pappas, G. & Genton, E. (1974) Platelet survival in patients with substitute heart valves. *New Eng. J. Med.*, **290**, 534.

Whaun, J. M., Urmson, J. & Oski, F. A. (1971) One year's experience with disseminated intravascular coagulation in a children's hospital. *Program. Am. Ped. Soc.*, p. 6. Quoted in Oski and Naiman (1972. p. 258.)

Willoughby, M. L. N., McMorris, S. & Goel, K. M. (1972A) Disseminated intravascular coagulation in meningococcal infection. *Arch. Dis. Childh.*, **47**, 324.

Willoughby, M. L. N., Murphy, A. V., McMorris, S. & Jewell, F. G. (1972B) Coagulation studies in haemolytic uraemic syndrome. *Arch. Dis. Childh.*, **47**, 766.

Winkelstein, A., Songster, C. L., Caras, T. S., Berman, H. H. & West, W. L. (1969) Fulminant meningococcemia and disseminated intravascular coagulation. *Archives of Internal Med.*, **124**, 55.

Winterborn, M. H., White, R. H. R. & Stuart, J. (1972) Fibrinolytic treatment of the haemolytic-uraemic syndrome. *Lancet*, **i**, 1071.

Witt, I., Muller, H. & Kunzer, W. (1969) Evidence for the existence of foetal fibrinogen. *Thromb. Diath. Haemorr.*, **22**, 107.

Wochner, D., Kulapongs, P. & Bachmann, F. (1967) ^{125}I-fibrinogen turnover and coagulation studies in a patient with Kasabach-Merritt syndrome. *J. Lab. Clin. Med.*, **70**, 997.

Yin, E. T., Wessler, S. & Stole, P. J. (1971) Biological properties of the naturally occurring plasma inhibitor to activated factor X. *J. Biol. Chem.*, **246**, 3703.

Yin, E. T., Giudice, L. C. & Wessler, S. (1973A) Inhibition of activated factor X-induced platelet aggregation by the plasma inhibitor to activated factor X and heparin. *IVth Int. Congress on Thrombosis and Haemostasis*, p. 270. Vienna: Springer Verlag.

Yin, E. T., Wessler, S. & Butler, J. V. (1973B) Plasma heparin: A unique practical, submicrogram-sensitive assay. *J. Lab. Clin. Med.*, **81**, 298.

Zetterqvist, E. & Francken, I. von (1963) Coagulation disturbances with manifest bleeding in extrahepatic portal hypertension and in liver cirrhosis. Preliminary results of heparin treatment. *Acta Med. Scand.*, **173**, 753.

20. Leukaemia and Related Disorders

Incidence of leukaemia in childhood / Aetiology of leukaemia / Cell kinetic considerations / Diagnosis of acute leukaemia / Haematological findings in acute leukaemia / Management of acute leukaemia, *Remission induction, Supportive treatment during remission induction, CNS prophylaxis, Treatment of overt meningeal leukaemia, Maintenance therapy* / Factors affecting prognosis, *Unusual types of childhood leukaemia, Non-leukaemic disorders with infiltration of the marrow.*

'Leukaemia is a major killer of children and is second only to accidents as a cause of death in children between one and fourteen years of age' (Lascari, 1973). It is a malignant proliferation of haemic precursor cells primarily affecting the bone marrow, but secondarily involving the peripheral blood and many other tissues, particularly those of the reticuloendothelial system. It is usually possible to classify a case of leukaemia according to the cell type involved in the malignant proliferation. When this is a 'blast' cell (e.g. myeloblast) the leukaemia is termed 'acute' since the untreated disease would be rapidly fatal. When the proliferation predominantly involves a more mature cell type (e.g. myelocyte) the leukaemia is classified as 'chronic'. In children, unlike adults, leukaemia is nearly always of the acute, blast cell type; and, again unlike adults, it is predominantly lymphoblastic rather than myeloblastic. The proportions of different types of leukaemia found in a survey of 1,770 children by Pierce, Borges, Heyn, Wolff and Gilbert (1969) were as follows:

Acute lymphoblastic or undifferentiated	77·96 per cent
Acute myeloblastic	8·47 per cent
Acute monocytic	8·25 per cent
Erythromyeloid (acute)	0·67 per cent
Chronic myelocytic	1·24 per cent
Leukaemic transformation of lymphosarcoma	1·80 per cent
Type not recorded	1·61 per cent

Acute lymphoblastic leukaemia (ALL) is the characteristic leukaemia of childhood. It is sometimes referred to as acute lymphocytic leukaemia, since in histology sections it is difficult to distinguish lymphoblasts from lymphocytes. It is also sometimes called 'stem cell' leukaemia (ASL) since the precise lymphoid origin of these cells is perhaps debatable. A proportion of blast cells remain unclassifiable or undifferentiated (AUL).

Since many cases of myeloblastic leukaemia show simultaneous monocytic or monoblastic proliferation in blood or marrow it is realistic to group these two together as myeloblastic (AML) and myelomonocytic (AMMoL), which together constitute 15–16 per cent of childhood leukaemia.

Tumours arising primarily from outside the bone marrow may on occasions enter a leukaemic phase with the malignant cells being found in the marrow and blood. Although this 'leukaemic transformation' is rare in adults (3 per cent) it is common in children with lymphosarcoma, occurring in around 30 per cent (Jones and Klingberg, 1963). The resultant disease is indistinguishable from ALL apart from the history of preceding localized tumour. Reticulum cell sarcoma can similarly give rise to a pure monocytic leukaemia referred to as the 'Schilling type' (Berkheiser, 1957), in contradistinction to the 'Naegeli type' of myelomonocytic leukaemia of haemic origin mentioned above. On rare occasions disseminated neuroblastoma may involve not only the marrow but also the peripheral blood. These and other rare causes of leukaemic manifestations such as Burkitt's lymphoma, leukaemic reticuloendotheliosis and familial erythrophagocytic lymphohistiocytosis are therefore included in this chapter.

INCIDENCE OF LEUKAEMIA IN CHILDHOOD

Iversen (1966) found the incidence in Danish children aged 0–14 years to be 4·4 for boys and 3·2 for girls per 100,000 of population. He calculated the risk of a child developing acute leukaemia during the first 14 years of life as 65 ± 4 per 100,000 for boys and 46 ± 3 per 100,000 for girls.

Miller (1967) calculated this chance as 1 in 2,880 (or 34·7 per 100,000 children) for white American children.

The peak incidence occurs between the ages of 2 and 4 years among white children (Cutler *et al.*, 1967; Zippin *et al.*, 1971), but it is only recently that a similar peak is beginning to appear in Japanese and black American children, at 3 and 4 years respectively (Fraumeni and Miller, 1967). In AML there is a much less pronounced peak at 2 years (Pierce *et al.*, 1969). Other relevant surveys include those by Court-Brown and Doll (1961) in the U.K., and Ederer *et al.* (1965) in the U.S. There is no great variation from country to country (Kessler and Lilienfeld, 1969).

After an apparent increase in incidence between 1940 and 1960 the incidence is now declining slightly, and cannot be attributed to increased survival from treatment (Miller, 1969).

AETIOLOGY OF LEUKAEMIA

In animals leukaemia can be induced by oncogenic viruses, chemical carcinogens or irradiation, with hereditary factors strongly determining the degree of susceptibility to these agents (Henderson, 1973). In man the cause of leukaemia remains unknown. Human leukaemogenesis is probably multifactorial in origin with environmental factors such as radiation and infection interacting upon a constitutional or genetic predisposition.

Clustering in time and space suggests an environmental, perhaps, infective, cause. In Niles, Illinois, 8 children developed ALL within a 3-year period. Three attended the same school and 4 others had older siblings who had attended the same school (Heath and Hasterlik, 1963). Other examples of similar clusters have occurred including a convincing recent report of 5 young patients with ALL and an older man with lymphosarcoma occurring in an Irish village within a period of 4½ years (Kemmoona, 1974). But prospective studies have given divergent results (Till *et al.*, 1967; Lock and Merrington, 1967; Powell, 1971). Present evidence suggests that apparent clustering may occasionally occur by pure chance.

Viruses are the main cause of leukaemia in mice, rats, chickens and cats, and probably also in cattle, dogs and monkeys (Aisenberg, 1973; Jarrett, 1973). These are predominantly RNA 'oncorna' viruses with C type morphology on electron microscopy (EM). It would be strange if the human disease failed to conform, but in spite of a considerable volume of research directed to this question the hypothesis remains unproven (Allen and Cole,

1972). Direct EM identification of C type particles in leukaemic cells or plasma as originally reported by Dmochowski *et al.* (1959) has subsequently been shown to be inconstant and no more frequent than in controls (Smith *et al.*, 1967; Murphy and Zarafonetis, 1968; Newell *et al.*, 1968). Neither have attempts at viral culture given consistent results (Todaro *et al.*, 1970). These negative findings do not, however, exclude the possibility that viral genome may be incorporated into the host DNA, resulting in the production of viral protein and virus-induced neoantigens without structural virus being identifiable (Allen and Cole, 1972). Since the majority of viral candidates for human leukaemia are RNA viruses this would necessitate transcription in the reverse direction from normal, i.e. from RNA to DNA. Specific biochemical and immunological techniques are necessary to distinguish reverse transcriptase of viral origin from that of cellular origin, viz. that present in normal lymphocytes (*Lancet*, 1973). Using these stringent newer criteria reverse transcriptase of apparently viral origin has been identified in at least some human leukaemic cells including lymphoblasts and myeloblasts (Baxt *et al.*, 1972; Sarngadharan *et al.*, 1972; Todaro and Gallo, 1973). The biochemical mechanism therefore exists in these cells for introduction of DNA corresponding to the RNA pattern of tumour (oncorna) viruses into their permanent genetic make-up. Although not proof of viral participation in human leukaemogenesis the presence of this enzyme may be regarded as 'a footprint left in the sand' (*Lancet*, 1973). The present state of knowledge regarding the apparent isolation of a 'human leukaemia virus' is described in an annotation in the *Lancet* (1975A).

Fialkow's observation (1971) of leukaemic transformation of engrafted male marrow cells in a female patient with leukaemia should also be mentioned as relevant to the possibility of cell-to-cell transfer of oncogenicity by viral or other agents.

It has also been widely appreciated that the demonstration of tumour specific surface antigens on leukaemic cells would support a common viral origin. In experimental animals virus-induced tumours show antigenic cross-reactivity but chemically induced tumours do not. A variety of techniques including immunofluorescein-labelled antisera to presumed viral antigen (Fink *et al.*, 1964), serum cytotoxicity tests (Dore *et al.*, 1967), mixed leucocyte culture and delayed skin hypersensitivity tests (Henderson, 1973) have given a high incidence of positive results supporting the existence of common neoantigens on human leukaemic cells, but some cross-reactivity with immature cells from normal marrow also occurred (Yohn and Grace, 1966). The results from this approach are therefore currently inconclusive, although highly relevant to the concepts underlying immunotherapy.

In order to illustrate the complexities of viral oncogenesis in man it is useful to consider another lymphoblastic tumour, Burkitt's lymphoma. The current state of the evidence that the Epstein-Barr virus (EBV) has an oncogenic role in this human tumour has recently been reviewed by Epstein and Achong (1973). They regard the chain of evidence as now almost complete. 100 per cent of these patients carry the virus and the EBV genome is present in all the tumour cells. EBV belongs to the class of DNA herpes viruses rather than RNA oncorna virus discussed above. The point is made by Epstein and Achong that this type of virus can produce two distinct types of infection, 'productive' and 'non-productive' (Table 20.1). Clinical

expressed virus genome (Table 20.2a), indirectly responsible for the blood picture. All patients with infectious mononucleosis subsequently develop antibodies to EBV. Similarly all patients with Burkitt's lymphoma have antibodies to EBV implying previous infection, usually subclinical. But in addition these patients harbour EBV both as a 'non-productive' unexpressed infection of peripheral lymphoid cells (Table 20.1) and as EB viral genome within the Burkitt's tumour cells (Table 20.2b). These cells do not contain capsulated virus particles but the viral genome induces the formation of specific membrane neoantigens. Complexities such as these may explain why it is difficult to obtain conclusive evidence of viral leukaemogenesis in man, where ethical considerations preclude the fulfilment of Koch's postulates.

To explain why EBV produces only the limited lymphoproliferation in infectious mononucleosis but malignant lymphoproliferation in Burkitt's

Table 20.1 Infection of cells by herpes viruses

1. Productive   —Virus replication leading to cell death
2. Non-productive —Virus genome present:
  (a) Unexpressed, but often activated to a productive cycle
  (b) Expressed in a malignant transformation but can be activated to a production cycle.

From Epstein and Achong (1973), Lancet, ii, 836, by permission.

Table 20.2   Genetic diseases associated with leukaemia

Disease	Type of leukaemia	Reference
Down's syndrome	ALL, AML	Rosner *et al.*, (1972) *Am. J. Med.*, **53**, 203
Bloom's syndrome	AML	Sawitsky *et al.* (1966) *Ann. Intern. Med.*, **65**, 487
Kleinfelter's syndrome	ALL, AML, CML	Fraumeni and Miller (1967) *J. Natl. Cancer Inst.*, **38**, 593
D-Trisomy syndrome	AML	Fraumeni and Miller (1967) *J. Natl. Cancer Inst.*, **38**, 593
Congenital agammaglobulinaemia	ALL, CML	{ Page *et al.* (1963) *Blood*, **21**, 197 { Gatti and Good (1971) *Cancer*, **28**, 89
Ataxia-telangiectasia	ALL	Hecht *et al.*, (1966) *Lancet*, **ii**, 1193
Osteogenesis imperfecta	ALL	Gilchrist and Shore (1967) *J. Pediat.*, **71**, 115
Fanconi's anaemia	AML, AMOL, AMMOL	Dosik *et al.* (1970) *Blood*, **36**, 341
Wiskott-Aldrich syndrome	AML	ten Bensel *et al.*, (1966) *J. Pediat.*, **68**, 761

Data from Lascari, André, D. (1973), *Leukaemia in Childhood.* Courtesy of Charles C. Thomas, Publisher, Springfield, Illinois and Prof. Lascari.

virus infections (e.g. herpes simplex) are examples of 'productive' infection, with destruction of the affected host cells. Infectious mononucleosis is a 'productive' infection with EBV affecting cells in the oropharynx with release of infectious virus particles into the buccal fluid (thus the transmission in adolescents by kissing). In addition these patients manifest a 'non-productive' infection of peripheral lymphoid cells containing the un-

lymphoma it is necessary to postulate a second factor in susceptible individuals. This might involve changes in the target cells or in immunological status (e.g. by chronic malarial infection), or might depend upon genetic factors. Experimental production of animal lymphomas by oncogenic viruses similarly depends upon certain secondary conditions. Thymectomy in AKR mice and bursectomy in chickens prevents lymphoma production by appropriate virus, presumably by removal of the susceptible lymphoid tissue (Aisenberg, 1973). Activation of the leukaemia virus of AKR mice by X-irradiation (Kaplan, 1967) is another example, which may have parallels in human leukaemia (*vide infra*). Recently it has been found that a major histocompatibility locus is a critical determinant for susceptibility to leukaemia viruses in mice (Pincus *et al.*, 1971). In children susceptibility to ALL could not be related to any particular HL-A phenotype or genotype (Lawler *et al.*, 1971). A later study by the same group, however, suggested that better survival and therefore perhaps 'resistance' to leukaemia may be associated with HL-A9 antigen (Lawler *et al.*, 1974).

If viral infection plays a part in human leukaemogenesis it could well be that the virus is widespread but that a number of additional environmental, immunological or genetic factors act as obligatory determinants. A practical question that may arise from consideration of the viral aetiology of leukaemia is whether cats, who are prone to viral leukaemia, constitute a hazard when kept as pets. At present evidence on this point is contradictory, Bross and Gibson (1970) finding a two-fold increase of leukaemia among children exposed to all cats, but Hanes *et al.* (1970) and Stewart (1970) finding no increase. This question is reviewed by Levy (1974).

Irradiation in relatively high doses is an undoubted cause of leukaemia in man. Evidence includes the high incidence of leukaemia among early radiologists, in patients with ankylosing spondylitis given spinal radiotherapy and in those exposed to the Hiroshima and Nagasaki atomic bombs (*B.M.J.*, 1972A). Those receiving an estimated 100 rads (whole body irradiation) or more showed an increase in AML, CML, and ALL, the latter being particularly increased among those under 15 years at the time of the bombing.

Alice Stewart and her colleagues in Oxford (1958) first drew attention to the relationship of low dose, diagnostic antenatal X-rays to later leukaemia in the infant. The subsequent incidence of childhood malignancy was nearly doubled in the first 10 years of life. Preconception diagnostic irradiation in the parents has also been claimed to increase the relative risk of leukaemia in the offspring to 1·6 for maternal and 1·4 for paternal exposure (Graham *et al.*, 1966). At variance with these conclusions is the fact that neither *in utero* nor parental preconception exposure to heavier irradiation in Hiroshima and Nagasaki led to increased incidence of leukaemia in the offspring (Jablon and Kato, 1970; Hoshino *et al.*, 1967). No

adequately sized prospective antenatal study has been reported and not all authorities accept the causal relationship between diagnostic X-rays and leukaemia (MacMahon, 1972). Alternative non-causal explanations attribute the high malignancy rate to an underlying abnormality in the mother leading to a greater chance that she will be given an X-ray examination.

A retrospective analysis by Bross and Natarajan (1972) suggested that the apparently harmful effects of antenatal exposure to X-rays was greatly increased in certain susceptible groups of infants including those with a liability to later viral or bacterial infections or allergic diseases. This work requires prospective confirmation. It once again suggests the multifactorial origin of leukaemia (*B.M.J.*, 1972B).

The extent to which the ubiquitous background radiation contributes to leukaemia is unknown, but it could account for up to $\frac{1}{8}$ of that seen in the 15–39 age group (*Lancet*, 1972).

Chemicals and drugs which suppress the bone marrow have also been incriminated as causing leukaemia, including AML following benzene (Vigliani and Saita, 1964), ALL in a child following chloramphenicol (Fraumeni, 1967) and AMMoL following cytotoxic chemotherapy (Catovsky and Galton, 1971). Similarly patients on chronic immunosuppressive therapy have a well recognized liability to lymphoma and other malignancies, perhaps due to breakdown of normal 'immunological surveillance' (*B.M.J.*, 1972C).

Genetic factors play an identifiable role in only a very small minority of patients with leukaemia. Multiple cases within a family have only been reported about 100 times (Zuelzer and Cox, 1969). Parental consanguinity was present in only 2 of these families. When one member of a family has leukaemia it has been calculated that the chances of leukaemia developing in a sibling or non-identical (dizygotic) twin are only four times that in the general population. In identical (monozygotic) twins, however, there is a 20 to 25 per cent incidence of concordance (MacMahon and Levy, 1964; Jackson, *et al.*, 1969) with leukaemia appearing in the second twin usually within a few months of the first. Clearly this information should only be given to parents if specifically requested. Other than in identical twins the incidence of concordance is so low as to be confidently disregarded. Progeny of survivors of childhood leukaemia or other malignancies do not show an excess of genetic or neoplastic disease (Li and Jaffe, 1974). Neither are infants born to mothers with leukaemia at increased risk (Miller, 1964), only two infants out of several hundred such pregnancies developing the disease.

A rather different situation is the increased incidence of acute leukaemia found in a number of genetically determined disorders (Table 20.2). Here the liability to leukaemia may be determined more by such factors as increased chromosome breakage, as in Fanconi's anaemia and Bloom's syndrome, or immune deficiency as in agammaglobulinaemia and ataxia telangiectasia (Sawitsky et al., 1966). Also an increased incidence of congenital defects in children with leukaemia has been noted, as well as in their siblings, and a greater than expected incidence of second primary tumours in patients with leukaemia (Regelson et al., 1965). Investigating 6 families where a child with acute leukaemia had a paternal grandparent with leukaemia or lymphoma, Till et al. (1975) found lower lymphocyte counts and higher serum IgA in the children's fathers. Atopy, repeated infections and rheumatic disease were common amongst the parents and sibs. They interpret these findings as suggesting an immunodeficiency basis for childhood ALL.

Estimates of the increased incidence of leukaemia in Down's syndrome vary between 3 times that in the general population (Krivit and Good, 1957) to 61 times (Wald et al., 1961). Stewart et al. (1958) in Great Britain gave a figure of twenty-fold increase. These are probably slight overestimates since leukaemoid reactions are particularly common in newborn mongol infants masquerading as a transient congenital leukaemia (Ross et al., 1963). Rosner et al. (1972) have recently reported the combined experience of Acute Leukaemia Group B between 1955 and 1970 in this field and have reviewed the world literature between 1930 and 1970. Their findings refute the commonly held view that the leukaemia that occurs in Down's syndrome is predominantly myeloblastic. When cases of transient neonatal leukamoid reaction are excluded they found that close to 70 per cent of the cases of leukaemia were lymphoblastic (Lancet, 1972).

A recent review on the aetiology of human and animal leukaemias is that of Roath (1972).

CELL KINETIC CONSIDERATIONS

The fundamental abnormality in behaviour of leukaemic blast cells is an arrest of maturation at a stage when the proliferative or multiplicative capacity is retained. Because of the arrested maturation normal end cells are not produced and there is a failure of the normal pathway of elimination. Combined with the continued potential for multiplication this results in progressive accumulation and replacement of normal marrow cells by leukaemic blast cells (Stuart, 1972). This leads to failure of production of normal haemic cells with neutropenia, thrombocytopenia and anaemia. Similar leukaemic proliferation in other tissues, particularly those of the reticuloendothelial system, results in the hepatosplenomegaly and lymphadenopathy characteristic of the disease in relapse. The rate of growth of the leukaemic tissue depends upon the balance between cell multiplication and death, either spontaneous or drug induced. The development of the powerful tool of autoradiography following tritiated thymidine (^{3}H-TDR) uptake by cells in DNA synthesis (S-phase) has greatly increased our knowledge of the kinetics of leukaemic cell growth. Excellent reviews on this topic are available (Cronkite, 1967; Killman, 1968; Lampkin, McWilliams and Mauer, 1972; Killmann, 1972). In essence it is only those cells in S-phase which are labelled when briefly exposed to ^{3}H-TDR in vivo or in vitro. (Fig. 20.1, flash labelling.)

Before these techniques were available it was generally supposed that the mass of leukaemic cells were engaged in rapid and continuous multiplications, outstripping the normal marrow cells. This has proved incorrect. By autoradiography on serial marrow aspirates it is possible to follow the fate of the resultant cohort of labelled cells until mitosis. From these and other considerations the duration of the cell cycle and its components can be estimated. The flash-labelling index (percentage of cells labelled 1 hour after injection of ^{3}H-TDR and therefore in DNA synthesis) of leukaemic myeloblasts in the marrow was very low (4·1 to 14·2 per cent) compared to the index of normal myeloblasts (40 to 70 per cent) (Killmann, 1968). Serial observations indicated a cell cycle time of 45 to 84 hours in leukaemic myeloblasts compared to approximately 15 hours in normal myeloblasts. It was concluded that leukaemic cells proliferate more slowly than their normal counterpart and that a large proportion of the leukaemic cells are in a non-dividing or 'resting state', sometimes referred to as G_0. Subsequent work has amply confirmed these points. Further calculations have shown that neither the relative nor absolute production rate of leukaemic blast cells exceeds that of normal granulocyte precursors (Killmann, 1968).

A similar low labelling index has been found in leukaemic lymphoblasts at diagnosis (15–35 per cent), but a somewhat higher index in early relapse (Foadi et al., 1968; Saunders et al., 1967), suggesting that the 'growth fraction' is inversely related

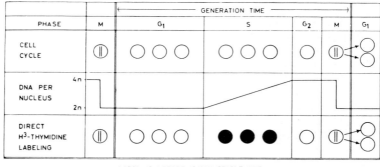

Fig. 20.1 Basic facts about ³H-thymidine cell labelling. (Reproduced from *Series Haematologica I* (1968), **3**, 38, by permission of the author Dr Killmann and the publisher Munksgaard).

to the total number of leukaemic cells, as in the Gompertzian growth curve of solid tumours. Mauer and Fisher (1966) found that it was only the larger leukaemic blast cells that labelled with ³H-TDR. When these large cells divided they gave rise to labelled small blast cells, apparently non-proliferative. Killmann (1965) noted that these smaller, resting cells had irregular nuclear outlines compared to the larger, more typical blast cells. Part of the relevance of these 'resting' cells is that they will be refractory to many of the antileukaemic drugs, most of which are active only during the S-phase or mitotic phase of the cell cycle (cycle active drugs, see Table 20.3) (Stuart, 1972). The magnitude of this problem is succinctly shown in the experiments of Clarkson (1969). Continuous infusion of ³H-TDR in patients with myeloblastic leukaemia in relapse still left 7 to 18 per cent of the blasts unlabelled after 8 to 10 days infusion, and 1 to 8 per cent unlabelled even after 20 to 21 days infusion.

Theoretically possible proliferative patterns for leukaemic blast cells are shown in Fig. 20.2. Whereas the average doubling time of individual blast cells is in the region of 60 hours, that of the whole population of leukaemic cells is 4–6 days in the untreated patient (Frei and Freireich, 1965). This difference is due to the small number of the leukaemic cells actually dividing. This figure also poses one of the unsolved problems concerning renewal of the proliferating pool, viz. is this permanently self-perpetuating or is it replenished

Table 20.3 Probable site of action of antileukaemic drugs in relation to cell cycle

Drug	Site of action	
	In-cycle	Out-of-cycle
Prednisolone	Prolongs late G_1 Blocks entry to S	General lymphocytolytic effect
Daunorubicin	S	Complexes with preformed DNA
Alkylating agents Cyclophosphamide Busulphan Chlorambucil	Non-specific	Non-specific
Vincristine	M	—
6-MP	S	—
MTX	S	—
Hydroxyurea	S	—
ARA-C	S	—

Data from Stuart (1972), by permission of the author and the editor of the British Medical Journal.

from a morphologically unidentified stem cell? (Gavosto *et al.*, 1967). Recent evidence is that it is the apparently 'resting' or 'non-proliferating' small blast cells which replenish the proliferating pool (Saunders and Mauer, 1969; Clarkson *et al.*, 1970; Stryckmans *et al.*, 1970; Wagner *et al.*, 1972). The distinction between proliferating and non-proliferating leukaemic blast cells is therefore relative rather than absolute. It is now realized that there is a wide range of cell cycle times around the *average* values commonly quoted.

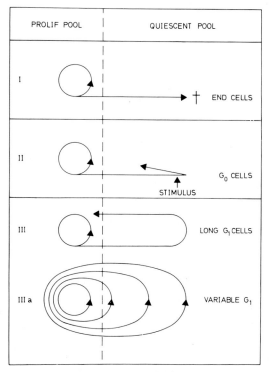

Fig. 20.2 Theoretical possibilities of leukaemic blast-cell kinetics. Available data could be explained by possibility IIIa, *i.e.* that there is a considerable spread in generation times of individual leukaemic cells; the major part of the variation in generation time would be accounted for by variation in G_1-duration. Distinction between 'resting'—and 'actively proliferating' cells would be arbitrary. (Reproduced from *Clinics in Haematology* (1972), **1**, 95, by permission of the author Dr Killmann).

This picture of cell kinetics emphasizes the need for better ways of eliminating the resting cells, this being obligatory for eradication of the cellular phase of the disease. Exploratory attempts to bring more of these cells into the dividing stage by the use of methotrexate (Gabutti *et al.*, 1969) or extracorporial irradiation (Chan and Hayhoe, 1971) are of interest. Fortunately a higher proportion of the residual leukaemic cells are in the sensitive dividing stage when the total tumour mass is reduced, justifying the use of intensive chemotherapy with antimetabolites (i.e. cycle active drugs) while in remission, and perhaps also re-induction with drugs such as vincristine.

Knowledge of the cell kinetics involved may also lead to improved timing in the use of existing antileukaemic drugs. Synchronization of a cohort of lymphoblasts has been shown to occur following a single dose of cytosine arabinoside apparently rendering them more sensitive to a dose of vincristine given 72 hours later (Lampkin, *et al.*, 1969). Other cytokinetically orientated drug schedules are likely to be evolved. It may also emerge that optimum drug combinations should include one cycle active drug and one active against resting cells (Table 20.3), e.g. vincristine plus prednisolone (in ALL) and cytosine arabinoside plus daunorubicin (in AML). When multiple drugs are used it may be preferable to select those that act at different points of the cell cycle (Stuart, 1972).

A new development in this field is the application of pulse cytophotometry, which is capable of determining the proportion of blast cells in S and other cycle phases during therapy (Hillen *et al.*, 1975). The likelihood of remission in AML was related to the percentage in S phase.

DIAGNOSIS OF ACUTE LEUKAEMIA

This is made by marrow examination. As emphasized by Henderson (1973) the main clinical problem is recognizing those signs, symptoms and laboratory findings that should lead to a marrow examination. In general this is indicated when there is clinical or laboratory evidence of progressive depression of platelet, granulocyte or haemoglobin levels, or in the presence of unexplained splenomegaly, hepatomegaly, generalized lymphadenopathy or bone involvement. Haematological depression (i.e. pancytopenia) without hepatosplenomegaly or lymphadenopathy may occur in leukaemia, but raises the possibility of aplastic anaemia. On rare occasions true aplastic anaemia may precede acute leukaemia by a number of months (Melhorn *et al.*, 1970). Characteristically such children show an unusually rapid and marked response of their aplastic anaemia to steroids, followed by the later development of leukaemia.

There is no single clinical feature that is pathognomonic of leukaemia. ALL and AML present similar clinical features. The most frequent symptoms leading to medical advice being sought by parents are pallor, bruising or bleeding, bone pain, fever, or any combination of these (Lascari, 1973). Although anorexia is often present marked weight loss is rare. Symptoms have usually been present for around 6 weeks before diagnosis. But the history can be as short as a few days or alternatively vague symptoms, especially skeletal, may antedate the diagnosis by 6 or more months.

The most common physical findings are:

	ALL (per cent)	AML (per cent)
Generalized lymphadenopathy	70	60
Splenomegaly	70	45
Hepatomegaly	60	60

Data from Lascari, 1973; and Freedman et al., 1971.

The liver and spleen are firm but smooth, and seldom tender. Lymph-glands are firm and discrete; seldom painful unless infected or enlarging unusually rapidly. Mediastinal gland enlargement may occur. Approximately 5 per cent of children have none of these signs at diagnosis.

The types of infection seen at diagnosis do not differ greatly from those occurring in the general paediatric population, otitis media, pneumonia and skin sepsis being common. More specifically occurring in leukaemia are staphylococcal or gram negative septicaemia and stomatitis or gingivitis. Certain infections including Pneumocystis carinii, Fungi, Cytomegalovirus and Toxoplasmosis characteristically occur in patients who are in remission but immunosuppressed as a result of long-continued chemotherapy. These are considered in the section on Management.

The haemorrhagic manifestations of leukaemia are similar to those of other forms of thrombocytopenia in childhood, closely mimicking that seen in ITP or aplastic anaemia, and consisting of purpura of skin and buccal mucosa, subconjunctival haemorrhages, bruising over bony prominences and skin punctures, sometimes with retinal haemorrhage, epistaxis, bleeding from the gums and haematuria. Deep haematomas do not occur except after intramuscular injections, which should be avoided in all types of thrombocytopenia.

The bone and joint involvement may lead to an initial clinical diagnosis of acute rheumatism. Radiological changes are present in almost all children at diagnosis. The most characteristic lesions are transverse radiolucent bands in the metaphysis adjacent to the epiphyseal line (X-ray Plate 1). Other changes include osteolytic lesions (X-ray Plate 2), generalized osteoporosis and periosteal elevation. These aspects are well described by Lascari (1973).

Unusual clinical findings include bilateral parotid or other salivary gland swelling, renal enlargement and subcutaneous skin nodules in ALL, gingival swelling in AMoL or AMMoL and proptosis due to orbital chloroma in AML. Priapism has also been recorded in chronic myelocytic leukaemia. It is noteworthy that intracranial leukaemia is rarely clinically apparent at diagnosis in ALL or AML, although we have noted that a group of patients with completely undifferentiated acute leukaemia (AUL) actually presented as serious neurological disorders (Graham Pole, 1973).

The reappearance of splenomegaly during the course of the disease usually indicates actual or impending relapse and is an indication for repeat marrow examination. Occasionally it can be secondary to portal hypertension due to drug-induced liver damage (Lascari et al., 1968). Hepatomegaly may likewise indicate relapse but may also occur due to fatty infiltration caused by corticosteroid therapy (Sharp et al., 1967), or due to liver toxicity from mercaptopurine (6-MP) (Einhorn et al., 1964) or methotrexate (MTX) (Sharp et al., 1969). Lymphadenopathy can be due to infection but posterior cervical or occipital enlargement is more suspicious of relapse. There is a tendency for the same tissue to be involved at relapse as at diagnosis. I have seen this to be so with joint involvement, salivary glands and certain groups of lymph glands. Reappearance of these manifestations may anticipate peripheral blood evidence of relapse.

Other extramedullary manifestations of leukaemia including in particular CNS leukaemia (meningeal leukaemia) and gonadal involvement differ from the above in that they characteristically develop at a time when the patient is otherwise in complete remission, in particular with the marrow free of leukaemic infiltration. They are discussed separately as their pathogenesis and prophylaxis are of particular importance in the long-term management of the disease.

HAEMATOLOGICAL FINDINGS IN ACUTE LEUKAEMIA

Peripheral blood findings in 95 cases of acute leukaemia diagnosed at the Royal Hospital for Sick Children, Glasgow, are shown in Table 20.4. It can be seen that blast cells were present in the peripheral blood in only 90 per cent of patients. Yet even although blast cells might be absent in the blood (aleukaemic leukaemia) there was always some definite abnormality in the peripheral blood values in this series, viz. thrombocytopenia

(< 100,000/mm³) in 90 per cent, neutropenia (< 1,000/mm³) in 63 per cent and anaemia (< 10 g/ 100 ml) in 86 per cent. Many patients showed several or all of these features. All patients had at least one of these abnormalities.

The identification of blast cells on a peripheral blood smear is not necessarily easy, and diagnosis should not be made on this basis alone. They may also be seen in the blood as part of a leukaemoid reaction to infection or haemolysis, particularly in the newborn, or as part of the leucoerythroblastic reaction to marrow replacement or fibrosis. Blast cells in the peripheral blood are not therefore diagnostic of leukaemia, and their absence most certainly does not exclude it. On the other hand an

sional case of disseminated neuroblastoma with circulating tumour cells (Plate G), in which the marrow will also be heavily involved, or the case of lymphosarcoma who has undergone leukaemic transformation, also usually with marrow infiltration. Consideration of the sequence of clinical events, radiological investigations including an IVP, and estimation of urinary VMA and HVA excretion are helpful in making the distinction from leukaemia. In the case of disseminated lymphosarcoma the distinction may be more semantic than real.

Marrow examination is, by definition, diagnostic of leukaemia at presentation and at relapse. The essential feature in the acute, blast cell leukaemias

Table 20.4 Peripheral blood findings at diagnosis in 95 children with acute leukaemia

Findings	Number of cases	Percentage
With blast cells in blood (50–700,000/mm³)	85	90
With anaemia (1.5–10.0 g/100 ml)	82	86
With thrombocytopenia (1,000–100,000/mm³)	85	90
With neutropenia (0–1,000/mm³)	60	63
Without either thrombocytopenia or neutropenia	6	6
Without anaemia, thrombocytopenia or neutropenia	3	3
Without anaemia, thrombocytopenia, neutropenia or blast cells	0	0

entirely normal peripheral blood picture must be extremely rare at a time when the marrow is infiltrated by leukaemia.

On occasions there is difficulty in distinguishing between the lymphocytosis of pertussis or infectious lymphocytosis, in which the cells are predominantly mature lymphocytes, and the type of blast cell classified as 'prolymphocytic' by Mathé (1972) (Fig. 20.10). 'Glandular fever cells' or 'atypical mononuclear cells' seen in infectious mononucleosis, CMV and glandular toxoplasmosis are less likely to cause confusion since at least some of these cells (Downey Type III) have abundant basophilic cytoplasm (Plate C), quite unlike that of leukaemic lymphoblasts (Plate D), or myeloblasts. This distinction, however, became critical in a recent case presenting with widespread purpura and generalized lymphadenopathy, due to concomitant ITP and infectious mononucleosis. When there is doubt a marrow examination will distinguish such cases from leukaemia since there will not be replacement of normal marrow cells by uniform blasts or lymphoid cells in the above mentioned infections. Positive diagnosis is achieved by associated features of the case, including serology.

More closely imitating leukaemia is the occa-

is that the normal haemic cells, myelocytes, normoblasts and megakaryocytes are largely 'crowded out' by infiltration with a relatively uniform population of blast cells. Occasional difficulty may be encountered in cases of the prolymphocytic variety of ALL since, again, many of these cells are morphologically indistinguishable from mature lymphocytes. However, there will be a number of typical lymphoblasts among this population of lymphoid cells (Fig. 20.10).

Technical factors may be critical to diagnosis by marrow examination. The posterior iliac crest is the optimum site for aspiration being both safe and harbouring a large volume of marrow. The sternum should *never* be used in children because of the danger of perforation and the psychological trauma involved with this approach. Smears, made in much the same fashion as a peripheral blood film, and quickly dried in air, provide infinitely more satisfactory material for identification of the fine morphological features necessary to distinguish exactly which cells are blasts and which are not. This is particularly true in the detection of early relapse, which may be impossible in 'squashes' of marrow particles because many cells are damaged or unidentifiable. Squashes, however, give a better assessment of the overall marrow

382 PAEDIATRIC HAEMATOLOGY

Table 20.5 'Defining characteristics' of value in the classification of acute leukaemia

Type	Romanowsky features*	Cytochemical features*
Acute lymphoblastic leukaemia (ALL)	Nuclear-cytoplasmic ratio high Nuclei not indented or twisted Erythroblasts not present in peripheral blood Erythroblasts not predominant in bone marrow	5 per cent or less of cells Sudan positive 5 per cent or less of cells peroxidase positive Neutrophil alkaline phosphatase (LAP) score normal or high PAS score in erythroblasts, polychromatophilic and oxyphilic, low
Acute myeloblastic leukaemia (AGL)	Cell outlines not irregular Nuclear-cytoplasmic ratio not high Monocytes form less than 1 per cent of nucleated cells of the peripheral blood Erythroblasts not predominant in the marrow	Neutrophil alkaline phosphatase (LAP) score is low Invariably more than 5 per cent and usually more than 85 per cent of cells are Sudan black positive which is of a strong local or heavy overall type More than 5 per cent of cells are peroxidase positive
Myelomonocytic leukaemia	Nuclei indented and twisted Monocytes form more than 1 per cent of the nucleated cells of the peripheral blood Nuclear-cytoplasmic ratio not high Erythroblasts not present in the peripheral blood Erythroblasts not predominant in the marrow	More than 5 per cent and less than 85 per cent of cells show Sudan black positivity which is of a more finely granular type than in myeloblastic leukaemia
Erythraemic myelosis	Cell outlines irregular Nuclear-cytoplasmic ratio not high Erythroblasts present in the peripheral blood Erythroblasts predominant in the marrow	PAS score high More than 5 per cent of cells Sudan black positive More than 5 per cent of cells peroxidase positive

*The features listed for each group are its 'group discriminating features',
Reproduced from Hayhoe and Cawley (1972) Clinics in Haematology, 1, 50, by permission of Professor Hayhoe and Saunders Company Ltd.

cellularity, which is useful to record in remission as an index of drug toxicity. The 'best of both worlds' can therefore be had by making a dozen or so 'smears', for cytology and cytochemistry, and a few 'squashes' for assessing cellularity and frequency of megakaryocytes. Histology of marrow fragments or of marrow trephine samples have little value in diagnosis of acute leukaemia since it is not possible to identify the different types of blast cell in histological sections. Histology may be helpful, however, in other types of marrow involvement which may enter into the differential diagnosis of acute leukaemia such as Hodgkin's disease, leukaemic reticuloendotheliosis, Letterer-Siwe disease, myelofibrosis and involvement by neuroblastoma or other secondary tumour.

Blast cells usually constitute 70 to 100 per cent of the cells present on marrow smears at the time of diagnosis. It would be unwise to make a firm diagnosis of acute leukaemia with less than 30 per cent of blast cells (Lascari, 1973). Leukaemic cells are relatively evenly spread throughout the field compared to neuroblastoma or other secondary 'non-haemic' tumour cells which show marked clumping (Plate F). The individual blast cells show a high nucleocytoplasmic ratio, more so in ALL than in AML, and a large nucleus with 'primitive' chromatin pattern and often nucleoli (Plate D). The exception to this nuclear pattern is the small prolymphocytic type of cell. In myeloblastic leukaemia there is often an admixture of monocytes or monoblasts among the myeloblasts denoted by term acute myelomonocytic leukaemia (AMMoL) to distinguish it from pure AML. A virtually pathognomonic feature of AML, AMMoL or AMOL is the presence of occasional Auer rods in the cytoplasm of the blast cells. It is probable, but not absolutely certain, that these inclusions only occur in leukaemia of the above types (Wintrobe, 1967).

Cytological features such as those described above can be determined from Leishman or May-

Grunwald-Geimsa stained smears (Romanowsky stains) and will often give a strong indication of the probable type of acute leukaemia. Cytochemical methods, particularly the periodic acid Schiff and Sudan Black stains, offer further help, especially in distinguishing between ALL on the one hand and the myeloblastic group (AML, AMMoL) on the other. Leukaemic lymphoblasts typically contain strongly PAS-positive bars or dots within the cytoplasm (Plate E) while myeloblasts usually show diffuse or granular Sudan Black positivity in the cytoplasm. Auer rods, if present, also stain with Sudan Black making it easier to spot them when present in small numbers. Neuroblastoma cells may show similar morphology to leukaemic blast cells but do not show PAS or SB positivity. The importance of achieving as accurate a distinction as possible between ALL and AML or AMMoL in relation to choice of chemotherapy is recognized by most of the co-operative Leukaemia Therapy groups. In M.R.C. trials, for instance, it is necessary to refer unstained marrow smears for cytochemical tests at the time a patient is entered upon a trial. The general validity of classification of blast cell type from cytological and cytochemical criteria was statistically evaluated by Hayhoe et al. (1964). The conclusions of this study are shown in Table 20.5. For a comprehensive recent review of cellular morphology, cytochemistry and fine structure of acute leukaemia as revealed by EM the reader is referred to the article of Hayhoe and Cawley (1972). The value of the lysosomal enzyme beta-glucuronidase in cytological classification has also been described (Mann et al., 1971). A diffuse cytoplasmic pattern is found in AML and strong, localized, granular positivity in ALL. This test is recommended in those cases of acute leukaemia in which the PAS is negative or equivocal.

During remission induction the bone marrow and the peripheral blood return to normal indicating a state of haematological remission. Sequential marrow examinations throughout the course of acute leukaemia play an important part in the present-day management of the disease, especially at times of unexplained marrow depression (i.e. peripheral neutropenia, thrombocytopenia or anaemia) in order to distinguish between relapse or depression from chemotherapy or infection. Relapse is indicated if the total number of blast cells exceed 5 per cent. In fact true relapse is usually associated with a return of 30 per cent or more of blasts, obviating the difficult problem of trying to decide whether small numbers of blast cells belong to the normal or leukaemic cell line.

MANAGEMENT OF ACUTE LEUKAEMIA

This entails not only the selection of appropriate antileukaemic therapy but also the use of supportive measures to correct or compensate for deficiencies of haemopoietic and immunological function caused by either the leukaemic process or its therapy. In addition, it also involves an element of personal support for the patient's family throughout what is usually a number of years (Willoughby, 1972).

The aim of therapy in childhood ALL has now shifted from palliation to cure. In other types of leukaemia the more limited objective of attaining a complete remission and maintaining this for a worthwhile period is generally all that can realistically be expected. With optimum management in ALL about 50 per cent of children can remain free of any leukaemic recurrence for 5 years or more (Simone, 1973) and perhaps half of these children may ultimately prove to be cured (B.M.J., 1973). No child should therefore be denied this possibility. If the necessary facilities and experience are not available locally then referral or close liaison with a special centre is advocated (Holland and Glidewell, 1972A). Because details of management are still in process of evolution today's therapeutic programmes will undoubtedly be improved upon in the future. The most fruitful arrangement is therefore to join a co-operative group, such as the M.R.C. in this country or similar groups (e.g. Acute Leukaemia Group B, Children's Cancer Study Group A, Southwest Oncology Group in the U.S.) if this is at all possible (Willoughby, 1974).

The basic plan of therapy that has emerged for ALL is shown in Fig. 20.3.

Remission induction

Modern therapy of leukaemia is largely based upon the concepts of combination chemotherapy. A recent review of this subject is that of De Vita and Schein (1973). Adoption of relatively uniform criteria for complete remission has permitted valid comparisons between different drug schedules used for remission induction (Bisel, 1956; National Criteria Committee, 1964). Blast cells usually disappear from the peripheral blood within a week, followed by a rise in platelet count and neutrophils at around 3 weeks from the beginning of therapy. Complete remission can be defined as:
1. No symptoms attributable to the disease
2. No hepatosplenomegaly, lymphadenopathy or other clinical evidence of residual leukaemia tissue infiltration

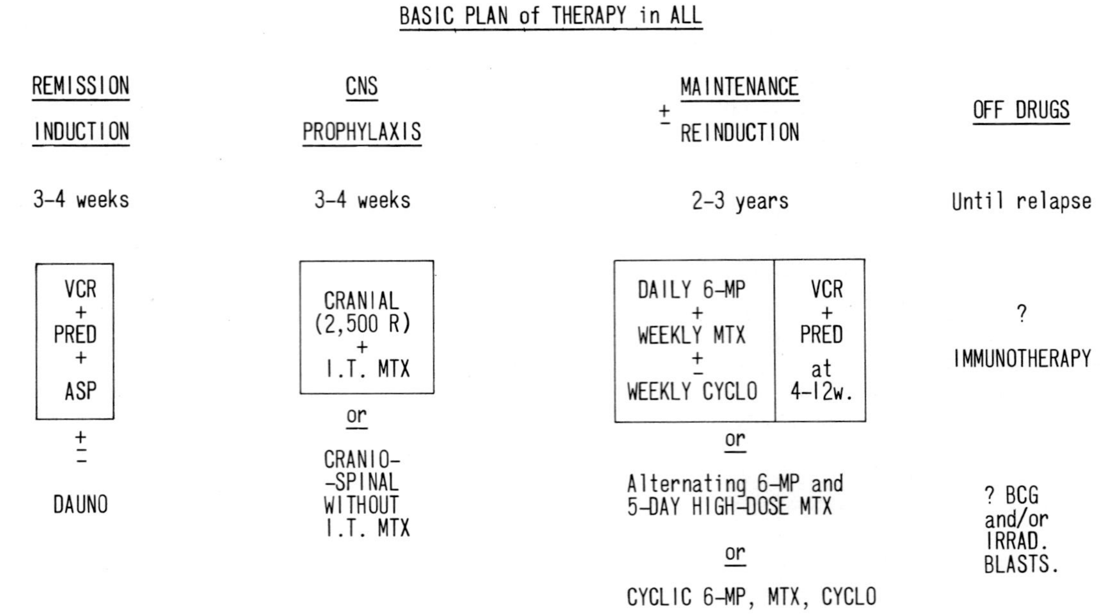

PAEDIATRIC HAEMATOLOGY

BASIC PLAN of THERAPY in ALL

REMISSION INDUCTION	CNS PROPHYLAXIS	MAINTENANCE ± REINDUCTION	OFF DRUGS
3–4 weeks	3–4 weeks	2–3 years	Until relapse

VCR + PRED + ASP	CRANIAL (2,500 R) + I.T. MTX	DAILY 6-MP + WEEKLY MTX ± WEEKLY CYCLO	VCR + PRED at 4–12w.	? IMMUNOTHERAPY

± DAUNO

or

CRANIO-SPINAL WITHOUT I.T. MTX

or

Alternating 6-MP and 5-DAY HIGH-DOSE MTX

? BCG and/or IRRAD. BLASTS.

or

CYCLIC 6-MP, MTX, CYCLO

Fig. 20.3 Basic plan of therapy in ALL. V VCR, vincristine (i.v.); PRED, prednisolone or prednisone (oral); ASP, 1-aspariginase (i.v.); DAUNO, daunorubicin (i.v.); MTX, methotrexate (oral or I.T.); 6-MP, 6-mercapto-purine (oral); CYCLO, cyclophosphamide (oral). 'Boxes' enclose the currently most favoured therapy in the author's opinion, but valid alternatives are also shown. (Reproduced from the *British Medical Journal* (1974), from a paper by Willoughby, by permission of the Editor).

3. A normal peripheral blood picture with minimal levels of 1,500/mm³ granulocytes, 150,000/mm³ platelets and 12 g/100 ml haemoglobin, with no blast cells seen on the peripheral blood film

4. A marrow smear of normal or nearly normal cellularity showing predominantly granulocytic and erythroid precursors together with adequate megakaryocytes and less than 5 per cent blast cells, none possessing frankly leukaemic features (A1 marrow status). Such features would include giant nucleoli, nuclear clefts (Reider Cells), Sudan Black positive Auer rods in myeloblasts or PAS positive 'blocks' or 'bars' in lymphoblasts.

In general, persistence of any clinical or haematological abnormality attributable to residual leukaemic infiltration precludes complete remission (CR) status: but manifestations of chemotherapeutic toxicity such as buccal ulceration, moderate degrees of marrow hypoplasia or megaloblastic erythropoiesis do not (Willoughby, 1972).

Complete remission (or disease-free state) is by definition terminated by the appearance of leukaemic blast cells in any tissue of the body including extramedullary sites such as the CNS or gonads.* *Haematological* remission is terminated when leukaemic cells reappear in the marrow. In the past it was the convention to consider only the length of haematological remission in evaluation of different therapeutic schedules but Pinkel (Simone *et al.*, 1972A) has pointed out that the measurement most related to ultimate survival in a group of patients is the duration of complete leukaemia-free remission. Those patients who show recurrence at any site are in general destined to finally perish of the disease, even although their first *haematological* remission may exceed 5 years as in Case 17.

Case 17. A little girl aged 2½ years (No. 103425) presented with pallor and listlessness in January, 1967. There was no splenomegaly or lymphadenopathy. Hb was 7·7 g/100 ml, WBC 2,450/mm³, neutrophils 170, platelets 42,000 with no circulating blast cells. Marrow examination showed 95 per cent blast cells with the cytological features of leukaemic lymphoblasts and strongly PAS +ve. The diagnosis was therefore ALL, but no adverse prognostic features were present. She was treated with weekly VCR plus daily oral prednisolone plus 6-MP. Complete clinical and marrow remission with a normal peripheral blood was attained by 4 weeks. Thereafter she was maintained on cyclic chemotherapy using 6-MP, MTX and Cyclo plus VCR and prednisolone 'pseudoreinduction' therapy at 5–6 month intervals.

* Testicular relapse, with painless swelling, can occur up to several years from diagnosis. Bilateral irradiation, including the inguinal canal, is the treatment of choice.

She remained in complete remission until July, 1970, $3\frac{1}{2}$ years from diagnosis, when she developed a meningeal relapse heralded by headaches and papilloedema. The CSF contained 25 blasts/mm³. She was given weekly IT MTX, which rapidly cleared the CSF of blasts. Following this she was given cranial irradiation (2,500 r) plus spinal (1,000 r) followed by a course of 10 weekly IT injections of MTX plus ARA-C (this was a pilot study for the first MRC Meningeal Trial). She tolerated this therapy exceedingly well, travelling some miles from home by train once per week for the IT drugs.

She remained on maintenance cyclic therapy in complete remission and without meningeal recurrence until $5\frac{1}{2}$ years from diagnosis when a marrow examination, performed because of pancytopenia, showed a relapse. A further remission was obtained, but a recurrence of the meningeal leukaemia occurred in November, 1973, nearly 7 years from diagnosis, or $3\frac{1}{2}$ years after the first meningeal relapse. This was followed one month later by a terminal marrow relapse and she died approximately 7 years from diagnosis.

It took $3\frac{1}{2}$ years for the first meningeal episode to occur (no CNS prophylaxis was given in 1967), and nearly a further $3\frac{1}{2}$ years for its recurrence to occur. It might be that the intensive CNS therapy reduced the number of blast cells in the CNS to a similar number as was present at diagnosis. Alternatively 'reseeding' of the CNS may have occurred at the time of the first marrow relapse. The final marrow relapse occurred shortly after the meningeal recurrence and may have represented spread from the CNS. All these protracted time relationships suggest a slowly growing leukaemic cell line, consistent with the absence of splenomegaly or circulating blast cells at diagnosis.

The great majority of newly diagnosed cases of childhood ALL can be brought into remission with VCR plus prednisolone alone (Table 20.6) and only seldom are additional drugs such as DAUNO, ASP or ARA-C required.

mission (Mathé et al., 1966; Nies et al., 1965). It is also established that the same chromosomal abnormalities are found in the marrow blast cells at relapse as were originally present in the same patient at diagnosis, suggesting persistence of the original cell line (Reisman et al., 1964). Presumably these residual foci are the source of later relapse, but could be reduced or eliminated by additional drugs or radiotherapy administered early in remission. The optimum use of a third 'inducer' drug asparaginase superimposed upon standard VCR plus prednisolone remission induction therapy has been studied by Acute Leukaemia Group B (Jones and Holland, 1973) and the M.R.C. (Johnston et al., 1974). In the ALGB protocol 7111 455 patients were randomized to receive:

1. VCR + prednisone without ASP
2. VCR + prednisone preceded by ASP
3. VCR + prednisone started simultaneously with ASP
4. VCR + prednisone followed by ASP started on DAY 21.

The dose of ASP was 1,000 units/kg/day IV × 10.

There was no significant difference in the remission induction rate, which was between 82 and 86 per cent in the different groups. The median duration of subsequent remission, however, was significantly longer in the three groups having ASP, than in the group without ASP. This was particularly so when ASP followed VCR + prednisolone (median not reached at 20 months), compared to no ASP (median 13 months). A striking finding was that an unacceptably high

Table 20.6 Incidence of complete remission in childhood ALL

Drugs	CR (per cent)	Author
VCR + prednisolone	85	Holland and Glidewell, 1972B
VCR + prednisolone	90	Pinkel et al., 1971
VCR + prednisolone	95·5	M.R.C., 1973
VCR + prednisolone + DAUNO	97	Bernard et al., 1968
VCR + prednisolone + DAUNO	100	Mathé et al., 1967

Currently chemotherapeutic investigations are being directed more to improving the *quality* of the remission, as judged by elimination of early relapses, rather than the percentage of remissions which are already high. This involves the concept of achieving a more profound degree of leukaemic cell kill than the 99 or 99·9 per cent (2- or 3-log kill corresponding to conventional complete remission) (Frei and Freireich, 1965). It is well established that small residual foci of leukaemic cells persist in between one to two thirds of patients fulfilling the conventional criteria of complete re-

mortality rate occurred when ASP was given before (8·9 per cent) or during VCR + prednisone (10·2 per cent), compared to the groups without ASP (3 per cent) or with late ASP (3 per cent). This higher mortality was also found in the M.R.C. trial UKALL II using simultaneous ASP, VCR and prednisolone. The increase in deaths was due to infection associated with more severe neutropenia in the early weeks and also a probable increase in immunosuppression. This was unexpected since, from its mechanism of action, ASP was thought to exert a selective inhibitory effect upon leukaemic lymphoblasts lacking asparagine synthetase, while sparing normal marrow cells (*B.M.J.*, 1969; Tallal *et al.*, 1970). Jones and Holland point out that the ASP effect on hepatic metabolism of VCR might have a bearing on these findings, since VCR neurotoxicity was greater in the groups having early ASP. On all grounds therefore, VCR + prednisolone followed by ASP appears superior, and at the present time probably constitutes the optimum induction therapy for ALL.

In relapsed patients there is less likelihood that VCR plus prednisolone will succeed in achieving a remission and ASP plus ARA-C (McElwain and Hardisty, 1969) or DAUNO plus VCR and prednisolone (Mathé *et al.*, 1967) may prove successful.

Remission induction in AML or AMMoL is less dependable with the complete remission rate lying between 44 and 65 per cent in predominantly adult series (Table 20.7). It is my impression that higher remission rates are obtainable in children with these forms of leukaemia. The drugs most active are ARA-C, TG and DAUNO.

Table 20.7 Remission induction rates in adult AML obtained with newer drug schedules

Drug combination	Complete remissions (per cent)	Authors
ARA-C + VCR + Pred + Cyclo (COAP)	17/39 (44)	Whitecar *et al.*, 1972
ARA-C + VCR + DAUNO	11/23 (48)	Rosenthal and Maloney, 1972
ARA-C + TG (Daily)	19/38 (50)	Gee *et al.*, 1969
ARA-C + DAUNO	39/72 (54)	Crowther *et al.*, 1973
ARA-C + TG (12-hourly) (L-6 Protocol)	28/42 (65)	Clarkson, 1972

Legend to Table:
ARA-C = Cytosine arabinoside (IV)
VCR = Vincristine (IV)
Pred = Prednisone or prednisolone (oral)
CYCLO = Cyclophosphamide (oral)
DAUNO = Daunorubicin (IV)
TG = Thioguanine (oral)

Reproduced from Willoughby (1974), by permission of the editor of the British Medical Journal.

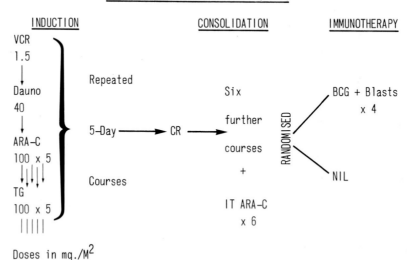

Fig. 20.4 MRC protocol for childhood AML. Abbreviations are as in Fig. 20.3. VCR, DAUNO and ARA-C are given i.v. on Day 1 of each course. ARA-C on Days 2–5 are s.c.; TG is oral. Systematic chemotherapy courses are given at 14-day intervals (9 days between courses), but the first two courses are given closer together, *e.g.* with a gap of 4 or 5 days. CNS prophylaxis consists of 6 doses of I.T. ARA-C (50 mg/m^2), commenced only after the peripheral blood is free of blasts, a single I.T. dose being given on Day 1 of six successive courses. *Caution:* ARA-C for I.T. use must not be dissolved in usual diluent.

The following remission induction schedule has been used in 7 children with AML or AMMoL aged 4 months to 9 years with 5 complete remissions, one partial remission later progressing to CR and one fatality due to leukaemic pericarditis and cardiac tamponade in the first week of treatment.

Day 1   DAUNO   40 mg/m²IV
Days 1–5   ARA-C   100 mg/m²IV or SC
Days 1–5   TG   100 mg/m² orally.

The 5-day courses are repeated at 7–10 day intervals for 2 to 4 courses. Fig. 20·4 shows the plan of the current MRC protocol for childhood AML, using VCR in addition to DAUNO, ARA-C and TG, together with IT ARA-C for CNS prophylaxis.

Since these drugs are more myelotoxic than those used in ALL the period and severity of neutropenia and thrombocytopenia is greater, demanding more meticulous supportive therapy.

Supportive treatment during remission induction

The potential cure of perhaps one quarter of children with ALL with modern therapy makes it doubly important that none are lost from infection, haemorrhage or metabolic disturbance during remission induction. Infection is the most serious of these hazards (Hersh et al., 1965) and is often present at the time of diagnosis. Although constituting a potentially fatal hazard during the first weeks of treatment it is unrelated to long-term prognosis, unlike factors such as the height of blast cell count or degree of splenomegaly at diagnosis. Great efforts are therefore justified both for the prevention and intensive treatment of infections during induction.

At presentation these patients may be dehydrated, infected, bleeding, anaemic and have impaired renal and hepatic function due to leukaemic infiltration. Blood urea, creatinine, electrolytes, SGPT, serum proteins and uric acid should be determined with blood culture if pyrexial. Most patients need packed red cell transfusion (approx. 4 ml packed cells/kg body wt/Hb g/100 ml deficit); those with overt bleeding and a platelet count below 20,000/mm³ need platelet transfusion (4 units for children aged 2–4, 6 units for older children) (Freireich, 1968). Allopurinol, 10 mg/kg/day, in divided doses, is currently advised for all cases and may with advantage be started before commencing antileukaemic drugs. It interferes with the metabolism of 6-MP and these two drugs must not be given together. This restriction does not apply to

TG. When the blast cell count is over 50,000/mm³ or there are large tumour masses (e.g. spleen or mediastinal shadow) allopurinol is obligatory, together with a fluid intake of 2–3 l./m² per day and oral bicarbonate 3 g/m² per day in divided doses to keep the urine neutral or alkaline. These measures are to prevent hyperuricaemic acidosis and uric acid nephropathy (Holland and Holland, 1968) which could otherwise be fatal. The pretreatment uric acid level may be elevated in the presence of gross tumour or renal impairment, and is further raised when effective tumouricidal therapy is instituted. Lactic acidosis, hyperkalaemia and hypocalcaemia may also occur during induction.

Every venepuncture must be performed with scrupulous asepsis. My own practice is to wear sterile surgical gloves; swab with Betadine in spirit, allow this to dry; wipe off with surgical spirit (to improve visualization of the vein) and to use a 'Butterfly' scalp vein set size 21 or 23. The freedom of movement that is possible with a scalp vein set allows one to draw off blood, inject drugs and set up a drip in succession, all with a single vene-puncture. Size 21 is adequate for giving packed cells and, being siliconed, is suitable for platelet transfusion (using a platelet-giving set). As these patients' veins are their 'life lines' this work should only be undertaken by experienced staff.

If high fever and possible septicaemia occur in the presence of neutropenia 'blind' antibiotic therapy will need to be instituted after taking one or more blood cultures, urine and other appropriate cultures and chest X-ray, etc. 80 per cent of febrile episodes in such children are due to infection (Rodriguez et al., 1973). A good first choice is IV Cloxacillin plus IV Gentamicin 6-hourly. In the more seriously ill patients or those not responding to these two drugs the five drug combination devised by Tattersal et al. (1972) is justified (Table 20.8). Hypokalaemia almost invariably develops, but is easily controlled with potassium supplements. Lincomycin is included in this schedule to cover Bacteriodes infections. An international trial under the auspices of EORTC is investigating different combinations of these antibiotics as initial treatment in this clinical context and it is anticipated that their conclusions will soon be available (Tattersal—personal communication). As soon as clinical or bacteriological evidence indicates the precise infection which is present then the 'blunderbuss' therapy is replaced by the antibiotic specifically indicated. By restricting the duration of Gentamicin and Cephalothin administration to 5–7 days, which is usually adequate, we have not

Table 20.8 Antibiotic combination for empirical treatment of patients with acute leukaemia and serious infection

SENSITIVITIES OF BACTERIA TO ANTIBIOTIC COMBINATION

	CARBENICILLIN	GENTAMICIN	CEPHALOTHIN	LINCOMYCIN
Clostridia	○		■	■
Streptococci	○	☆	■	■
Staphylococci	▲	■	■	■
Enterococci	○	☆	○	■
Neisseria	○	■	■	
Haemophilus	○	■	○	
Escherichia	■	■	■	
Proteus	▲	■	▲	
Klebsiella		■	■	
Enterobacter		■	▲	
Pseudomonas	■	■		
Bacteroides				■

Mycobacteria
Candida
Other Fungi
Viruses
Rickettsia
Protozoa
} This régime has no useful activity against the organisms in these groups.

■ = Fully sensitive.
○ = Adequate activity in the high dosage used.
▲ = Only some species fully sensitive.
☆ = Active only in synergistic combination with another drug.

Cephalothin	4 g/m²/day	IV 6-hourly
Carbenicillin	20 g/m²/day	,,
Gentamicin	140 mg/m²/day	,,
Lincomycin	1,500 mg/m²/day	,,

Notes: Gentamicin injected into drip tubing by IV 'push' and flushed through; the other antibiotics can be mixed with 70–100 ml of infusion fluid (usually half-strength saline) in chamber of infusion set. Thus *in vitro* mixing of gentamicin and other drugs is avoided.

Hypokalaemia very common with use of carbenicillin. Daily monitoring of plasma potassium necessary. KC1 supplements usually needed after Day 1.

Gentamicin and cephalothin are nephrotoxic and course is preferably limited to 5 days, after which time sensitivity results may indicate use of a single antibiotic, or infection may be fully resolved.

Lincomycin is only component active against bacteroides.

From Tattersal et al. (1972) Lancet, i, 162, by permission.

encountered the complication of renal failure that has been reported when these two drugs are given together (Kleinknecht *et al.*, 1973; Noone *et al.*, 1973). In patients failing to respond to a combination of these antibiotics plus granulocyte transfusions the possibility of a fungal infection should be considered. I have seen several dramatic responses to the antifungal drug 5-Fluorocytosine in this situation (100–200 mg/kg/day, 6 hourly).

Granulocyte transfusions obtained either by conventional plasmapheresis of chronic myeloid leukaemia donors or, better, by the use of an Aminco or IBM cell separator with healthy donors such as parents, may also be available in special centres.

These have a proven value in patients with septicaemia and severe neutropenia due to leukaemia (Graw et al., 1972; Boggs, 1974). Irradiation with 1,500 rads to the bag of leucocytes is advised so as to reduce the chance of a graft versus host reaction from the donor lymphocytes (Graw et al., 1970). After transfusion of around 10^{10} leucocytes there is frequently a rapid resolution of the fever even although the elevation of granulocytes in the peripheral blood is only minimal and transient. The benefit from granulocyte transfusions is particularly apparent when there has been a failure to respond to adequate antibiotic therapy. A recent review (Boggs, 1974) and annotation (*Lancet*, 1975B) on the use of granulocyte transfusions is available. The liability to infection is closely related to the granulocyte level (Table 20.9).

reduction in the incidence of severe and fatal infections was found in the group having both protective environment plus gut sterilization and a topical antiseptic régime (Table 20.10). Similar results have been reported by Schimpff et al. (1973). The patients in these studies were predominantly adults with myeloblastic leukaemia and therefore at far greater risk of infection during remission induction than is the case in childhood ALL. Superficially there is more justification for these elaborate measures in AML than in ALL, but the possibility of cure in childhood ALL in fact makes it doubly important that they do not perish from infection during the early weeks of treatment. Although many cases of childhood ALL respond smoothly and without complication to VCR plus prednisolone, often without admission

Table 20.9   Incidence of infection related to granulocyte count

Granulocyte count	Incidence of infection (per cent patient days)
100/mm³	53
100–500/mm³	36
500–1,000/mm³	20
1,000/mm³	10

Data derived from Bodey et al., 1966.

Table 20.10   Value of protective isolation during remission induction

	Total patients	Severe infections	Life threatening infections	Fatal infections
Open ward	28	22	16	6
Gut sterilization (GVN) only	38	30	17	9
Gut sterilization, sterile food, topical antiseptic régime plus protective isolation (isolator or laminar flow)	22	8	3	0

Data reprinted, by permission, from Levine et al. (1973) New England Journal of Medicine, **288**, 477.

In addition there may be defective granulocyte function and impaired ability to migrate from the vascular compartment to the site of infection (Spivak et al., 1969) especially in AML (Holland et al., 1971). Protective isolation by laminar flow or plastic 'Life Island' coupled with reduction of the endogenous bacterial flora of gut, skin and oral cavity during the limited period of remission induction, when these patients are at maximal risk of neutropenia and infection, have been investigated (Levine et al., 1973). Topical and unabsorbable antibiotics are used for this purpose, and not systemically absorbed antibiotics. A striking

to hospital, others still die during remission induction, figures of 8·9 and 10·2 per cent having already been mentioned in the ALGB cases having early ASP as well as VCR and prednisolone (Jones and Holland, 1973). Hughes and Smith (1973) from Pinkel's group reported the incidence of infection during the first 6 weeks of therapy in 100 children with ALL. Only 30 remained free of infection. Seven had severe infections including Pseudomonas, Proteus, Staphylococcus, sepsis, systemic candidiasis and haemophilus meningitis. The overall mortality rate from infection was 3 per cent. Döhman, Plüss and Hitzig, (1973) have shown that sterile reverse isolation in laminar flow cabinets with complete eradication of the endogenous bacterial flora can be achieved during remission induction in children (aged 3 and 6) with ALL or AML without major psychological problems. A similar investigation comparing laminar flow modules (Figs. 20.5 and 6) with cubicles is in progress in Glasgow. From these trials the place of pathogen free nursing during the initial stages of treatment in childhood leukaemia may be defined.

For a more complete discussion of the management of infections during antileukaemic therapy the reader is referred to the articles of Levine *et al*.

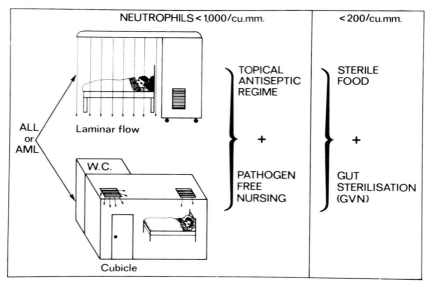

Fig. 20.5 Trial comparing Laminar Flow with Reverse-Barrier Nursed Cubicle isolation in childhood acute leukaemia. Those with severe neutropenia also had gut sterilization by means of unabsorbable oral antibiotics, plus sterile food. The results of this trial showed that Laminar-Flow isolation was superior to Cubicle on psychological, social and practical nursing grounds. A satisfactory degree of protection from exogenous infection was obtained with either method of isolation.

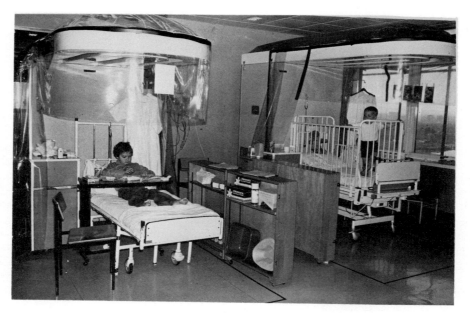

Fig. 20.6 General view of a paediatric ward containing two Laminar-Flow isolation modules.

LEUKAEMIA AND RELATED DISORDERS

(1972) and Bodey (1972). Infections occurring late in the course of the disease are more often due to the immunosuppressive effects of prolonged exposure to drugs such as 6-MP, MTX or cyclophosphamide (Borella and Webster, 1971), and show a different pattern from those described during remission induction. *Pneumocystis carinii* (Hughes *et al.*, 1973), herpes virus, cytomegalovirus (Cangir *et al.*, 1966) and fungi are the commonest cause of fatal infections at this later stage of the disease (Simone *et al.*, 1972B). Acute toxoplasmosis can also occur (Abell and Holland, 1969).

CNS prophylaxis

Without early CNS prophylaxis there is recurrence of leukaemia in the CNS (meningeal leukaemia) in up to 50 per cent of children with ALL while still in systemic (marrow) remission. Their state of remission is terminated by this recurrence and ultimate cure becomes improbable. Cytogenetic studies have shown exactly corresponding chromosome abnormalities to be present in the leukaemic blast cells appearing in the CSF as in those that are in the same patient's marrow at diagnosis or relapse, suggesting that the CNS disease arises by metastatic spread (Mastrangelo *et al.*, 1970). Histological studies (Price and Johnson, 1973) suggest that passage of leukaemic cells takes place from the walls of small arachnoid veins with later spread to the CSF and finally perivascular 'cuffing' deep into the neural tissue. Only after rupture of the pia-glial membrane does the leukaemic process spread into the brain tissue. If seeding of the CNS with blast cells occurs around the time of diagnosis the cells are subsequently protected from adequate concentrations of systemically administered drugs which fail to cross the blood CSF barrier in adequate concentrations (Rall and Zubrod, 1962).

The incidence of CNS leukaemia is directly correlated with the height of the blast cell count, the degree of lymph node enlargement, and the severity of thrombocytopenia at diagnosis (West *et al.*, 1972), as recently reviewed by Graham Pole and Willoughby (1974).

In a series of trials between 1962 and 1972 Pinkel's group at St. Jude's, Memphis, explored progressively increasing doses of craniospinal radiotherapy and latterly cranial radiotherapy plus IT MTX administered early in remission in an attempt to prevent the subsequent development of CNS leukaemia. It has been conclusively and repeatedly shown that *either craniospinal* radiotherapy at a dose of 2,400 rads *or cranial* radiotherapy 2,400 rads plus a simultaneous course of 5 doses of IT MTX (12 mg/m^2/dose) will reduce the incidence of initial CNS relapse from around 50 per cent to as low as 4 to 6.6 per cent (Simone *et al.*, 1972; Aur *et al.*, 1973). Since the cranial and spinal CSF are in continuity and the CSF may be seeded it is essential that both areas should be 'attacked' simultaneously, but the spinal area appears to be equally 'sterilized' of blast cells by either radiotherapy or a course of IT MTX. There is accumulating evidence, however, that spinal irradiation at this dose gives rise to a greater degree of marrow depression with resulting interruption of systemic chemotherapy (Aur *et al.*, 1973) as well as lymphopenia due to deficiency of thymus-dependent T lymphocytes as long as a year after the radiotherapy (Campbell *et al.*, 1973). This finding may have been related to deaths due to infection while in remission in the M.R.C. study (M.R.C. 1973). A transient defect of phagocytic bactericidal activity has also been described during cranial or craniospinal radiotherapy (Baehner *et al.*, 1973). It has not yet been shown that IT MTX alone can achieve a comparable degree of prophylaxis of CNS leukaemia. Cranial radiotherapy 2,400 rads plus 5 doses of IT MTX are currently thought to be the optimal method (Aur *et al.*, 1973). Unfortunately no study has so far demonstrated a reduced incidence of marrow relapse among patients given CNS prophylaxis, which might have been expected from the reasonable hypothesis that overt CNS leukaemia could 'reseed' the marrow (Frei *et al.*, 1965). Unfortunately a few instances of encephalopathy after CNS prophylaxis in childhood ALL have been reported (McIntosh and Aspnes, 1973). Price *et al.* (1974) have suggested that cranial irradiation (2,400 r) increases permeability of the blood-brain barrier to subsequent systemically administered MTX. With improving long-term results in childhood AML the place of CNS prophylaxis in this form of leukaemia is also currently under consideration.

Treatment of overt meningeal leukaemia

In spite of the efficacy of CNS prophylaxis cases of meningeal leukaemia still occur, more commonly among cases diagnosed before prophylaxis was widely practised.

The most common clinical presentation is with headache and vomiting and papilloedema. Progressive weight gain due to the hypothalamic syndrome may also be a clue to early meningeal involvement. A wide range of other neurological manifestations including cranial nerve palsies, cerebellar signs, autonomic symptoms, behaviour disorders, coma and hypertension may also occur in a minority of patients. The neurological features have been reviewed by Pierce (1962). X-rays of the skull show spreading of the sutures in about 50 per cent of children with meningeal leukaemia (Hyman et al., 1965).

Diagnostic lumbar puncture in meningeal leukaemia is relatively safe in spite of the signs of are the typical findings with florid meningeal leukaemia it should also be remembered that even with 1 cell/mm^3 there could still be 1,000 per ml, which is a considerable number of tumour cells to have in the CSF! This state of affairs may exist at an early stage of the evolution of meningeal leukaemia or in a partially treated patient. I have seen a boy with ALL who had developed the hypothalamic syndrome and whose CSF findings were normal until one examined a stained concentrate. Precisely one indisputable blast cell could

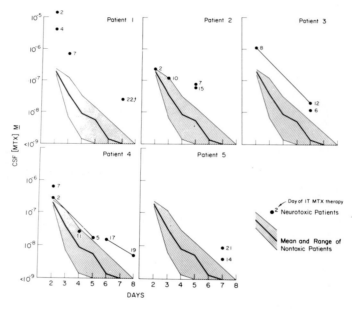

Fig. 20.7 CSF-methotrexate concentration in patients with neurotoxicity (●) as compared to range in asymptomatic patients (shaded areas). The abscissa represents the days elapsed since the last intrathecal methotrexate treatment. The number beside each dot designates days elapsed since the first intrathecal methotrexate treatment. Successive samples after a single treatment are shown by ●———●. The †in patient 1 signifies a post-mortem specimen obtained from the cistera magna. (Reproduced from the *New England Journal of Medicine* (1973), **289**, 770, from a paper by Bleyer et al. by permission of the authors).

raised intracranial pressure, since there is no localized supratentorial or posterior fossa tumour liable to produce 'coning' (Pochedly, 1973). Nevertheless it is a wise policy to use a manometer, not only to record the pressure but also because it allows one to withdraw fluid without too sudden a drop in pressure. It is, of course, from the post LP leak following badly performed punctures that the greatest danger of 'coning' arises (*New Eng. J. Med.*, 1974).

CSF findings show a variable pleocytosis up to several 1,000 cells/mm^3 with elevated protein (> 40 mg/100 ml) in nearly 50 per cent and a decreased glucose level (< 50 mg/100 ml) in nearly 70 per cent (Sullivan et al., 1969). Although these be found. His hypothalamic syndrome completely disappeared after a course of IT MTX. Because of the much finer diagnostic sensitivity achieved by examining a concentrate of several millilitres of CSF for morphologically identifiable blast cells it is now recommended standard practice to examine all CSF samples from leukaemic patients by the cytocentrifugation technique (Komp, 1972; Evans et al., 1974).

Treatment of overt meningeal leukaemia is conventionally with IT MTX at a dose of 10–12 mg/m^2 given at weekly or twice-weekly intervals. The m^2 dose should not be exceeded because the size of the brain does not continue to grow beyond the age of 3 to 4 years. A course of 6 weeks IT MTX injections, 10 mg/m², achieved meningeal remission in 29 out of 31 children in a recent MRC trial. The concentration of MTX in the CSF after the standard dose is around 1,000 times that ever achieved in other tissue fluids during systemic therapy with this drug, explaining its remarkable efficacy in the treatment of meningeal leukaemia in both ALL and AML. There is considerable variation in the rate of subsequent fall in concentration (Fig. 20.7), and there is some evidence that the occasional cases of severe neurotoxicity seen after IT MTX are due to slower than normal elimination of the drug (Bleyer et al., 1973). This seems to occur only during the treatment of active meningeal leukaemia, not in prophylaxis. This finding may account for the cases of severe dementia reported by Kay et al. (1972), also more common in patients treated for meningeal disease and sometimes responding to systemic folic or folinic acid. A high single dose 52 mg, administered accidentally caused no complications (Lampkin et al., 1967). Preservative-free MTX for IT use is now available from Lederle. It may be diluted further with normal saline so as to give a final concentration of 1 mg MTX per ml of solution given IT. Whenever IT MTX is given there is always the possibility of some degree of systemic toxicity which can be treated by giving systemic folinic acid. Plasma levels of MTX are more sustained after IT administration than after oral or IV administration of the same dose (Jacobs et al., 1975).

Other drugs such as IT ARA-C (Wang and Pratt, 1970; Band et al., 1973) or combinations of IT MTX (10–15 mg/m²) plus IT ARA-C (30 mg/m²) plus IT hydrocortisone (10–15 mg/m²) Sullivan et al., 1971) should be reserved for cases failing to respond to an adequate course of IT MTX. The neurotoxicity of commonly used antineoplastic drugs has been reviewed by Weiss et al. (1974). For IT use ARA-C must not be dissolved in its normal diluent which contains benzyl alcohol. Normal saline or Elliot's B solution should be used, and the advice of the hospital pharmacist sought. Omaya reservoirs have also been recommended as a simple way of giving drugs into the ventricular CSF (Spiers, 1972), but this may not be entirely free of complications. Pyrimethamine has also been recommended but appears to be too toxic.

Following a normal course of 6 or more IT doses the neurological signs and symptoms and the CSF return to complete normality and blast cells can no longer be found after cytocentrifugation. But this state of meningeal remission lasts for only a median duration of around 3 months unless

* See also B.M.J. i, 864, (1976).

further antimeningeal therapy is given. Selawry and Odom (1968) pointed out that there were 10⁸ to 10⁹ blast cells in the CSF at diagnosis of meningeal leukaemia, and that each dose of IT MTX on average reduced the cell count by 1 log. They therefore suggested that a total of 10 doses might eliminate the meningeal disease. Although longer meningeal remissions were obtained by the extra doses these failed to achieve eradication, probably because IT drugs cannot reach all the cells in situations such as perivascular cuffing deep within the brain substance. A recent M.R.C. trial, however, has shown that the addition of *craniospinal* irradiation to a course of IT MTX greatly improves the duration of subsequent control (Fig. 20.8) (Willoughby, 1974). This dose of radio-

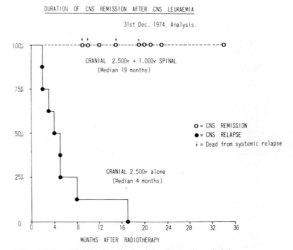

Fig. 20.8 MRC meningeal leukaemia trial.*

therapy may not be entirely safe to give to those who have received previous cranial irradiation. Sullivan and Haggard (1970) showed that 8-weekly injections of IT MTX after CSF remission had been obtained produced a four-fold prolongation of control of the CNS disease. This would provide a reasonable form of palliative control for those patients unable to have a repeat dose of radiotherapy. Sullivan et al. (1971) also showed that systemic BCNU was ineffective at controlling human meningeal leukaemia, although active in experimental animals. Experience in the treatment of myeloblastic meningeal leukaemia is too limited for definitive recommendations but IT ARA-C deserves prime consideration. On the other hand, I have treated one case with IT MTX followed by cranial irradiation without recurrence over a period of 3½ years.

Maintenance therapy

It has been well established that the great majority of children with ALL will relapse if chemotherapy is stopped within $1\frac{1}{2}$ to 5 months after remission (Henderson, 1969). The median duration of this unmaintained remission was greater after intensive consolidation chemotherapy, this being a reflection of the greater leukaemic cell kill, but did not exceed 20–22 weeks. Intermittent high-dose chemotherapy (POMP) given for 5 days in every month and continued for 14 months gave a median unmaintained remission of only 8 months, and intensive 5-day courses of MTX given fortnightly for 8 months together with 'reinforcement' pulses of VCR plus prednisolone after every 3 courses extended this to 10 months. Greatly superior remission duration has been obtained by chemotherapy continued for $2\frac{1}{2}$ to 3 years, indicating that 8 months of intensive chemotherapy is inadequate for the majority of children with ALL.

Multidrug continuous chemotherapy with superimposed VCR plus prednisolone 'reinforcement' has been used by ALGB, Group A and Pinkel's group with good long-term results, particularly when preceded by early CNS prophylaxis (Holland and Glidewell, 1972B; Simone et al., 1972A). Careful monitoring of haematological or other toxicity is needed at weekly or fortnightly clinic visits, with adjustment of dosage if necessary.

VCR + prednisolone) was stopped after $2\frac{1}{2}$ to 3 years with only 12 per cent of the patients subsequently relapsing while off drugs (Aur, 1975). The early part of the remission duration curve of ALGB protocol 6801, similar to Pinkel's Protocol V but omitting cyclophosphamide, appears to be giving similarly good results, with 21 out of 27 patients (78 per cent) still in their first remission at $2\frac{1}{2}$ to $3\frac{1}{2}$ years (Holland and Glidewell, 1972A).

A multidrug intensive intermittent schedule (L-2 protocol) has recently been shown to be giving good results (Haghbin et al., 1974). Ten out of 12 children entered on this trial 3 years ago are free of recurrence. Future long-term results are awaited with interest.

Unfortunately these good long-term results are not obtained without a considerable degree of chronic immunosuppression (Borella and Webster, 1971) leading to the tragic occurrence of deaths in remission due to opportunist infections. Simone et al. (1972B) reported 26 out of 499 (5·2 per cent) such deaths in childhood ALL over a 10-year period. Chicken pox can be fulminating and fatal in children on antileukaemic drugs. If a susceptible patient becomes a close contact of this disease protection is possible by giving gamma globulin prepared from convalescent zoster immune serum (Brunel et al., 1969). Likewise protection from measles with normal gamma globulin is possible in contacts (Robertson, 1970). Pneumonitis due to

Table 20.11   6-MP and MTX dosage during maintenance therapy

	ALGB*	Pinkel†	MRC‡
Daily oral 6-MP plus	90 mg/m²	50 mg/m²	75 mg/m²
Once per week oral MTX	15 mg/m²	20 mg/m²	15 mg/m²

*ALGB protocol 6801 (Holland and Glidewell, 1972).
†Plus once per week oral cyclophosphamide, 200 mg/m² (Aur et al., 1973).
‡MRC Protocol UKALL III.
Reproduced from Willoughby (1974), by permission of the editor of the British Medical Journal.

The basic drug schedule used by ALGB, Pinkel, Cancer Study Group A and currently the M.R.C. consists of daily oral 6-MP plus weekly oral MTX (Table 20.11). Pinkel's group also added weekly cyclophosphamide and lowered the dose of 6-MP. VCR plus prednisolone reinforcement pulses are superimposed upon the other drug schedules.

Of 31 patients entered on Pinkel's Protocol V 18 (58 per cent) are still in their first remission without recurrence of leukaemia in any site at over 5 years from diagnosis (Simone, 1973). The 5-drug chemotherapy as shown above (daily 6-MP, weekly MTX and cyclophosphamide, 3-monthly

cytomegalovirus (Cangir et al., 1967), MTX toxicity or associated virus (Robbins et al., 1973) or *Pneumocystis carinii* (Fig. 20.9) constitute particular hazards requiring a high index of suspicion (Repsher et al., 1972; Sedaghatian and Singer, 1972). Treatment is with pentamidine (150 mg/m² per day × 5, then 75 mg/m²/day × 5), together with fresh or fresh frozen plasma as a source of gamma globulin. Renal function must be monitored throughout the course. Reducing the dose of drugs so as to lessen the degree of immunosuppression results in distinctly inferior remission duration and survival (Pinkel et al., 1971). This dilemma

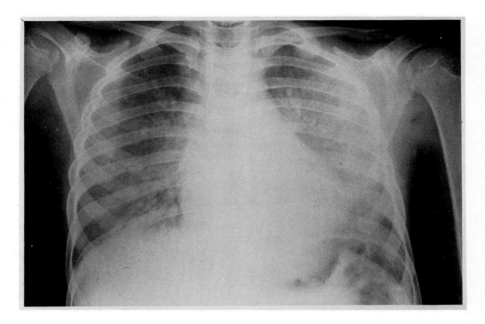
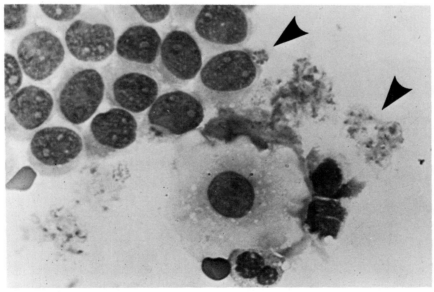

Fig. 20.9 Pneumocystis Carinii. A, Chest X-ray showing patchy pneumonitis; B, Lung Aspirate showing numerous pulmonary macrophages, free-living pneumocystis organisms (*rt. arrow*) and diagnostic octocyst (*upper arrow*). Note size of red cell at bottom of field for comparison. (Cytospin preparation, Leishman stain, x 2,700).

highlights an important currently unanswered question first posed by Krivit *et al.* (1970), viz. 'What is the optimum duration of multidrug chemotherapy?' Is there a point at which all susceptible leukaemic cells have already been killed or rendered non-proliferative by the chemotherapy and beyond which time the hazards of opportunist infection (viral, fungal, *Pneumocystis carinii*) from immunosuppression outweigh any antileukaemic benefit? Present evidence would suggest that this optimum time lies in the region of $2\frac{1}{2}$ to 3 years. This point is being deliberately investigated in the current M.R.C. trials. It has been shown that cessation of chemotherapy after $2\frac{1}{2}$ to 3 years is followed by rapid lymphocytic and immunological rebound within 8 to 10 weeks in children under 5 but not in those over 5 years (Borella *et al.*, 1972). This return to normal would be expected to remove the hazards of infection.

Prognosis in optimally treated ALL is shown in Fig. 20.10, which gives the percentage of children

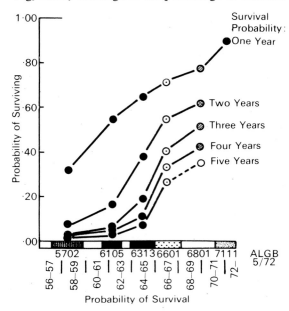

Fig. 20.10 Survival probabilities in childhood ALL, based on ALGB studies. Points are plotted at mid-study, and the actual period when the study was conducted is shown across the abscissa. (Reproduced from *Cancer* (1972), **30**, 1480, from a paper by Holland and Glidewell, by permission of the authors).

surviving for 1, 2, 3, 4 and 5 years respectively. The steadily improving prognosis with successive trials over recent years is clearly demonstrated. For children treated in 1971–2 there is a 90 per cent probability of surviving one year. Over 50 per cent remain free of disease for over 5 years after optimum therapy. It is also gratifying that no excess of inherited defects have been detected in the offspring of long-term survivors of childhood cancer or leukaemia (Li and Jaffe, 1974).

The optimum type of maintenance therapy for AML or AMMoL is not yet established. In some groups in the U.S. all types of childhood acute leukaemia are given the same treatment. In adults the 'Hammersmith' régime employs repeated 5-day courses of TRAP (TG, Rubidomycin, ARA-C, Pred), COAP (Cyclo, Oncovin, ARA-C, Pred) and POMP (Purinethol, Oncovin, MTX, Pred) at 2–3 week intervals according to tolerance for at least 2 years (Spiers, 1972). The median duration of 'complete' remission in adults given similarly repeated courses of COAP was $10\frac{1}{4}$ months (White-

car *et al.*, 1972). The large number of IV injections necessary for these particular drug schedules makes them unsuitable for children.

Currently the best long-term survival in adult AML has been obtained with the L-6 protocol from the Memorial Hospital, New York (Clarkson, 1972). This employs a complex sequence of drugs consisting of four-day courses of 'cycle-active' drugs followed on the fifth day of the course by a 'non-cycle active' drug, rather similar to the L-2 protocol mentioned above for ALL.

In 43 previously untreated patients entered on the trial a 50 per cent survival for 2 years is predicted from the life-table curve. Of those obtaining a complete remission the projection indicates that 70 per cent will survive for 2 years. Both the L-6 and L-2 schedules would require considerable experience, and could not yet be recommended for general use.

A simple form of maintenance chemotherapy that I have found valuable in children with AML consists of daily oral TG, 60 mg/m², plus weekly SC ARA-C 100 mg/m², omitting the latter at times of neutropenia, thrombocytopenia or infection.

Immunotherapy may also come to play an important part in the treatment of AML. Powles *et al.* (1973) have reported recent results of a combined trial conducted at St. Bartholomew's Hospital and the Royal Marsden Hospital in London in 107 patients with AML aged 14 to 59 years. The 45 patients obtaining complete remission with ARA-C plus DAUNO were randomized to receive monthly 5-day courses of chemotherapy (ARA-C + DAUNO alternating with ARA-C + TG) with or without weekly immunotherapy with BCG plus irradiated allogeneic myeloblasts. With chemotherapy alone 7 out of 19 are surviving (median 7 months). With chemotherapy plus immunotherapy 16 out of 23 are surviving (median 18 months). Part of the improved survival with immunotherapy may be due to a greater chance of obtaining a second remission, which is otherwise rare in AML. Hersh *et al.* (1971) have also shown that the chance of obtaining an initial complete remission in adult AML is greater in those patients who retain intact immunological reactivity during this phase of treatment. It therefore appears that immunological factors play a greater part in controlling leukaemic growth in AML than in ALL, presumably related to stronger 'neoantigens'. The work of Gutterman *et al.* (1973, 1974) and an annotation in the *Lancet* (1974) should be consulted for an account of recent advances in this field. In childhood ALL, by contrast, a randomized trial of BCG immunotherapy following intensive cytoreductive chemotherapy showed no improvement in duration of remission (M.R.C., 1971), similar negative results having been found in a randomized trial by Group A (Heyn et al., 1973); but BCG plus irradiated myeloblasts are being tested in the current MRC trial for childhood AML (Fig. 20.4). Bone-marrow transplantation from identical twins has given good results in otherwise refractory patients (Fefer, 1974) and may have a place in the future.

For further details of the treatment of childhood leukaemia, including in particular a detailed description of the pharmacology and toxic side effects of antileukaemic drugs the reader is referred to the text book by Lascari, Leukaemia in Childhood (1973). Other recent reviews include those of Lampkin et al. (1972); Spiers (1972); De Vita and Schein (1973); Henderson (1973); McIntosh and Pearson (1973); Willoughby (1974) and the book of Pochedly (1973). A recent development is the concept that more intensive chemotherapy is needed in the minority of ALL patients having 'bad' prognostic features at the time of diagnosis (*vide infra*).

FACTORS AFFECTING PROGNOSIS

Before the introduction of effective chemotherapy the average survival of children with ALL was 3 months from the time of diagnosis (Tivey, 1954). With optimal 'total therapy' over 50 per cent are free of recurrence at 5 years (Simone, 1973). Treatment in special centres also gives longer survival (M.R.C., 1971). Not all cases of ALL do equally well, however, and there is a statistical relationship between the duration of remission and a number of prognostic features present at the time of diagnosis. This relationship is not absolute and exceptions occur, with individual patients showing better than average survival in spite of initially bad prognostic features.

AGE AT DIAGNOSIS

The prognosis is better for ALL diagnosed between 1 and 10 years than for infants and older children (Iversen, 1966; Pierce et al., 1969; Zippin et al.[7] 1971). In AML children do better than adults (Henderson, 1968).

RACE

Negro children have remission duration less than half that of Caucasian children (Walters et al., 1972).

WHITE-CELL COUNT AT DIAGNOSIS

Zuelzer (1964) showed that children with total white cell counts below 20,000/mm^3 had double the mean survival of those with higher counts. This was independently shown with respect to both remission duration and survival in ALL by Freireich et al. (1961) and Acute Leukaemia Group B (1963), and many times since (M.R.C., 1973). Children with AML also do worse if the count is above 25,000/mm^3 at diagnosis.

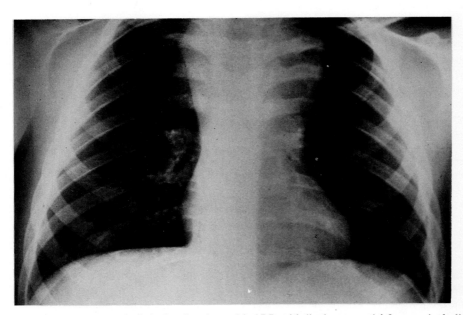

Fig. 20.11 Broadening of Mediastinal shadow in a boy with ALL with 'bad prognostic' features including a white cell. count of 39,000/mm^3 at diagnosis. In spite of intensive chemotherapy he relapsed in 7 months.

DEGREE OF TISSUE INFILTRATION

Hardisty and Till (1968) showed that not only the height of the circulating blast cell count ($> 10,000/mm^3$) but also the degree of splenomegaly, the presence of hepatomegaly and presence of lymphadenopathy, especially hilar, had adverse prognostic significance. It is clear that all these features reflect the total mass of tumour tissue in the body at diagnosis, and may also reflect the rate of leukaemic proliferation in the individual patient (Hardisty and Norman, 1967). The presence of thrombocytopenia ($< 100,000/mm^3$) was also an adverse feature, but not the severity of the anaemia.

CYTOLOGICAL FEATURES

Mathé et al. (1971) has recently proposed classification of ALL into the following 4 cytological types: (a) prolymphoblastic, (b) macrolymphoblastic, (c) microlymphoblastic, and (d) prolymphocytic, in order of increasing morphological differentiation and decreasing nuclear size. These cell types are illustrated in Fig. 14 in the article by Mathé in *Clinics in Haematology* (1972). Only the microlymphoblastic (mLbAL) and prolymphocytic (PLcAL) varieties show remission and survival curves which form a plateau for 50 per cent or more of the patients, the prognosis for microlymphoblastic cases being particularly good. Patients with the prolymphoblastic form had the worst prognosis.

Pantazopoulos and Sinks (1974) have independently shown a relationship between the proportion of macrolymphoblasts (i.e. $> 12\mu$) in the pretreatment marrow and the duration of remission in ALL. Ten children with less than 10 per cent of macrolymphoblasts had no relapses within 57 months of observation; in 16 children with 11–25 per cent macrolymphoblasts 14 had relapses with a median first remission of 15 months; and of 12 children with over 26 per cent macrolymphoblasts 11 relapsed with a median remission of 12 months.

The percentage of lymphoblasts in the marrow at diagnosis showing PAS-positive staining also appears to be correlated with remission duration, at least in patients on cyclic chemotherapy (Laurie, 1968). A more recent analysis of the same patients confirmed this finding (Vowels and Willoughby, 1973), but this relationship has not uniformly been confirmed by other workers.

Great interest has recently been focused upon the occurrence of T- or B-lymphocyte surface markers on lymphoblasts in ALL. In one study 4 out of 22 cases of ALL had T-cell markers (Brown et al., 1974), and in another series of 11 cases

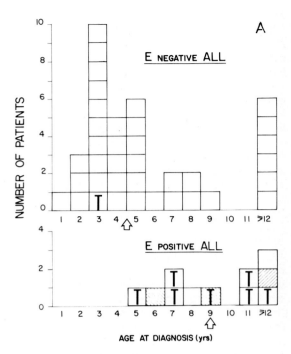

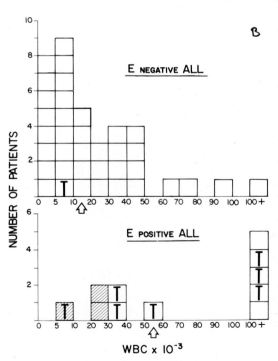

Fig. 20.12 A, Relationship of E-positive ALL to age at diagnosis; B, white-cell count at diagnosis. E-positive blast cells, by possessing T-cell characteristics, form rosettes with sheep erythrocytes. (Reproduced from the *New England Journal of Medicine* (1975), **292**, 828, from a paper by Sen and Borella, by permission of the authors).

1 had T- and 1 B-surface markers (Haegert et al., 1975). Catovsky et al. (1974) suggested that T-cell ALL had a worse prognosis, perhaps indicating that the disease has arisen from leukaemic transformation of a thymic lymphosarcoma (Fig. 20.11).

Sen and Borella (1975) have shown that T-cell markers (E-positive ALL) are associated with a high proportion of older children, predominantly boys, a thymic mass and a high white count at diagnosis (Fig. 20.12). HL-A9 phenotype has also been found to be associated with a better prognosis in childhood ALL (Lawler et al., 1974).

Conflicting evidence exists as to whether a lymphocytosis (>20 per cent) during remission is a favourable (Skeel et al., 1968) or unfavourable (Breslow et al., 1970) feature. It might reflect an immunological reaction against the leukaemic cells.

In AML the presence of Auer rods is associated with higher remission rate and longer survival (Levin and Kundel, 1964).

Although the prognostic features of white cell count, blast cell count, platelet count and degree of organ involvement are related to the chance of survival for up to 4 years they no longer seem to be relevant to the chance of very long-term survival e.g. for over 9 years (Till et al., 1973). The best indicator of an exceptionally favourable prognosis in ALL seems to be survival for 4 years without relapse. Likewise Burchenal (1968) found that 50 per cent of acute leukaemia patients who survive for 5 years will go on to survive for 15 years.

Unusual types of childhood leukaemia

CHRONIC MYELOCYTIC LEUKAEMIA (CML)

This constitutes between 2 and 5 per cent of all cases of childhood leukaemia, and occurs in two distinct forms; 'juvenile' usually presenting under the age of 4, and 'adult' usually presenting in older children (Fig. 20.13). Cytogenetic evidence suggests that the 'adult' form is the same disease as is seen in adults, the childhood cases merely representing one end of the broad age distribution curve of Philadelphia chromosome-positive (Ph^1 +ve) CML. The 'juvenile' form has several unique features raising the possibility that it is congenital in origin (Weatherall et al., 1968).

Juvenile CML. Common presenting symptoms are pallor, recurrent infections, bleeding or bruising and a protuberant abdomen. Clinical features include prominent generalized lymphadenopathy, firm hepatosplenomegaly with the spleen more markedly enlarged than the liver, and a characteristic facial rash described as eczematous or pustular in appearance particularly on the cheeks and forehead. The general course of juvenile CML is rapid with

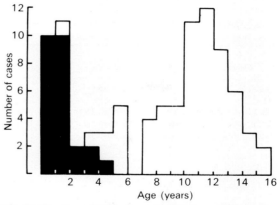

Fig. 20.13 Age distribution of 25 cases of juvenile CML (black) and 66 cases of 'adult' CML in children (white). (Reproduced from the *British Journal of Haematology* (1964), **10**, 551, by permission of the authors Hardisty et al.).

prominent haemorrhagic features and the need for frequent blood transfusions. Overall survival is distinctly poor, with a median duration of 9 months, compared to 2 years, 9 months in the 'adult' form of childhood CML.

Haematological features include severe anaemia (normochromic or slightly macrocytic), marked thrombocytopenia and moderate leukocytosis with increased numbers of myelocytes, promyelocytes, myeloblasts (up to 8 per cent), and normoblasts as well as plentiful neutrophils, eosinophils and basophils. Typical findings at diagnosis are shown for 6 personally observed patients in Table 20.12. On occasions this picture may be confused with a 'leucoerythroblastic' anaemia secondary to marrow infiltration or to a 'leukaemoid' reaction to infection. A useful feature distinguishing CML from the latter is cytochemical assessment of the leucocyte alkaline phosphatase reaction. This is increased in a myeloid leukaemoid reaction and is usually, but not always, low in juvenile CML (Table 20.12).

Marrow examination shows increased cellularity with preponderance of the myeloid series with up to 10 per cent blast cells and a decrease in megakaryocytes and erythroid precursors (Hardisty et al., 1964).

Additional investigations show elevation of Hb F both as judged on a Kleihauer film (Weatherall et al., 1968) or by the Singer alkaline denaturation test, when levels of between 40 and 55 per cent are found in the juvenile, but not the adult, form (Hardisty et al., 1964). As the disease progresses there is an increase, both in the percentage of cells staining by the Kleihauer technique (e.g. from 20 per cent at diagnosis to over 80 per cent terminally) and as the percentage of Hb (e.g. from

Table 20.12 Haematological data in chronic myelocytic leukaemia

Juvenile type

Case	Age	Survival	Hb	WBC	Platelets	Ph$_1$	HbF	A'Ptase	Se B$_{12}$ pg/ml
S.McF.	1 year	2 weeks	6·8	13,800	36,000	—ve	/	/	/
D.C.	1 year	2 years	6·5	150,000	30,000	—ve	+++	+++	2,000
M.F.	1½ years	3 months	8·5	26,000	9,000	—ve	+++	—ve	1,400
K.N.	2 years	5 months	5·4	129,000	2,600	/	40%	weak	2,160
A.G.	2½ years	20 months	3·8	20,400	22,000	—ve	+++	—ve	1,400
I.O.	3 years	3 months	9·4	27,000	29,000	—ve	43%	weak	1,650

Adult type

Case	Age	Survival	Hb	WBC	Platelets	Ph$_1$	HbF	A'Ptase	Se B$_{12}$ pg/ml
J.M.	7 months	2 months	6·8	400,000	300,000	+ve	±	—ve	1,200
D.M.	5 years	Alive	7·0	292,000	286,000	+ve	—	—ve	1,800
A.A.	9 years	Alive	7·4	960,000	150,000	+ve	—	—ve	/
D.T.	12 years	Alive	10·8	308,000	600,000	+ve	—	—ve	2,010

20 to 65·5 per cent) (Weatherall *et al.*, 1968). Transfusions would, of course, affect these results. Only slight increases in Hb F level were found in ALL (1–3 per cent) or AML (2–6 per cent) (Weatherall *et al.*, 1968), and no increase in children with adult CML (Hardisty *et al.*, 1964). Weatherall also found a reduction in carbonic anhydrase levels in the red cells in juvenile CML, both the electrophoretic pattern of the isoenzymes and the total activity being identical to those of a newborn infant. Together with the reversion to synthesis of Hb F these findings indicate a return to foetal erythropoiesis, supporting the suggestion of Hardisty *et al.* (1964) that this is a congenital disorder, or that it arises from a 'nest' of stem cells in which normal differentiation has not occurred.

Serum B$_{12}$ levels are excessively high in both forms of CML, this being due to liberation of a B$_{12}$-binding protein from the cytoplasm of effete myeloid cells (Chikkappa *et al.*, 1971), and merely reflecting the increased mass and turnover of these cells in tissues and blood.

In 90 per cent of adults with CML cytogenetic examination of direct marrow preparations show a normal diploid number of chromosomes (46) but, included among the small achrocentric G21 or G22 group, is the very small Ph[1] chromosome whose arms have lost around 50 per cent of their length (Nowell and Hungeford, 1960; Sandberg and Hossfeld, 1970). It is not found in PHA-cultured lymphocytes or skin fibroblasts in this disease, but is present in erythroblasts and megakaryocytes as well as the pathological myeloid series. Other diseases in which Ph[1] has been found include myelofibrosis, myeloid metaplasia, polycythaemia rubra vera and thrombocythaemia.

Whereas children with the adult form of CML have shown diploid marrow karyotypes with Ph[1] in 32 to 94 per cent of dividing blood or marrow cells 2 out of 4 children with the juvenile form showed aneuploidy with 47 chromosomes, the extra chromosome being minute (Reisman and Trujillo, 1963). Hardisty *et al.* (1964) similarly found the Ph[1] chromosome in normal diploid cells in all 4 of their adult type patients, but in none of their 3 juvenile cases. In two of these juvenile cases, although diploid, there was a structural abnormality of one of the small acrocentric chromosomes (21 or 21). This consisted of condensation of the chromatin of the long arm resulting in a smaller chromosome than normal, but lacking the characteristic morphology of Ph[1]. Neither aneuploidy nor structural abnormalities have been found in 6 personally observed patients.

Treatment of juvenile CML has been relatively unsatisfactory. Responses to oral 6-MP (2·5 mg/kg/day) occur, but not to busulphan (Reisman and Trujillo, 1963). No reports are available on the use of the newer antileukaemic drugs such as ARA-C, TG or DAUNO and perhaps these are worthy of cautious assessment, bearing in mind the poor natural history of the disease. Splenectomy has been followed by remission of over 5 years in an atypical case (Holton and Johnson, 1968). Local radiotherapy to the spleen has been of temporary value when gross splenomegaly has been producing abdominal distress. Frequent transfusions of packed cells are necessary, and with platelet concentrates at times of overt bleeding.

The adult form of CML in children presents more insidiously than the juvenile form. Initial symptoms may be of simple lethargy and pallor with later abdominal distension. Priapism has been a presenting symptom in boys (Graw *et al.*, 1969). Haemorrhagic manifestations do not occur. On examination the most striking feature is gross splenomegaly, sometimes extending to the pelvis or across the midline. The liver is also enlarged, but not so markedly. Lymphadenopathy is minimal or absent. Bone or joint symptoms may also be present.

Peripheral blood examination shows a grossly elevated white cell count without thrombocytopenia (Table 20.12). Myelocytes and promyelocytes are abundant, as well as neutrophils, eosinophils and basophils, but myeloblasts and normoblasts are present in much smaller numbers than in the juvenile form. Leucocyte alkaline phosphatase reaction is consistently absent or very weak. There is no increase in Hb F. Serum B_{12} levels are extremely high. The Ph^1 chromosome is consistently present in direct marrow preparations. It is present in the myeloid, erythroid and megakaryocytic cell lines, but not in lymphocytes, skin fibroblasts or bone marrow fibroblasts (Maniatis *et al.*, 1969). Marrow smears show increased cellularity due to hyperplasia of the myeloid series and, by contrast with the juvenile form, megakaryocytes are plentiful. Conventional treatment of adult type CML is with busulphan (Myeleran) 0·06 mg/kg/day (2 mg tablets) which usually causes the total white cell count to fall in 2–4 weeks (Turesson, 1957) and to reach normal levels in 12–20 weeks (Galton, 1969). Allopurinol should also be given because of the hazard of hyperuricaemia. Blood counts are carried out weekly and the results plotted on semilogarithmic graphs as extrapolation will then indicate when the count is likely to reach around $15,000/mm^3$. Busulphan is stopped when the count falls below $20,000/mm^3$ or the platelet count below $100,000/mm^3$, and is later restarted at a dose of 0·03 mg/kg to stabilize the white cell count at around $10,000/mm^3$. Radiotherapy to the spleen may be of value when gross splenomegaly is causing distressing symptoms but is no longer regarded as a primary mode of therapy for the systemic disease (Spiers, 1974). Hydroxyurea (30–50 mg/kg/day) and dibromannitol (125–250 mg/day in adults) are 'second line' drugs of value in patients developing unacceptable thrombocytopenia on busulphan.

A constant long-term hazard in adult type CML is the development of 'blastic crises' which are acute transformations into myeloblastic leukaemia of a particularly refractory variety, seldom responding to therapy (Karanas and Silver, 1968). It has been suggested that this develops in children with this form of CML even more frequently than in adults (Ghose *et al.*, 1965). Transformation to promyelocytic leukaemia can also occur.

Both the hazards of long-term busulphan, including pulmonary fibrosis, and the inability of conventional treatment to eliminate the Ph^1 leukaemic clone, with the ever-present hazard of AML transformation, are encouraging exploration of more radical methods of treatment (Spiers, 1974).

The M.R.C. are conducting a controlled clinical trial of elective splenectomy performed shortly after remission has been obtained by busulphan. A pilot study of this approach has shown a halving of the expected incidence of AML transformation (Spiers *et al.*, 1975A). There were no deaths after the operation.

In an attempt to eliminate the Ph^1 marrow clone alternative chemotherapy is being investigated. Spiers *et al.* (1975B) used oral thioguanine, given 8-hourly, at an initial total daily dose of 3–4 mg/kg (approx. 100 mg/m^2) and found that this drug was at least as effective as busulphan, and had the advantage of rapid reversibility of haemopoietic depression when discontinued. It could conveniently be combined with allopurinol for prevention of hyperuricaemia. Unfortunately, even the use of intensive high dose thioguanine plus ARA-C failed to eradicate the Ph^1 clone in spite of the temporary production of severe neutropenia.

ERYTHROLEUKAEMIA (DI GUGLIELMO'S SYNDROME)

Traditionally considered to be an acute leukaemia arising from the erythroblast cell line or more commonly a mixed myeloblastic-erythroblastic leukaemia the clinical presentation is indistinguishable from AML. It is a considerable rarity in paediatric practice, only 4 cases being seen over a ten-year period. Few reports of children with this form of leukaemia are available (Megalini and Åhström, 1958; Dyment *et al.*, 1968; Schwartz *et al.*, 1970).

Haematological findings include severe anaemia, thrombocytopenia and neutropenia, together with large numbers of circulating erythroblasts. Marrow smears similarly show extensive replacement of normal marrow elements with erythroblasts many of which are polyploid with megaloblastic features and strongly PAS-positive cytoplasm (Quaglino and Hayhoe, 1960). In addition there is usually a pathological increase in myeloblasts, which sometimes possess leukaemic stigmata such as Auer rods. Megakaryocytes are reduced in parallel with the thrombocytopenia.

This disease proves more refractory to treatment than AML or AMMoL and complete remissions are seldom attained. But perhaps few cases have been given present-day combination chemotherapy. Cytosine arabinoside produced a 'good partial' remission in one personally observed case, and 'TRAMPCO' a complete remission.

Schwartz *et al.* (1970) have shown that transfusion alone was followed by disappearance of the erythroblastic abnormalities in blood and marrow, suggesting that they were under normal humoral control. There was no suppression of myeloblastic proliferation though. These authors proposed that secondary haemolysis or ineffective erythropoiesis might be responsible for the erythroblastic picture and challenged the concept of a primary malignancy of the erythroid cell line. On the other hand there is recent evidence that red cell precursors can be directly involved in the leukaemic process in AML, sharing the same chromosomal abnormalities, suggesting a common stem cell origin (Blackstock and Garson, 1974).

PROMYELOCYTIC LEUKAEMIA

This is an uncommon variant of AML characterized by marked haemorrhagic manifestations and absence of hepatosplenomegaly or lymphadenopathy. More than half the patients in one series of 25 were children (Bernard *et al.*, 1963). The peripheral blood showed from zero to 98 per cent of promyelocytes and the marrow 50 to 100 per cent. These cells differ from myeloblasts in having abundant cytoplasm containing numerous red granules. Auer rods and also PAS-positive cytoplasmic masses have occasionally been found (Didisheim *et al.*, 1964).

The unusually marked haemorrhagic tendency is due to associated consumptive coagulopathy with low fibrinogen and Factor V levels, and secondary fibrinolysis (Didisheim *et al.*, 1964; Rand *et al.*, 1969; Albarracin and Haust 1971). It is thought that DIC is triggered by release of the promyelocytic granules. Correction of the coagulation disturbance can be obtained by heparin treatment or if leukaemic remission is achieved.

Treatment of promyelocytic leukaemia should probably be with the same drug schedules as used in AML. In the past remission has seldom been obtained (Bernard *et al.*, 1963), but this situation might improve with more modern combination chemotherapy and supportive care, including correction of the DIC.

CHRONIC LYMPHOCYTIC LEUKAEMIA (CLL)

Only 3 probable cases of CLL in childhood have been recorded (Holowach, 1948; Casey, 1968; Sardeman, 1973). Clinical and haematological features were similar in each case. Young children,

aged under 3 years, presented primarily with chronic gross splenomegaly without lymphadenopathy or other prominent clinical feature except pallor. Only one had mild haemorrhagic symptoms and thrombocytopenia was not a feature. Anaemia was only moderate (8·8 to 10·2 g/100 ml). Total white cell counts were elevated to the 20,000–30,000/mm³ level for much of their clinical course, with 80 to 90 per cent mature small or medium sized lymphocytes. Marrow infiltration was present with around 90 per cent of the cells small lymphocytes. One would be reluctant to accept the diagnosis on morphological grounds alone since the leukaemic cells in 'prolymphocytic' types of ALL closely resemble mature lymphocytes, and even typical lymphoblasts may be indistinguishable from lymphocytes in blood or marrow smears that have been made too thickly, or in histological sections. It is the fact that the clinical and other haematological features of these reported cases, as well as their relatively protracted course, differ from ALL that suggests that they were, in fact, a different disease. One wonders if they may have been leukaemic transformation from lymphosarcoma of the spleen. Although this usually results in ALL in children (*vide supra*), in adults it is more often CLL.

No therapeutic response to prednisone, 6-MP or splenectomy was found by Sardeman (1973) and cyclophosphamide probably had an inadequate trial, the patient dying of sudden overwhelming infection. Chlorambucil produced a good response with reduction in white cell count from 120,000/mm³ to 20,000/mm³ in another patient (Casey, 1968) with current maintenance at a dose of 2 mg/day (Lascari, 1973).

EOSINOPHILIC AND BASOPHILIC LEUKAEMIA

This is a variety of myeloid leukaemia and may occur as either blast cell or mature eosinophilic leukaemia, running an acute or chronic course (Bentley *et al.*, 1961). It is a rare disease but about one third of reported cases have been in children. Distinction has to be made from the eosinophilia that occurs in CML (both juvenile and adult types), Hodgkin's disease or other forms of eosinophilic leukaemoid reaction (Rickles *et al.*, 1972) including visceral larvae migrans, trichinosis, tropical eosinophilia, eosinophilic pneumonitis, metastatic carcinoma, polyarteritis nodosa and familial eosinophilia (Lascari, 1973).

The clinical picture is similar to other types of acute leukaemia but additional features include a high incidence of pulmonary manifestations, including chronic cough, cyanosis and transient radiological infiltration (Bentley *et al.*, 1961). Myocardial involvement and mural thrombi may also occur.

Anaemia and thrombocytopenia are usually present together with a white cell count in the range seen in CML but with a preponderance of mature or immature cells of the eosinophil series. Occasional aleukaemic cases occur. Marrow and other tissues are heavily infiltrated by eosinophils in all forms; eosinophilic blast cells or myelocytes in the acute form, mature eosinophils in the chronic form (Lascari, 1973).

Basophilic leukaemia is even more rare than eosinophilic forms and few childhood cases have been reported (Quattrin *et al.*, 1959). Acute and chronic forms exist with clinical manifestations and treatment similar to AML and CML. True basophilic leukaemia has to be distinguished from CML with a raised basophil count and mast cell leukaemia in which superficially similar cells may appear in blood and marrow as part of systemic mastocytosis, associated with urticaria pigmentosa (Waters *et al.*, 1957).

CHRONIC MONOCYTIC LEUKAEMIA (CMOL)

This is also excessively rare in children, only 2 cases occurring in a series of 900 leukaemic children (Pearson and Diamond, 1958). In addition to hepatosplenomegaly, anaemia and thrombocytopenia a widespread infiltrated maculopapular skin rash is characteristic. Skin histology shows infiltration by monocytes. Gingival hypertrophy is less common than in AMOL. A progressive monocytosis develops in both blood and marrow. The clinical course is protracted with liability to recurrent infections and anaemia.

LEUKAEMIC RETICULOENDOTHELIOSIS

Essentially a reticulum cell leukaemia of either acute or chronic course this is currently often referred to as 'hairy cell leukaemia' since short villi can be seen projecting from the cell surface by phase contrast (Schrek and Donnelly, 1966). Recent evidence is that these cells are lymphoid in origin (Haak *et al.*, 1974). On conventionally stained blood or marrow films the cells are large with abundant cytoplasm showing pseudopodlike-projections. A specific tartrate-resistant isoenzyme of acid phosphatase has been found in the cells of leukaemic reticuloendotheliosis (Yam *et al.*, 1971).

Clinical presentation is insidious with anaemia, infection, and sometimes bleeding. Splenomegaly is virtually always present, hepatomegaly in over half, and lymphadenopathy in a third of the patients (Bouroncle *et al.*, 1958). Pancytopenia develops with or without reticulum cells in the peripheral blood. Bone marrow aspiration is difficult but marrow biopsy shows increased cellularity with 30 to 90 per cent of reticulum cells (Bouroncle *et al.*, 1958). Childhood cases have been reported by Vaithianathan *et al.* (1962) and Fuduka (1966). The course of the disease in children has been acute with survival of 3–10 months, contrasting with the disease in adults where only a third have an acute course (Bouroncle *et al.*, 1958). Temporary improvement has been obtained in adults after irradiation or removal of the spleen, and with VCR and corticosteroids.

LEUKAEMIC TRANSFORMATION OF RETICULOSES

In children lymphosarcoma undergoes leukaemic transformation to a disease distinguishable from ALL in approximately 30 per cent of patients (Jones and Klingberg, 1963), compared to a figure nearer 3 per cent in adults, where the leukaemic phase is usually CLL. These children present with hepatosplenomegaly, generalized lymphadenopathy and evidence of marrow failure just as do ordinary cases of ALL. If the apparent transformation occurs only a month or so after the localized lesion it becomes arguable whether or not the disease was ALL from the start. Only if a marrow examination was performed at the time of initial diagnosis can this possibility be reasonably excluded. This practice is therefore advocated in all patients with lymphosarcoma.

Not only do the blast cells in blood and marrow appear similar to the blasts in ALL, but they also respond to the same chemotherapy, with comparable remission duration to similarly treated children with ALL (Jones *et al.*, 1967). This has certainly been my own experience (Cases 18 and 19).

Since 30 per cent of children with leukaemic transformation of lymphosarcoma develop meningeal involvement (Jones *et al.*, 1967), prophylactic CNS therapy is recommended as in ALL. Because of the liability to leukaemic transformation in children and because of the demonstrable efficacy of antileukaemic drugs against lymphosarcoma cells Pinkel (1968) and Aur *et al.* (1971) recommend a chemotherapy schedule similar to that used in ALL in addition to local surgery and/or radiotherapy in all but the most localized forms of lymphosarcoma. This is the current policy at the Royal Hospital for Sick Children, Glasgow, but CNS prophylaxis is reserved for those cases where leukaemic transformation has occurred.

In Burkitt's lymphoma marrow involvement occurs in around 8 per cent of patients (Wright and Pike, 1968). A leucoerythroblastic blood picture is then usual, but on rare occasions circulating lymphoma cells have been reported producing a picture indistinguishable from ALL (Clift *et al.*, 1963).

By contrast with lymphosarcoma localized reticulum cell sarcoma undergoes leukaemic transformation in less than 5 per cent of cases (Zeffren and Ultmann, 1960), giving rise to a pure monocytic leukaemia of the Schilling type. This differs from the more usual Naegeli type of AMMoL in that it lacks the concomitant myeloblastic proliferation. The clinical and haematological picture in such cases is that of an acute leukaemia due to primitive monocytes or monoblasts (Belding *et al.*, 1955). Gingival hypertrophy due to leukaemic infiltration is common. There is a fulminant and refractory clinical course although a response to methotrexate has been recorded (Dubowitz, 1964).

Hodgkin's disease very occasionally undergoes apparent leukaemic transformation, giving rise to Reed-Sternberg cell leukaemia (Scheerer *et al.*, 1964). Good photomicrographs are shown in the paper of Bouroncle (1966) who used white cell concentrates on peripheral blood. Conventional marrow aspiration is virtually useless for the *diagnosis* of Hodgkin's disease since its involvement is usually focal (Kadin *et al.*, 1971). For staging purposes open wedge biopsy is needed (Kaplan, 1972).

Case 18. This little girl (No. 83649) presented at the age of 6 months with a subcutaneous lump above her left eyebrow. Biopsy showed this to be a lymphosarcoma. The tumour was excised and local radiotherapy given to the surrounding area. Six months later she became ill with hepatosplenomegaly, generalized lymphadenopathy, 7,500 circulating blast cells per mm³ in the blood and a marrow which showed replacement by PAS +ve blast cells indistinguishable from ALL. This was in May, 1965. She was treated as if she had ALL. This involved prednisolone and 6-MP for remission induction, followed by cyclic chemotherapy using 6-MP, MTX and cyclophosphamide with VCR plus prednisolone 'pseudo-reinduction' introduced in August, 1968. There was no recurrence of the disease either local or systemic and chemotherapy was stopped in May, 1973, after 8 years. Fortunately she remains well now 2 years later and 10 years from diagnosis of generalized lymphosarcoma with leukaemic transformation.

Case 19. A girl aged 4 (No. 132331) developed a cough and was referred to the chest physicians who found a thymic mass on chest X-ray. Transferred to a Thoracic Surgery Unit a thoracotomy and biopsy were performed, confirming the diagnosis of lymphosarcoma of the thymus. The tumour was too extensive for surgical removal and she was referred to the Radiotherapy Department. By this time she had become anaemic and we were consulted. She did not have hepatosplenomegaly or lymphadenopathy but the peripheral blood contained blast cells (700/mm³). The marrow showed replacement with blast cells very similar in morphology to leukaemic lymphoblasts. Since the marrow had not been examined at the time of appearance of the thymic tumour some 6 weeks earlier, it remains arguable whether she had disseminated lymphosarcoma or ALL with thymic involvement. We transferred her to a laminar flow isolation unit and commenced chemotherapy with VCR, daunorubicin and prednisolone. The blast cells rapidly disappeared from the blood, she became moderately neutropenic and developed acute 'gout' of a big toe. This responded to allopurinol. In 4 weeks she was in complete clinical and marrow remission, with a normal peripheral blood. Prednisolone was tailed off and she was given a 5-day course of MTX (15 mg/m²/day) as consolidation therapy. The thymic shadow progressively disappeared during this time. Thereafter she was given maintenance chemotherapy consisting of daily 6-MP, weekly oral MTX and weekly oral cyclophosphamide, plus VCR and prednisolone at 12-week intervals. With the object of eradicating possible residual thymic tumour we gave her local thymic irradiation 5 months from initial chemotherapy. Shortly afterwards we gave a course of cranial radiotherapy (2,400 r) plus IT MTX in case the CNS had been seeded at the time there were circulating blast cells. Subsequently she has remained free of recurrence, but she developed dyspnoea and cyanosis with striking changes on chest X-ray 11 months after the thymic irradiation. A lung aspirate failed to demonstrate *Pneumocystis carinii* but nevertheless we treated her with IM pentamidine, fresh plasma, O₂ and temporarily stopped her antileukaemic drugs. She gradually recovered although developing moderate renal impairment during the second week of pentamidine. Thereafter we omitted the weekly cyclophosphamide from her chemotherapy. After a further two years on daily 6-MP, weekly MTX and monthly VCR plus prednisolone we stopped chemotherapy (3 years from its initiation). Latterly she had been having considerable trouble from recurrent otitis media and upper respiratory tract infections. Since stopping chemotherapy 18 months ago she has been in better health. There has been no recurrence of the tumour.

CONGENITAL LEUKAEMIA

The term congenital leukaemia implies that the disease is overtly manifest on the first day of life. It does not refer to those cases of leukaemia arising in later childhood that are thought to have a genetic or congenital aetiology. Since infants are liable to show myeloid leukaemoid reactions, even with a few blast cells in the peripheral blood, as a reaction to infection (Holland and Mauer, 1963) or haemolysis it is wise to regard the diagnosis of leukaemia in the newborn with considerable scepticism, as pointed out by Kauffman and Hess (1962).

Clinically infants with congenital leukaemia show characteristic skin nodules in sites such as the scalp, cheeks, ear lobes, nose and trunk, ranging from 0·2 to 3 cm in diameter (Reimann *et al.*, 1955;

Fortina and Petrocini, 1953). These are firm but mobile, with bluish discoloration of the overlying skin. Hepatosplenomegaly is usual, but lymphadenopathy and jaundice uncommon. Thrombocytopenic bleeding may occur from the umbilical stump, mucous membranes and gastrointestinal tract (Oski and Naiman, 1972).

Neonatal leukaemia also occurs but does not show such a uniform clinical picture. The infants may present with unexplained fever, diarrhoea, poor weight gain, pallor and petechiae. Nodular skin infiltration is unusual. Differential diagnosis includes bacterial infection, erythroblastosis foetalis, syphilis, cytomegalovirus, toxoplasmosis, neuroblastoma and Letterer-Siwe disease (Oski and Naiman, 1972).

AML is 7 to 8 times more common than ALL in the newborn. Anaemia may not develop until after birth but thrombocytopenia is invariable (Pierce, 1959). Neutropenia may be present and the peripheral blood and marrow findings are similar to those of AML or ALL in older children. Therapy in this age group presents considerable practical problems and it is known that the prognosis is poor for children under one year. Nevertheless it is possible to obtain worthwhile complete remissions in infants of 4 months or so with AMMoL using modern chemotherapy and supportive measures.

In infants with mongolism the diagnosis of neonatal leukaemia is particularly thwart with difficulties. Engel, Hammond, Eitzman, Pearson and Krivit (1964) described 7 infants with Down's syndrome in whom the diagnosis of AML (5), AMOL (1) or ASL (1) had been made within the first 10 days of life. Splenomegaly was present in all as well as white cell counts between 25,000 and 387,000/mm³ with blast cells between 36 and 95 per cent. The marrow also suggested leukaemia in the 3 patients in which it was examined. All recovered without residual evidence of leukaemia, only 2 receiving antileukaemic drugs.

In a review of the world literature Rosner *et al.* (1972) collected 18 newborn mongoloid infants who had clinical and haematological features resembling leukaemia but disappearing spontaneously over weeks or months. These apparently leukaemoid reactions to which the newborn mongol are prone are predominantly of the myeloid or myeloblastic type, giving rise to the false impression that the *true* leukaemia to which mongoloid infants also have an increased susceptibility is also usually myeloid in type. In fact the ratio of ALL:AML in later life is the same in mongols as in other children (Rosner *et al.*, 1972). The transient leukaemia-like disturbances shown by these infants is attributed to disturbed control of not only myelopoiesis but also megakaryocyte proliferation (Okada *et al.*, 1972). In two out of three infants with translocation mongolism Behrman *et al.* (1966) found thrombocytopenia, myeloid metaplasia, infiltrative lesions resembling myelocytic leukaemia and disordered erythropoiesis. It is clear that more than usual reservations must be made in making the diagnosis of leukaemia in mongol infants.

Congenital leukaemia has recently been reviewed by Pochedly (1971).

Non-leukaemic disorders with infiltration of the marrow

METASTATIC MALIGNANT INFILTRATION OF THE MARROW

Involvement of the marrow can occur with a number of childhood tumours giving rise to a leucoerythroblastic anaemia and eventual pancytopenia. Marrow aspiration shows a picture that may range from occasional tumour cell clumps found among normal marrow after prolonged search to almost total replacement of normal marrow elements by tumour cells. The main morphological feature distinguishing this appearance from acute leukaemic infiltration of the marrow is the fact that the tumour cells are predominantly arranged in 'clumps' or 'sheets', unlike tumours of haemic or reticuloendothelial origin.

In paediatric practice neuroblastoma is the most frequent metastatic tumour involving the marrow. On rare occasions neuroblastoma cells may also appear in the peripheral blood (Plate F) closely simulating leukaemia. It is a helpful feature that neuroblastoma cells give neither the PAS reaction of leukaemic lymphoblasts nor the Sudan Black staining of myeloblasts. Taken together with the usual clinical features of neuroblastoma such as displacement of the kidney seen in an IVP, calcification in the tumour and increased urinary excretion of VMA or HVA no confusion with leukaemia usually arises. The radiological bone changes, however, may be similar.

Delta and Pinkel (1964) and Finkelstein *et al.* (1970) have reported the incidence of marrow infiltration as detected by aspiration in children. Their findings are shown in Table 20.13. Neuroblastoma, rhabdomyosarcoma, retinoblastoma and ganglioneuroblastoma involve the marrow relatively frequently; Wilm's tumour does not.

Finkelstein *et al.* (1970) describe the neuroblastoma cell as of similar size to a small lymphocyte (10 microns), whereas rhabdomyosarcoma and

PAEDIATRIC HAEMATOLOGY

Table 20.13   Incidence of marrow infiltration

	Delta and Pinkel (1964)	Finkelstein et al. (1970)
Neuroblastoma	21/30	49/70
Rhabdomymyosarcoma	3/18	5/25
Retinoblastoma	1/2	3/13
Ganglioneuroblastoma	—	2/5
Ganglioneuroma	—	0/2
Osteogenic Sarcoma	2/6	0/4
Ewing's Tumour	1/8	0/7
Wilm's Tumour	0/12	0/53
Miscellaneous Sarcoma	—	1/13
Miscellaneous Carcinoma	—	0/27
Total children in series	76	213

Fractions indicate the number of patients with positive marrow findings/number of patients tested.

retinoblastoma cells are more the size of promyelocytes (20 microns). A syncytium is characteristic of neuroblastoma, with rhabdomyosarcoma and retinoblastoma as clumps. Four out of 5 rhabdomyosarcoma patients showed PAS positivity of the tumour cells in the marrow, but other tumours were PAS negative. Delta and Pinkel (1964) describe the appearance of rhabdomyosarcoma cells in marrow as either fusiform and binucleated or anaplastic.

A source of possible confusion is that up to 21 per cent of blast cells, which are actually lymphoblasts, may be found in marrows of children with localized neuroblastoma who are doing well and presumably represent an immunological reaction against the tumour (Evans and Hummeler, 1973).

MYELOMATOSIS

Excessively rare in childhood there are, however, reports of myelomatous involvement of lumbar spine, pelvis and skull in a boy of 4 (Slavens, 1934) and of marrow replacement by myeloma cells producing pancytopenia and hyperglobulinaemia in a boy of $7\frac{1}{2}$ (Porter, 1963).

LETTERER-SIWE DISEASE

This is the infantile form of histiocytosis X, other forms being Hand-Schuller-Christian disease and eosinophilic granuloma of bone which occur in older children, are less widely disseminated and have a better prognosis. A unifying pathological feature is non-lipid reticulum cell or histiocytic proliferation of unknown cause (Avery et al., 1957).

In Letterer-Siwe disease many different tissues may be involved including skin, marrow, lung, liver, spleen, skull and skeleton; whereas in Hand-Schiller-Christian disease it is usually only the skull, skeleton and lungs, and in eosinophilic granuloma only the skull and skeleton that are involved. Exceptions occur, however, and it is clear that histiocytosis X includes a continuous spectrum of disorders.

Even within the category of Letterer-Siwe disease the clinical course can vary between one similar to acute leukaemia at one extreme and one showing spontaneous remission without recurrence at the other (Doede and Rappaport, 1967). Lahey (1962) has shown that adverse prognostic features are: (a) an early age of onset, particularly if under age of 6 months; (b) multiple system involvement. If 3 or 4 tissues (e.g. skin, bone, lung or spleen) are infiltrated the mortality is around 35 per cent; if 5 or 6 tissues are involved it approaches 100 per cent.

Presentation is commonly in the first year of life or even at birth (Hertz and Hambrick, 1968), but it may also occur in older children. Early manifestations are often a characteristic, slightly infiltrated apparently seborrheic dermatitis, with associated purpura involving the scalp, palms and trunk (Fig. 20.14). This is often accompanied by anaemia, fever, bleeding, prominent generalized lymphadenopathy, firm hepatosplenomegaly and discharge from the ear due to otitis media or externa. Histiocytes are found in the ear discharge and are also responsible for the skin infiltrate (Fig. 20.14). Skin biopsy is a valuable confirmatory diagnostic procedure. Radiological examination typically shows 'punched out' areas (X-ray Plate 3), especially of skull, ribs and pelvis, and sometimes 'honeycomb' changes in the lung fields consisting of areas of overinflation superimposed upon a ground glass background due to pulmonary infiltration. Pneumomediastinum or pneumothorax may also develop (X-ray Plate 4).

Haematological changes are relatively nonspecific and may present diagnostic difficulties in

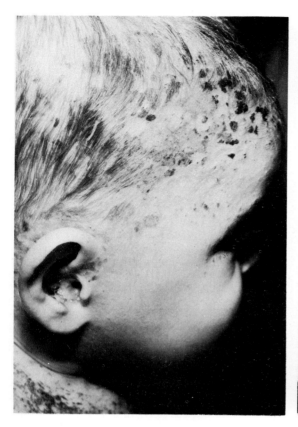
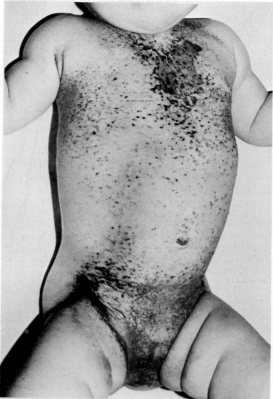

A

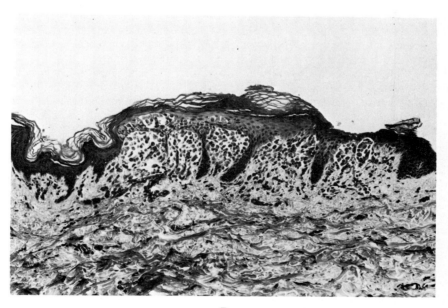

B

Fig 20.14 Rash of Letterer-Siwe Disease. A, Head and body of a child with purpura plus eczematous eruption; B, histology showing superficial haemorrhages plus histiocytic infiltration. (x 40).

the early stages before the syndrome becomes fully developed. Anaemia is usually severe and is normocytic with rouleaux formation and a high ESR. Sometimes a haemolytic or leucoerythroblastic picture may also be present. Neutropenia and thrombocytopenia occur when either the spleen is grossly enlarged or there is heavy infiltration of the marrow. Thrombocytopenia due to DIC has also been recorded (Mauger, 1971). Eosinophilia is not a feature.

Marrow examination may show infiltration with large, foamy reticulum cells (Plate G) (Baber, 1960), some of which may show erythrophagocytosis. They do not contain lipid or vacuoles. But it is only in around 20 per cent of cases that marrow examination proves diagnostic (Mauer, 1969), although more frequently becoming infiltrated as the disease progresses.

Treatment of the disseminated variety of Letterer-Siwe disease is unsatisfactory but corticosteroids, vinca alkaloids, cyclophosphamide (Beier et al., 1963; Hertz and Hambrick, 1968; Starling et al., 1972) and methotrexate are of temporary benefit. Bone pain can be controlled with local irradiation. Less disseminate disease may respond well to steroids alone.

FAMILIAL ERYTHROPHAGOCYTIC LYMPHOHISTIOCYTOSIS (FEL)

This is a rare disorder originally described by Farquhar and Claireaux (1952) in two siblings (one male, one female) each presenting at around 9 weeks with hepatosplenomegaly, pancytopenia and lymphoid 'smear' cells in the peripheral blood. Subsequent reports such as those of MacMahon et al. (1963) and Bell et al. (1968) have likewise been of successive infants presenting at between 9 weeks and 9 months with severe anaemia, fever and gross hepatosplenomegaly but insignificant lymphadenopathy. Peripheral blood findings showed a haemolytic anaemia, sometimes spherocytic, with polychromasia, reticulocytosis and circulating normoblasts, and moderate neutropenia plus thrombocytopenia. Marrow smears showed erythroid hyperplasia with reduced myeloid and megakaryocyte series and, in one case, large basophilic erythrophagocytic histiocytes ingesting normoblasts of all stages of maturity, but not red cells, leucocytes or platelets. The disease has seldom been diagnosed in life, as was done by Varadi et al. (1964).

Histologically the disease is characterized by proliferation of reticulum cells throughout the reticuloendothelial system with extreme erythrophagocytosis. The proliferating reticulum cells do not show features of malignancy as in Letterer-Siwe disease, nor do they contain lipid as in the storage diseases (McMahon et al., 1963). Cases have been reported where the disease has been confined to the CNS (Price et al., 1971), with convulsions, meningeal irritation and spasticity as the manifestations.

Splenectomy has been of temporary value in one patient, correcting the haemolytic anaemia, and thrombocytopenia, but followed later by death from infection at the age of 10 months (McMahon et al., 1963). This has been the usual outcome in other cases.

A recent report of a single case diagnosed during life and without other family members being affected gives evidence suggesting that an immune reaction is the pathogenetic mechanism, rather than a neoplastic histiocytic proliferation (Blennow et al., 1974). An autosomal recessive mode of inheritance has been suggested, first cousins sometimes being affected (Buist et al., 1971).

HISTIOCYTIC MEDULLARY RETICULOSIS (HMR)

This shows a rather similar histiocytic infiltration of the reticuloendothelial system with haemophagocytosis but occurring predominantly in adults and only rarely in children, and without a familial tendency. The haemophagocytosis involves not only red cells but also neutrophils and platelets (Natelson et al., 1968).

Clinical presentation is usually with fever, weight loss, hepatosplenomegaly with lymphadenopathy in about half the patients (Vaithianathan et al., 1967). Jaundice, purpura, pleural effusions and ascites may also occur.

Blood findings show pancytopenia with shortened red cell survival and reticulocytosis. Histiocytes and atypical mononuclear cells are present in the peripheral blood in around 50 per cent of cases (Greenberg et al., 1962; Clark and Dawson, 1969). Marrow examination shows a variable and progressive increase in histiocytes (5 to 15 per cent) which can be seen to be phagocytosing red cells, white cells and platelets (Lynch and Alfrey, 1965).

The course is rapidly down-hill with little benefit from splenectomy, antibiotics or steroids. Vincristine plus prednisone, however, has produced a brief remission (Kingdon et al., 1970). A case of this disease in a child has been described by Fowler (1960).

A closely related disorder terminating in histiocytic leukaemia has been described by Johnson et al. (1973). A 9-year-old girl had a life-long susceptibility to infection and thrombocytopenia with abnormal histiocytes present in the marrow for at least 4 years before the onset of histiocytic leukaemia. The patient's histiocytes phagocytosed bacteria but did not kill them; a situation analogous to CGD in blood phagocytes and accounting for the history of recurrent pneumonia, otitis and other infections. Splenectomy hastened progression of the disease.

Histiocytosis confined to the lymph nodes and marrow has also been described under the term 'sinus histiocytosis'. The clinical presentation may be similar to HMR but the course is benign. Hypergammaglobulinaemia, testicular involvement and rheumatoid arthritis may also be present (Azoury and Reed, 1966). A transient immunological defect in a child with mediastinal involvement and massive lymphadenopathy due to benign sinus histiocytosis has also been reported (Becroft et al.[7] 1973).

STORAGE DISEASES

Although their clinical manifestations are predominantly in the CNS, skeleton, connective tissues and viscera, haematological stigmata are also present in many of these hereditary disorders. Circulating leucocytes may contain vacuoles or inclusions and the marrow histiocytes, reticulum cells or even plasma cells may show characteristic morphological or staining reactions due to accumulation of the specific pathological material (Plates H, I, K, L). In certain instances (e.g. Gaucher's disease) the presence of large numbers of these 'storage' cells in the marrow produces secondary haematological changes due to marrow encroachment and/or phagocytic ingestion of blood cells and platelets.

Each storage disease is probably due to hereditary deficiency of a different enzyme resulting in intracellular accumulation of a specific metabolite. A recent classification is as follows:

Mucopolysaccharidoses
I	Hurler
II	Hunter
III	Sanfilippo
IV	Morquio
V	Scheie
VI	Maroteaux-Lamy
VII	Thompson-Nelson-Grobelny
Others	

Mucolipidoses
GM_1 Type I	Gangliosidosis	
GM_1 Type II	Gangliosidosis	
Fucosidosis		
Mannosidosis		
Sulphatidosis	(Austin)	
Mucolipidosis	Type I	(Spranger-Wiedeman)
Mucolipidosis	Type II	(Leroy-Opitz)
Mucolipidosis	Type III	(Pseudopolydystrophy)
Others		

Sphyngolipidoses
Tay-Sachs disease, and other forms of amaurotic familial idiocy
Niemann-Pick's disease
Gaucher's disease
Metachromatic leukodystrophy
Fabry's disease

After Hansen (1972), McKusick (1969) and Maroteaux (1970)

Gargoylism, dysostosis, neuronal and visceral storage are common among the mucopolysaccharidoses and mucolipidoses, with urinary excretion of mucopolysaccharides in the former group. Hepatosplenomegaly and neuronal storage without gargoylism is more characteristic of the sphyngolipidoses. Definitive diagnosis is made from a combination of biochemical, clinical and radiological findings, but haematological features may give an early clue to diagnosis.

Reilly or Alder-Reilly bodies are characteristic of the mucopolysaccharidoses. Originally described as an increase in the number and density of granules of neutrophils and monocytes by Adler (1939) and Reilly (1941) the presence of similar inclusions, consisting of a purple or red dot within a white halo (Plate K) in lymphocytes (Mittwoch, 1961) constitutes a more characteristic finding since the visual contrast with the normal cell is greater. Gasser in 1950 described similar inclusions in the marrow reticulum cells (Gasser cells) in these disorders and Pearson and Lorincz (1964) found marrow examination more sensitive than the peripheral blood showing abnormal granules in 17 out of 18 patients with Hurler's syndrome. The different varieties of mucopolysaccharidoses show minor variations in the distribution and appearances of Reilly bodies described by Hansen (1972) as follows:

Hurlers: Consistent diffuse inclusions in lymphocytes.
Hunters: Similar but less consistent than in Hurlers.
Sanfilippo: Lymphocyte inclusions are of a brighter red and more localized. Marrow plasma cells increased and contain impressive inclusions with giant halos, (Buhot Cells) (Royer, 1959). Reticulum cells have similar inclusions.
Morquio: Lymphocyte inclusions absent or rare but 50 to 90 per cent of neutrophils contain 1–3 large inclusions (up to 1 μm). Reticulum cells have variable fine granules.
Scheie: Haematologically least rewarding! Variable inclusions in up to 10 per cent of lymphocytes (McKusick et al. 1965). Occasional reticulum cells have fine granules.
Maroteaux: 'Haematologically a real bonus!' Coarse, closely packed granules in neutrophils of blood and marrow (what Adler (1939) and Reilly (1941) described). Also characteristic black-grey eosinophils.
Thompson-Nelson-Grobelny: Few lymphocytes have inclusions. Marrow shows variable number of reticulum cells containing coarse granules in vacuoles.

410   PAEDIATRIC HAEMATOLOGY

May-Grunwald-Giemsa stain is preferable to Wright's stain for showing up all these abnormalities and impeccable blood and marrow smears are necessary. Toluidine blue shows staining of the granules in Morquio and metachromatic, reddish staining in Thompson-Neslon-Grobelny.

Vacuolated lymphocytes (Plate L) and marrow reticulum cells are characteristic of the gangliosidoses and cerebroretinal degenerative diseases (Harlem, 1960). They are accompanied by characteristic changes in the marrow reticulum cells (Hansen, 1972).

GM_1 Type I: Striking grape-like clusters of vacuoles of uniform size in blood lymphocytes (Plate L). As disease progresses marrow becomes heavily infiltrated with vacuolated reticulum cells and pancytopenia may develop.

GM_1 Type II: Striking large (40 μm) reticulum cells in marrow with light blue (sky blue) cytoplasm (Hansen, 1972). These cells are non-granular but stain strongly with PAS.

Fucosidosis: Peripheral blood unhelpful. Marrow shows 'foamy' reticulum cells, some containing Hurler-like inclusions, others with coarse vacuoles.

Sulphatidosis: Very similar findings to Maroteaux mucopolysaccharidosis. Plasma cells strikingly involved.

Mucolipidosis Type I: Vacuoles plus inclusions in lymphocytes. Foamy reticulum cells in marrow.

Mucolipidosis Type II: Lymphocytes in blood and marrow show multiple inclusions (I-cell disease). Osteoblasts 'motheaten'.

Mucolipidosis Type III: Marrow shows increased plasma cells having coarse, pinkish-red inclusions and vacuoles.

Tay-Sachs: Vacuolated lymphocytes.

In Gaucher's and Niemann-Pick disease there are no morphological changes in the peripheral blood but marrow reticulum cells show characteristic changes. Gaucher cells result from the accumulation of a cerebroside-protein complex (Uzman, 1951). An inherited deficiency of the enzyme glucocerebrosidase causes an accumulation of its substrate, glucocerebroside in reticuloendothelial cells (Brady *et al.*, 1966). This results in their characteristic morphology with a tendency to linear striation and PAS positivity. Iron metabolism in Gaucher cells suggest that phagocytosed red cells are the source of the cerebroside (Lee *et al.*, 1967). Electron microscopy studies support this theory (Pennelli *et al.*, 1969). These cells appear to phagocytose not only red cells but also platelets, contributing to the thrombocytopenia seen in this disease (Green *et al.*, 1971). Similar cells are found in thalassaemia (Zaino *et al.* 1971) and chronic myelocytic leukaemia (Kattlove *et al.*, 1969) resulting from excessive ingestion of red cells and

granulocytes respectively, presumably exceeding the capacity of the normal enzyme with respect to catabolism of cerebrosides from these cells. The same morphological abnormality can therefore arise from either inherited or acquired causes. By contrast the Niemann-Pick cells have a vacuolated foamy rather than fibrillary appearance, due to accumulation of a phospholipid, sphyngomyelin, which reacts with fat stains.

Clinically Gaucher's disease presents as a recessive disorder occurring predominantly in Jewish stock. There is gradual accumulation of cerebroside in reticulum cells of spleen, liver, bone marrow and lymph glands. It occurs in two forms. The commonest is the chronic or adult type with gross splenomegaly, cutaneous pigmentation, pinguecula and bone lesions in mid-childhood or later and often followed by many years of survival into adult life. A less common acute form occurs in infancy with neurological manifestations, fever and pulmonary infiltration as well as infiltration of the reticuloendothelial system. This form is usually fatal before 2 years of age.

Niemann-Pick disease has many features in common with the infantile form of Gaucher's disease. It is inherited as a recessive character and is again more common in Jewish stock. Instead of isolated splenomegaly as in Gaucher's disease there is a similar degree of hepatomegaly. Other clinical features include severe mental and physical retardation from infancy, a cherry-red spot at the macular (as in Tay-Sachs disease), a brownish skin discoloration, spasticity, deafness, blindness and usually a fatal outcome by the age of 2 years. Hypersplenism is usually less marked than in Gaucher's disease. Survival is too short for marked bone changes to occur. There is no specific treatment.

Foamy cells similar to those in Niemann-Pick disease may be found in cases of chronic hyperlipaemia, corticosteroid therapy, Wolman's disease (Marshall *et al.*, 1969) and in the usual form of reticuloendotheliosis (Vitale *et al.*, 1970). Fat containing vacuoles in the granulocytes, monocytes and occasional lymphocytes have been found in two sisters with ichthyosis (Jordan's anomaly) (Rozenszajn *et al.*, 1966).

Interest in Gaucher's disease and other hereditary lysosomal enzyme deficiencies has been stimulated by the possibility of enzyme replacement therapy, which may play an increasing role in their management in future (Erbe, 1974).

SEA BLUE HISTIOCYTE SYNDROME

Silverstein *et al.* (1970) collected a series of 9 patients, of whom one was a girl of 6, who had hepatosplenomegaly, haemolytic anaemia and characteristic bright blue staining histiocytes in the marrow (Plate H) and were accumulating mucopolysaccharides in the liver and excreting them in the urine. Lake *et al.* (1970) described a similar syndrome in a group of children associated with a neurological disorder. Progressive liver failure may also occur. There are clearly some features in common with the mucopolysaccharide group of storage diseases. However, there is no clear hereditary tendency and recent work suggests that the 'Sea blue histiocyte' as seen in Romanowsky stained smears is a ceroid-containing phagocyte resulting from ingestion of oxidized unsaturated lipids, and is seen in a wide variety of acquired or congenital diseases, including ITP, CGD, hyper-lipoproteinaemia, sickle cell disease, and cirrhosis of the liver as well as in a number of well recognized storage diseases (Rywlin *et al.*, 1971). The ceroid is probably derived from long continued phagocytosis of platelets, granulocytes or red cell membranes in the above-mentioned diseases. Ceroid gives a blue colour in Romanowsky stains (Plate H). The Sea blue histiocyte syndrome is therefore probably not a single entity.

MYELOFIBROSIS

Fibrosis of the marrow, an entirely different entity from marble bone disease (Chap. 13), is excessively rare in childhood unlike its relative frequency in adult patients with myeloproliferative disorders. The peripheral blood usually shows a normochromic, normocytic anaemia with distorted 'teardrop' red cells, a leucoerythroblastic blood picture with reticulocytosis and circulating normoblasts, and sometimes thrombocytopenia. There is a neutrophil leucocytosis, up to 50,000/mm³, together with circulating myelocytes and a few blast cells. Marrow aspiration is very difficult, often resulting in a 'dry tap'. Histology of marrow fragments or trephine specimens shows hyperplasia of all marrow elements. An early finding is an increase in reticulin fibres, as shown by silver stains, which may precede the development of actual fibrosis.

Clinical features include symptoms of anaemia and thrombocytopenia, infections and bone pain. Splenomegaly, often gross, is almost always present. Extramedullary haemopoiesis is usually present, especially in the spleen. An authoritative account of the clinical and haematological findings is that of Bouroncle and Doan (1962).

Rosenberg and Taylor (1958) reported details of 2 infants presenting at 13 and 23 months with anaemia (Hb 5·9 and 4·4 g/100 ml) splenomegaly (5 and 3 cm below costal margin), myelofibrosis of the marrow and myeloid metaplasia of the spleen. The marrow progressed to hypoplasia in one. Megakaryocytes were prominent in both cases and death was due to disseminated agranulocytic abscesses. They collected 8 other cases of myelofibrosis in children in the literature.

Say and Berkel (1964) described a $7\frac{1}{2}$-month-old infant presenting with similar haematological and clinical features terminating with infection. They reviewed the literature and concluded that the prognosis for paediatric patients seemed to be more serious than in the adult form, 12 out of 13 reported childhood cases having died. Krasilnikoff (1967) reported a single case of myelofibrosis in a boy of $3\frac{3}{4}$ years terminating in AML a year after diagnosis.

FAMILIAL MYELOPROLIFERATIVE DISEASE

Randall *et al.* (1965) have reported a unique disease affecting 9 related children living in Colorado, Texas and Nebraska. Onset was between 5 months and 4 years. Gross splenomegaly was present and the haematological features were similar to myelofibrosis although the presence of myeloid leukocytosis initially suggested chronic myelocytic leukaemia. Chromosome studies showed many aneuploid cells but excluded the Philadelphia chromosome. Leucocyte alkaline phosphatase was low. Early death occurred in 3 of the children, but 6 had a chronic course with 2 of these apparently recovering after 10 to 12 years, who had been treated with a folic acid antagonist.

Lascari (1973) considers that this was a distinct entity not fitting the criteria of known myeloproliferative disorders such as CML, myeloid metaplasia, polycythaemia rubra vera nor leukaemoid reaction. He advises that antileukaemic therapy should be withheld in the present state of knowledge.

REFERENCES

Abell, C. & Holland, P. (1969) Acute toxoplasmosis complicating leukemia. Diagnosis by bone marrow aspiration. *Am. J. Dis. Child.*, **118**, 782.

Acute Leukaemia Group B (1963) The effect of 6-Mercaptopurine on the duration of steroid induced remissions in acute leukaemia: A model for evaluation of other potentially useful therapy. *Blood*, **21**, 699.

Adler, A. (1939) Über konstitutionell bedingte granulationsveränderungen der Leukozyten. *Dtsch. Arch. Klin. Med.*, **183**, 372.

Aisenberg, A. C. (1973) Malignant lymphoma. *New Eng. J. Med.*, **288**, 883.

Albarracin, N. S. & Haust, M. D. (1971) Intravascular coagulation in promyelocytic leukemia. *Am. J. Clin. Path.*, **55**, 677.

Allen, D. W. & Cole, P. (1972) Viruses and human cancer. *New Eng. J. Med.*, **286**, 70.

Aur, R. J. A., Hustu, H. O., Simone, J. V., Pratt, C. B. & Pinkel, D. (1971) Therapy of localised and regional lymphosarcoma of childhood. *Cancer*, **27**, 1328.

Aur, R. J. A., Simone, J. V., Hustu, O. & Verzosa, M. S. (1973) A comparative study of central nervous system irradiation and intensive chemotherapy early in remission of childhood acute lymphocytic leukemia. *Cancer*, **29**, 381.

Aur, R. J. (1975) Reply to letter: Relapses in children with ALL off treatment. *New Eng. J. Med.*, **292**, 431.

Avery, M. E., McAfee, J. G. & Guild, H. G. (1957) The course and prognosis of reticuloendotheliosis (eosinophilic granuloma, Schüller-Christian disease and Letterer-Siwe disease', *Am. J. Med.*, **22**, 636.

Azoury, F. J. & Reed, R. J. (1966) Histiocytosis. Report of an unusual case. *New Eng. J. Med.*, **274**, 928.

Baber, M. D. (1960) Two cases of reticuloendothelioses—Letterer-Siwe syndrome. *Arch. Dis. Childh.*, **35**, 613.

Baehner, R. L., Neiburger, R. G., Johnson, D. E. & Murrmann, S. M. (1973) Transient bactericidal defect of peripheral blood phagocytes from children with acute lymphoblastic leukaemia receiving craniospinal irradiation. *New Eng. J. Med.*, **289**, 1209.

Band, P. R., Holland, J. F., Bernard, J., Weil, M., Walker, M. & Rall, D. (1973) Treatment of central nervous system leukaemia with intrathecal cytosine arabinoside. *Cancer*, **32**, 744.

Baxt, W., Hehlmann, R. & Spiegelman, S. (1972) Human leukaemic cells contain reverse transcriptase associated with a high molecular weight virus-related RNA. *Nature New Biol.*, **240**, 72.

Becroft, D. M. O., Dix, M. R., Gillman, J. C., MacGregor, B. J. L. & Shaw, R. L. (1973) Benign sinus histiocytosis with massive lymphadenopathy: transient immunological defects in a child with mediastinal involvement. *J. Clin. Path.*, **26**, 463.

Behrman, R. E., Sigler, A. T. & Patchefsky, A. S. (1966) Abnormal hematopoiesis in 2 of 3 siblings with mongolism. *J. Pediat.*, **68**, 569.

Beier, F. R., Thatcher, L. G. & Lahey, M. E. (1963) Treatment of reticuloendotheliosis with vinblastine sulphate. *J. Pediat.*, **63**, 1087.

Belding, H. W., Daland, G. A. & Parker, F. (1955) Histiocytic and monocytic leukemia. A clinical, hematological and pathological differentiation. *Cancer*, **8**, 237.

Bell, R. J. M., Brafield, A. J. E., Barnes, N. D. & France, N. E. (1968) Familial haemophagocytic reticulosis. *Arch. Dis. Childh.*, **43**, 601.

Bentley, H. P., Reardon, A. E., Knoedler, J. P. & Krivit, W. (1961) Eosinophilic leukaemia. *Am. J. Med.*, **30**, 310.

Berkheiser, S. W. (1957) Studies on the comparative morphology of monocytic leukemia, granulocytic leukemia, and reticulum-cell sarcoma. *Cancer*, **10**, 606.

Bernard, J., Lasneret, J., Chome, J., Levy, J. P. & Boiron, M. (1963) A cytological and histological study of acute promyelocytic leukaemia. *J. Clin. Path.*, **16**, 319.

Bernard, J., Boiron, M., Jacquillat, C. *et al.* (1968) Rubidomycin in 400 patients with leukaemias and other malignancies. Abstracts of XII Congress Int. Soc. Hematol., p. 5. New York: Grune & Stratont.

Bisel, H. F. (1956) Criteria for the evaluation of the response to treatment in acute leukemia. *Blood*, **11**, 676.

Blackstock, A. & Garson, M. (1974) Direct evidence for involvement of erythroid cells in acute myeloblastic leukaemia. *Lancet*, **ii**, 1178.

Blennow, G., Berg, B., Brandt, L., Messeter, L., Low, B. & Söderström (1974) Haemophagocytic reticulosis: A state of chimerism? *Arch. Dis. Childh.*, **49**, 960.

Bleyer, W. A., Drake, J. C. & Chabner, B. A. (1973) Neurotoxicity and elevated cerebrospinal-fluid methotrexate concentration in meningeal leukemia. *New Eng. J. Med.*, **289**, 770.

Bodey, G. P., Buckley, M., Sathe, Y. S. & Freireich, E. J. (1966) Quantitative relationships between circulating leukocytes and infection in patients with acute leukemia. *Ann. Intern. Med.*, **64**, 328.

Bodey, G. P. (1972) Management of infectious complications during cancer chemotherapy. In *Cancer Chemotherapy II*, p. 293. Edited by Brodsky, I., Kahn, S. B. and Moyer, J. H. New York: Grune and Stratton.

Boggs, D. R. (1974) Transfusion of neutrophils to prevent or treat infection in neutropenic patients. *New Eng. J. Med.*, **290**, 1055.

Borella, L. & Webster, R. G. (1971) The immunosuppressive effects of long-term combination chemotherapy in children with acute leukemia in remission. *Cancer Research*, **31**, 420.

Borella, L., Green, A. A. & Webster, R. G. (1972) Immunologic rebound after cessation of long-term chemotherapy in acute leukemia. *Blood*, **40**, 42.

Bouroncle, B. A., Wiseman, B. K. & Doan, C. A. (1958) Leukemic reticuloendotheliosis. *Blood*, **13**, 609.

Bouroncle, B. A. & Doan, C. A. (1962) Myelofibrosis: Clinical, haematologic and pathologic study of 110 patients. *Am. J. Med. Sci.*, **243**, 697.

Bouroncle, B. A. (1966) Sternberg-Reed cells in the peripheral blood of patients wtih Hodgkin's disease. *Blood*, **27**, 544.

Brady, R. O., Kanfer, J. N., Bradley, R. M. & Shapiro, D. (1966) Demonstration of a deficiency of glucocerebroside-cleaving enzyme in Gaucher's disease. *J. Clin. Invest.*, **45**, 1112.

Breslow, N. & Zandstra, R. (1970) A note on the relationship between bone marrow lymphocytosis and remission duration in acute leukemia. *Blood*, **36**, 246.

British Medical Journal (1969) Editorial: Asparaginase. *Brit. med. J.*, **ii**, 465.

British Medical Journal (1972A) Editorial: Irradiation and leukemia. *Brit. med. J.*, **iii**, 485.

British Medical Journal (1972B) Editorial: Multiple factors in leukaemogenesis. *Brit. med. J.*, **iii**, 128.

British Medical Journal (1972C) Immunosuppression and malignancy. *Brit. med. J.*, **iii**, 713.

British Medical Journal (1973) Editorial: Better results in childhood acute leukaemia. *Brit. med. J.*, **ii**, 624.

Bross, I. D. J. & Gibson, R. (1970) Cats and childhood leukemia. *J. Med.*, **1**, 180.

Bross, I. D. J. & Natarajan, N. (1972) Leukemia from low-level radiation. Identification of susceptible children. *New Eng. J. Med.*, **287**, 107.

Brown, G., Greaves, M. F., Lister, T. A., Rapson, N. & Papamichael, M. (1974) Expression of human T and B lymphocyte cell-surface markers on leukaemic cells. *Lancet*, **ii**, 753.

Brunell, P. A., Ross, A., Miller, L. H. & Kuo, B. (1969) Prevention of varicella by zoster immune globulin. *New Eng. J. Med.*, **280**, 1191.

Buist, N. R. M., Jones, R. N. & Cavens, T. R. (1971) Familial haemophagocytic reticulosis in first cousins. *Arch. Dis. Childh.*, **46**, 728.

Burchenal, J. H. (1968) Long-term survivors in acute leukemia and Burkitt's tumor. *Cancer*, **21**, 595.

Campbell, A. C., Hersey, P., MacLennan, I. C. M., Kay, H. E. M., Pike, M. C. & M. R. C. Working Party on Leukaemia in Childhood (1973) Immunosuppressive consequences of radiotherapy and chemotherapy in patients with acute lymphoblastic leukaemia. *Brit. med. J.*, **ii**, 385.

Cangir, A. & Sullivan, M. P. (1966) The occurrence of cytomegalovirus infections in childhood leukemia. Report of three cases. *J.A.M.A.*, **195**, 616.

Cangir, A., Sullivan, M. P., Sutow, W. W. & Taylor, G. (1967) Cytomegalovirus syndrome in children with acute leukemia. *J.A.M.A.*, **201**, 612.

Casey, T. P. (1968) Chronic lymphocytic leukemia in a child presenting at the age of two years and eight months. *Aust. Ann. Med.*, **17**, 70.

Catovsky, D. & Galton, D. A. G. (1971) Myelomonocytic leukaemia supervening on chronic lymphocytic leukaemia. *Lancet*, **i**, 478.

Catovsky, D., Goldman, J. M., Okos, A., Frisch, B. & Galton, D. A. G. (1974) T-lymphoblastic leukaemia: A distinct variant of acute leukaemia. *Brit. med. J.*, **ii**, 643.

Chan, B. W. B. & Hayhoe, F. G. J. (1971) Changes in proliferative activity of marrow leukaemic cells during and after extracorporeal irradiation of blood. *Blood*, **37**, 657.

Chikkappa, G., Corcino, J., Greenberg, M. L. & Herbert, V. (1971) Correlation between various blood white cell pools and the serum B_{12}-binding capacities. *Blood*, **37**, 142.

Clark, B. S. & Dawson, P. J. (1969) Histiocytic medullary reticulosis presenting with a leukemic blood picture. *Am. J. Med.*, **47**, 314.

Clarkson, B. (1969) Review of recent studies of cellular proliferation in acute leukemia. National Cancer Institute Monograph No. 30. Human Tumor Cell Kinetics, p. 81. U.S. Dept. of Health, Education and Welfare.

Clarkson, B., Fried, J., Strife, A., Sakai, Y., Ota, K. & Ohkita, T. (1970) Studies of cellular proliferation in human leukemia. III. Behaviour of leukemic cells in three adults with acute leukemia given continuous infusion of ³H-thymidine for 8 and 10 days. *Cancer*, **25**, 1237.

Clarkson, B. D. (1972) Acute myelocytic leukemia in adults. *Cancer*, **30**, 1572.

Clift, R. A., Wright, D. H. & Clifford, P. (1963) Leukemia in Burkitt's lymphoma. *Blood*, **22**, 243.

Court Brown, W. M. & Doll, R. (1961) Leukaemia in childhood and young adult life. Trends in mortality in relation to aetiology. *Brit. med. J.*, **i**, 981.

Cronkite, E. P. (1967) Kinetics of leukemic cell proliferation. *Seminars in Hematology*, **4**, 415.

Crowther, D., Powles, R. L., Bateman, C. J. T., Beard, M. E. J., Gauci, C. L., Wrigley, P. F. M., Malpas, J. S., Hamilton Fairley, G. & Bodley Scott, Sir R. (1973) Management of adult acute myelogenous leukaemia. *Brit. med. J.*, **i**, 131.

Cutler, S. J., Axtell, H. & Heise, H. (1967) Ten thousand cases of leukemia. *J. Natl. Cancer Inst.*, **39**, 993.

Delta, B. G. & Pinkel, D. (1964) Bone marrow aspiration in children with malignant tumors. *J. Pediat.*, **64**, 542.

Didisheim, P., Thrombold, J. S., Vandervourt, R. L. E. & Mibashan, R. S. (1964) Acute promyelocytic leukemia and fibrinogen and factor V deficiencies. *Blood*, **23**, 717.

Dmochowski, L., Grey, C. E., Sykes, J. A., Shullenberger, C. C. & Howe, C. D. (1959) Studies on human leukemia. *Proc. Soc. Exp. Biol. Med.*, **101**, 686.

Doede, K. G. & Rappaport, H. (1967) Long-term survival of patients with acute differentiated histiocytosis (Letterer-Siwe disease). *Cancer*, **20**, 1782.

Döhmann, U., Plüss, H. J. & Hitzig, W. H. (1973) Sterile Pflege als hilfsmittel bei der Therapie der akuten Leukämie des Kindesalters. *Helv. Paediat. Acta.*, **28**, 145.

Dore, J. F., Motta, R., Marholev, L., Hrsak, I., Colas De La Noue, H., Seman, G., Vassal, F. & Mathé, G. (1967) Preliminary results of researches for new antigens in human leukaemic cells, and antibody in the serum of leukaemic patients. *Lancet*, **ii**, 1396.

Dubowitz, V. (1964) Acute monocytic leukaemia with response to methotrexate. *Arch. Dis. Childh.*, **39**, 289.

Dyment, P. G., Melnyk, J. & Brubaker, C. A. (1968) A cytogenetic study of acute erythroleukemia in children. *Blood*, **32**, 997.

Ederer, F., Miller, R. W. & Sotto, J. (1965) U.S. childhood cancer mortality patterns. *J.A.M.A.*, **192**, 593.

Einhorn, M. & Davidsohn, I. (1964) Hepatotoxicity of mercaptopurine. *J.A.M.A.*, **188**, 802.

Engel, R. R., Hammond, D., Eitzman, D. V., Pearson, H. & Krivit, W. (1964) Transient congenital leukemia in 7 infants with mongolism. *J. Pediat.*, **65**, 303.

Epstein, M. A. & Achong, B. G. (1973) Various forms of Epstein-Barr virus infection in man: Established facts and a general concept. *Lancet*, **ii**, 836.

414 PAEDIATRIC HAEMATOLOGY

Erbe, R. W. (1974) Therapy in genetic disease. *New Eng. J. Med.*, **291**, 1028.

Evans, A. E. & Hummeler, K. (1973) The significance of primitive cells in marrow aspirates of children with neuroblastoma. *Cancer*, **32**, 906.

Evans, D. I. K., O'Rourke, C. & Morris Jones, P. (1974) The cerebrospinal fluid in acute leukaemia of childhood: Studies with the cytocentrifuge. *J. Clin. Path.*, **27**, 226.

Farquhar, J. W. & Claireaux, A. E. (1952) Familial haemophagocytic reticulosis. *Arch. Dis. Childh.*, **27**, 519.

Fefer, A., Eeinstein, A. B., Thomas, E. D., Buckner, C. D., Clift, R. A., Glucksberg, H., Neiman, P. E. & Storb, R. (1974) Bone-marrow transplantation for hematologic neoplasia. *New Eng. J. Med.*, **290**, 1389.

Fialkow, P. J. (1971) Leukaemic transformation of engrafted cells. *Lancet*, ii, 101.

Fink, M. A., Malmgren, R. A., Rauscher, F. J., Orr, H. C. & Karon, M. (1964) Application of immunofluorescence to the study of human leukemia. *J. Natl. Cancer Inst.*, **33**, 581.

Finklestein, J. Z., Ekert, H., Isaacs, H. & Higgins, G. (1970) Bone marrow metastases in children with solid tumors. *Am. J. Dis. Child.*, **119**, 49.

Foadi, M. D., Cooper, E. H. & Hardisty, R. M. (1968) Proliferative activity of leukaemic cells at various stages of acute leukaemia of childhood. *Brit. J. Haemat.*, **15**, 269.

Fortina, A. & Petrocini, S. (1953) Contributo alto studio della manifestazoni cutanee delle leucemie del' infanzia. *Pediatrica*, **61**, 199.

Fowler, M. (1960) Histiocytic medullary reticulosis in a child. *Arch. Dis. Childh.*, **35**, 591.

Fraumeni, J. F. (1967) Bone marrow depression induced by chloramphenicol or phenylbutazone. Leukemia and other sequelae. *J.A.M.A.*, **201**, 828.

Fraumeni, J. F. & Miller, R. W. (1967) Epidemiology of human leukemia: Recent observations. *J. Natl. Cancer Inst.*, **38**, 593.

Freedman, M. H., Finklestein, J. Z., Hammond, G. D. & Karon, M. (1971) The effect of chemotherapy on acute myelogenous leukemia in children. *J. Pediat.*, **78**, 526.

Frei, E. & Freireich, E. J. (1965) Progress and perspectives in the chemotherapy of acute leukemias. In *Advances in Chemotherapy*, p. 286. Edited by Goldin, A., Hawking, F. and Schnitzer, R. J. New York: Academic Press.

Frei, E. & A.L.G.B. (1965) The effectiveness of combinations of antileukemic agents in inducing and maintaining remissions in children with acute leukemia. *Blood*, **26**, 642.

Freireich, E. J., Gehan, E. A., Sulman, D., Boggs, D. R. & Frei, E. (1961) The effect of chemotherapy on acute leukemia in the human. *J. Chronic. Dis.*, **14**, 593.

Freireich, E. J. & Platelet Transfusion Sub-Committee of the Acute Leukemia Task Force (1968) Platelet transfusion procedures. *Cancer Chemotherapy Rep. Part I.*, 1.

Fukuda, T. (1966) Leukemic reticulosis. *J. Reticuloendothel. Soc.*, **3**, 117.

Gabutti, V., Pileri, A., Tarocco, R. P., Gavosto, F. & Cooper, E. H. (1969) Proliferative potential of out-of-cycle leukaemic cells. *Nature*, **224**, 375.

Gallo, R. C. (1972) Analytical review: RNA-dependant DNA polymerase in viruses and cells: Views on the current state. *Blood*, **39**, 117.

Galton, D. A. G. (1969) Chemotherapy of chronic myelocytic leukemia. *Sem. Hematol.*, **6**, 323.

Gasser, C. (1950) Konstitutionelle bedingte granulations-veranderungen der Leukocyten und Knochenveranderungen. *Schweiz. med. Wschr.*, **80**, 1095.

Gavosto, F., Pileri, A., Gabutti, V. & Masera, P. (1967) Cell population kinetics in human acute leukaemia. *Eur. J. Cancer*, **3**, 301.

Gee, T. S. G., Yu, K. P. & Clarkson, B. D. (1969) Treatment of adult acute leukemia with arabinosyl cytosine and thioguanine. *Cancer*, **23**, 1019.

Ghose, S., Ray, R. N. & Chatterjea, J. B. (1965) Observations on blastic crisis in chronic myeloid leukaemia. *J. Indian Med. Assoc.*, **45**, 525.

Graham, S., Levin, M. L., Lilienfeld, A. M. *et al.* (1966) Preconception, intrauterine, and postnatal irradiation as related to leukemia. *Natl. Cancer Inst. Monograph.*, **19**, 347.

Graham Pole, J. (1973) Childhood leukaemia presenting in the central nervous system. *Arch. Dis. Childh.*, **48**, 867.

Graham Pole, J. R. & Willoughby, M. L. N. (1975) Acute childhood leukaemia. *Mod. Probl. Paediat.*, **16**, 59. Basel: Karger.

Graw, R. G., Skeel, R. T. & Carbone, P. P. (1969) Priapism in a child with chronic granulocytic leukaemia. *J. Pediat.*, **74**, 788.

Graw, R. G., Buckner, C. D. & Whang-Peng, J. (1970) Complication of bone-marrow transplantation: graft-versus: host disease resulting from chronic-myelogenesis-leukaemia leucocyte transfusions. *Lancet*, ii, 338.

Graw, R. G., Herzig, G., Perry, S. & Henderson, E. S. (1972) Normal granulocyte transfusion therapy: Treatment of septicemia due to gram-negative bacteria. *New Eng. J. Med.*, **287**, 367.

Green, D., Battifora, H. A., Smith, R. T. & Rossi, E. C. (1971) Thrombocytopenia in Gaucher's disease. *Ann. Int. Med.*, **74**, 727.

Greenberg, E., Cohen, D. M., Pease, G. L. & Kyle, R. A. (1962) Histiocytic medullary reticulosis. *Mayo Clin. Proc.*, **37**, 271.

Gutterman, J. U., Rossen, R. D., Butler, W. T., McCredie, K. B., Bodey, G. P., Freireich, E. J. & Hersh, E. M. (1973) Immunoglobulin on tumor cells and tumor-induced lymphocyte blastogenesis in human acute leukemia. *New Eng. J. Med.*, **288**, 173.

Gutterman, J. U., Rodriguez, V., Mavligit, G., Burgess, M. A., Gehan, E., Hersh, E. M., McCredie, K. B., Reed, R., Smith, T., Bodey, G. P., Sr. & Freireich, E. J. (1974) Chemoimmunotherapy of adult acute leukaemia. Prolongation of remission in myeloblastic leukaemia with BCG. *Lancet*, ii, 1405.

Haak, H. L., Man, J. C. H. de, Hijmans, W., Knapp, W. & Speck, B. (1974) Further evidence for the lymphocytic nature of leukaemic reticuloendotheliosis (Hairy cell leukaemia). *Brit. J. Haemat.*, **27**, 31.

Haegert, D. G., Stuart, J. & Smith, J. L. (1975) Acute lymphoblastic leukaemia: A heterogenous disease. *Brit. med. J.*, **i**, 312.

Haghbin, M., Tan, C., Clarkson, B. D., Miké, V., Burchenal, J. H. & Murphy, M. L. (1974) Intensive chemotherapy in children with acute lymphoblastic leukaemia (L-2 Protocol). *Cancer*, **33**, 1491.

Hanes, B., Gardner, M. B., Loosli, C. G., Heidbreder, G., Kogan, B., Marylander, H. & Huebner, R. J. (1970) Pet association with selected human cancers: A household questionnaire survey. *J. Natl. Cancer Inst.*, **45**, 1155.

Hansen, H. G. (1972) Hematologic studies in mucopolysaccharidoses and mucolipidoses, p. 115. In *Birth Defects: Original Article Series*, Vol. VIII, No. 3. Edited by Bergsma, D. Baltimore: Williams and Wilkins.

Hardisty, R. M., Speed, D. E. & Till, M. (1964) Granulocytic leukaemia in childhood. *Brit. J. Haemat.*, **10**, 551.

Hardisty, R. M. & Norman, P. M. (1967) Meningeal leukaemia. *Arch. Dis. Childh.*, **42**, 441.

Hardisty, R. M. & Till, M. M. (1968) Acute leukaemia 1959–64: Factors affecting prognosis. *Arch. Dis. Childh.*, **43**, 107.

Harlem, O. K. (1960) Juvenile cerebroretinal degeneration (Spielmeyer-Vogt). Blood and EEG findings in a family of ten members. *Am. J. Dis. Child.*, **100**, 918.

Hayhoe, G. F. J., Quaglino, D. & Doll, R. (1964) The cytology and cytochemistry of acute leukaemias. A study of 140 cases. *M.R.C. Special Report Series, No. 304*. London: H.M.S.O.

Hayhoe, F. G. J. & Cawley, J. C. (1972) Acute leukaemia: Cellular morphology, cytochemistry and fine structure. *Clinics in Haematology*, **1**, 49.

Heath, C. W. & Hasterlik, R. J. (1963) Leukemia among children in a suburban community. *Am. J. Med.*, **34**, 796.

Henderson, E. S. (1968) Treatment of acute leukemia. *Ann. Intern. Med.*, **69**, 628.

Henderson, E. S. (1969) Treatment of acute leukemia. *Seminars in Hematology*, **6**, 285.

Henderson, E. S. (1973) Acute lymphoblastic leukemia. In *Cancer Medicine*. Edited by Holland, J. F. and Frei, E. Philadelphia: Lea and Febiger.

Hersh, F. M., Bodey, G. P., Nies, B. A. & Freireich, E. J. (1965) Causes of death in acute leukemia. *J.A.M.A.*, **193**, 105.

Hersh, E. M., Whitecar, J. P., McCredie, K. B., Bodey, G. P. & Freireich, E. J. (1971) Chemotherapy, immuno-competence, immunosuppression and prognosis in acute leukemia. *New Eng. J. Med.*, **285**, 1211.

Hertz, C. G. & Hambrick, G. W. (1968) Congenital Letterer-Siwe disease. A case treated with vincristine and corti-costeroids. *Am. J. Dis. Child.*, **116**, 553.

Heyn, R., Borges, W., Joo, P., Karon, M., Nesbit, M., Shore, N., Breslow, J., Weiner, J. & Hammond, D. (1973) BCG in the treatment of acute lymphocytic leukaemia. *Proc. Am. Ass. Cancer. Res.*, **14**, 45.

Hillen, H., Wessels, J. & Haanen, C. (1975) Bone marrow proliferation patterns in acute myeloblastic leukaemia determined by pulse cytophotometry. *Lancet*, **i**, 609.

Holland, P. & Mauer, A. M. (1963) Myeloid leukemoid reactions in childhood. *Am. J. Dis. Child.*, **105**, 569.

Holland, P. & Holland, N. H. (1968) Prevention and management of acute hyperuricemia in childhood leukemia. *J. Pediat.*, **72**, 358.

Holland, J. F., Senn, H. & Banerjee, T. (1971) Quantitative studies of localized leukocyte mobilization in acute leukemia. *Blood*, **37**, 499.

Holland, J. F. & Glidewell, O. (1927A) Oncologists' reply: Survival expectancy in acute lymphocytic leukemia. *New Eng. J. Med.*, **287**, 769.

Holland, J. F. & Glidewell, O. (1972B) Chemotherapy of acute lymphocytic leukemia of childhood. *Cancer*, **30**, 1480.

Holowach, J. (1948) Chronic lymphoid leukemia in children. *J. Pediat.*, **32**, 84.

Holton, C. P. & Johnson, W. W. (1968) Chronic myelocytic leukemia in infant siblings. *J. Pediat.*, **72**, 377.

Hoshino, T., Kato, H., Finch, S. C. & Hrubec, Z. (1967) Leukaemia in offspring of atomic bomb survivors. *Blood*, **30**, 719.

Hughes, W. T., Price, R. A., Kim, H. K., Coburn, T. P., Grigsby, D. & Feldman, S. (1973) Pneumocystis carinii pneumonitis in children with malignancies. *J. Pediat.*, **82**, 404.

Hughes, W. T. & Smith, D. R. (1973) Infection during induction of remission in acute lymphocytic leukemia. *Cancer*, **31**, 1008.

Hyman, C. B., Bogle, J. M., Brubaker, C. A., Williams, K. & Hammond, D. (1965) Central nervous system involve-ment by leukemia in children: I. Relationship to systemic leukemia and description of clinical and laboratory manifestations. *Blood*, **25**, 1.

Iversen, T. (1966) Leukaemia in infancy and childhood. *Acta Paediatrica Scand.*, Supplement 167.

Jablon, S. & Kato, H. (1970) Childhood cancer in relation to prenatal exposure to atomic bomb radiation. *Lancet*, **ii**, 1001.

Jackson, E. W., Norris, F. D. & Klauber, M. R. (1969) Childhood leukemia in California-born twins. *Cancer*, **23**, 913.

Jacobs, S. A., Bleyer, W. A., Chabner, B. S. & Johns, D. G. (1975) Altered plasma pharmacokinetics of methotrexate administered intrathecally. *Lancet*, **i**, 465.

Jarrett, W. F. H. (1973) Annotation: Viruses and leukaemia. *Brit. J. Haemat.*, **25**, 287.

Johnson, D. E., Griep, J. A. & Baehner, R. L. (1973) Histiocytic leukemia following life-long infection and thrombo-cytopenia: Histologic, metabolic and bactericidal studies. *J. Pediat.*, **82**, 664.

Johnston, P. G. B., Hardisty, R. M., Kay, H. E. M. & Smith, P. G. (1974) Myelosuppressive effect of Colaspase (L-Asparaginase) in initial treatment of acute lymphoblastic leukaemia. *Brit. med. J.*, **iii**, 81.

Jones, B. & Klingberg, W. G. (1963) Lymphosarcoma in children. A report of 43 cases and review of the recent literature. *J. Pediat.*, **63**, 11.

Jones, B., Kung, F., Nyhan, W. L., Hananian, J. *et al.* (1967) Chemotherapy of the leukemic transformation of lymphosarcoma. *J. Pediat.*, **70**, 442.

Jones, B. & Holland, J. (1973) Optimal use of Asparaginase in acute lymphocytic leukemia of childhood. *Blood*, **42**, 1015.

Kadin, M. E., Glatstein, E. & Dorfman, R. F. (1971) Clinical-pathological studies of 117 untreated patients subjected to laparotomy for the staging of Hodgkin's disease. *Cancer*, **27**, 1277.

Kaplan, H. S. (1967) On the natural history of murine leukemias: Presidential Address. *Cancer Res.*, **27**, 1325.

Kaplan, H. S. (1972) *Hodgkin's Disease,* p. 84. Cambridge, Massachusetts: Harvard University Press.

Karanas, A. & Silver, R. T. (1968) Characteristics of the terminal phase of chronic granulocytic leukemia. *Blood*, **32**, 445.

Kattlove, H. E., Williams, J. C., Gaynor, E., Spivack, M., Bradeley, R. M. & Brady, R. O. (1969) Gaucher cells in chronic myelocytic leukemia: An acquired abnormality. *Blood*, **33**, 379.

Kauffman, H. J. & Hess, R. (1962) Does congenital leukaemia exist? *Brit. med. J.*, **i**, 867.

Kay, H. E. M., Knapton, P. J., O'Sullivan, J. P., Wells, D. G., Harris, R. F., Innes, E. M., Stuart, J., Schwartz, F. C. M. & Thompson, E. N. (1972) Encephalopathy in acute leukaemia associated with methotrexate therapy. *Arch. Dis. Childh.*, **47**, 344.

Kemmoona, I. (1974) Direct contact clusters of acute lymphatic leukaemia. *Lancet*, **i**, 994.

Kessler, I. J. & Lilienfeld, A. M. (1969) Perspectives in the epidemiology of leukemia. *Advances in Cancer Res.*, **12**, 225.

Killmann, S.-Aa (1965) Proliferative activity of blast cells in leukemia and myelofibrosis. *Acta Med. Scandinav.*, **178**, 263.

Killmann, S.-Aa (1968) Acute leukemia: the kinetics of leukemic blast cells in man. An analytic review. *Series Haematologica*, **I**, 38.

Killmann, S.-Aa (1972) Kinetics of leukaemic blast cells in man. *Clinics in Haematol.*, **i**, 95.

Kingdon, H. S., Baron, J. M., Byrne, G. E. & Rappaport, H. (1970) Malignant histiocytosis. Results of combination vincristine-prednisone therapy. *Ann. Intern. Med.*, **72**, 705.

Kleinknecht, D., Ganeval, D. & Droz, D. (1973) Acute renal failure after high doses of gentamicin and cephalothin. *Lancet*, **i**, 1129.

Komp, D. M. (1972) Cytocentrifugation in the management of central nervous system leukemia. *J. Pediat.*, **81**, 992.

Krasilnikoff, P. A. (1967) Myelofibrosis and myeloid leukemia. *Acta. Paediat. Scand.*, **56**, 424.

Krivit, W. & Good, R. A. (1957) Simultaneous occurrence of mongolism and leukemia. *Am. J. Dis. Child.*, **94**, 289.

Krivit, W., Gilchrist, G. & Beatty, E. C. (1970) The need for chemotherapy after prolonged complete remission in acute leukemia in children. *J. Pediat.*, **76**, 138.

Lahey, M. E. (1962) Prognosis in reticuloendotheliosis in children. *J. Pediat.*, **60**, 664.

Lake, B. D., Stephens, R. & Neville, B. G. R. (1970) Syndrome of the sea-blue histiocyte. *Lancet*, **ii**, 309.

Lampkin, B., Higgins, G. R. & Hammond, D. (1967) Absence of neurotoxicity following massive administration of methotrexate. Case report. *Cancer*, **20**, 1780.

Lampkin, B. C., Nagao, T. & Mauer, A. M. (1969) Synchronization of the mitotic cycle in acute leukemia. *Nature*, **222**, 1274.

Lampkin, B. C., McWilliams, N. B. & Mauer, A. M. (1972) Cell kinetics and chemotherapy of acute leukemia. *Seminars in Hematology*, **9**, 211.

Lampkin, B. C., McWilliams, N. B. & Mauer, A. M. (1972) Treatment of acute leukemia. *Pediat. Clin. N. Amer.*, **19**, 1123.

Lancet (1972) Epidemiology of leukaemia. *Lancet*. **i**, 82.

Lancet (1972) Down's syndrome and acute leukaemia. *Lancet*, **ii**, 1187.

Lancet (1973) Reverse transcriptase in acute leukaemia. *Lancet*, **ii**, 542.

Lancet (1974) Immunotherapy for acute myeloid leukaemia. *Lancet*, **i**, 846.

Lancet (1975A) A human-leukaemia virus? *Lancet*, **i**, 670.

Lancet (1975B) Granulocyte transfusions. *Lancet*, **i**, 377.

Lascari, A. D., Givler, R. L., Soper, R. T. & Hill, L. F. (1968) Portal hypertension in a case of acute leukaemia treated with antimetabolites for ten years. *New Eng. J. Med.*, **279**, 303.

Lascari, A. D. (1973) *Leukemia in Childhood.* Springfield, Illinois: Thomas.

Laurie, H. C. (1968) Duration of remissions in lymphoblastic leukaemia in childhood. *Brit. med. K.*, **ii**, 95.

Lawler, S. D., Klouda, P. T., Hardisty, R. M. & Till, M. M. (1971) The HL-A system in lymphoblastic leukaemia: A study of patients and their families. *Brit. J. Haemat.*, **21**, 595.

Lawler, S. D., Klouda, P. T., Smith, P. G., Till, M. M. & Hardisty, R. M. (1974) Survival and the HL-A system in acute lymphoblastic leukaemia. *Brit. med. J.*, **i**, 547.

Lee, R. E., Balcerzak, S. P. & Westerman, M. P. (1967) Gaucher's disease. A morphologic study and measurement of iron metabolism. *Amer. J. Med.*, **42**, 891.

Levin, R. H. & Kundel, D. (1964) Prognostic implications of bone marrow morphology in acute myelocytic leukemia. *Proc. Am. Ass. Cancer. Res.*, **5**, 40.

Levine, A. S., Graw, R. G. & Young, R. C. (1972) Management of infections in patients with leukemia and lymphoma: Current concepts and experimental approaches. *Seminars in Hematology*, **9**, 14.

Levine, A. S., Siegel, S. E., Schreiber, A. D., Hauser, J., Preisler, H., Goldstein, I. M., Seidler, F., Simon, R., Perry, S., Bennet, J. E. & Henderson, E. S. (1973) Protected environments and prophylactic antibiotics in therapy of leukemia. *New Eng. J. Med.*, **288**, 477.

Levy, S. B. (1974) Cat leukemia: A threat to man? *New Eng. J. Med.*, **290**, 513.

Li, F. P. & Jaffe, N. (1974) Progeny of childhood—cancer survivors. *Lancet*, **ii**, 707.

Lock, S. P. & Merrington, M. (1967) Leukaemia in Lewisham. *Brit. med. J.*, **iii**, 759.

Lynch, E. C. & Alfrey, C. P. (1965) Histiocytic medullary reticulosis. *Ann. Intern. Med.*, **63**, 666.

McElwain, T. J. & Hardisty, R. M. (1969) Remission induction with cytosine arabinoside and L-asparaginase in acute lymphoblastic leukaemia. *Brit. med. J.*, **iv**, 596.

McIntosh, S. & Aspnes, G. T. (1973) Encephalopathy following CNS prophylaxis in childhood lymphoblastic leukemia. *Pediatrics*, **52**, 612.

McIntosh, S. & Pearson, H. A. (1973) Treatment of childhood leukemia. *J. Pediatrics*, **83**, 899.

McKusick, V. A., Kaplan, D., Wise, D., Hanley, W. B., Suddarth, S. B., Sevick, M. E. & Maumanee, A. E. (1965) The genetic mucopolysaccharidoses. *Medicine*, **44**, 445.

McKusick, V. A. (1969) The nosology of the mucopolysaccharidoses. *Amer. J. Med.*, **47**, 730.

MacMahon, H. E., Bedizel, M. & Ellis, C. A. (1963) Familial erythrophagocytic lymphohistiocytosis. *Pediatrics*, **32**, 868.

MacMahon, B. & Levy, M. A. (1964) A prenatal origin of childhood leukemia. *New Eng. J. Med.*, **270**, 1082.

MacMahon, B. (1972) Susceptibility to radiation-induced leukemia? *New Eng. J. Med.*, **287**, 144.

Maniatis, A. K., Amsel, S., Mitus, W. J. & Coleman, N. (1969) Chromosome pattern of bone marrow fibroblasts in patients with chronic granulocytic leukaemia. *Nature*, **222**, 1278.

Mann, J. R., Simpson, J. S., Munkley, R. M. & Stuart, J. (1971) Lysosomal enzyme cytochemistry in acute leukaemia. *J. Clin. Path.*, **24**, 831.

Maroteaux, P. (1970) Nomenclature internationale des maladies osseuses constitutionelles. *Ann. Radiol.*, **13**, 455.

Marshall, W. C., Ockenden, B. G., Fosbrooke, A. S. & Cummings, J. N. (1969) Wolman's disease, a rare lipoidosis with adrenal calcification. *Arch. Dis. Childh.*, **44**, 331.

Mastrangelo, R., Zuelzer, W. W., Ecklund, P. S. & Thompson, R. I. (1970) Chromosomes in the spinal fluid: Evidence for metastatic origin of meningeal leukemia. *Blood*, **35**, 227.

Mathé, G., Schwarzenberg, L., Mery, A. M., Cattan, A., Schneider, M., Amil, J. L., Schlumberger, J. R., Poisson, J. & Wajchner, G. (1966) Extensive histological and cytological survey of patients with acute leukaemia in 'complete remission'. *Brit. med. J.*, **i**, 640.

Mathé, G., Hayat, M., Schwarzenberg, L., Amiel, J. L., Schneider, M., Cattan, A., Schlumberger, J. R. & Hasmin, C. (1967) Acute lymphoblastic leukaemia treated with combination of prednisone, vincristine and rubidomycin. *Lancet*, **ii**, 380.

Mathé, G., Pouillart, P., Sterescu, M., Amiel, J. L., Schwartzenberg, L., Schneider, M., Hayat, M., Vassae, F. de, Jasmin, C. & Lafleur, M. (1971) Subdivision of classical varieties of acute leukemia: correlation with prognosis and cure expectancy. *European J. Clin. Biol. Res.*, **16**, 554.

Mathé, G. (1972) Immunological approaches to the treatment of acute leukaemia. *Clinics in Haematology*, **1**, 165.

Mauer, A. M. & Fisher, V. (1966) Characteristics of cell proliferation in four patients with untreated acute leukemia. *Blood*, **28**, 428.

Mauer, A. M. (1969) *Pediatric Hematology*. Philadelphia: McGraw-Hill.

Mauger, D. C. (1971) Letterer-Siwe's disease (acute disseminated histiocytosis X): A case complicated by disseminated intravascular coagulation and responding to heparin therapy. *Pediatrics*, **47**, 435.

Medical Research Council (1968) Chronic granulocytic leukaemia: Comparison of radiotherapy and busulphan therapy. *Brit. med. J.*, **i**, 201.

Medical Research Council (1971) Duration of survival of children with acute leukaemia. *Brit. med. J.*, **iv**, 7.

Medical Research Council (1971) Treatment of acute lymphoblastic leukaemia. Comparison of immunotherapy (BCG), intermittent methotrexate, and no therapy after a five-month intensive cytotoxic regimen (Concord Trial). *Brit. med. J.*, **iv**, 189.

Medical Research Council (1973) Treatment of acute lymphoblastic leukaemia: Effect of prophylactic radiotherapy against central nervous system leukaemia. *Brit. med. J.*, **ii**, 381.

Megalini, S. I. & Åhström, L. (1958) Clinical and hematological aspects of acute erythromyelosis. *J. Pediat.*, **52**, 501.

Melhorn, D. K., Gross, S. & Newman, A. J. (1970) Acute childhood leukemia presenting as aplastic anemia: The response to corticosteroids. *J. Pediat.*, **77**, 647.

Miller, R. W. (1964) Radiation, chromosomes and viruses in the etiology of leukemia: evidence from epidemiological research. *New Eng. J. Med.*, **271**, 30.

Miller, R. W. (1967) Persons with exceptionally high risk of leukemia. *Cancer Res.*, **27**, 2420.

Miller, R. W. (1969) Decline in U.S. childhood leukaemia mortality. *Lancet*, **ii**, 1189.

Mittwoch, U. (1961) Inclusions of mucopolysaccharide in the lymphoctyes of patients with gargoylism. *Nature*, **191**, 1315.

Murphy, W. H. & Zarafonetis, C. J. D. (1968) Viral studies in human leukaemia. Proceedings of the International Conference on Leukemia-Lymphoma, p. 127. Edited by Zarafonetis, C. J. D. Philadelphia: Lea and Febiger.

Natelson, E. A., Lynch, E. C., Hettig, R. A. & Alfrey, C. P. (1968) Histiocytic medullary reticulosis: The role of phagocytosis in pancytopenia. *Arch. Intern. Med.*, **122**, 223.

National Criteria Committee (1964) Criteria for evaluating chemotherapy in acute leukemia. *Cancer Chemotherapy Reports*, **42**, 27.

New England Journal of Medicine (1974) Editorial: The lumbar puncture. *New Eng. J. Med.*, **290**, 225.

Newell, G. R., Harris, W. W., Bowman, K. O., Boone, C. W. & Anderson, N. G. (1968) Evaluation of 'virus-like' particles in the plasma of 255 patients with leukemia and related diseases. *New Eng. J. Med.*, **278**, 1185.

Nies, B. A., Bodey, G. P., Thomas, L. B., Brecher, G. & Freireich, E. J. (1965) The persistence of extramedullary leukemic infiltrates during bone marrow remission of acute leukemia. *Blood*, **26**, 133.

Noone, P., Pattison, J. R. & Shafi, M. S. (1973) Acute renal failure after high doses of gentamicin and cephalothin. *Lancet*, **i**, 1387.

Nowell, P. C. & Hungerford, D. A. (1960) Chromosome studies on normal and leukaemic human leukocytes. *U.S. Nat. Cancer Inst. J.*, **25**, 85.

Okada, H., Liu, P. I., Hoshino, T., Yamamoto, T., Yamaoka, H. & Murakami, M. (1972) Down's syndrome associated with a myeloproliferative disorder. *Amer. J. Dis. Child.*, **124**, 107.

Oski, F. A. & Naiman, J. L. (1972) *Hematologic Problems in the Newborn*, p. 316. Philadelphia: Saunders.

Pantazopoulos, N. & Sinks, L. (1974) Morphological criteria for prognostication of acute lymphoblastic leukaemia. *Brit. J. Haemat.*, **27**, 25.

Pearson, H. A. & Diamond, L. K. (1958) Chronic monocytic leukemia in childhood. *J. Pediat.*, **53**, 259.

Pearson, H. A. & Lorincz, A. E. (1964) A characteristic bone marrow finding in the Hurler syndrome. *Pediatrics*, **34**, 280.

Pennelli, N., Scaravilli, F. & Zazzhello, F. (1969) Themorphogenesis of Gaucher cells investigated by electron microscopy. *Blood*, **34**, 331.

Pierce, M. I. (1959) Leukemia in the newborn infant. *J. Pediat.*, **54**, 691.

Pierce, M. I. (1962) Neurological complications in acute leukemia in children. *Pediat. Clin. N. Amer.*, **9**, 425.

Pierce, M. I., Borges, W. H., Heyn, R., Wolff, J. A. & Gilbert, E. S. (1969) Epidemiological factors and survival experience in 1,770 children with acute leukemia. *Cancer*, **23**, 1296.

Pincus, T., Hartley, J. W. & Rowe, W. P. (1971) A major genetic locus affecting resistance to infection and murin leukemia viruses. I. Tissue culture studies of naturally occurring viruses. *J. Exp. Med.*, **133**, 1219.

Pinkel, D. (1968) Letter. *J.A.M.A.*, **206**, 1091.

Pinkel, D., Hernandez, K., Borella, L., Holton, C., Aur, R., Samoy, G. & Pratt, C. (1971) Drug dosage and remission duration in childhood lymphocytic leukemia. *Cancer*, **27**, 247.

Pochedly, G. (1971) Thrombocytopenic purpura of the newborn. *Obst. and Gynec. Survey*, **26**, 63.

Pochedly, C. (1973) *The Child with Leukemia*. Springfield, Illinois: Thomas.

Graham Pole, J. & Willoughby, M. L. N. (1975) Leukaemia in the nervous system: Factors in pathogenesis. In *Modern Problems in Pediatric Series*. Basel/New York: Karger. In press.

Porter, F. S. (1963) Multiple myeloma in a child. *J. Pediat.*, **62**, 602.

Powell, D. F. B. (1971) Incidence and distribution of acute leukaemia in one district general hospital area. *Lancet*, **ii**, 350.

Powles, R. L., Crowther, D., Bateman, C. J. T., Beard, M. E. J., McElwain, T. J., Russell, J., Lister, T. A., Whitehouse, J. M. A., Wrigley, P. F. M., Pike, M., Alexander, P. & Hamilton Fairley, G. (1975) Immunotherapy for acute myelogenous leukaemia. *Brit. J. Cancer*, **28**, 365.

Price, D. L., Woolsey, J. E., Rosman, N. P. & Richardson, E. P. (1971) Familial lymphohistiocytosis of the nervous system. *Arch. Neurol.*, **24**, 270.

Price, R. A. & Johnson, W. W. (1973) The central nervous system in childhood lymphocytic leukemia: I. The arachnoid. *Cancer*, **31**, 520.

Price, R. A., Jamieson, P. A. & Pitner, S. E. (1974) Degenerative changes in the brain following irradiation and methotrexate therapy for childhood lymphocytic leukaemia. *Blood*, **44**, 929.

Quaglino, D. & Hayhoe, F. (1960) Periodic-acid-Schiff positivity in erythroblasts with special reference to Di Gugliemo's disease. *Brit. J. Haemat.*, **6**, 26.

Quattrin, V. N., Dini, E. & Palumbo, E. (1969) Basophile Leukämien. *Blut.*, **5**, 166.

Rall, D. P. & Zubrod, C. G. (1962) Mechanisms of drug absorption and excretion. *A. Rev. Pharmac.*, **2**, 109.

Rand, J. J., Maloney, W. C. & Sise, H. S. (1969) Coagulation defects in acute promyelocytic leukemia. *Arch. Intern. Med.*, **123**, 39.

Randall, D. L., Reiquam, C. W., Githens, J. H. & Robinson, A. (1965) Familial myeloproliferative disease. *Am. J. Dis. Child.*, **110**, 479.

Regelson, W., Bross, I. D. J., Hananian, J. & Nigogosyan, G. (1965) Incidence of second primary tumors in children with cancer and leukemia: seven-year survey of 150 consecutive autopsied cases. *Cancer*, **18**, 58.

Reilly, W. A. (1941) The granules in the leukocytes in gargoylism. *Am. J. Dis. Child.*, **62**, 489.

Reimann, D. L., Clemmens, R. L. & Pillsbury, W. A. (1955) Congenital acute leukemia. *J. Pediat.*, **46**, 415.

Reisman, L. E. & Trujillo, J. M. (1963) Chronic granulocytic leukemia of childhood. *J. Pediat.*, **62**, 710.

Reisman, L. E., Mitani, M. & Zuelzer, W. W. (1964) I. Evidence for the origin of leukemic stem lines from aneuploid mutants. *New Eng. J. Med.*, **270**, 590.

Repsher, L. H., Schröter, G. & Hammond, W. S. (1972) Diagnosis of pneumocytosis carinii pneumonitis by means of endobronchial brush biopsy. *New Eng. J. Med.*, **287**, 340.

Rickles, F. R. & Miller, D. R. (1972) Eosinophilic leukemoid reaction. *J. Pediat.*, **80**, 418.

Roath, S. (1972) Observation on the aetiology of acute leukaemia. *Clinics in Haematology*, **1**, 23.

Robbins, K. M., Gribertz, I., Strauss, L., Leonidas, J. C. & Sanders, M. (1973) Pneumonitis during methotrexate therapy. *J. Pediat.*, **82**, 84.

Robertson, J. H. (1970) Pneumonia and methotrexate. *Brit. med. J.*, **ii**, 156.

Rodriguez, V., Burgess, M. & Bodey, G. P. (1973) Management of fever of unknown origin in patients with neoplasms and neutropenia. *Cancer*, **32**, 1005.

Rosenberg, H. S. & Taylor, F. M. (1958) The myeloproliferative syndrome in children. *J. Pediat.*, **52**, 407.

Rosenthal, D. S. & Maloney, W. C. (1972) Treatment of acute granulocytic leukemia in adults. *New Eng. J. Med.*, **286**, 1176.

Rosner, F., Lee, S. L. & Acute Leukemia Group B. (1972) Down's syndrome and acute leukemia: Myeloblastic or lymphoblastic? Report of forty-three cases and review of the literature. *Am. J. Med.*, **53**, 203.

Ross, J. D., Maloney, W. C. & Desforges, J. F. (1963) Ineffective regulation of granulopoiesis masquerading as congenital leukemia in a mongoloid child. *J. Pediat.*, **63**, 1.

Royer, P. (1959) La cellule de Buhot de le diagnostic du gargoylisme. *Sang.*, **30**, 37.

Rozenszajn, L., Klajman, A., Yaffe, D. & Efratti, P. (1966) Jordan's anomaly in white blood cells. Report of a case. *Blood*, **28**, 258.

Rywlin, A. M., Hernandez, J. A., Chastain, D. E. & Pardo, V. (1971) Ceroid histiocytosis of spleen and bone marrow in idiopathic thrombocytopenic purpura (ITP): A contribution to the understanding of the sea-blue histiocyte. *Blood*, **37**, 587.

Sandberg, A. A. & Hossfeld, D. K. (1970) Chromosomal abnormalities in human neoplasia. *Ann. Rev. Med.*, **21**, 379.

Sardeman, H. (1973) Chronic lymphocytic leukemia in an infant. *Acta Paediat. Scand.*, **61**, 213.

Sarngadharan, M. G., Sarin, P. S., Reitz, M. S. & Gallo, R. C. (1972) Reverse transcriptase activity of human acute leukaemic cells: Purification of the enzyme, response to AMV 70S RNA, and characterization of the DNA product. *Nature New Biol.*, **240**, 67.

Saunders, E. F., Lampkin, B. C. & Mauer, A. M. (1967) Variation of proliferative activity in leukemic cell populations of patients with acute leukemia. *J. Clin. Invest.*, **46**, 1356.

Saunders, E. F. & Mauer, A. M. (1969) Re-entry of non-dividing leukemic cells into a proliferative phase in acute childhood leukemia. *J, Clin. Invest.*, **48**, 1299.

Sawitsky, A., Bloom, D. & German, J. (1966) Chromosomal breakage and acute leukemia in congenital telangiectatic erythema and stunted growth. *Ann. Intern. Med.*, **65**, 487.

Say, B. & Berkel, I. (1964) Idiopathic myelofibrosis in an infant. *J. Pediat.*, **64**, 580.

Scheerer, P. P., Pierre, R. V., Schwartz, D. L. & Linman, J. W. (1964) Reed-Steinberg-cell leukemia and lactic acidosis. *New Eng. J. Med.*, **270**, 274.

Schimpff, S. C., Green, W. H., Young, V. M., Fortner, C. L., Jepsen, L., Cusack, N. E. & Wiernik, P. H. (1973) Infection prevention in acute nonlymphocytic leukemia with consequent improved remission rates and survival duration. *Blood*, **42**, 1015.

Schrek, R. & Donnelly, W. J. (1966) 'Hairy' cells in blood in lymphoreticular neoplastic disease and 'flagellated' cells of normal lymph nodes. *Blood*, **27**, 199.

Schwartz, A. D., Zelson, J. H. & Pearson, H. A. (1970) Acute myelogenous leukemia with compensatory but ineffective erythropoiesis: Di Gugliemo's syndrome. *J. Pediat.*, **77**, 653.

Scott, A. J., Nicholson, G. I. & Kerr, A. R. (1973) Lincomycin as a cause of pseudomembranous colitis. *Lancet*, **ii**, 1232.

Sedaghatian, M. R. & Singer, D. B. (1972) Pneumocystis carinii in children with malignant disease. *Cancer*, **29**, 772.

Selawry, O. S. & Odom, S. (1968) On eradication of leukemic meningopathy. *Proc. Am. Ass. Cancer Res.*, **9**, 62.

Sen, L. & Borella, L. (1975) Clinical importance of lymphoblasts with T markers in childhood acute leukemia. *New Eng. J. Med.*, **292**, 828.

Sharp, H. L., Nesbit, M. E., White, J. G. & Krivit, W. (1967) Renal and hepatic pathology following initial remission of acute leukemia induced by prednisone. *Cancer*, **20**, 1395.

Sharp, H., Nesbit, M., White, J. & Krivit, W. (1969) Methotrexate liver toxicity. *J. Pediat.*, **74**, 818.

Silverstein, M. N., Ellefson, R. D. & Ahern, E. J. (1970) The syndrome of the sea-blue histiocyte. *New Eng. J. Med.*, **282**, 1.

Simone, J., Aur, R. J. A., Hustu, O. & Pinkel, D. (1972) Total therapy studies of acute lymphocytic leukemia in children. *Cancer*, **30**, 1488.

Simone, J., Aur, R. J. A., Hustu, H. O. & Pinkel, D. (1972A) 'Total therapy' studies of acute lymphocytic leukemia in childhood: Current results and prospects for cure. *Cancer*, **30**, 1488.

Simone, J. V., Holland, E. & Johnson, W. (1972B) Fatalities during remission of childhood leukaemia. *Blood*, **39**, 759.

Simone, J. V. (1973) Editorial: Preventive central-nervous-system therapy in acute leukaemia. *New Eng. J. Med.*, **289**, 1248.

Skeel, R. T., Henderson, E. S. & Bennett, J. M. (1968) The significance of bone marrow lymphocytosis of acute leukemia patients in remission. *Blood*, **32**, 767.

Smith, J. W., Freeman, A. I. & Pinkel, D. (1967). Search for a human leukaemic virus. *Archiv. für die gesamte Virus forschung*, **22**, 294.

Spiers, A. S. D. (1972) Chemotherapy of acute leukaemia. *Clinics in Haematology*, **1**, 127.

Spiers, A. S. D. (1974) Chronic granulocytic leukaemia and chronic lymphocytic leukaemia. *Brit. med. J.*, **iv**, 460.

Spiers, A. S. D., Baikie, A. G., Galton, D. A. G., Richards, H. G. H., Wiltshaw, E., Goldman, J. M., Catovsky, D., Spencer, J. & Peto, R. (1975A) Chronic granulocytic leukaemia: Effect of elective splenectomy on the course of the disease. *Brit. med. J.*, **i**, 175.

Spiers, A. S. D., Galton, D. A. G., Kaur, J. & Goldman, J. M. (1975B) Thioguanine as primary treatment for chronic granulocytic leukaemia. *Lancet*, **i**, 829.

Spivak, J. L., Brubaker, L. H. & Perry, S. (1969) Intravascular granulocyte kinetics in acute leukemia. *Blood*, **34**, 582.

Starling, K. A., Donaldson, M. H., Haggard, M. E., Vietti, T. J. & Sutow, W. W. (1972) Therapy of histiocytosis X with vincristine, vinblastine, and cyclophosphamide. *Am. J. Dis. Child.*, **123**, 105.

Stewart, A., Webb, J. & Hewitt, D. (1958) A survey of childhood malignancies. *Brit. med. J.*, **i**, 1495.

Stewart, A. (1970) Cat leukaemia. *Brit. med. J.*, **ii**, 49.

Stryckmans, P., Delalieux, G., Manaster, J. & Socquet, M. (1970) The potentiality of out-of-cycle acute leukemic cells to synthesise DNA. *Blood,* **36,** 697.

Stuart, J. (1972) Scientific basis of clinical practice: Disordered leucocyte proliferation in leukaemia. *Brit. med. J.,* **ii,** 152.

Sullivan, M. P., Vietti, T. J., Fernbach, D. J., Griffith, K. M., Haddy, T. B. & Watkins, W. L. (1969) Clinical investigations in the treatment of meningeal leukemia: Radiation therapy regimens vs conventional intrathecal methotrexate. *Blood,* **34,** 301.

Sullivan, M. P. & Haggard, M. E. (1970) Comparison of the prolongation of remission in meningeal leukaemia with maintenance intrathecal methotrexate and I.V. BCNU. *Proc. Am. Ass. Cancer Res.,* **11,** 77.

Sullivan, M. P., Sutow, W. W., Taylor, H. G. & Wilbur, J. R. (1971) Intrathecal (IT) combination chemotherapy for meningeal leukemia using methotrexate (MTX) Cytosine arabinoside (CA), and Hydrocortisone (HDC). *Proc. Am. Ass. Cancer Res.,* **12,** 45.

Sullivan, M. P., Vietti, T. J., Haggard, M. E., Donaldson, M. H., Krall, J. M. & Gehan, E. A. (1971) Remission maintenance therapy for meningeal leukemia: Intrathecal methotrexate vs intravenous bis-nitrosourea. *Blood,* **38,** 680.

Tallal, L., Tan, C., Oettgen, H., Wollner, N., McCarthy, M., Helson, L., Burchenal, J., Karnofsky, D. & Murphy, M. L. (1970) *E. coli* L-asparaginase in the treatment of leukemia and solid tumors in 131 children. *Cancer,* **25,** 306.

Tattersal, M. H., Spiers, A. S. & Darrell, J. H. (1972) Initial therapy with combination of five antibiotics in febrile patients with leukaemia and neutropenia. *Lancet,* **i,** 162.

Till, M. M., Hardisty, R. M., Pike, M. C. & Doll, R. (1967) Childhood leukaemia in Greater London: A search for evidence of clustering. *Brit. med. J.,* **iii,** 755.

Till, M. M., Hardisty, R. M. & Pike, M. C. (1973) Long survivals in acute leukaemia. *Lacnet,* **i,** 534.

Till, M. M., Jones, L. H., Pentycross, C. R., Hardisty, R. M., Lawler, S. D., Harvey, B. A. M. & Soothill, J. F. (1975) Leukaemia in children and their grandparents: Studies of immune function in six families. *Brit. J. Haemat.,* **29,** 575.

Tivey, H. (1954) The natural history of untreated acute leukaemia. *Ann. N.Y. Acad. Sci.,* **60,** 322.

Todaro, G. J., Zeve, V. & Aaronson, S. A. (1970) Virus in cell culture derived from human tumor patients. *Nature,* **226,** 1047.

Todaro, G. J. & Gallo, R. C. (1973) Immunological relationship of DNA polymerase from human acute leukaemia cells and primate and mouse leukaemia virus reverse transcriptase. *Nature,* **244,** 206.

Turesson, D. (1957) Myleran treatment in chronic granulocytic leukaemia. *Brit. J. Haemat.,* **3,** 220.

Uzman, L. L. (1951) The lipoprotein of Gaucher's disease. *Arch. Path.,* **51,** 329.

Vaithianathan, T., Bolonik, S. J. & Gruhn, J. G. (1962) Leukemic reticuloendotheliosis. *Am. J. Clin. Path.,* **38,** 605.

Vaithianathan, T., Fishkin, S. & Gruhn, J. G. (1967) Histiocytic medullary reticulosis. *Am. J. Clin. Pathol.,* **47,** 160.

Varadi, S., Gordon, R. R. & Abbott, D. (1964) Haemophagocytic reticulosis diagnosed during life. *Acta Haematol.,* **31,** 349.

Vigliani, E. C. & Saita, G. (1964) Benzene and leukemia. *New Eng. J. Med.,* **271,** 872.

Vita, V. T. de & Schein, P. S. (1973) The use of drugs in combination for the treatment of cancer. *New Eng. J. Med.,* **288,** 998.

Vitale, L. F., Shahidi, N. T. & Abtshuler, C. H. (1970) Reticuloendotheliosis with Neiman-Pick type foam cells in bone marrow and spleen. *Arch. Pathol.,* **90,** 218.

Vowels, M. R. & Willoughby, M. L. N. (1973) Cyclic chemotherapy in acute lymphoblastic leukaemia of childhood. *Arch. Dis. Childh.,* **48,** 436.

Wagner, H. P., Cottier, H. & Cronkite, E. P. (1972) Variability of proliferative patterns in acute lymphoid leukaemia of children. *Blood,* **39,** 176.

Wald, N., Borges, W. L., Li, C. C., Turner, J. H. & Harnois, M. C. (1961) Leukaemia associated with Mongolism. *Lancet,* **i,** 1228.

Walters, T. R., Bushore, M. & Simone, J. (1972) Poor prognosis in negro children with acute lymphoblastic leukemia. *Cancer,* **29,** 210.

Wang, J. J. & Pratt, C. B. (1970) Intrathecal arabinosyl cytosine in meningeal leukemia. *Cancer,* **25,** 531.

Waters, W. J. & Lacson, P. S. (1957) Mast cell leukemia presenting as urticaria pigmentosa. *Pediatrics,* **19,** 1033.

Weatherall, D. J., Edwards, J. A. & Donohoe, W. T. A. (1968) Haemoglobin and red cell enzyme changes in juvenile myeloid leukaemia. *Brit. med. J.,* **i,** 679.

Weiss, H. D., Walker, M. D. & Wiernik, P. H. (1974) Neurotoxicity of commonly used antineoplastic agents (two parts). *New Eng. J. Med.,* **291,** 75, 127.

West, R. J., Graham Pole, J., Hardisty, R. M. & Pike, M. C. (1972) Factors in the pathogenesis of central-nervous-system leukaemia. *Brit. med. J.,* **III,** 311.

Whitecar, J. P., Bodey, G. P., Freireich, E. J., McCredie, K. B. & Hart, J. S. (1972) Cyclophosphamide (NSC-26271), Vincristine (NSC-67574), Cytosine Arabinoside (NSC-63878), and Prednisone /NSC-10023) (COAP) Combination Chemotherapy for acute leukaemia in adults. *Cancer Chemother. Rep.,* **56,** 543.

Willoughby, M. L. N. (1972) Management of childhood leukaemia, p. 71. In *Recent Advances in Cancer and Radiotherapeutics.* Edited by Halnan, K. E. London: Churchill Livingston.

Willoughby, M. L. N. (1974) Treatment of overt meningeal leukaemia. *Lancet,* **1,** 363.

Willoughby, M. L. N. (1974) Blood and neoplastic diseases: Acute lymphoblastic leukaemia. *Brit. med. J.,* **4,** 282.

Willoughby, M. L. N. (1974) Blood and neoplastic diseases: Acute myeloblastic leukaemia. *Brit. med. J.,* **4,** 337.

Willoughby, M. L. N., Al-Janabi, S., Shannon, V., Jones, J. B., Brewis, E. A., Robertson, H. J., Porteus, J. &

Disbrey, M. (1974B) Evaluation of pathogen free nursing for children with acute leukaemia. Proceedings of European Society for Paediatric Haematology and Immunology, Genoa. *Z. Kinderheilk*, **117**, 291.

Wintrobe, M. M. (1967) *Clinical Hematology*, p. 1018. London: Henry Kimpton.

Wright, D. H. & Pike, P. A. (1968) Bone marrow involvement in Burkitt's tumour. *Brit. J. Haemat.*, **15**, 409.

Yam, L. T., Li, C. Y. & Lam, K. W. (1971) Tartrate-resistant acid phosphatase isoenzyme in the reticulum cells of leukemic reticuloendotheleiosis. *New Eng. J. Med.*, **284**, 357.

Yates, J. W. & Holland, J. F. (1973) A controlled study of isolation and endogenous microbial suppression in acute myelocytic patients. *Cancer*, **32**, 1490.

Yohn, D. S. & Grace, J. T. (1966) Immunofluorescent studies in human leukemia. *Proc. Am. Assoc. Cancer. Res.*, **7**, 78.

Zaino, E. C., Rossi, M. B., Pham, T. D. & Azar, H. A. (1971) Gaucher's cells in thalassemia. *Blood*, **38**, 457.

Zeffren, J. L. & Ultmann, J. E. (1960) Reticulum cell sarcoma terminating in acute leukaemia. *Blood*, **15**, 277.

Zippin, C., Cutler, S. J., Reeves, W. J. & Lum, D. (1971) Variations in survival among patients with acute lymphocytic leukemia. *Blood*, **37**, 59.

Zuelzer, W. W. (1964) Implications of long-term survival in acute stem leukemia of childhood treated with composite cyclic therapy. *Blood*, **24**, 477.

Zuelzer, W. W. & Cox, D. E. (1969) Genetic aspects of leukemia. *Sem. Hematol.*, **6**, 228.

Index

ABO Haemolytic Disease of New-born (ABO HDNB)
clinical features, 182
exchange transfusion in, 182
laboratory findings, 182
late anaemia in, 182
management, 183
pathogenesis, 181
phenobarbitone therapy, 183
phototherapy, 183
Acanthocytosis, 83, 148
Acute Leukaemias
ALL, 382
AML, 382
AMMoL, 382
AMOL, 382
AUL, 382
ASL, 382
Acute rheumatic fever and anaemia, 206
Addison's disease anaemia, 208
Adenosine triphosphatase deficiency, 105
Albinism and platelet defect, 294
Alkali treatment in sickle-cell disease, 123
Alpha-thalassaemia, 130, 131
Amniocencesis in,
anti-c̄ immunisation, 185
anti-D immunisation, 165
anti-E immunisation, 185
hazards of, 167
lecithin: sphingomyelin ratio, 170, 172
prediction of Rh disease, 165
Anaemia
aplastic, 43 (*See also* Aplastic anaemia)
autoimmune, 150 (*See also* Autoimmune haemolytic anaemia)
B_{12} deficiency, 36 (*See also* Vitamin B_{12} deficiency)
chronic infection, 204
chronic inflammation, 206
copper deficiency, 204
Felty's syndrome, 206
folate deficiency
anticonvulsants, 26
clinical features, 29
due to increased loss, 29
haematological changes, 18
haemolysis, 24
Howell-Jolly bodies, 18
hypersegmentation of polymorphs, 18
infection, 22

Anaemia—*continued*
macrocytes, 18
malabsorption, 23
marrow findings, 18
megaloblasts, 19
nutritional, 25
prematurity, 20, 21
sickling states, 123
treatment, 29
Haemoglobinopathies, 116
Haemolytic
autoimmune, 150
hereditary elliptocytosis, 80
hereditary spherocytosis, 78
infectious mononucleosis, 243
non-spherocytic (enzyme deficiencies), 89
secondary to systemic disease, 203
Hypochromic
chronic infection, 6, 7, 204
chronic inflammation, 6, 7, 206
congenital metabolic defect, 6, 7
congenital transferrin deficiency, 6, 7
copper deficiency, 6, 7, 204
iron deficiency, 5
lead poisoning, 6, 7, 154, 212
pulmonary haemosiderosis, 6
sideroblastic anaemia, 6, 7
thalassaemia, 6, 7, 132
Iron deficiency
biochemical tests of, 7
blood transfusion, 10
chelated iron preparations, 9
clinical features, 4
gastro-intestinal function, 3
hookworm, 3
haematological findings, 5
incidence, 1, 4
infection, 5
intestinal blood loss, 3 4
iron deficiency, 1
marrow iron, 6
Meckel's diverticulum, 4, 7
marrow iron, 6
occult intestinal blood loss, 7
oral iron therapy, 9
parenteral iron, 10
pathogenesis of, 1
platelet count, 280
pseudomacrocytosis, 6
red-cell survival, 6
response, 9, 10
serum ferritin, 7
serum iron, 7

Anaemia—*continued*
TIBC, 7
treatment, 8
Megaloblastic
anticonvulsants, 26
B_{12} deficiency, 36, 38
congenital, 28
cyclohydrase deficiency, 28
folate deficiency, 16, 18
folinic acid responsive, 28
formimino transferase, 28
hereditary, 28
inborn errors, 25, 28
isolated folate malabsorption, 24
leukaemia, 384
orotic aciduria, 28
thiamine responsive, 28
Microangiopathic, 146
Neonatal, 189
physiological, of newborn, 204
prematurity, 203
renal failure, 207
secondary anaemias, 203
thalassaemias, 129
Anaesthesia in Sickle cell States, 124
Anaphylactoid Purpura, 302
Aplastic Anaemia
acquired forms, 53
aetiology, 43, 53
androgens, 58
associated with PNA, 57
classification, 44
clinical features, 46, 49, 56
constitutional forms, 45
laboratory diagnosis, 48, 56
prognosis, 58, 60
treatment, 50, 58
Aplastic crises
hereditary spherocytosis, 79
sickle-cell disease, 122
Anti-c̄ antibodies and neonatal jaundice, 164, 165, 167, 184, 185
Anti-D gamma globulin, 164
Anti-E antibodies and neonatal jaundice, 184, 185
Asparaginase in ALL, 385
Aspirin
avoidance in Haemophilia, 299
gastrointestinal bleeding, 298
platelet dysfunction, 298
post-tonsillectomy bleeding, 298
purpura, 299
Auer rods
AML and AMMoL, 382
erythroleukaemia, 401

424 PAEDIATRIC HAEMATOLOGY

Autoimmune haemolytic anaemia (AHA)
clinical manifestations, 152
cold types, 153
DLE, 151
evan's syndrome, 265
following infections, 152
haematological features, 152
I antigen, 153
infectious mononucleosis, 243
lymphomas, 151
pathogenesis, 151
treatment, 153
underlying disease, 151
Autosplenectomy in sickle-cell disease, 123, 124

B_{12} deficiency (See Vit. B_{12} deficiency
Bacterial killing by granulocytes
biochemistry of, 235
Benign inherited neutropenia (Glansslen), 227
Bernard-Soulier syndrome, 294
Beta-thalassaemia, 130, 131
Bilirubin, serum
albumen binding, 171
indirect reacting, 169
Blackfan-Diamond syndrome, (See Pure red-cell aplasia)
Bleeding time, 288
Blood coagulation, 309
capillary tests of, 311, 312
cascade hypothesis, 309
consumptive coagulopathy, 311, 343
disorders of, 311
extrinsic system, 310
FDPs, 310, 344
fibrinolytic system, 310
intrinsic system, 310
investigation of, 311
physiology, 309
Bone marrow in aplastic anaemia, 43, 44, 49, 56
Burkitt's tumour
EBV, 375
Marrow involvement, 403
Burr cells, 145, 146, 147, 345
congenital virus infections, 191
DIC, 345
hypothyroidism, 208
MAHA, 146
renal failure, 207

Capillary blood samples
techniques, i,
Cardiac and vascular diseases
haematological changes, 354, 355
platelet survival, 355
Carotid body tumours and factor VII and X deficiency, 328
Cell-kill in leukaemia, 385
CNS leukaemia, see Meningeal leukaemia
CSF folate, 24, 27
Chédiak-Higashi Disease
defective bacterial killing, 236, 238

Chloramphenicol and aplastic anaemia, 54
Christmas disease. See Haemophilia and Xmas Disease
Chromosome breakage
Bloom's syndrome, 46
Fanconi's, 46
Chronic benign granulocytopenia of childhood (CG), 227
Chronic granulomatous disease
biochemical defect, 235
clinical features, 236
inheritance, 237
NBT test, 236
pathology, 236
See also G-6-PD deficiency in leucocytes, Job's syndrome, Leukocyte glutathione peroxidase deficiency, Myeloperoxidase deficiency
Chronic myelocytic leukaemia, 399
adult form, 401
chromosomes, 399, 401
Hb. F, 399
juvenile, 399
serum B_{12} levels, 400
splenectomy, 401
Clot retraction, 292
Coagulation factor levels in neonate, 335, 336
related to birthweight, 336
related to gestation, 336
liver disease, 342
premature infants, 335, 336
Cold agglutinins in sickle-cell disease, 123
Cold haemagglutinin syndrome in AHA, 152, 153
I antigen, 153
infective mononucleosis, 153
mycoplasmal infection, 153
Collagen diseases and anaemia, 206
Combined factor VIII and V deficiency, 329
Compensatory marrow activity, 73
Congenital afibrinogenaemia
coagulation defect, 329
platelet dysfunction, 298
Congenital dyserythropoietic anaemias (CDA)
Type I, 84
Type II, 84
Type III, 84
Congenital hypoplastic anaemia, see Pure red-cell aplasia
Congenital megaloblastic anaemia, 28
Consumptive coagulopathy, see also DIC, 343
'balanced' DIC, 344
FDPs, 344
Cooley's anaemia see Thalassaemia
Copper deficiency
anaemia, 204
neutropenia, 204
premature infants, 204

Cyanate therapy in sickle-cell disease, 124
Cyclic neutropenia, 229
Cyclohydrase deficiency
congenital, 29
Cystic fibrosis and B_{12}, 40
Cytomegalovirus (CMV and neonatal haemolysis, 190
Cytosine arabinoside in acute leukaemia, 386

Daunorubicin in acute leukaemia, 386
Dehydrated red cells
congenital haemolytic anaemia due to, 82
Delta-beta thalassaemia, 130
Delta thalassaemia, 131
Desferrioxamine, 64
DIC, 312, 343
'balanced' DIC, 344
burr cells, 345
capillary screening tests, 345
circulating 'fibrin', 345
clinical features, 345
coagulation changes, 345
cryofibrinogen, 345
diagnosis, 345
ethanol gelation test, 345
exchange transfusion, 347
FDPs, 344
heparin therapy, 347, 349
MAHA, 345
plateletand fibrinogen survival, 346
shock, 345
specific therapy, 346
therapeutic considerations, 346
DIC in neonatal period, 349
asphyxia and acidosis, 350
hypothermia, 350
infection, 350
maternal causes, 352
prematurity, 350
RDS, 352
severe Rh disease, 350
DIC in later childhood
acute liver failure, 362
congenital heart disease, 354
disseminated malignant disease, 362
fungal septicaemia, 361
giant haemangioma, 353
haemolytic uraemic syndrome (HUS), 356
homocystinaemia, 355
hypertonic dehydration, 352
incompatible blood transfusion, 363
kwashiorkor, 361
malaria, 361
materno-foetal transfusion, 363
meningococcal Septicaemia, 360
miscellaenous causes, 363
neuroblastoma, 362
post cardiotomy bleeding, 355
promyelocytic leukaemia, 362
purpura fulminans, 361

DIC—continued
prosthetic heart valves, 355
protozoal septicaemia, 361
renal vein thrombosis, 352
rheumatic heart disease, 355
rickettsial septicaemia, 361
septicaemia, 359
Thrombotic thrombocytopenci purpura (TTP), 359
ventriculojugular shunts, 355
viraemia, 361
rickettsial, 361
septicaemia, 359
thrombotic thrombocytopenic purpura (TTP), 359
ventriculojugular shunts, 355
viraemia, 361
Dihydroxybenzoic acid in iron overload, 64
2, 3-diphosphoglyceromutase deficiency, 105
Diphyllobothrium latum and B_{12} deficiency, 40
Dipyrrole pigments
thalassaemia, 130
unstable haemoglobins, 124, 126
Direct Coombs test
ABD HD, 182
AHA, 152
drug-induced haemolysis, 156
Evans's syndrome, 265
Rh disease, 169
DLE
Anaemia, 206
Thrombocytopenia, 259, 265
Döhle Bodies
EM findings, 274
May-Hegglin, 238, 274
severe bacterial infections, 239
Donath-Landsteiner antibody, 151, 153
Drug haptene disease, 156, 277
haemolytic anaemia, 156
neutropenia, 156
thrombocytopenia, 156
Drug-induced haemolysis, 93, 154, 155
autoimmune type, 156
defects of GSH synthesis, 99
GSH-Px deficiency, 99
GSSG-R deficiency, 98
G-6-PD deficiency, 94
6-PGD deficiency, 98
Hb Zurich, 117
immune or drug-haptene type, 156
red cell enzyme defects, 94
unstable haemoglobins, 124, 126
unstable haemoglobinopathies, 126
drug-induced neutropenia, 232
Dubin-Johnson syndrome
coagulation changes in, 343
Duffy antibodies and neonatal jaundice, 184, 185
Dyserythropoiesis in aplastic anaemia, 49, 56

Ehler-Danlos syndrome, 303
Marfan's syndrome, 304
defect in collagen, 303
Electron Microscopy (EM) of leukaemic cells, 382
Embden-Meyerhof pathway, 89, 100
Eosinophilia
causes of, 244, 245
ITP, 261
eosinophilic leukaemia, 402
Erythroblastosis foetalis, see Rh disease
Erythrogenesis imperfecta, see Pure red-cell aplasia
Erythropoietic porphyria
haemolytic anaemia, 157
Erythropoietin
androgens, 53
aplastic anaemia, 53
chronic renal failure, 207
endocrine disorders, 208
haemolytic anaemia, 74
postnatal changes, 203
pure red cell aplasia, 62
renal tumours, 219
Evans's syndrome, 258, 265
Exchange transfusion
ABO HD, 183
DIC, 347, 350, 352
enzyme deficiencies, 195
G-6-PD deficiency, 193
hazards of, 171
HS, 194
hypoglycaemia after, 172
hyperkalaemia, 172
indications for, 170, 171
infantile pycnocytosis, 199
PK deficiency, 195
Rh disease, 170
use of albumen, 171
use of bicarbonate, 172
use of tham, 172
Extramedullary leukaemia, see Meningeal and Testicular
Factor II (Prothrombin) deficiency hereditary, 327
Factor V deficiency, hereditary, 328
Factor VII deficiency hereditary, 327
Factor VIII deficiency, hereditary— see Haemophilia
Factor X deficiency, hereditary, 328
Factor XI (PTA) deficiency, hereditary, 327
Factor XII (hageman) deficiency, hereditary, 327
Failure to gain weight in folate deficiency, 29
Failure to thrive in B_{12} deficiency, 36
Familial erythrophagocytic lymphohistiocytosis (FEL), 408
CNS, 408
haemolytic blood picture, 408
hepatosplenomegaly, 408
pancytopenia, 408

Familial haemophagocytic reticulosis
haemolytic anaemia, 157
Familial myeloproliferative disease, 411
Fanconi's aplastic anaemia—see Aplastic anaemia, constitutional
Felty's syndrome
anaemia, 206
neutropenia, 206
splenomegaly, 206
Ferritin
serum, 7
FDPs
assays, 344
'balanced' DIC, 344
DIC, 343, 345
FDPs, 310, 312, 344
fragments, X, Y, D, E, 344
levels, 344
MAHA, 147
thrombosis, 345
Fibrinogen and platelet survival
intravascular coagulation, 346
response to dipyridamole, 346
response to heparin, 346
selective platelet sequestration, 346
Fibrinogen Titre, 312
DIC, 346
Fibrinolysis
chronic liver disease, 342
DIC, 343
fibrinolysis, 310, 313
study of, in RDS, 351
Wilson's disease, 342
Fibrinolytic Activator, 310, 313
chronic liver disease, 342
Wilson's disease, 342
FIGLU test, 17
Foeto-maternal haemorrhage
chronic and foetal anaemia, 2
Rh immunisation, 163
Folate, see also Anaemia, Folate deficiency
absorption, 15, 23
assays, 16, 17
biochemistry of derivatives, 13
CSF level, 24, 27
daily requirements, 19
dietary sources, 14
FIGLU metabolism, 17
hyperfolicaemia, 28
inborn errors of metabolism, 25, 28
metabolism, 13
methyl folate 'trap', 14
red-cell level, 16, 17
serum level, 16, 17
sickle-cell states, 124
status in newborn, 20
thalassaemia, 132
whole-blood level, 16, 17
Folinic acid responsive anaemia, 28
Formimino transferase deficiency congenital, 28

426 PAEDIATRIC HAEMATOLOGY

Fy antibodies, and neonatal jaundice, 184, 185

G-6-PD deficiency in leucocytes, 236, 238
Gamma-beta thalassaemia, 130, 134
Gamma globulin inhibition test, 152
Gaucher cells
chronic myeloid leukaemia, 410
hempas, 84
storage disease, 410
thalassaemia, 410
Gaucher's disease, 410
Giant haemangioma
coagulation changes, 353
intravascular coagulation, 352
MAHA, 354
Prednisone, 352
Thrombocytopenia, 262
Gilbert's syndrome
low factor VII, 343
Glanzmann's thrombasthenia, 293
Glucose-6-phosphate dehydrogenase
deficiency, 92
clinical manifestations, 94
drug-induced haemolysis, 94
favism, 96
genetics, 94
infantile pycnocytosis, 188
kernicterus, 96
neonatal jaundice, 96
neurological disorder, 97
sickle-cell disease, 124
vitamin K, 95
Glutathione peroxidase deficiency
hereditary, 99
neonatal jaundice, 99
newborn infants, 98
premature infants, 98
Glutathione reductase deficiency, 98
neurological disorder, 98
pancytopenia, 98
Glutathione synthesis
defects, 99
neurological defect, 100
Glyceraldehyde-3-phosphate dehy-drogenase deficiency, 104
Glycogen storage disease, platelet defect, 294
Glycolytic pathway, disorders, 100
Goat's milk anaemia, 25
Gonadal leukaemia, *see* Testicular leukaemia
Granulocyte function, acquired dis-orders
acute leukaemia, 238
acquired disorders, 238
diabetes, mellitus, 238
Down's syndrome, 238
drugs, 238
dysproteinaemia, 239
hyperalimentation, 239
leukaemia, 389
after radiotherapy, 391
See also Chronic granulomatous disease

Granulocyte transfusions in leu-kaemia, 388
Granulocytes
kinetics, 223
maturation, 223
physiology, 224, 234
Growth hormone in Fanconi's anaemia, 46
Gum infiltration in leukaemia, 380, 404

Haemodialysis anaemia, 207
Haemodialysis and folate loss, 29
Haemoglobin
alpha chains, 112
beta chains, 112
chemical structure, 111
foetal, 112, 113
genetically determined variants, 116
normal variants, 112
normal values, ii
oxygen dissociation, 114, 115
post-natal changes, 115
types present at birth, 113
Haemoglobinopathies
geographic distribution, 117
inheritance, 117
methaemoglobins, 127
M-Haemoglobinopathies, 127
sickling states, 118
unstable haemoglobins, 124
Haemolytic anaemia
bossing of skull, 74
compensatory marrow activity, 73
folate utilisation, 74
pigment metabolism, 74
red-cell fragmentation, 73
red-cell survival, 73
spherocytes, 71
urobilinogen excretion, 75
Haemolytic disease of the newborn (HDNB). *See* Rh disease, and ABO haemolytic disease
Haemolytic uraemic syndrome (HUS), 356
age incidence, 356
anti-platelet drugs, 259
clinical features, 356
coagulation investigations, 357
haematological findings, 357
pathogenesis, 356
platelet and fibrinogen kinetics, 357
treatment, 358
Haemophilia and Christmas disease, 313
alleviation with age, 317
calculation of dosage, 320, 321
CNS bleeding, 323
circumcision, 316
clinical manifestations, 316
concentrates, 321
cryoprecipitate, 320
cuts and lacerations, 321
diagnosis, 317
dental treatment, 323

Haemophilia and Christmas disease
—*continued*
detection of carriers, 316
education, 319
factor VIII antigen, 315
in females, 315
fibrinolytic inhibitors, 323, 325
fresh-frozen plasma, 320
gastrointestinal bleeding, 323
haemarthrosis, 317, 322
haematomata, 317
haematuria, 323
half-life of activity, 320
historical associations, 314
home transfusion and prophylaxis, 324
incidence, 314
inheritance, 315
inhibitors, 326
injections and immunisations, 324
intracranial haemorrhage, 317
joint aspiration, 322
management, 319
newborn, 316
nosebleeds, 322
physiotherapy, 322
prophylactic dental care, 319
pseudotumour, 317
relation to factor VIII levels, 316
replacement therapy, 319
soft tissue, bleeding, 322
surgery, 324
transmission, 314
treatment of pain, 325
Haemorrhagic disease of newborn, 338
anticonvulsants, 340
breast feeding, 338
diagnosis, 340
incidence, 338
intrapartum and perinatal bleed-ing, 339
maternal drug ingestion, 339
prevention, 339
primary and secondary, 338
prothrombin complex, 338
Quick's prothrombin time, 338
subaponeurotic haematoma, 339
treatment, 340
vitamin K deficiency, 338
Hb. C
clinical manifestations, 123
haematological features, 119, 121
Hb. Chesapeake
polycythaemia, 125, 219
Hb. D
clinical manifestations, 123
haematological features, 119, 121
Hb. E
clinical manifestations, 123
haematological features, 119, 121
Hb. F
ALL, 400
AML, 400
aplastic anaemia, 50, 56, 57
juvenile CML, 399
Schwachman's syndrome, 231

INDEX 427

Haemoglobin H inclusions, 130
  technique, 133
Hb. Köln, 125, 126
Hb. S, *see* Sickle-cell anaemia
Hb. Zurich, 125, 126
Hand-foot syndrome (in Hb. S), 122
Heinz bodies, 72, 91, 127
  alpha thalassaemia, 193
  aniline dyes, 192
  asplenia, 192
  chloramphenicol, 192
  congenital H.B. haemolytic anaemia, 192
  defects of pentose shunt, 96
  gamma-GC synthetase deficiency, 100
  G-6-PD deficiency, 96
  GSH-Px deficiency, 99
  GSSG-R deficiency, 98
  hyposplenia, 191
  methaemoglobinaemia, 194
  moth balls, 192
  newborn, 191
  PK (Post Splenectomy) deficiency, 101
  premature infants, 191
  situs inversus, 192
  sulphonamides, 192
  synthetic vitamin K, 192
  toxic methaemoglobinaemia, 127
  unstable haemoglobins, 124, 126
  unstable haemoglobinopathies, 124, 126
Hempas, 84
Henoch-Schönlein syndrome, 302
Heparin
  assay, 348
  capillary clotting time, 349
  continuous vs intermittent, 349
  control, 348
  DIC, 347
  dosage, 349
  purpura fulminans, 362
  renal vein thrombosis, 353
Hepatic stores
  B_{12}, 37
  folate, 16
Hereditary elliptocytosis (HE), 80
  aetiology, 80
  clinical features, 81
  laboratory findings, 81
  treatment, 81
Hereditary factor XIII deficiency 330
Hereditary haemorrhagic telangiectasia, 303
Hereditary megaloblastic anaemia, 28
Hereditary spherocytosis (HS), 78
  aetiology, 78
  clinical features, 78
  laboratory findings, 79
  pathogenesis, 78
  treatment, 80
Hermansky-Pudlak syndrome, 294
  platelet defect, 294

Hexokinase deficiency, 102
  neonatal jaundice, 102
  pancytopenia, 103
Hexose monophosphate shunt, 97
  disorders, 92, 97
Histiocytic medullary reticulosis (HMR)
  hepatosplenomegaly, 408
  marrow, 408
  mononucleosis, 408
  pancytopenia, 408
Hodgkin's disease
  marrow infiltration, 209
Hydrops foetalis, due to:
  alpha thalassaemia, 135
  chronic foeto-maternal haemorrhage, 198
  congenital neuroblastoma, 198
  congenital syphilis, 190
  infections, 190
  placental chorioangioma, 198
  Rh disease, 165, 168
Hyperbaric oxygen treatment
  sickle-cell disease, 123, 124
Hypercoagulable states, *see also* DIC
  familial elevated factor V, 329
  favism, 363
  HUS, 357
  liver disease, 362
Hypersplenism
  anaemia, 157
  chronic malaria, 157
  Gaucher's disease, 410
  hypersplenism, 157
  other infections, 157
  liver disease, 208
  Neiman-Pick disease, 410
  neutropenia, 233
  portal hypertension, 157
  reticulosis, 157
  storage disease, 157
  thalassaemia, 157
  thrombocytopenia, 279
Hypertonic dehydration
  coagulation changes, 353
  MAHA, 353
Hypophosphataemia
  haemolysis, 149
Hypopituitarism
  anaemia, 208
Hypothyroidism
  anaemia, 208
  B_{12} deficiency, 208
  contracted RBCs, 208
  response to thyroxine, 209

I antigen, in AHA, 153
i-antigen, in aplastic anaemia, 57
Icterus gravis neonatorum. *See* Rh disease
Idiopathic thrombocytopenic purpura (ITP) 257
  antiplatelet antibodies, 258
  following chickenpox, 260
  clinical course, 260

ITP—*continued*
  clinical features, 260
  detection of anti-platelet antibodies, 259
  diagnosis, 261
  differential diagnosis, 261
  effect of plasma transfusion, 278
  haematological findings, 261
  infectious mononucleosis, 260
  immune nature, 258
  immunosuppressive drug therapy, 264
  intracranial haemorrhage, 260
  management, 262
  maternal and neonatal, 264
  following measles, 260
  following measles vaccine, 260
  following mumps, 260
  pathogenesis, 257
  platelet survival, 261
  retinal haemorrhage, 261
  following rubella, 260
  site of sequestration, 259
  following smallpox vaccination, 260
  splenectomy, 262
  steroids, 262
  following URTI, 260
  vincristine therapy, 264
  viruses, 258
Ileal malabsorption of B_{12}
  associated with proteinuria
  imerslund's syndrome, 39
Imerslund's syndrome, 39
Immunoneutropenias
  autoimmune, neonatal, 233
  chlorothiazide, neonatal, 233
  DLE, neonatal, 233
  isoimmune, neonatal, 233
Immunosuppressive therapy
  AHA, 153
  chicken-pox, during, 394
  CMV, 391, 394
  fungi, 391, 395
  giant cell pneumonia, 394
  herpes virus, 391
  ITP, 264
  leukaemia therapy, 385, 394
  leukaemogenesis, 376
  measles, during, 394
  pneumocystis carinii, 391, 394
  toxoplasmosis, 391
Inborn errors of metabolism
  neutropenia, 232
  thrombocytopenia, 232
Ineffective myelopoiesis, 229
Infantile genetic agranulocytosis (IGA) (Kostman), 225
Infantile pycnocytosis, 188
Infection
  anaemia in septicaemia, 157
  chronic and anaemia, 204
  haemolytic anaemi, 152, 156
  Lederer's anaemia, 157
  neonatal haemolysis, 190, 191
Infectious lymphocytosis, 245

428 PAEDIATRIC HAEMATOLOGY

Infectious mononucleosis
  adenovirus, 244
  clinical features, 243
  CMV, 244
  EBV, 243, 375
  herpes simplex, 244
  infectious mononucleosis, 242
  open-heart surgery, 244
  rubella, 244
  toxoplasmosis, 244
  treatment, 244
Inherited disorders of platelet function
  Bernard Soulier syndrome, 294
  congenital afibrinogenaemia, 298
  Glanzmann's thrombasthenia, 293
  inherited disorders of platelet function, 293
  May-Hegglin anomaly, 295
  thrombopathia, 293
  Von Willebrand's disease, 295
Inherited vascular disorders, 303
  Ehler-Danlos syndrome 303
  hereditary haemorrhagic telangiectasia, 303
  osteogenesis imperfecta, 304
  pseudoxanthoma elasticum, 304
  Rendu-Osler-Weber disease, 303
Inhibitors of coagulation
  Christmas disease, 326
  DLE, 363
  haemophilia, 326
  idiopathic, 363
  inhibitors of coagulation, 363
Intestinal resection and B_{12} malabsorption, 39
Intrauterine transfusion
  cord blood results, 169, 173
  indications in Rh disease, 166, 172
  intrauterine transfusion, 172
  technique, 173
Intrinsic factor deficiency
  associated endocrine deficiencies, 39
  associated immunological abnormality, 39
Involuntary movements in infantile B_{12} deficiency, 40
Iron. See also Anaemia, Iron deficiency
  dietary, 2
  effect on gastro-intestinal function, 3
  endowment at birth, 1
  malabsorption, 4
  mucosal cell loss, 4
  red-cell survival, 6
  serum, 7
  stores, 6
  TIBC, 7

Jk antibodies and neonatal jaundice, 184, 185
Job's syndrome, 237

Kaolin clotting time (KCT), 312

KPTT test (kaolin PTT or APTT), 312
  heparin control, 347
  newborn, 335, 336
Kell antibodies and neonatal jaundice, 184, 185
Kernicterus
  ABO HD, 182
  G-6-PD deficiency, 193
  heinz body haemolytic anaemia, 192
  hereditary spherocytosis, 78, 194
  relation to hyperbilirubinaemia, 168
  other blood group incompatibilities, 184
  other disorders, 168
  PK deficiency, 195
  relation to albumen saturation, 168
  relation to bilirubin level, 168
  relation to duration of, 168
  Rh disease, 165, 168
Kidd antibodies and neonatal jaundice, 184, 185

Late anaemia
  ABO HD, 182
  other blood group incompatibilities, 184
  phototherapy, 184
  prematurity, 203, 204
  Rh disease, 172
Lazy-leucocyte syndrome, 231
Le antibodies and neonatal jaundice, 184, 185
Lead intoxication, 154
Lederer's anaemia, 157
Leterer-Siwe disease (histiocytosis X)
  clinical features, 406
  haematological findings, 209, 408
  marrow examination, 209, 408
  prognostic features, 406
  rash, 407
  skeletal changes, 406
  treatment, 408
Leucocyte changes in infection
  bacterial, 239
  CMV, 244
  Döhle bodies, 239
  fungal, 239
  infectious mononucleosis, 243
  NBT reaction, 239
  toxic granulations, 239
  toxoplasmosis, 244
  Turk cells, 239, 242
  viral, 239
Leucocytes
  normal values, ii
Leucoerythroblastic anaemia, 209
  osteopetrosis, 210
Leukaemia
  aetiology
    cats, 376
    chemicals and drugs, 376
    clusters, 374
    diagnostic X-rays, 376

Leukaemia—continued
  Down's syndrome, 277
  genetic disorders associated with, 377
  HL-A type, 376, 399
  irradiation, 376
  maternal leukaemia, 376
  multifactorial, 376
  neoantigens, 374
  progeny, 376
  reverse transcriptase, 374
  sibs, 376
  twins, 376
  viruses, 374
  ALL therapy, 384
  AML therapy, 387, 396
  antibiotics in septicaemia, 388
  antifungal drugs, 388
  auer rods, 382
  basic plan of therapy of ALL, 384
  basophilic, 402
  bone marrow transplant, 397
  cell cycle and drug action, 379
  cell kinetics, 377
  CNS prophylaxis, 391
  chronic lymphocytic leukaemia, 402
  chronic monocytic, 403
  chronic myelocytic (CML), 399
  clinical findings, 380
  congenital, 404
  criterial of remission, 383
  cytochemical stains, 382
  cytological diagnosis, 382
  cytological types, 373
  diagnosis, 379
  eosinophilic, 402
  erythroleukaemia, 401
  factors affecting prognosis, 397
    age at diagnosis, 397
    cytology, 398
    hepatosplenomegaly, 398
    HL-A9 type, 399
    mediastinal mass, 397
    PAS-positivity, 398
    race, 397
    T-cell markers, 398
    white cell count, 397
  granulocyte transfusions, 388
  Gut sterilization, 389
  haematological findings, 380
  improving survival, 395
  immunosuppression, 394
  immunotherapy, 396
  incidence, 373
  juvenile CML, 399
  leukaemic cell kill, 385
  leukaemic reticuloendotheliosis, 403
  leukocyte glutathione peroxidase deficiency, 236, 238
  maintenance therapy, 394
  management, 383
  marrow examination, 381
  meningeal leukaemia, 391
  metabolic support, 387
  neonatal, 405

INDEX   429

Leukaemia—*continued*
  neuroblastoma, 405
  promyelocytic leukaemia, 402
  protective isolation, 389
  remission induction, 383, 385
  supporve therapy, 387
  transfotirmation of reticuloses, 403
  Lewis antibodies and neonatal jaundice, 184, 185
Liability to infection in folate deficiency, 29
Lipid accumulation on RBCs haemolysis and, 83, 147
Lipid peroxidation haemolysis and, 149
Liver disease
  anaemia, 208
  due to antileukaemic drugs, 380
  coagulation deficiency, 342
  DIC, 362
  fibrinolysis, 342
  folate loss, 29
  spur cells, 208
Lymphadenopathy
  CG, 227
  CGD, 235
  IGA, 226
  ITP, 261
  infectious lymphocytosis, 245
  infectious mononucleosis, 243
  juvenile CML, 399
  leukaemia, 377, 379
  mediastinal in leukaemia, 380
  secondary infections, 380
  TAR, 269
Lymphocytosis
  infectious lymphocytosis, 245
  pertussis, 381
Lysosomal enzymes
  cytochemical classification of leukaemia, 383
  storage diseases, 409

Malabsorption and folate deficiency, 23
Malignant disease
  anaemia, 209
  hypochromic type, 209
  leucoerythroblastic anaemia, 209
  reticulocytosis, 209
Malignant infiltration of marrow
  ganglioneuroblastoma, 405
  letterer-Siwe, 406
  leukaemia, 381, 384
  metastatic, 405
  myelomatosis, 406
  neuroblastoma, 405
  retinoblastoma, 405
  rhabdomyosarcoma, 405
Management of acute leukaemia, 383
Marble bone disease. *See* osteopetrosis
Marrow
  examination, 381
  leukaemia, 381, 384
  myelofibrosis, 411
  non-leukaemic infiltrations, 405

Marrow—*continued*
  normal values, iii
  stainable iron, 6
  storage diseases, 409
  marrow encroachment anaemia, 209
Marrow transplantation
  aplastic anaemia, 60
  leukaemia, 397
Maternal antibody titre
  measurement as micrograms, 167
  relation to foetal outcome, 165
  relation to titre in foetal serum, 169
May-Hegglin anomaly
  bleeding, 274
  giant platelets, 290
  inclusions, 238, 274
  May-Hegglin anomaly, 238
  platelet dysfunction, 295
  thrombocytopenia, 274
MCV
  normal values, ii
Mediterranean anaemia. *See* Thalassaemia
Megakaryocytes
  morphological classification, 256
Megaloblastic changes
  aplastic anaemia, 49
  B_{12} deficiency, 36
  folate deficiency, 19
  haemodialysis, 207
  haemoglobinopathies, 120
  liver disease, 208
  Rh disease, 169
  rheumatoid arthritis, 206
  sideroblastic anaemia, 212
  thalassaemia, 135
Meningeal leukaemia, 380, 384
  CNS prophylaxis, 391
  CSF findings, 392
  CSF methotrexate levels, 392
  Cytocentrifuge in examination of CSF, 392
  encephalopathy, 391
  I.T. methotrexate, 392
  long-term control, 393
  lumbar puncture, 392
  treatment of overt, 391
Meningococcal septicaemia
  DIC, 361
Mental retardation. *See also* Neurological disorder
  acanthocytosis, 83
  CSF folate, 27
  congenital B_{12} dependent reactions, 35
  cyclohydrase deficiency, 29
  Fanconi's aplastic anaemia, 48
  FIGLU excretion, 28
  formimino transferase deficiency, 28
  G-6-PD deficiency, 97
  glutathione reductase deficiency, 98
  hempas, 84
  hereditary spherocytosis, 78

Mental retardation—*continued*
  hyperfolicacidaemia, 28
  infantile B_{12} deficiency, 40
  isolated folate malabsorption, 24
  megaloblastic changes, 28
  methaemoglobin reductase deficiency, 128
  orotic aciduria, 28
  PGK deficiency, 105
  RBC membrane disorder, 150
6-mercaptopurine in Acute Leukaemia, 394
Methaemoglobinaemia
  ascorbic acid, 128, 129
  cyanosis, 128
  grey cyanosis, 194
  Heinz body anaemias, 194
  M-Haemoglobinopathies, 128
  Methaemoglobin reductase deficiency, 128
  methylene blue, 127, 129
  neonatal, 128
  toxic, 128
  unstablehaemoglobinopathies, 126
Methods
  capillary, i
Methotrexate
  leukaemia, 394
  meningeal leukaemia, 392
Microangiopathic Haemolytic Anaemia (MAHA)
  causes of MAHA, 146
  diagnosis, 146
  mechanism of burr cell formation, 146
  pathogenesis of MAHA, 146
  renal failure, 207
Mongolism (Down's syndrome)
  incidence of leukaemia, 277
  leukaemoid reactions, 405
  neonatal leukaemia, 405
  thrombocytopenia, 275, 405
  type of leukaemia, 277, 405
Monocytosis
  CG, 228
  IGA, 226
Myelofibrosis
  marrow, 411
Myelomatosis, 406
Myeloperoxidase deficiency, 236, 237

Nieman-Pick disease, 410
NBT reduction, 235
Neonatal anaemia. *See also* Neonatal haemolysis
  acute foetal blood loss, 196
  causes, 197
  chronic foetal blood loss, 196
  chronic foeta-maternal haemorrhage, 198
  congenital neuroblastoma, 198
  foeto-maternal haemorrhage, 196
  HE, 195
  HS, 194
  intrapartum foetal blood loss, 197
  Kleihauer film in diagnosis, 197
  osteopetrosis, 199

430 PAEDIATRIC HAEMATOLOGY

Neonatal anaemia—*continued*
  other enzyme deficiencies, 195
  PK deficiency, 195
  pure red-cell aplasia, 199
  Singer's test in diagnosis, 197
  subaponeurotic haematoma, 198
  twin-transfusion syndrome, 197
Neonatal haemolysis
  ABO HDNB, 181
  alpha thalassaemia, 193, 195
  bacterial infections, 191
  Coxsackie B, 191
  cytomegalovirus, 190
  Hb. F Poole, 193
  Hb. H disease, 193, 195
  Heinz body anaemias, 191
  hereditary elliptocytosis, 195
  hereditary enzyme deficiencies, 195
  hereditary spherocytosis, 194
  herpes simplex, 191
  infantile pycnocytosis, 188
  malaria, 191
  other antibodies, 184
  Rh disease, 163
  rubella, 191
  syphilis, 190
  table of causes, 187
  toxoplasmosis, 190
Neonatal jaundice
  ABO HD, 182
  delayed clamping of cord, 198, 220
  galactosaemia, 195
  gamma-beta thalassaemia, 134, 196
  G-6-PD deficiency, 93, 96
  GSH-Px deficiency, 99
  HE, 195
  hereditary enzyme deficiencies, 195
  HK deficiency, 102
  hereditary spherocytosis, 78, 80, 194
  infantile pycnocytosis, 188
  infections, 190
  neonatal polycythaemia, 220
  other blood group incompatibilities, 184
  6-PGD deficiency, 98
  PHI deficiency, 103
  PK deficiency, 101
  Rh disease, 168
  table of causes, 187
Neonatal neutropenia
  autoimmune, 233
  chlorothiazide, 233
  DLE, 233
  isoimmune, 233
Nephrotic syndrome
  low factor IX, 343
Neuroblastoma
  marrow involvement, 209
Neurological disorder. *See also*
    Mental retardation
  acanthocytosis, 83
  cranial radiotherapy, 391
  FEL, 408

Neurological disorder—*continued*
  gamma-glutamyl-cysteine synthetase deficiency, 100
  Gaucher's disease, 410
  G-6-PD deficiency, 97
  GSSG-R deficiency, 98
  Hempas, 84
  I.T. Methotrexate, 393
  leukaemia, 380, 391
  Nieman-Pick disease, 410
  PGK deficiency, 105
  sea-blue histiocyte syndrome, 411
  sickle-cell disease, 122
  storage diseases, 409
  TPI deficiency, 104
Neuromuscular disorder
  triosephosphate isomerase deficiency, 104
Neutropenia
  AHA, 152
  ataxia telangiectasia, 231
  agammaglobulinaemia, 231
  B_{12} deficiency, 36
  Chediak-Higashi syndrome, 234, 238
  chronic benign, 227
  classification, 225
  copper deficiency, 204, 234
  cyclic, 229
  drug-induced, 232
  Felty's syndrome, 206
  haemodialysis, 233
  hereditary forms, 225
  hypersplenism, 157, 233
  immunoneutropenias, 233
  inborn errors of metabolism, 232
  lazy-leucocyte syndrome, 231
  leukaemia, 381
  osteopetrosis, 234
  pancreatic insufficiency, 231
  relationship to infection, 389
  sideroblastic anaemia, 212
Non-spherocytic haemolytic anaemias
  2, 3-DPG ase deficiency, 105
  gamma-glutamyl-cysteine-synthetase deficiency, 100
  G-3-PD deficiency, 104
  G-6-PD deficiency, 97
  GSH-Px deficiency, 99
  GSH synthetase deficiency, 99
  GSSG-R deficiency, 98
  HK deficiency, 102
  Non-spherocytic haemolytic anaemias, 90
  PFK deficiency, 103
  PGK deficiency, 104
  PHI deficiency, 103
  PK deficiency, 101
  TPI deficiency, 104
  unstable haemoglobins, 124, 126
Non-thrombocytopenic purpura
  allergic, 303
  anaphylactoid purpura, 302
  Henoch-Schönlein, 302
  scurvy, 303
Normal values, ii

Opsonization, 234
Orotic aciduria, 28
Osteogenesis imperfecta, 304
  platelet defect, 294
Osteopetrosis (marble bone disease)
  facies, 211
  haemolytic anaemia, 157
  marrow encroachment, 210
  skeletal changes, 211
Ovarian tumours and AHA, 152
Overwhelming post-splenectomy infection (OPSI), 263
Oxygen dissociation curve
  foetal RBCs, 115
  Hb. Barts, 132

PCV
  normal values, ii
Pancreatic insufficiency and neutropenia, 231
Pancytopenia
  aplastic anaemia, 48
  aplastic crises in HS, 79
  Chediak-Higashi disease, 238
  FEL, 408
  GSSG-R deficiency, 98
  hexokinase deficiency, 103
  HMR, 408
  leukaemia, 377, 379, 381
  marrow examination, 383
  megaloblastic anaemia, 19
  osteopetrosis, 210
  PNH, 150
  transcobalamin II deficiency, 40
Paroxysmal cold haemoglobinuria, 152
Paroxysmal nocturnal haemoglobinuria (PNH), 150
  aplastic anaemia, 57
PTT test (Partial thromboplastin time), 312
  newborn, 337
PAS stain in ALL, 383
  erythroleukaemia, 401
  Gaucher's cells, 410
Peritoneal dialysis and folate loss, 29
Phagocytosis, 234
Phenobarbitone
  ABO HD, 183
  neonatal G-6-PD deficiency, 183
  prematurity, 183
  Rh disease, 172
Philadelphia chromosome, 399, 400
phosphofructokinase deficiency, 103
6-phosphoglucose dehydrogenase deficiency, 97
  neonatal jaundice, 98
phosphoglycerate kinase deficiency, 104
  neurological disorder, 105
Phosphohexose isomerase deficiency, 103
  neonatal jaundice, 103
Phototherapy, 183, 184
  ABO HD, 183
  prematurity, 184
  Rh disease, 172

Physiological anaemia of newborn, 204
'Physiological' doses of B_{12} and folate, 36
Pigment metabolism in haemolytic anaemia, 74
Pigmentation in infantile B_{12} deficiency, 40
Plasma exchange in polycythaemia, 220, 221
Plasminogen, 310, 313
  DIC, 345
  newborns, 351
  RDS, 351
  therapy within RDS, 352
Plasticity of RBCs
  haemolysis, 149
Platelet adhesion to glass beads, 291
Platelet aggregation, 290
Platelet factor 3 availability, 292
Platelet function, acquired defects
  aspirin, 298
  carbenicillin, 300
  congenital heart disease, 355
  drug ingestion, 298
  dysproteinaemia, 300
  FDPs, 301
  liver disease, 300
  neonatal, 299
  uraemia, 300
Platelet function, congenital defects
  Bernard-Soulier syndrome, 294
  congenital afibrinogenaemia, 298
  Glanzmann's thrombasthenia, 293
  May-Hegglin anomaly, 295
  thrombasthenia, 293
  thrombopathia, 293
  Von Willebrand's disease, 295
  Wiskott-Aldrich syndrome, 294
Platelet function in newborn, 299
  sensitivity to drugs, 299
Platelet function tests, 288
  adhesion to glass beads, 291
  aggregation in vitro, 290
  bleeding time, 288
  clot retraction, 292
  PF-3 availability, 292
  size and morphology, 289
Platelet kinetics, 254, 255
  patterns in thrombocytopenia, 255
  patterns in thrombocytosis, 255
Platelet life span and sequestration, 254
  ITP, 259
Platelet size and morphology, 289
Platelet transfusion, 301
  aplastic anaemia, 302
  Bernard-Soulier syndrome, 295
  dose calculation, 302
  Glanzmann's thrombasthenia, 293
  HL-A compatibility, 302
  ITP, 302
  leukaemia, 301
  transmission of infection, 302
Platelets
  aggregation, 287
  function, 287

Platelets—continued
  haemostatic function, 287
  inhibition by drugs, 288
  normal values, iii, 253
  pre-term infants, 253
  reaction with ADP, 288, 290
  reaction with collagen, 287, 290
  release reaction, 288, 290
  size related to age, 256
  small, in WAS, 271
  term infants, 253
Polycythaemia
  Hb Chesapeake, 125
  M-Haemoglobinopathy, 127
  neonatal, 219
    congenital adrenal hyperplasia, 220
    Down's syndrome, 220
    intrauterine anoxia, 220
    materno-foetal, 198, 220
    placental insufficiency, 220
    twin transfusion, 220
  primary
    benign familial polycythaemia, 218
    polycythaemia rubra vera, 217
  secondary
    abnormal haemoglobins, 219
    cyanotic congenital heart disease, 218
    renal disease, 219
    tumours, 219
  small-for-dates babies, 203
  twin transfusion syndrome, 198
Poor weight gain in B_{12} deficiency, 36
Portsmouth syndrome, 294
Premature infants
  serum B_{12} changes, 37
Prematurity
  anaemias, 203
  copper deficiency, 204
  early, 1, 203
  folate deficiency, 21, 203
  iron deficiency, 2, 203
  late, 2, 203
  vitamin E. deficiency, 149, 203
Primary red-cell aplasia. See Pure red-cell aplasia
Prothrombin complex (II, VII, IX, X), 335
  Haemolytic disease of the newborn, 340
  hepatocellular disease, 342
  newborn, 335, 336
  Reye's syndrome, 342
  therapeutic concentrate, 342
  first year of life, 337
P and P Test
  Haemolytic disease of the newborn, 340, 341
  P and P test, 312
  first year of life, 337
Prothrombin time, 312
  Haemolytic disease of the newborn, 341
  liver disease, 342
  newborn, 335, 338

Pseudoxanthoma elasticum, 304
Pulmonary infarction in sickle-cell disease, 122
Pure red-cell aplasia
  aetiology, 61
  ascorbic acid, 64
  clinical features, 62
  course, 64
  desferrioxamine, 64
  dihydroxybenzoic acid, 64
  growth, 63
  laboratory diagnosis, 63
  marrow, 63
  nitrogen-stored red cells, 65
  treatment, 64
Purpura fulminans, 361
  heparin, 362
Pyruvate kinase deficiency, 101
  neonatal jaundice, 101

Quick's one-stage prothrombin time, 312
  haemorrhagic disease of the newborn, 341
  liver disease, 342
  newborn, 335, 338

Raynaud phenomena, in AHA, 152
Red-cell folate, 16, 17
Red-cell aplasia. See Pure red-cell aplasia
Red-cell fragmentation, 73, 146, 147
  congenital virus infections, 191
  drug-induced haemolysis, 193
  Heinz body haemolytic anaemia, 192
Red-cell membrane disorders, 147
Red-cell survival, 73
Renal failure anaemia, 207
  androgen treatment, 207
  folate deficiency, 207
  haemodialysis, 207
  histidine therapy, 207
  iron deficiency, 207
  MAHA, 207
  renal transplantation, 207
Renal involvement in leukaemia, 380
Renal vein thrombosis
  coagulation changes, 353
  heparin, 353
  intravascular clotting, 353
  MAHA, 353
Rendu-Osler-Weber disease, 303
Reticular dysgenesis (congenital aleucocytosis), 227
Retinoblastoma
  marrow involvement, 209
Reye's syndrome
  coagulation deficiency, 342
Rhabdomyosarcoma
  marrow involvement, 209
Rhesus disease (Rh disease)
  late anaemia, 172
  antenatal detection, 164
  clinical findings, 168
  intrauterine transfusion, 172
  laboratory findings, 169

432 PAEDIATRIC HAEMATOLOGY

Rhesus disease—*continued*
management and treatment, 170
pathogenosis, 163
plasmapheresis, 173
prediction of severity, 165
prevention, 164
synonyms, 163
Rh isoimmunization. *See* Rh disease
Rheumatoid arthritis and anaemia, 206
Ristocetin aggregation test, 291
von Willebrand's disease, 296

Salivary glands involvement in leukaemia, 380
Scleroderma
intestinal and B_{12} malabsorption, 39
Scurvy
anaemia, 25
haemorrhagic manifestations, 303
Sea-blue histiocyte syndrome, 410
ceroid-containing phagocytes, 411
ITP, CGG, etc., 411
storage disease, 411
Septicaemia
causing DIC, 350, 359
causing thrombocytopenia, 268
haemolysis, 157
haemolysis in newborn, 191
leukaemia, 387
leucocyte changes, 240
vacuolation of neutrophils, 240
Serum B_{12} in CML, 400
Serum ferritin in anaemia of chronic infection, 205
Serum folate, 16, 17
Sickle-cell anaemia disease
autosplenectomy, 123
clinical manifestations, 121, 122
cold agglutinins, 123
haematological diagnosis, 120
manifestations in infancy, 122
other sickling states, 119, 123
pathogenesis of haemolysis, 118
pathogenesis of sickling phenomena, 118
renal function, 123
treatment, 123, 124
Sideroblastic anaemia, 212
folate therapy, 212
hereditary, 212
lead poisoning, 212
pyridoxine therapy, 212
Skeletal changes
CGD, 237
constitutional aplastic anaemia, 48
haemolytic anaemia, 74
hereditary spherocytosis, 78
Letterer-Siwe disease, 406
leukaemia, 380
osteopetrosis, 210
regression with hypertransfusion, 135
sickling states, 122, 123
storage diseases, 409
thalassaemia, 134

Skin involvement
congenital leukaemia, 404
juvenile CML, 399
Letterer-Siwe disease, 406, 407
leukaemia, 380
Smooth tongue in B_{12} deficiency, 36
Specific leucocyte granule defect (congenital), 238
Spherocytes, 71
Spherocytosis
ABO HDNB, 182
autoimmune, HA, 151, 152
congenital rubella, 191
drug-induced haemolysis, 156
Heinz body haemolytic anaemia, 192
HS, 78, 194
hypophosphataemia, 149
Lederer's anaemia, 157
Lewis HDNB, 185
M HDNB, 185
MAHA, 146
spherocytosis (general), 71
Spitz-Holter valves and anaemia, 157
Splenectomy
aplastic anaemia, 51, 60
AHA, 153
Bernard-Soulier syndrome, 295
causing thrombocytosis, 280
cyclic neutropenia, 230
FEL, 408
HE, 81
hereditary spherocytosis, 80
hereditary thrombocytopenia, 273, 274
hypersplenism, 279
ITP, 262
increase in burr cells, 146
iron overload, 135
neutropenia, 223
osteopetrosis, 210
overwhelming infection, 135
overwhelming infection after (OPSI), 263
platelet transfusion, 263
pure red-cell aplasia, 65
sideroblastic anaemia, 212
spur cell anaemia, 148
thalassaemia, 135
WAS, 272, 273
Splenomegaly
ABO HD, 182
absent radii syndrome (TAR), 269
adult-type CML, 401
AHA, 152
Chediak-Higashi disease, 238
chronic benign granulocytopenia, 227
CGD, 235
chronic lymphocytic L., 402
chronic monocytic leukaemia, 403
congenital CMV, 190
congenital leukaemia, 377, 379, 380
congenital malaria, 191
congenital syphilis, 190
congenital toxoplasmosis, 190

Splenomegaly—*continued*
congenital virus infections, 191
eosinophilic leukaemia, 403
FEL, 408
familial myeloproliferative disease, 411
Felty's syndrome, 206
Gaucher's disease, 410
HE, 81
HS, 78
HMR, 408
ITP, 261
infantile pycnocytosis, 188
infectious lymphocytosis, 245
infectious mononucleosis, 243
juvenile CML, 399
Lederer's anaemia, 157
Letterer-Siwe disease, 406
leukaemia, 377, 379, 380
leukaemic reticuloendotheliosis, 403
myelofibrosis, 411
Nieman-Pick disease, 410
neonatal leukaemia, 405
osteopetrosis, 210
PNH, 156
platelet sequestration, 254
polycythaemia rubra vera, 217
PK deficiency, 195
Rh disease, 168, 169
sea-blue histiocyte syndrome, 411
sickle-cell disease, 124
storage diseases, 409
thalassaemia, 134
unstable haemoglobins, 125, 126
Spur cell haemolytic anaemia, 148
liver disease, 208
Steroid treatment
AHA, 153
ALL, 385
aplastic anaemia, 51, 59
ITP, 262
pure red-cell aplasia, 64
Stomatocytosis, 81
autohaemolysis, 82
Storage diseases, 409
classification, 409
enzyme replacement therapy, 410
enzymes, 409
Gaucher's disease, 410
hepatosplenomegaly, 409
marrow histiocytes, 409
Nieman-Pick disease, 410
Reilly bodies, 409
sea-blue histiocyte syndrome, 410
vacuolated lymphocytes, 409
Storage pool disease, 294
Sudan black stain in AML, 383
Surgical blind loops and B_{12} malabsorption, 39
Syphilis and neonatal haemolysis, 190

Tapeworm and B_{12} deficiency, 40
Target cells
Hb. C, 120
Hb. H disease, 134, 193

INDEX 433

Target cells—*continued*
  Hb. S disease, 120
  iron deficiency, 133
  jaundice, obstructive, 133, 148
  lead poisoning, 133
  LCAT deficiency, 148
  liver disease, 133, 148, 208
  after splenectomy, 133
  thalassaemias, 132, 193
Technitium pertechnetate in diagnosis of Meckel's diverticula, 7
Testicular leukaemia, 384
Thalassaemia syndromes, 129
  age at presentation, 133
  biochemical lesion, 129
  clinical features, 134
  diagnosis, 132
  genetics, 130
  haematological findings, 132
  management, 135
  pathogenesis of anaemia, 131
Thiamine-responsive anaemia, 28
Thioguanine in acute leukaemia, 386
Thrombin Time, 313
  DIC, 346
  newborn, 337
Thrombocytopathia, 293
Thrombocytopenia
  absent radii syndrome (TAR), 268
  AHA, 152
  autosomal, 273
  B_{12} deficiency, 36
  Chediak-Higashi, 238
  classification, 257
  congenital CMV, 190
  congenital leukaemia, 275, 405
  congenital syphilis, 190
  congenital toxoplasmosis, 190
  congenital virus infections, 191
  cyclical, 278
  DIC, 279
  drug-Haptene type, 275
  drug-induced, 275
  Evans's syndrome, 258, 265
  folate deficiency, 29
  Gaucher's disease, 279
  giant haemangioma, 268
  Hb. Köln disease, 126
  hereditary, 271, 272
    autosomal, 273, 274
    hereditary forms, 271
    May-Hegglin, 273
    sex-linked recessive, 272
    Wiscott-Aldrich (WAS), 271
  hyperglycinaemia, 232, 275
  hypersplenism, 157, 279
  ITP, 257
  ineffective thrombopoiesis, 275
  infectious mononucleosis, 243
  iron deficiency, 280
  leukaemia, 380
  marrow encroachment, 279
  marrow infiltration, 279
  May-Hegglin, 238

Thrombocytopenia—*continued*
  metabolic disorders, 275
  methyl malonic acidaemia, 232
  MAHA, 147, 279
  neonatal, 199, 264
    absent radii (TAR), 268
    congenital amegakaryocytic, 268
    congenital leukaemia, 275
    Fanconi's anaemia, 271
    giant haemangioma, 268
    infections, 267
    isoimmune, 265
    maternal drugs, 267
    maternal Evans's, 265
    maternal ITP, 264
    metabolic causes, 275
    renal vein thrombosis, 268
    severe Rh disease, 170, 267
    trisomy syndromes, 271
  nephritis and deafness, 273
  osteopetrosis, 210
  platelet kinetics, 255
  platelet size, 256
  post-transfusion, 278
  renal-vein thrombosis, 268
  Schwachman's syndrome, 231
  Sedormid purpura, 275
  septicaemia, 240, 268
  severe Rh disease, 170, 267
  sex-linked recessive, 273
  sideroblastic anaemia, 212
  thrombopoietin deficiency, 278
  translocation mongols, 275, 405
  trisomy syndromes, 271
  uraemia, 300
  values, 199, 264
  viral infections, 242
  Wiskott-Aldrich syndrome (WAS) 271
Thrombocytosis, 279
  causes of, 280
  infantile cortical hyperostosis, 279
  iron deficiency, 280
  platelet kinetics, 255
  platelet size, 256
  polycythaemia rubra vera, 217
  post-splenectomy, 280
  primary, 280
  vitamin E deficiency, 149
Thrombopathia, 293
TGT (thromboplastin generation test), 318
TPST test, 312
  DIC, 346
  newborn, 340
Thrombosis in familial elevated factor V, 329
Thrombosis in polycythaemia rubra vera, 218
Thrombotest, 312, 340
  haemorrhagic disease of newborn, 340, 341
  hepatic disease, 342
  newborn, 336
Thymectomy in AHA, 154

Toxoplasmosis and neonatal haemolysis, 190
Transcobalamins
  physiology, 36
  TC II deficiency, 40
Transfusion
  blood, 10
  calculation of volume, 10
  diuretics, 10
  granulocytes, 388
  packed cells, 10
  platelets, 301
  severe anaemia, 10
Triophosphate isomerase deficiency, 104
  neuromuscular disorder, 104

Urea treatment in sickle-cell disease, 123
Urinary folate loss
  neonatal, 29
Urobilinogen in haemolytic anaemia (faecal excretion index), 75

Vacuolation in polymorphs in septicaemia, 240
Vincristine
  remission induction in ALL, 385
Viscosity of blood
  related to Hct, 218
  polycythaemia, 218
Vitamin B_{12}
  absorption, 35
  biochemistry, 35
  breast milk content, 37
  deficiency, causes, 38
  Imerslund-Gräsbeck syndrome, 39
  intestinal disease, 40
  intrinsic factor, 38
  megaloblastic anaemia, 36
  nutritional, 40
  proteinuria, 39
  requirements, 37
  serum levels, 36
  subacute combined degeneration of cord, 35
  transcobalamins, 36, 40
  transport, 36
  vegetarianism, 40
Vitamin E deficiency
  haemolysis, 149
  Heinz body anaemia, 192
  prematurity, 149
Vitamin E
  lipid peroxidation, 149
Vitamin K
  breast feeding, 336
  dietary content, 336
  deficiency in haemolytic disease of the newborn, 338
  deficiency in later childhood, 341
  malabsorption, 34
  physiology, 335
  prophylactic dose, 338

434 PAEDIATRIC HAEMATOLOGY

Vitamin K—*continued*
  stores at birth, 337
  therapy, 340
Vitamin K dependent coagulation
    factors
  beyond neonatal period, 341
  hepatocellular disease, 342
  newborn, 336, 339
Von Willebrand's disease, 295

Von Willebrand's disease—*continued*
  clinical manifestations, 297
  cryoprecipitate, 298
  diagnostic criteria, 297
  factor VIII antigen, 296
  haemarthroses, 298
  management, 298
  prophylactic dental care, 298
  ristocetin aggregation, 296

Von Willebrand's disease—*cantinued*
  variants, 296, 297

Whole-blood folate, 16, 17
Wilson's disease
  haemolytic anaemia, 157

Xmas disease. *See* Haemophilia and
    Xmas disease